Advances in Experimental Medicine and Biology

Volume 1152

More information about this series at http://www.springer.com/series/5584

Advances in Experimental Medicine
and Biology

Volume

Aamir Ahmad
Editor

Breast Cancer Metastasis and Drug Resistance

Challenges and Progress

Second Edition

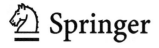 Springer

Editor
Aamir Ahmad
Mitchell Cancer Institute
University of South Alabama
Mobile, AL, USA

ISSN 0065-2598   ISSN 2214-8019   (electronic)
Advances in Experimental Medicine and Biology
ISBN 978-3-030-20300-9   ISBN 978-3-030-20301-6   (eBook)
https://doi.org/10.1007/978-3-030-20301-6

© Springer Nature Switzerland AG 2013, 2019
This work is subject to copyright. All rights are reserved by the Publisher, whether the whole or part of the material is concerned, specifically the rights of translation, reprinting, reuse of illustrations, recitation, broadcasting, reproduction on microfilms or in any other physical way, and transmission or information storage and retrieval, electronic adaptation, computer software, or by similar or dissimilar methodology now known or hereafter developed.
The use of general descriptive names, registered names, trademarks, service marks, etc. in this publication does not imply, even in the absence of a specific statement, that such names are exempt from the relevant protective laws and regulations and therefore free for general use.
The publisher, the authors, and the editors are safe to assume that the advice and information in this book are believed to be true and accurate at the date of publication. Neither the publisher nor the authors or the editors give a warranty, express or implied, with respect to the material contained herein or for any errors or omissions that may have been made. The publisher remains neutral with regard to jurisdictional claims in published maps and institutional affiliations.

This Springer imprint is published by the registered company Springer Nature Switzerland AG
The registered company address is: Gewerbestrasse 11, 6330 Cham, Switzerland

Preface

It is indeed an honor to be called upon by Springer Publishers to edit this second volume of *Breast Cancer Metastasis and Drug Resistance: Challenges and Progress*. The first volume was published in 2013, and, as with the original volume, the main objective of this follow-up volume is to comprehensively summarize breast cancer as the disease, the factors that make it particularly lethal, and the current state of breast cancer research. As outlined in the first volume, to successfully treat breast cancer, it is imperative to (a) fully understand the disease with all its heterogeneity; (b) understand the underlying processes that lead to the phenomenon of drug resistance, making breast cancer particularly incurable; and (c) understand factors that influence the metastasis of breast cancer to distant organs making it lethal.

We begin this volume by looking at the breast cancer statistics trends. Chapter 1 provides the perspectives with regard to the numbers associated with breast cancer incidence and mortality, over the last 10 years. Epidemiology of breast cancer is discussed in Chapter 2 with a focus on the various risk factors. Chapter 3 evaluates the racial disparity in breast cancer, which remains an area of concern given the wealth of information on how breast cancer mortality rates differ between women from different ethnic backgrounds. Chapter 4 provides a snapshot of breast cancer as a disease, with an overview of the current practices for the diagnosis and treatment, while Chapter 5 discusses fundamentals of breast cancer development and progression. Finally, Chapter 6 rounds up the first part of this volume by discussing heterogeneity associated with primary as well as metastatic breast cancers.

The next nine chapters (Chapters 7, 8, 9, 10, 11, 12, 13, 14, and 15) detail our most up-to-date knowledge on the mechanisms of metastasis and drug resistance in breast cancer, the central theme of this volume. Chapter 7 deals with bone metastasis of breast cancer. Bone is one of the earliest and most common sites of breast cancer metastasis. Breast cancer metastasizes to bones in approximately three-fourths of the patients with advanced disease, and bone is also the first site of breast cancer metastases in 26–50% of clinical cases. The therapeutic options for breast cancer patients with a metastatic disease are discussed in Chapter 8. Effects of chemotherapy on cytokine production with implications on drug efficacy within the tumor microenvironment are the subject of discussion in Chapter 9. Clearly, acquired drug resistance remains a major clinical concern. Targeted therapies are available for breast cancer patients with the expression of ER, PR or the overexpression of HER2/neu. Many patients respond to the targeted therapy initially but eventually develop resistance to the therapy, with the passage of time and continued administration of therapeutic agent. Such drug-resistant breast cancers are comparatively much more aggressive, and difficult to treat. They are invariably linked to poor prognosis as well as overall poor survival. Chapter 10 provides an updated account of trastuzumab (herceptin) resistance, as relevant to HER2 overexpressing breast cancers, while Chapter 11 discusses the problem of tamoxifen resistance, as relevant to ER expressing breast cancers, with a focus on the emerging role of noncoding RNAs. Chapters 12, 13, 14, and 15 focus on various strategies to overcome breast cancer drug resistance and/or metastasis. Chapter 12 discusses TRAIL signaling, Chapter 13 focuses on platinum-based drugs, while Chapters 14 and 15 discuss JAK-STAT and mTOR signaling, respectively. The chapters in the second part integrate knowledge from basic and translational research with clinical implications, resulting in a better understanding of the developments in basic research laboratories as well as in the clinics.

The last part of this volume, comprising of Chapters 16, 17, 18, 19, 20, 21, and 22, provides an insight into some of the very innovative ideas and methodologies that can help unravel the mystery associated with breast cancer metastasis and drug resistance. Chapter 16 discusses the evolving knowledge on epigenetic regulation of breast cancer, Chapter 17 details the updated information on the role of cancer stem cells in aggressive breast cancers, and Chapter 18 focuses on the potential of miRNAs in regulating breast cancer drug resistance and metastasis. Chapter 19 provides information on novel therapeutic targets in breast cancer, and Chapter 20 details the emerging knowledge on targeted therapies against triple negative breast cancer, a particularly aggressive breast cancer subtype. Chapter 21 provides a fresh look at breast cancer cells' proteolysis and migration as therapeutic targets, and, finally, Chapter 22 details the current and emerging 3D models to better study and understand breast cancer progression in research laboratories without compromising on the clinical relevance.

The first volume was very well received because of its comprehensive coverage of topics. With the ever-evolving research, technology, and knowledge, it was imperative to provide updated information on many of the original topics. This was the primary objective of this volume. In addition, several new topics have been covered in this volume that are reflective of the progress and current topics of interest in the field. Approximately half of the chapters in this volume are contributed by experts who also contributed to the first volume. These chapters by returning contributors provide updated information on respective topics. At the same time, the other half of this volume comes from experts who are new to the team. These chapters, and the new topics covered therein, provide fresh perspective on our overall understanding of breast cancer metastasis and drug resistance.

I remain thankful to all the authors who contributed their knowledge to this book. Thanks again to Springer Publishers for entrusting me with this project, and to the many talented and dedicated team members and collaborators with whom I worked at different stages of the production of this volume. It is my distinct pleasure to present this volume to the scientific community with the hope that recent advancements in our knowledge translate into a better future for all breast cancer patients.

Mobile, AL, USA   Aamir Ahmad

Contents

Contributors

Mohammad Aatif Department of Public Health, College of Applied Medical Sciences, King Faisal University, Al-Ahsa, Kingdom of Saudi Arabia

Rashda Abbasi Institute of Biomedical and Genetic Engineering (IBGE), Islamabad, Pakistan

Aamir Ahmad Mitchell Cancer Institute, University of South Alabama, Mobile, AL, USA

Nafees Ahmad Institute of Biomedical and Genetic Engineering (IBGE), Islamabad, Pakistan

Misbah Akram Department of Bioinformatics and Biotechnology, International Islamic University, Islamabad, Pakistan

Nataly Naser Al Deen Department of Biology, Faculty of Arts and Sciences, American University of Beirut, Beirut, Lebanon

Richard A. Alo Natural Chemotherapeutics Research Laboratory, NIH/NIMHD RCMI-Center for Environmental Health, College of Science, Engineering and Technology, Jackson State University, Jackson, MS, USA

Aliye Aras Department of Botany, Faculty of Science, Istanbul University, Istanbul, Turkey

Rukset Attar Department of Obstetrics and Gynecology, Faculty of Medicine, Yeditepe University Hospital, Istanbul, Turkey

Cigir Biray Avci Medical Faculty, Department of Medical Biology, Ege University, Izmir, Turkey

Bakiye Goker Bagca Medical Faculty, Department of Medical Biology, Ege University, Izmir, Turkey

Bin Bao Department of Oncology, School of Medicine, Wayne State University, Detroit, MI, USA

Oznur Bayraktar Ekmekcigil Faculty of Medicine, Department of Medical Biology and Genetics, Okan University, Istanbul, Turkey

Bernhard Biersack Organic Chemistry Laboratory, Bayreuth, Germany

Yelda Birinci Faculty of Engineering and Natural Sciences, Sabanci University, Istanbul, Turkey

Takae M. Brewer Genomic Medicine Institute, Cleveland Clinic, Cleveland, OH, USA

Ghazala Butt Department of Botany, GCU, Lahore, Pakistan

Steven S. Coughlin Division of Epidemiology, Department of Population Health Sciences, Medical College of Georgia, Augusta University, Augusta, GA, USA

Prasad Dandawate ISTRA, Abeda Inamdar Senior College, Pune, India

Derek W. Edwardson Graduate Program in Biomolecular Sciences, Laurentian University, Sudbury, ON, Canada

Mohammad Fahad Ullah Department of Medical Laboratory Technology, Faculty of Applied Medical Science, University of Tabuk, Tabuk, Saudi Arabia

Mohd Farhan Department of Biology, College of Basic Sciences, King Faisal University, Al-Ahsa, Kingdom of Saudi Arabia

Ammad Ahmad Farooqi Institute of Biomedical and Genetic Engineering (IBGE), Islamabad, Pakistan
Laboratory for Translational Oncology and Personalized Medicine, RLMC, Lahore, Pakistan

Duber D. Fonseca Natural Chemotherapeutics Research Laboratory, NIH/NIMHD RCMI-Center for Environmental Health, College of Science, Engineering and Technology, Jackson State University, Jackson, MS, USA

Maria Luisa Gasparri Department of Gynecology and Obstetrics, University Hospital of Bern and University of Bern, Bern, Switzerland
Surgical and Medical Department of Translational Medicine, Department of Gynecology and Obstetrics, "Sapienza" University of Rome, Rome, Italy

William Harless Encyt Technologies Inc., Membertou, NS, Canada

Kyungmin Ji Department of Pharmacology and Barbara Ann Karmanos Cancer Institute, Wayne State University School of Medicine, Detroit, MI, USA

Lauren Kalinowski Faculty of Medicine, The University of Queensland, Centre for Clinical Research, Royal Brisbane and Women's Hospital, Herston, QLD, Australia
Pathology Queensland, Royal Brisbane and Women's Hospital, Herston, QLD, Australia

Gokce Seker Karatoprak Department of Pharmacognosy, Faculty of Pharmacy, Erciyes University, Kayseri, Turkey

Sumbul Khalid Department of Bioinformatics and Biotechnology, International Islamic University, Islamabad, Pakistan

A. Thomas Kovala Graduate Program in Biomolecular Sciences, Laurentian University, Sudbury, ON, Canada

Department of Chemistry and Biochemistry, Laurentian University, Sudbury, ON, Canada

Division of Medical Sciences, Northern Ontario School of Medicine, Sudbury, ON, Canada

Department of Biology, Laurentian University, Sudbury, ON, Canada

Sunil R. Lakhani Faculty of Medicine, The University of Queensland, Centre for Clinical Research, Royal Brisbane and Women's Hospital, Herston, QLD, Australia

Pathology Queensland, Royal Brisbane and Women's Hospital, Herston, QLD, Australia

Leroy Lowe Getting to Know Cancer (NGO), Truro, NS, Canada

Tomas G. Lyons Breast Medicine Service, Memorial Sloan Kettering Cancer Center, New York, NY, USA

Raymond R. Mattingly Department of Pharmacology and Barbara Ann Karmanos Cancer Institute, Wayne State University School of Medicine, Detroit, MI, USA

Amy E. McCart Reed Faculty of Medicine, The University of Queensland, Centre for Clinical Research, Royal Brisbane and Women's Hospital, Herston, QLD, Australia

Syed Musthapa Meeran Laboratory of Cancer Epigenetics, Department of Biochemistry, CSIR-Central Food Technological Research Institute, Mysore, India

Lucio Miele LSU Health Sciences Center, School of Medicine, Department of Genetics, New Orleans, LA, USA

Priya Mondal Laboratory of Cancer Epigenetics, Department of Biochemistry, CSIR-Central Food Technological Research Institute, Mysore, India

Rihab Nasr Department of Anatomy, Cell Biology and Physiological Sciences, Faculty of Medicine, American University of Beirut, Beirut, Lebanon

Farah Nassar Department of Internal Medicine, Faculty of Medicine, American University of Beirut, Beirut, Lebanon

Felicite Noubissi Natural Chemotherapeutics Research Laboratory, NIH/NIMHD RCMI-Center for Environmental Health, College of Science, Engineering and Technology, Jackson State University, Jackson, MS, USA

Kingsley O. Osuala Department of Pharmacology and Barbara Ann Karmanos Cancer Institute, Wayne State University School of Medicine, Detroit, MI, USA

Ulku Ozbey Department of Genetics, Health High School, Munzur University, Tunceli, Turkey

Amadeo M. Parissenti Graduate Program in Biomolecular Sciences, Laurentian University, Sudbury, ON, Canada

Department of Chemistry and Biochemistry, Laurentian University, Sudbury, ON, Canada

Division of Medical Sciences, Northern Ontario School of Medicine, Sudbury, ON, Canada

Health Sciences North Research Institute, Sudbury, ON, Canada

Division of Oncology, Faculty of Medicine, University of Ottawa, Ottawa, ON, Canada

Marinelle Payton Department of Epidemiology and Biostatistics, College of Public Service, Jackson State University, Jackson Medical Mall - Thad Cochran Center, Jackson, MS, USA

Dhanamjai Penta Laboratory of Cancer Epigenetics, Department of Biochemistry, CSIR-Central Food Technological Research Institute, Mysore, India

Sally Peyman School of Physics and Astronomy, University of Leeds, Leeds, UK

Ananda S. Prasad Department of Oncology, School of Medicine, Wayne State University, Detroit, MI, USA

Jelena Purenovic Faculty of Technical Sciences, Cacak University of Kragujevac, Cacak, Serbia

Bessi Qorri Department of Biomedical and Molecular Sciences, Queen's University, Kingston, ON, Canada

Muhammad Zahid Qureshi Department of Chemistry, GCU, Lahore, Pakistan

Sophie Roberts Leeds Institute of Cancer and Pathology, University of Leeds, Leeds, UK

Mirna Azalea Romero Facultad de Medicina, Universidad Autónoma de Guerrero, Laboratorio de Investigación Clínica, Av. Solidaridad S/N, Colonia Hornos Insurgentes, Acapulco, Guerrero, Mexico

Uteuliyev Yerzhan Sabitaliyevich Kazakhstan Medical University "KSPH", Almaty, Kazakhstan

Manpreet Sambi Department of Biomedical and Molecular Sciences, Queen's University, Kingston, ON, Canada

Jodi M. Saunus Faculty of Medicine, The University of Queensland, Centre for Clinical Research, Royal Brisbane and Women's Hospital, Herston, QLD, Australia

Rainer Schobert Organic Chemistry Laboratory, Bayreuth, Germany

Durray Shahwar Lahore College for Women University, Lahore, Pakistan

Samriddhi Shukla Department of Paediatrics, Cincinnati Children's Hospital Medical Center, Cincinnati, OH, USA

Jennifer N. Sims Department of Epidemiology and Biostatistics, College of Public Service, Jackson State University, Jackson Medical Mall - Thad Cochran Center, Jackson, MS, USA

Bonnie F. Sloane Department of Pharmacology and Barbara Ann Karmanos Cancer Institute, Wayne State University School of Medicine, Detroit, MI, USA

Valerie Speirs Leeds Institute of Cancer and Pathology, University of Leeds, Leeds, UK

Myron R. Szewczuk Department of Biomedical and Molecular Sciences, Queen's University, Kingston, ON, Canada

Sobia Tabassum Department of Bioinformatics and Biotechnology, International Islamic University, Islamabad, Pakistan

Rie K. Tahara Department of Breast Medical Oncology, The University of Texas MD Anderson Cancer Center, Houston, TX, USA

Rabih Talhouk Department of Biology, Faculty of Arts and Sciences, American University of Beirut, Beirut, Lebanon

Paul B. Tchounwou Natural Chemotherapeutics Research Laboratory, NIH/ NIMHD RCMI-Center for Environmental Health, College of Science, Engineering and Technology, Jackson State University, Jackson, MS, USA

Richard L. Theriault Department of Breast Medical Oncology, The University of Texas MD Anderson Cancer Center, Houston, TX, USA

Tiffany A. Traina Breast Medicine Service, Memorial Sloan Kettering Cancer Center, New York, NY, USA

Department of Medicine, Weil Medical College of Cornell University, New York, NY, USA

Naoto T. Ueno Department of Breast Medical Oncology, The University of Texas MD Anderson Cancer Center, Houston, TX, USA

Ilhan Yaylim Department of Molecular Medicine, Aziz Sancar Institute of Experimental Medicine, Istanbul University, Istanbul, Turkey

Clement G. Yedjou Natural Chemotherapeutics Research Laboratory, NIH/NIMHD RCMI-Center for Environmental Health, College of Science, Engineering and Technology, Jackson State University, Jackson, MS, USA

Liu Yi Department of Cancer Biology, Mayo Clinic Comprehensive Cancer Center, Jacksonville, FL, USA

Ning Yin Department of Cancer Biology, Mayo Clinic Comprehensive Cancer Center, Jacksonville, FL, USA

Tokmurziyeva Gulnara Zhenisovna Kazakhstan Medical University "KSPH", Almaty, Kazakhstan

Chapter 1
Breast Cancer Statistics: Recent Trends

Aamir Ahmad

Abstract Breast Cancer is the leading cancer, in terms of incidence, that affects women. Better prognosis is still associated with detection at early stages, resulting in increased emphasis on timely and improved screening strategies. More data is now available on the incidence as well as mortality of almost all cancers, including breast cancer. This article discusses the trends in incidence as well as mortality of breast cancer in the US over last ten reportings i.e. years 2009 through 2018, along with an overview of recently reported numbers globally. The incidence rate is clearly on rise, which is indicative of aggressive screenings and detections. The mortality rate has not increased at the same pace, suggesting better clinical management of breast cancer patients, but the numbers are still too high. While screenings and early diagnoses should still be a point of focus, particularly in developing and poor countries, more efforts are needed to improve the prognosis of patients diagnosed at a later stage.

Keywords Breast cancer statistics · Breast cancer trends · Breast cancer incidence · Breast cancer mortality

1.1 Introduction

Breast cancer (BC) continues to abruptly disrupt the lives of millions of women. Just this year (2018), 2.1 million new cases of BC are expected to be diagnosed worldwide [3]. In US alone, this number is expected to be more than a quarter of million [20]. For many years, BC has consistently ranked among the top cancers in the women, both in terms of incidence and mortality. However, with the changing population dynamics, screening methods, therapies etc., the relative rankings of some cancers have changed. This introductory chapter in this volume will discuss

A. Ahmad (✉)
Mitchell Cancer Institute, University of South Alabama, Mobile, AL, USA
e-mail: aahmad@health.southalabama.edu

© Springer Nature Switzerland AG 2019

A. Ahmad (ed.), *Breast Cancer Metastasis and Drug Resistance*,
Advances in Experimental Medicine and Biology 1152,
https://doi.org/10.1007/978-3-030-20301-6_1

the most recent BC statistics and will compare statistical data over the last 10 years in the US, for which the most comprehensive figures are available, with the aim to get a sense of the changings trends, if any, as they relate to BC.

1.2 Breast Cancer in the US over Last 10 Years

The estimated total (men and women combined) new BC cases and BC-related deaths in the US for the current year are 268,670 and 41,400, respectively [20]. About a decade back, for the year 2009, these numbers were 194,280 and 40,610, respectively [9] (Table 1.1). Looking at just the raw numbers in the Table, the one thing that stands out is the big jump in estimated new cases – a 38.29% increase in total cases. In contrast, the increase in estimated deaths over this decade has been relatively low, just 1.95%. The increase in new cases is alarmingly. Or maybe it might not be a such a bad news and might just be reflective of more aggressive screening efforts and the resulting diagnoses. The silver lining among these numbers is the comparative lower increase in deaths. Even though it should be realized that even a single death is one too many, the ability to keep these numbers in check through the last decade is a feat to be proud of. An even better way to look at these results would be to look at deaths as a fraction of incidence. Whereas in 2009, estimated deaths were 21.11% of estimated new cases, they are 15.41% for the current year. This represents a 27% reduction in the estimated deaths, relative to estimated new cases, over the last decade.

A more detailed analysis over these years, with year-to-year changes in incidence and deaths are presented in Figs. 1.1 and 1.2 [6, 9, 10, 14–20]. Years 2009 through 2011 witnessed a tremendous increase in estimated new cases. The estimated new cases then actually declined for the year 2012 [14]. Though surprising in the current representation, this was not a huge surprise at the time given that the BC incidence declined initially in the early 2000s. This was largely attributed to the findings of Women's Health Initiative (WHI) study which resulted in significant reduction in the use of postmenopausal hormone therapy, and, with it, the incidence of BC in the year 2003, compared to the preceding year [5, 11]. The decline, as

Table 1.1 Change in breast cancer incidence and mortality over last decade

| Year | Estimated new cases | | | Estimated deaths | | |
	Females	Males	Total	Females	Males	Total
2018	266,120 (30%, Rank1)	2550	268,670	40,920 (15%, Rank2)	480	41,400
2009	192,370 (27%, Rank1)	1910	194,280	40,170 (14%, Rank2)	440	40,610
Change (%)	38.34	33.51	38.29	1.87	9.09	1.95

The numbers are extracted from Cancer Statistics for the years 2018 [20] and 2009 [9]. Change (%) is the change (increase) in the year 2018, relative to year 2009. Numbers in parenthesis in the Females columns represent the percentage share of breast cancer among the women, relative to all cancers and its rank

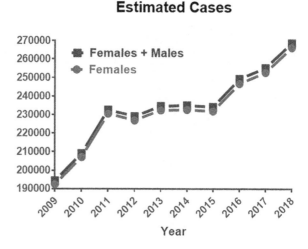

Fig. 1.1 Breast cancer incidence trend in the US. The estimated new cases of breast cancer in the US, as reported by American Cancer Society, for the years 2009 through 2018

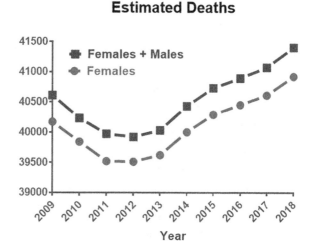

Fig. 1.2 Estimated breast cancer-related deaths trend in the US. The estimated breast cancer-related deaths in the US, as reported by American Cancer Society, for the years 2009 through 2018

witnessed just after the WHI study, however, did not sustain. The incidence of BC did not change much between the years 2003 through 2007, but then started increasing [5]. This is evident in our analysis as well (Fig. 1.1). The estimated death rates over the last decade have also witnessed interesting trend. They first decreased from year 2009 through 2012 but have been on an upward trend ever since (Fig. 1.2).

In terms of how BC in women stands among all the different cancers that are diagnosed in women, the percentage share of BC has ranged between 27% and 30% during the last decade (Fig. 1.3). It currently stands at 30% [20]. With such high numbers, accounting for more than a quarter of all diagnosed cancers, BC has consistently ranked the number 1 cancer diagnosed in women in the US. In terms of

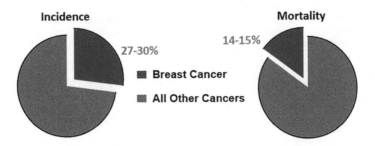

Fig. 1.3 Breast cancer burden among female cancer patients. The percentage share of breast cancer among all the different cancers diagnosed in females, as calculated from the data for years 2009 through 2018. The range (27–30% for incidence and 14–15% for mortality) represents the range reported over this period of reporting

deaths, the share of BC has altered between 14% and 15% during the last ten cancer statistics (Fig. 1.3). It now stands at 14% [20]. With these numbers, BC has consistently ranked number 2 in terms of cancer-related deaths in US women, second only to lung cancer.

1.3 Breast Cancer in Men

BC is men is a rare disease and accounts for just about 1% of the total BC incidence and BC-related deaths in the US (Table 1.1). However, compared to the women, the mortality rate in men has gone up significantly in 2018 (9.09% in men, compared to 1.87% in women). This is attributed to limited information on the men BC. Almost all the studies on BC and the clinical trials are focused on women and the knowledge gained is extrapolated to manage male BC patients in clinics [12]. This is not an optimum approach given the hormonal difference between the two genders. For example, male BC is typically hormone receptor positive with presence of androgen receptor and *BRCA1* mutations [8]. Though relatively much less abundant, male BC is very poorly understood, and studies exclusively focused on this BC subset are needed.

1.4 Trends in Breast Cancer Survival Rates

As expected, the best prognosis for BC is when it is diagnosed at an early stage and when it has not yet metastasized [1]. The 5-year survival of BC patients in the US was a poor 63% in the early 1960s but improved to 89% by the year 2009 [9]. In 2009, the 5-year survival for locally advanced BC that had spread to nearby organs was 84% and the same for BC that had spread to distant organs was 27% [9]. This clearly highlighted the poor prognosis of BC patients with advanced and metastatic disease. In 2018, it is estimated that a majority of cases (62%) are diagnosed when they have not yet metastasized and such patients have a 5-year survival rate of 99% [20]. The patients with invasive BC have 5-year survival rate of 90% and a 10-year survival rate of 83% [20]. The improvements in survival rates have been documented for women representing all major racial groups but they remain about 10% lower in African American women, compared to the White Caucasian women [20]. The reasons behind these racial disparities are not well-understood and a number of molecular as well as epigenetic factors are currently under investigation [2, 7]. The improvement in survival rates can be appreciated by the fact that mortality rate has gone down from 33.2 in 1989 to 20.3 in 2015 (per a population size of 100,000) resulting in prevention of approximately 322,600 BC-related deaths [20].

1.5 Global Trends in Breast Cancer Statistics

Globally, both the cancer incidence as well as cancer-related deaths are increasing rapidly [3]. For BC, 2088849 new cases are expected to be diagnosed and 626679 BC patients are estimated to die, worldwide, in the current year 2018 [3]. This corresponds to 11.6% of all cancers in terms of incidence which is statistically equal to the lung cancer incidence and ranks a co-number 1. Deaths-wise, BC's share is 6.6% of all cancer-related deaths worldwide and ranks number 1 for women.

As would probably be expected, the trends in individual countries/regions of the world vary. BC is the most frequently diagnosed cancer in women in 154 of 185 countries and is also the leading cause of cancer-related deaths in more than 100 countries. A list of top 25 US states and the top 25 countries globally, in terms of BC incidence, is provided in Table 1.2. An interesting observation is the overwhelming presence of developed countries in the list which could possibly be due to increased awareness and aggressive screenings.

1.6 Factors Influencing Differential Breast Cancer Incidence and Mortality

Even though a lot of factors are being investigated to explain these trends and the different incidence rates of BC in various populations, there is yet no consensus. Mutation in *BRCA1* and *BRCA2* have been investigated for long time and are risk factors for BC [21]. Other risk factors include changes in menstruation (early menarche age and delayed menopause), reproduction (late age at first birth), hormonal and alcohol intake and obesity [4]. Breastfeeding and more physical activity, on the contrary, are protective factors against BC. Interestingly, it has been reported that individuals migrating from low-incidence locations to high-incidence locations eventually report high incidence [22] thus supporting a role of environmental, dietary factors etc. in BC risk.

Table 1.2 US (states) and global (countries) ranking by breast cancer incidence

US		Global	
States	*Incidence Rate*[a]	*Countries*	*Incidence Rate*[b]
Dist. of Columbia	143.5	Belgium	113.2
New Hampshire	140.4	Luxembourg	109.3
Connecticut	139.2	Netherlands	105.9
Massachusetts	136.1	France (metropolitan)	99.1
Hawaii	136	New Caledonia (France)	98
Washington	134.9	Lebanon	97.6
Delaware	133.1	Australia	94.5
New Jersey	132	UK	93.6
Maryland	131	Italy	92.8
South Dakota	130.7	New Zealand	92.6
Rhode Island	130.3	Ireland	90.3
Minnesota	130.2	Sweden	89.8
Vermont	130.1	Finland	89.5
Illinois	130	Denmark	88.8
Pennsylvania	129.8	Switzerland	88.1
North Carolina	129.4	Montenegro	87.8
New York	129	Malta	87.6
Wisconsin	127.9	Norway	87.5
South Carolina	127.2	Hungary	85.5
Virginia	126.9	Germany	85.4
Oregon	126	Iceland	85.2
Missouri	125.9	US	84.9
Maine	125.5	Canada	83.8
Alaska	125.4	Cyprus	81.7
Colorado	123.7	Samoa	80.1

All numbers are per a population size of 100,000
[a]Incidence rate for US states is for the Years 2010–2014, age-adjusted to 2000 US population. **Source:** NAACCR 2017. Data are collected by cancer registries participating in the National Cancer Institute's SEER program and the Centers for Disease Control and Prevention's National Program of Cancer Registries
[b]Global Incidence rate is for the year 2018. **Source:** https://www.wcrf.org/dietandcancer/cancer-trends/breast-cancer-statistics

1.7 Conclusions

In terms of incidence, BC ranks number 1 in the US as well as globally. When counting for deaths, it ranks number 2 in the US but number 1 globally. Clearly, the best prognosis is when BC diagnosis is made at an early stage. In this era of personalized medicine, a personalized approach for cancer screening has been discussed recently in an attempt to improve BC diagnoses and early detections for better prognosis, however, there are clearly challenges associated with personalized approaches when dealing with large populations [13]. Progress has been made in the detection of BC at early stages resulting in better management and prognosis of patients, however, diagnosis at late stages still presents a challenge and more needs to be done for such patients.

References

1. Ahmad A (2013) Pathways to breast cancer recurrence. ISRN Oncol 2013:290568
2. Ahmad A, Azim S, Zubair H, Khan MA, Singh S, Carter JE, Rocconi RP, Singh AP (2017) Epigenetic basis of cancer health disparities: looking beyond genetic differences. Biochim Biophys Acta Rev Cancer 1868(1):16–28
3. Bray F, Ferlay J, Soerjomataram I, Siegel RL, Torre LA, Jemal A (2018) Global cancer statistics 2018: GLOBOCAN estimates of incidence and mortality worldwide for 36 cancers in 185 countries. CA Cancer J Clin 68(6):394–424
4. Brinton LA, Gaudet MM, Gierach GL (2018) Breast cancer. In: Thun MJ, Linet MS, Cerhan JR, Haiman CA, Schottenfeld D (eds) Cancer epidemiology and prevention, 4th edn. Oxford University Press, New York, pp 861–888
5. DeSantis C, Howlader N, Cronin KA, Jemal A (2011) Breast cancer incidence rates in U.S. women are no longer declining. Cancer Epidemiol Biomark Prev 20(5):733–739
6. DeSantis C, Siegel R, Bandi P, Jemal A (2011) Breast cancer statistics, 2011. CA Cancer J Clin 61(6):409–418
7. Deshmukh SK, Srivastava SK, Tyagi N, Ahmad A, Singh AP, Ghadhban AAL, Dyess DL, Carter JE, Dugger K, Singh S (2017) Emerging evidence for the role of differential tumor microenvironment in breast cancer racial disparity: a closer look at the surroundings. Carcinogenesis 38(8):757–765
8. Gucalp A, Traina TA, Eisner JR, Parker JS, Selitsky SR, Park BH, Elias AD, Baskin-Bey ES, Cardoso F (2019) Male breast cancer: a disease distinct from female breast cancer. Breast Cancer Res Treat 173(1):37–48
9. Jemal A, Siegel R, Ward E, Hao Y, Xu J, Thun MJ (2009) Cancer statistics, 2009. CA Cancer J Clin 59(4):225–249
10. Jemal A, Siegel R, Xu J, Ward E (2010) Cancer statistics, 2010. CA Cancer J Clin 60(5):277–300
11. Krieger N, Chen JT, Waterman PD (2010) Decline in US breast cancer rates after the women's health initiative: socioeconomic and racial/ethnic differentials. Am J Public Health 100(Suppl 1):S132–S139
12. Leon-Ferre RA, Giridhar KV, Hieken TJ, Mutter RW, Couch FJ, Jimenez RE, Hawse JR, Boughey JC, Ruddy KJ (2018) A contemporary review of male breast cancer: current evidence and unanswered questions. Cancer Metastasis Rev 37:599–614
13. Narod SA (2018) Personalised medicine and population health: breast and ovarian cancer. Hum Genet 137(10):769–778
14. Siegel R, Naishadham D, Jemal A (2012) Cancer statistics, 2012. CA Cancer J Clin 62(1):10–29
15. Siegel R, Naishadham D, Jemal A (2013) Cancer statistics, 2013. CA Cancer J Clin 63(1):11–30
16. Siegel R, Ma J, Zou Z, Jemal A (2014) Cancer statistics, 2014. CA Cancer J Clin 64(1):9–29
17. Siegel RL, Miller KD, Jemal A (2015) Cancer statistics, 2015. CA Cancer J Clin 65(1):5–29
18. Siegel RL, Miller KD, Jemal A (2016) Cancer statistics, 2016. CA Cancer J Clin 66(1):7–30
19. Siegel RL, Miller KD, Jemal A (2017) Cancer statistics, 2017. CA Cancer J Clin 67(1):7–30
20. Siegel RL, Miller KD, Jemal A (2018) Cancer statistics, 2018. CA Cancer J Clin 68(1):7–30
21. Winters S, Martin C, Murphy D, Shokar NK (2017) Breast cancer epidemiology, prevention, and screening. Prog Mol Biol Transl Sci 151:1–32
22. Ziegler RG, Hoover RN, Pike MC, Hildesheim A, Nomura AM, West DW, Wu-Williams AH, Kolonel LN, Horn-Ross PL, Rosenthal JF, Hyer MB (1993) Migration patterns and breast cancer risk in Asian-American women. J Natl Cancer Inst 85(22):1819–1827

Chapter 2
Epidemiology of Breast Cancer in Women

Steven S. Coughlin

Abstract Epidemiologic studies have contributed importantly to current knowledge of environmental and genetic risk factors for breast cancer. Worldwide, breast cancer is an important cause of human suffering and premature mortality among women. In the United States, breast cancer accounts for more cancer deaths in women than any site other than lung cancer. A variety of risk factors for breast cancer have been well-established by epidemiologic studies including race, ethnicity, family history of cancer, and genetic traits, as well as modifiable exposures such as increased alcohol consumption, physical inactivity, exogenous hormones, and certain female reproductive factors. Younger age at menarche, parity, and older age at first full-term pregnancy may influence breast cancer risk through long-term effects on sex hormone levels or by other biological mechanisms. Recent studies have suggested that triple negative breast cancers may have a distinct etiology. Genetic variants and mutations in genes that code for proteins having a role in DNA repair pathways and the homologous recombination of DNA double stranded breaks (*APEX1, BRCA1, BRCA2, XRCC2, XRCC3, ATM, CHEK2, PALB2, RAD51, XPD*), have been implicated in some cases of breast cancer.

Keywords Alcohol · Breast cancer · Diet · Epidemiology · Genetics · Physical activity

S. S. Coughlin (✉)
Division of Epidemiology, Department of Population Health Sciences, Medical College of Georgia, Augusta University, Augusta, GA, USA
e-mail: scoughlin@augusta.edu

© Springer Nature Switzerland AG 2019   9
A. Ahmad (ed.), *Breast Cancer Metastasis and Drug Resistance*,
Advances in Experimental Medicine and Biology 1152,
https://doi.org/10.1007/978-3-030-20301-6_2

2.1 Introduction

The global burden of breast cancer in women, measured by incidence or mortality, is substantial and rising in several countries [1, 2]. Breast cancer is the most commonly diagnosed invasive cancer in the United States for women of all racial and ethnic groups, with an estimated 231,840 new cases diagnosed in 2015 [3]. Breast cancer accounts for more cancer deaths among United States women than any site other than lung cancer. Breast cancer also occurs in men [4], but the disease is rare among men and there is a pronounced female-to-male disparity in breast cancer incidence. This chapter provides a summary of the distribution and determinants of breast cancer in women including both the descriptive epidemiology of the disease and an up-to-date review of risk factors identified in epidemiologic studies.

2.1.1 Incidence and Mortality Rates in the US

Breast cancer incidence and death rates increase with age; about 95% of new cases occur in women 40 years of age and older [3]. Breast cancer incidence rates in the United States continue to rise after menopause and are highest in the older age categories. Age-standardized incidence rates are higher among white women than black women, although black women in the United States have a higher mortality rate than white women. Incidence rates for Asian/Pacific Islander, American Indian/ Alaska Native, and Hispanic women in the United States are generally lower than those for white or black women [5, 6]. Mortality rates from breast cancer have decreased in recent years but racial disparities persist [7]. Whitman et al. [8] examined disparities in breast cancer mortality for the period 2005–2007 in the 25 largest cities in the United States. Almost all the non-Hispanic black rates were greater than almost all the non-Hispanic white rates. In an updated analysis of data from Chicago and nine other cities, the racial disparity in breast cancer mortality decreased in Chicago by 13.9% but, in the remaining nine cities, the mortality disparity either grew or remained the same.

The incidence of breast cancer in the United States increased until about 2000 then decreased from 2002 to 2003 [9]. Most of the decrease in that period was among women with estrogen receptor positive cancers [10]. From 2004 to 2012, overall breast cancer incidence rates remained stable [3].

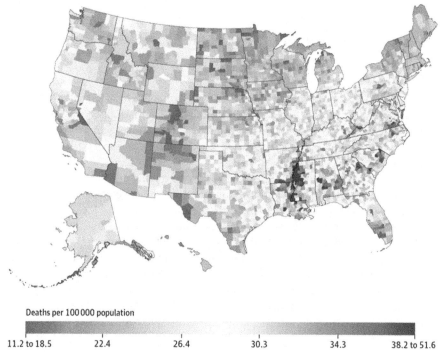

Deaths per 100 000 population

| 11.2 to 18.5 | 22.4 | 26.4 | 30.3 | 34.3 | 38.2 to 51.6 |

Age-standardized mortality rate from breast cancer (females only), 2014. (Mokdad et al. [113])

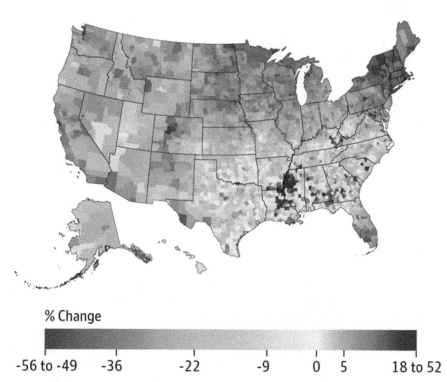

% Change

| -56 to -49 | -36 | -22 | -9 | 0 | 5 | 18 to 52 |

Percent change in age-standardized mortality rate from breast cancer (females only), 1980–2014. (Mokdad et al. [113])

2.1.2   International Trends in Breast Cancer Incidence and Mortality

Worldwide, an estimated 1.7 million women were diagnosed with breast cancer in 2012 and about 521,900 women died from the disease that same year [2]. Breast cancer incidence rates tend to be higher among more affluent women, both within countries and internationally. More than two-thirds of breast cancer cases are diagnosed in women aged 50 years and older; the majority of these cases are in developed countries [11]. For women aged 15–49 years, twice as many breast cancer cases are diagnosed in developing countries than in developed countries [9]. Between 1980 and the late 1990s, breast cancer incidence rates rose about 30% in westernized countries [2]. This trend was likely due to changes in reproductive patterns and increased screening. Since about 2000, rates in several countries have stabilized or decreased [2]. In many low- and middle-income countries, incidence rates have continued to increase [2]. In countries where mammography is available or affordable, adherence to recommendations for routine screening is associated with reduced mortality from breast cancer. Since about 1990, breast cancer mortality has been decreasing in many countries in Europe and North America [2].

2.2   Risk Factors

A variety of risk factors for breast cancer have been well-established by epidemiologic studies carried out to date, in addition to increasing age and female sex. These risk factors include nonmodifiable factors such as race, ethnicity, and genetics, as well as modifiable exposures related to diet, physical inactivity, exogenous hormones, and certain female reproductive factors. Circulating levels of endogenous sex steroid hormones such as estradiol have been associated with increased risk of breast cancer among postmenopausal women [12]. Sex hormone levels are strongly associated with some risk factors for breast cancer (for example, obesity and higher alcohol consumption) and may mediate the effects of these factors on breast cancer risk [13].

2.2.1   Race

Several factors may account for racial differences in breast cancer mortality including socioeconomic factors, access to screening mammography and timely treatment, and biological factors. In the United States, Hispanic ethnicity and black race have been associated with later stage at breast cancer diagnosis [7, 14, 15]. Compared with white women in the United States, black women tend to have more aggressive breast cancers that present more frequently as estrogen receptor (ER) negative tumors [16]. Among premenopausal women, tumors that are ER negative, progesterone receptor (PR) negative, and HER2 negative ("triple negative" tumors) are more common among black women than among white women.

2.2.2 Age at Menarche, Parity, and Age at First Live Birth

Younger age at menarche, parity, and older age at first full-term pregnancy are well-established risk factors for breast cancer. These risk factors may influence breast cancer risk through long-term effects on sex hormone levels in premenopausal women, through long-lasting changes in breast tissue, or by other biological mechanisms [17]. Reproductive hormones may influence breast cancer risk by increasing cell proliferation and increasing the likelihood of damage to DNA or by promoting cancer growth [3]. In a pooled analysis of control group data from 13 studies of postmenopausal women, circulating levels of estradiol were 6% lower in women who had menarche at ages 14 years or older than in women who had menarche before 12 years [13].

Nulliparity increases breast cancer risk in older women [18]. Results from a cohort study of Norwegian women indicated that nulliparity and obesity may have a synergistic effect on breast cancer risk among older women [19]. In the Black Women's Health Study in the United States [20], higher parity was associated with a reduced risk of ER positive/PR positive breast cancer (hazard ratio = 0.53, 95% CI 0.39–0.73 for 3 vs. 0 births, p-trend = 0.0002). Pregnancy may reduce breast cancer risk by bringing about persistent changes in the mammary gland that make the breast less susceptible to carcinogenic factors [19]. Younger age at first live birth is protective.

2.2.3 Breastfeeding

Breastfeeding reduces a woman's risk of breast cancer and is an important modifiable preventive behavior. Longer duration of breastfeeding has been associated with a greater reduction in breast cancer risk. The higher incidence of ER negative/PR negative breast cancer among black women in the United States may be partly explained by their lower prevalence of breastfeeding relative to white women [20].

2.2.4 Menopausal Status and Age at Menopause

Older age at menopause is also a well-recognized risk factor for breast cancer. Both early menarche and older age at menopause increase lifetime exposure of breast tissue to hormones. Menopause hormone therapy is discussed below in Sect. 2.2.6.

2.2.5 Oral Contraceptives

Epidemiologic studies of oral contraceptive use and breast cancer risk have generally shown little or no increased risk [21]. Recent use of oral contraceptives may slightly increase the risk of breast cancer [3]. Using data from the Alberta Cancer Registry, Grevers et al. [22] estimated that about 6.3% of breast cancers diagnosed in Alberta in 2012 were attributable to the use of oral contraceptives. In an analysis of data from a multicenter, population-based case–control study, Marchbanks et al. found that breast cancer risk did not vary by oral contraceptive formation [21]. No formulation was significantly associated with an increased risk of breast cancer.

2.2.6 Hormone Therapy

Results from observational studies and the Women's Health Initiative Randomized Trial indicate that hormone replacement therapy after menopause increases breast cancer risk [23–25]. Use of a regimen that includes both estrogen and progesterone has been associated with a higher risk of breast cancer than the use of estrogen alone [23]. In the Carolina Breast Cancer Study, DeBono et al. [26] found that black women were less likely than white women to use any hormone therapy (HT) and were more likely to use an unopposed-estrogen formulation. Combined estrogen-progestin HT use was associated with a greater odds of breast cancer in white (adjusted OR = 1.48, 95% CI 1.03–2.13) and black women (OR = 1.43, 95% CI 0.76–2.70). Studies of breast cancer incidence in the United States, Canada, and European countries showed a 5–10% decline in breast cancer incidence following reductions in HT use after 2002 [27]. In several countries, however, temporal changes in screening mammography are also likely to have played a role in the decline in breast cancer incidence. Women who do not currently use HT may also undergo screening mammography less frequently [27, 28].

2.2.7 Diet

A wide variety of dietary factors have been examined as potential breast cancer risk factors in case–control and prospective studies, including increased consumption of alcohol [29–31], red meat, processed meat, and animal fat, and decreased consumption of fruits and vegetables, calcium, vitamin D, soy, and antioxidants such as beta-carotene and other carotenoids, vitamin C, and vitamin E [32–35]. The ratio of omega-3 to omega-6 fatty acids has also been examined in relation to breast cancer risk. Although initial studies suggest that a higher ratio of omega-3 to omega-6 fats may reduce breast cancer risk, more research is warranted [36]. For most dietary factors, epidemiologic studies of breast cancer have provided inconsistent or inconclusive results. A notable exception is alcohol consumption, which is discussed separately below.

Foods with a high glycemic index and glycemic load and dietary carbohydrates, which can influence blood glucose and insulin concentrations, have also been examined in relation to breast cancer risk [37–40]. Low-energy dense diets are generally high in fiber and fruits and vegetables and low in fat [41]. The glycemic index is an indicator of the blood sugar response of the body to a standardized amount of carbohydrate in food. The glycemic load takes into account the amount of food consumed [36]. A meta-analysis by Mulholland et al., which focused on cohort study results, showed no overall association between postmenopausal breast cancer risk and glycemic load intake (RR = 1.03, 95 % CI 0.94–1.12) [42].

In a meta-analysis of prospective studies (14 studies of breast cancer incidence and 4 studies of breast cancer recurrence), Dong and Qin found that soy isoflavones consumption was inversely associated with breast cancer risk (RR = 0.89, 95% CI 0.79–0.99). However, the protective effect of soy was only observed among studies conducted in Asian populations [32].

Recent studies have examined dietary patterns in relation to breast cancer risk [43–46]. Harris et al. [44] examined whether adolescent and early adulthood inflammatory dietary pattern (high intake of sugar-sweetened and diet soft drinks, refined grains, red and processed meat, and margarine, an low intake of green leafy vegetables, cruciferous vegetables, and coffee) was associated with breast cancer among 45,204 women in the Nurses' Health Study II. Women in the fifth quintile of the inflammatory pattern score had adjusted hazard ratios for premenopausal breast cancer of 1.35 for adolescent diet (95% CI 1.06–1.73, p-trend = 0.002) and 1.41 for early adulthood diet (95% CI 1.11–1.78, p-trend = 0.0006) compared with women in the first quintile. Similar associations were not observed for postmenopausal breast cancer. In the Netherlands Cohort Study, van den Brandt and Schulpen [46] found a significant inverse association between Mediterranean diet adherence and risk of ER negative breast cancer (hazard ratio = 0.60, 95% CI 0.39–0.93, for high vs. low Mediterranean diet adherence, p-trend = 0.032). Mediterranean diet adherence showed only weak inverse associations with ER positive or total breast cancer risk. In the European Prospective Investigation into Cancer and Nutrition Cohort Study [45], which recruited women from ten countries, adherence to the Mediterranean diet was inversely associated with breast cancer risk overall (high vs. low adapted relative Mediterranean diet score hazard ratio = 0.94, 95% CI 0.88–1.00, p-trend = 0.048) and in postmenopausal women (high vs. low adapted relative Mediterranean diet score hazard ratio = 0.93, 95% CI 0.87–0.99, p-trend = 0.037). In a study of 20,009 cases and 2086 controls of the Canadian National Enhanced Cancer Surveillance System [43], consumption of the highest quartile of the "healthy" dietary pattern was related to a 22% decreased in risk of breast cancer (95% CI 0.61–1.00) compared to the lowest quartile.

2.2.8 Alcohol

An increasing number of epidemiologic studies have implicated alcohol consumption as a risk factor for breast cancer [29–31, 47]. Studies have shown a linear dose–response relation between alcohol consumption and breast cancer risk. Chen et al. [29] examined the association of breast cancer with alcohol consumption among 105,986 women enrolled in the Nurses' Health Study, of whom 7690 developed invasive breast cancer over the period 1980 through June 2008. Alcohol consumption was significantly associated with increased breast cancer risk even at levels as low as 5.0–9.9 g per day, or about three to six drinks per week (RR = 1.15, 95% CI 1.06–1.24). Cumulative average alcohol consumption over long periods of time was found to be the most relevant measure [29]. The possible biological mechanisms include alcohol's effects on circulating estrogen levels. Ja Kim et al. [47] examined the association between alcohol consumption and breast cancer risk in younger women in the Nurses' Health Study II. Alcohol consumption was not associated with breast cancer risk overall (multivariate hazard ratio = 1.07, 95% CI 0.94–1.22 for 10 g/day intake vs. nondrinkers). However, when the association was stratified by family history and folate intake, a positive association between alcohol consumption and breast cancer was found among those with a positive family history and folate intake of <400 µg/day (multivariate hazard ratio = 1.82, 95% CI 1.06–3.12, p-trend = 0.08).

2.2.9 Physical Activity

There is considerable evidence from epidemiologic studies that high levels of physical activity reduces breast cancer risk in women [48]. The possible biological mechanisms include the influences of physical activity on body composition, insulin resistance, and circulating levels of sex steroid hormones [49]. In the Women's Health Initiative Cohort Study, which involved 74,171 women aged 50–79 years recruited by 40 United States clinical centers, women who engaged in regular strenuous physical activity at age 35 had a 14% decreased risk of breast cancer (RR = 0.86, 95% CI 0.78–0.95) compared to inactive women [50]. Similar but attenuated findings were observed for strenuous physical activity at ages 18 years and 50 years. The study results also indicated that longer duration of physical activity provides the most benefit [50]. The majority of epidemiologic studies that have examined associations between physical activity and breast cancer risk have evaluated activity during adulthood. Recent studies have found that physical activity during childhood and adolescence may also be inversely related to breast cancer risk [51–53].

2.2.10 Anthropometric Factors

Anthropometric factors such as body height, weight, and adiposity have been extensively studied in epidemiologic studies of breast cancer [54, 55]. Body fat provides
a substrate for the production of estrogen from androgen in adipose tissue [56]. In
the Cancer Prevention Study II cohort (n = 495,477 women), Calle et al. found that
women with higher values of body mass index had an increased risk of dying from
breast cancer and certain other cancers [57]. Welti et al. [58] examined weight-
change patterns during early to mid-adulthood and risk of postmenopausal breast
cancer using data from the Women's Health Initiative Observational Study.
Compared with weight stability, weight gain was associated with risk of breast cancer (hazard ratio = 1.11, 95% CI 1.03–1.20) after adjustment for body mass index.
Although overweight and obesity are important modifiable risk factors for breast
cancer among postmenopausal women, epidemiologic studies have shown that high
body mass index and other measures of adiposity are associated with a reduced risk
of breast cancer among premenopausal women [59, 60]. The age at which body
mass or adiposity is assessed (childhood, adolescence, or adulthood) is important.
In some studies, body mass index at age 18 years and body fatness during youth
have been inversely associated with breast cancer risk in both pre- and postmenopausal women [60].

Obesity and physical inactivity are important determinants of hyperinsulinemia
and insulin resistance. Hyperinsulinemia with insulin resistance has been reported
to be an independent risk factor for breast cancer [61]. Higher insulin levels may
contribute to increased tumor growth [62].

Obesity influences the amount of free insulin-like growth factor I (IGF-I) available to cells. Breast cancer has been related to cell proliferation in response to
growth factors such as IGF-1 and sex hormones [63]. The IGF-1 system is involved
in breast cancer development, progression, and metastasis [62, 64]. Increases in
serum or plasma levels of IGF-I have been observed in some epidemiologic studies
of premenopausal breast cancer [65] but results to date have been inconsistent.
Schernhammer et al. [66] conducted a nested, case-control study of IGF-I, insulin-
like binding protein-1 (IGFBP-1) and IGFBP-3 and breast cancer incidence in the
Nurses Health Study II cohort, which mainly consists of premenopausal women.
Plasma levels of IGF-I and its binding proteins were measured using prediagnostic
samples obtained from 317 women diagnosed with invasive or in situ breast cancer
and 634 matched controls. Overall, plasma levels of IGF-I, IGFBP-1 and IGFBP-3
were not associated with breast cancer risk. To examine the relationships between
IGF-I and breast cancer incidence among premenopausal women. The relationship
between prediagnostic IGF-I and insulin-like growth factor binding protein-3
(IGFBP-3) levels and breast cancer risk was examined in a meta-analysis of data
from 17 prospective studies conducted in 12 countries [67]. The overall odds ratio
for breast cancer for women in the highest versus the lowest quintile of IGF-I concentration was 1.28 (95% CI 1.14–1.44). The positive association with IGF-I, which

was not substantially modified by IGFBP-3 or menopausal status, was limited to estrogen receptor positive breast cancers.

In general, results from epidemiologic studies do not support an association between IGFBP-1 and breast cancer risk. Although results from some epidemiologic studies support an association between IGFBP-3 and risk of breast cancer among younger women, results to date have been inconsistent. Rinaldi et al. conducted a pooled analysis of data from three prospective studies in New York, Northern Sweden, and Milan, Italy [68]. Statistically nonsignificant, positive associations were observed between IGF-I and IGFBP-3 and breast cancer risk among younger women.

2.2.11   Mammographic Breast Density

Breast density is one of the strongest established risk factors for breast cancer. Women with more extensive mammographic density have over a fourfold increased risk of breast cancer [69]. Recent studies have suggested that interactions between mammographic breast density and breast cancer are modified by tumor characteristics such as ER status and grade [70, 71]. Mammographic density likely reflects the amount of epithelial and stromal cells in the breast and the proliferation of these cells but does not indicate any histological abnormality [72]. Mammographic breast density is less extensive in women who are parous and in those with a larger number of life births, and changes in response to exposure to hormones [72]. Mammographic breast density decreases throughout menopause and increases with combined hormone therapy [73]. Longitudinal epidemiologic studies have shown that mammographic density declines as women get older [74]. The change in mammographic density with age reflects a reduction in glandular tissue and increase in fat [72]. Although influenced by changes in exposure to hormones, mammographic density is also a heritable quantitative trait [73].

2.2.12   Environmental and Occupational Exposures

Exposure to ionizing radiation (as a result of nuclear explosions, diagnostic fluoroscopy, or radiotherapy in adolescence) is an established breast cancer carcinogen [75, 76]. The biological mechanism is likely to be induction of DNA mutations. A variety of chemical exposures have been purported to be associated with breast cancer. In epidemiologic studies, organochlorines, which included polychlorinated biphenyls (PCBs), dioxins, and pesticides such as dichlorodiphyenyl-trichlorethane (DDT), lindane and hexachlorobenzene, have not been consistently associated with breast cancer [77–79]. The risks of breast cancer associated with a wide variety of environmental exposures were reviewed by the Institute of Medicine at the request of Susan G.Komen for the Cure [80]. The IOM concluded that the evidence associating individual chemicals with breast cancer risk is not conclusive, and also recognized the need for further research in this area. The IOM noted that exposure to chemicals with estrogenic or other properties relevant to sex steroid activity, such as bisphenol A (BPA), polybrominated diphenyl ethers (PBDEs), and certain dioxins or dioxin-like compounds, may possibly influence breast cancer risk. The risk of breast cancer from exposure to 2, 3, 7, 8-tetrachlorodibenzo-*p*-dioxin (TCDD) has been reviewed by several authors and expert panels with no consistent evidence of an increased risk [81]. Despite the lack of conclusive evidence from epidemiologic studies, exposures to chemicals with estrogenic or other properties relevant to sex steroid activity could influence breast cancer risk if the exposures occur at critical life stages or in combination with exposure to other similar chemicals [80]. Body mass and weight change may also modify associations between environmental exposures and breast cancer. In a population-based study of 10,006 post-menopausal women with in situ or invasive breast cancer and 990 age-frequency matched controls, Niehoff et al. [82] found that body mass index modified the polycyclic aromatic hydrocarbons-DNA adduct and breast cancer association. The odds ratio for detectable vs. non-detectable adducts was increased among women with a body mass index ≥ 25 (OR = 1.34, 95% CI 0.94–1.92), but not in those with a body mass index <25 (OR = 0.86, 95% CI 0.57–1.28). Sources of polycyclic aromatic hydrocarbons included cigarette smoking, grilled or smoked meat intake, residential synthetic log burning, and vehicle exhaust.

Shift work (evening or night work, rotating shifts, and working on-call) has an important influence on the body's sleep-wake rhythm. Results from several studies support an association between shift work and disruption of the circadian rhythm with breast cancer risk. In 2007, the International Agency for Research on Cancer concluded that shift work was probably associated with breast cancer, based on studies in animals and humans. However, some epidemiologic studies that have not found an association between shift work and breast cancer risk. In the Nurses' Health Study [83] a moderate increase in breast cancer risk was observed among women who worked 1–14 years (adjusted RR = 1.08, 95% CI 0.99–1.18) or 15–29 years on rotating night shifts (adjusted RR = 1.08, 95% CI 0.90–1.30). Levels of serum melatonin, which may have a protective effect, decrease when people are exposed to light at night. In experimental studies, the disruption of the nocturnal melatonin signal has been shown to activate human breast cancer growth, metabolism, and signaling [84].

Epigenetic changes such as DNA methylation have been associated with breast cancer in epidemiologic studies [85]. DNA methylation, which has been associated with environmental exposures such as cigarette smoke and persistent organic pollutants, may play a role in cancer causation by silencing genes through hypermethylation or, conversely, by activating genes through hypomethylation [85].

2.3 Risk Factors According to ER, PR, and HER2 Expression

As detailed in other chapters in this book, breast cancer subtypes are biologically distinct and may have distinct etiologies [86, 87]. This includes cases that express estrogen and/or progesterone receptors and those that overexpress the tyrosine kinase human epidermal growth factor receptor-2 (HER2) due to amplification of its encoding oncogene *ERBB2*. Using data from the Breast Cancer Surveillance Consortium (n = 743,623 women), Phipps et al. [88] examined associations between reproductive history and breast cancer cases classified according to tumor marker expression: estrogen receptor (ER) positive (n = 8203 cases), ER negative/proges- terone receptor (PR) negative/HER2 positive (n = 288), or ER negative, PR nega- tive, and HER2 negative (triple negative, n = 645). Nulliparity was most strongly associated with risk of ER positive breast cancer (hazard ratio = 1.31, 95% CI 1.23–1.39). Late age at first birth was most strongly associated with risk of ER negative/PR negative/HER2 positive disease (hazard ratio = 1.83, 95% CI 1.31– 2.56). Neither parity nor age at first birth was associated with triple negative breast cancer. About 12% of breast cancers are triple negative [3]. The most consistent evidence from epidemiologic studies for associations with reproductive risk factors exists for ER positive breast cancers [89]. The single protective factor most consis- tently associated with triple negative breast cancer was longer duration of breast- feeding [89]. In a pooled analysis of data from three population-based case-control studies, Ma et al. [90] examined associations of reproductive factors and risk of triple negative breast cancer in white women and African-American women. Risk of triple negative breast cancer decreased with increasing duration of breastfeeding (p-trend = 0.006), but age at menarche, age at first live birth, and nulliparity were not associated with risk of triple negative breast cancer. The association between breastfeeding and risk of triple negative breast cancer was modified by age and race; the decrease in risk was greater for younger African-American women. Studies have shown that female reproductive factors such as early age at menarche, nulliparity, and older age at first live birth are most clearly associated with hormone receptor positive tumors, suggesting that triple negative breast cancer may have a distinct etiology [89–91]. Shi et al. [92] examined the relationship of moderate-to- vigorous physical activity (MVPA) with ER/PR/HER-defined post-menopausal breast cancer risk. Total lifetime leisure-time MVPA was associated with reduce risk of ER negative/PR negative breast cancer (p-trend = 0.014), regardless of HER2 status. In contrast, total lifetime household MVPA was associated with reduced risk of ER positive and/or PR positive breast cancer (p-trend <0.001), regardless of HER2 status. Recent studies, including emerging areas of research, have focused on central obesity and the metabolic syndrome as predictors of triple negative breast cancer [93].

2.4   Genetic Factors

Population-based epidemiologic studies and family-based studies have identified a number of low-penetrance genetic variants and rare, moderate-to-high penetrance genetic mutations including *BRCA1* and *BRCA2* gene mutations. As discussed in other chapters in this book, breast cancer is a heterogeneous disease and genetic factors likely account for pathological subtypes and much of the heterogeneity of the disease [94].

2.4.1   Family History of Cancer

Having a positive family history of breast cancer is an established risk factor for the disease. Women who have one first degree relative with breast cancer have about a twofold increased risk of developing breast cancer [95, 96]. Risk increases the younger the relative was at the time of diagnosis and with increasing number of first-degree relatives with breast cancer [3]. About 20% of breast cancer patients have a family history of the disease in a first degree relative. Only about 5–10% of breast cancer cases associated with a family history of the disease in a first-degree relative are inherited in an autosomal dominant fashion. These cases have features such as bilaterality, early age at onset, and occurrence in multiple generations [97]. Most breast cancer cases are sporadic and not associated with high penetrance gene mutations.

2.4.2   Genetic Polymorphisms

Genetic polymorphisms may account for why some people are more sensitive than others to environmental carcinogens such as exogenous estrogens and alcohol. A large number of genetic variants have been reported to be associated with breast cancer risk but relatively few low-penetrance polymorphisms have been consistently associated with the disease [98]. Most breast cancer susceptibility loci identified in candidate gene studies have not been confirmed [94]. Single nucleotide polymorphisms (SNPs) of the *XRCC2* and *XRCC3* genes, which code for proteins that play a role in the homologous recombination of DNA double strand breaks, have been shown to influence breast cancer risk. These include *XRCC2* rs3218536 and rs3218536 [98–100]. A variant of the caspase 8 gene (*CASP8*) has been convincingly associated with breast cancer risk [94]. Caspase 8 is a protease that is involved in the initiation of programmed cell death (apoptosis) following DNA damage [101].

2.4.3 BRCA Gene Mutations

Mutations in the *BRCA1 gene*, which is located on chromosome 17q, have been identified as causes of predisposition to breast, ovarian, and other cancers. The *BRCA2* gene is located on chromosome 13q. BRCA1 and BRCA2 are expressed in breast, ovarian, and other tissues and play a key role in the repair of double-stranded DNA breaks in the cell nucleus. Most of the deleterious mutations in the *BRCA1* and *BRCA2* genes are small deletions or insertions that result in the translation of a truncated protein [94]. *BRCA1* and *BRCA2* mutations account for about 15–20% of familial breast cancers [102]. Women who carry *BRCA1* and *BRCA2* mutations have an estimated 40–87% risk of breast cancer by age 70, although these risks are modified by other factors [103, 104]. There is considerable variability in the age of onset of cancer and the site of cancer across populations [105]. Kuchenbaecker et al. [106] examined risks of breast and contralateral breast cancer for *BRCA1* and *BRCA2* mutation carriers using data from the International BRCA1/2 Carrier Cohort Study, the Breast Cancer Family Registry, and the Kathleen Cuningham Foundation Consortium for Research into Familial Breast Cancer. The cumulative breast cancer risk by age 80 years was 72% (95% CI 65–79%) for *BRCA1* and 69% (95% CI 61–77%) for *BRCA2* carriers. For contralateral breast cancer, the cumulative risk 20 years after breast cancer diagnosis was 40% (95% CI 35–45%) for *BRCA1* and 26% (95% CI 20–33%) f for *BRCA2* carriers.

Genetic variants and gene–gene interactions that account for inter-individual variation in DNA repair capacity influence risk of breast cancer [105]. These include variants in the APEX1, *CHEK2, PALB2, ATM, and XPD* genes, which, like *BRCA1* and *BRCA2*, play a role in DNA repair mechanisms and help to maintain chromosomal stability [94]. Studies have suggested that genomic variation at multiple loci modify breast cancer risk in women who carry *BRCA1* mutations [107]. Some of these loci are known to encode proteins that interact biologically with *BRCA1* [94]. Candidate gene studies suggest that homozygosity for the *RAD51* 135G [C allele is associated with breast cancer risk in women who carry *BRCA2* gene mutations [108]. Interacting with *BRCA1, BRCA2*, and *ATM* at the cellular level, *RAD51* is part of a protein complex that plays a role in the repair of double strand DNA breaks. Genome-wide association studies carried out in general populations have identified additional genetic variants that are associated with breast cancer risk among *BRCA1* and *BRCA2* mutation carriers.

Other high-penetrance genetic mutations that increase breast cancer risk, and which are rare in the general population, include *TP53* germ-line mutations (found in Li-Fraumeni cancer syndrome), *PTEN* mutations (Cowden syndrome), and *STK1* mutations (Peutz-Jegher syndrome) [94].

2.5 Summary and Conclusions

This chapter has summarized the substantial epidemiologic literature on environmental and genetic risk factors for breast cancer in women. Breast cancer risk factors that have been well-established by epidemiologic studies include race, ethnicity, family history of cancer, and genetic variants, as well as modifiable exposures such as increased alcohol consumption, physical inactivity, exogenous hormones, and certain female reproductive factors such as younger age at menarche, nulliparity, and older age at first full-term pregnancy. Based upon attributable risks, about 30–35% of breast cancers could potentially be prevented by addressing obesity, physical inactivity, alcohol consumption, and hormone replacement therapy [109–112]. There is increasing evidence that breast cancer is a heterogeneous disease and that subtypes such as triple negative breast cancers may have a distinct etiology. Epidemiologic studies, family studies, and genome-wide association studies have identified several genetic variants and rare but moderate-to-high penetrance gene mutations that account for some cases of breast cancer. These include genetic variants of genes involved in DNA repair and the homologous recombination of DNA double-stranded breaks. However, the etiology of many breast cancer cases in the population remains unknown.

References

1. Coughlin SS, Ekwueme DU (2009) Breast cancer as a global health concern. Cancer Epidemiol 33:315–318
2. American Cancer Society (2011) Global cancer facts and figures, 2nd edn. American Cancer Society, Atlanta
3. American Cancer Society (2011) Breast cancer facts and figures 2011–2012. American Cancer Society, Atlanta
4. Miao H, Verkooijen HM, Chia KS, Bouchardy C, Pukkala E, Laronningen S, Mellemkjaer L, Czene K, Hartman M (2011) Incidence and outcome of male breast cancer: an international population-based study. J Clin Oncol 29:4381–4386
5. Joslyn SA, Foote ML, Nasseri K, Coughlin SS, Howe HL (2005) Racial and ethnic disparities in breast cancer rates by age: NAACCR breast cancer project. Breast Cancer Res Treat 92:97–105
6. Wingo PA, King J, Swan J, Coughlin SS, Kaur JS, Erb-Alvarez JA, Jackson-Thompson J, Arambula Solomon TG (2008) Breast cancer incidence among American Indian and Alaska native women: US, 1999–2004. Cancer 113(5):1191–1202
7. Yedjou CG, Tchounwou PB, Payton M, Miele L, Fonseca DD, Lowe L, Alo RA (2017) Assessing the racial and ethnic disparities in breast cancer mortality in the United States. Int J Environ Res Publ Health 14:486
8. Whitman S, Orsi J, Hurlbert M (2011) The racial disparity in breast cancer mortality in the 25 largest cities in the United States. Cancer Epidemiol 36:e147–ee51
9. DeSantis C, Howlader N, Cronin KA, Jemal A (2011) Breast cancer incidence rates in US women are no longer declining. Cancer Epidemiol Biomark Prev 20:733–799
10. Anderson WF, Katki HA, Rosenberg PS (2011) Incidence of breast cancer in the United States: current and future trends. J Natl Cancer Inst 21:1397–1402

11. Forouzanfar MH, Foreman KJ, Delossantos AM, Lozano R, Lopez AD, Murray CJL, Naghavi M (2011) Breast and cervical cancer in 187 countries between 1980 and 2010: a systematic analysis. Lancet 378:1461–1484

12. James RE, Lukanova A, Dossus L et al (2011) Postmenopausal serum sex steroids and risk of hormone receptor-positive and -negative breast cancer: a nested case-control study. Cancer Prev Res 4:1626–16311

13. Endogenous Hormones and Breast Cancer Collaborative Group (2011) Circulating sex hormones and breast cancer risk factors in postmenopausal women: reanalysis of 13 studies. Br J Cancer 105:709–722

14. Coughlin SS, Yoo W, Whitehead MS, Smith SA (2015) Advancing breast cancer survivorship among African-American women. Breast Cancer Res Treat 153:253–261

15. Coughlin SS, Richardson LS, Orelien J, Thompson T, Richards TB, Sabatino SA, Wu W, Conney D (2009) Contextual analysis of breast cancer stage at diagnosis among women in the United States, 2004. Open Health Services Policy J 2:45–46

16. Dunn BK, Agurs-Collins T, Browne D, Lubet R, Johnson KA (2010) Health disparities in breast cancer: biology meets socioeconomic status. Breast Cancer Res Treat 121:281–292

17. Russo J, Moral R, Balogh GA, Mailo D, Russo IH (2005) The protective role of pregnancy in breast cancer. Breast Cancer Res 7:131–142

18. Jatoi I, Anderson WF (2010) Qualitative age interactions in breast cancer studies: a mini-review. Future Oncol 6:1781–1788

19. Opdahl S, Alsaker MD, Jansky I, Romundstad PR, Vatten LJ (2011) Joint effects of nulliparity and other breast cancer risk factors. Br J Cancer 105:731–736

20. Palmer JR, Boggs DA, Wise LA, Ambrosone CB, Adams-Campbell LL, Rosenberg L (2011) Parity and lactation in relation to estrogen receptor negative breast cancer in African American women. Cancer Epidemiol Biomark Prev 20:1883–1891

21. Marchbanks PA, Curtis KM, Mandel MG, Wilson HG, Jeng G, Folger SG, McDonald JA, Daling JR, Bernstein L, Malone KE, Wingo PA, Simon MS, Norman SA, Strom BL, Ursin G, Weiss LK, Burkman RT, Spirtas R (2012) Oral contraceptive formulation and risk of breast cancer. Contraception 85:342–350

22. Grevers X, Grundy A, Poirier AE, Khandwala F, Feldman M, Friedenreich CM, Brenner DR (2016) Cancer incidence attributable to the use of oral contraceptives and hormone therapy in Alberta in 2012. CMAJ Open 4:E754–EE59

23. Calle EE, Feigelson HS, Hildebrand JS, Teras LR, Thun MJ, Rodriguez C (2009) Postmenopausal hormone use and breast cancer associations differ by hormone regimen and histologic subtype. Cancer 115:936–945

24. Reeves GK, Beral V, Green J, Gathani T, Bull D, Million Women Study Collaborators (2006) Hormonal therapy for menopause and breast-cancer risk by histological type: a cohort study and meta-analysis. Lancet Oncol 7:910–918

25. Chlebowski RT, Hendrix SL, Langer RD et al (2003) Influence of estrogen plus progestin on breast cancer and mammography in healthy postmenopausal women: the women's health initiative randomized trial. JAMA 289:3243–3253

26. DeBono NL, Robinson WR, Lund JL, Tse CK, Moorman PG, Olshan AF, Troester MA (2017) Race, menopausal hormone therapy, and invasive breast cancer in the Carolina Breast Cancer Study. J Womens Health (Larchmt) 27:377–386

27. Pelucchi C, Levi F, La Vecchia C (2010) The rise and fall in menopausal hormone therapy and breast cancer incidence. Breast 19:198–201

28. Breen N, Cronin KA, Tiro JA, Meissner HI, McNeel TS, Sabatino SA, Tangka FK, Taplin SH (2011) Was the drop in mammography rates in 2005 associated with the drop in hormone therapy use? Cancer 117:5450–5460

29. Chen WY, Rosner B, Hankinson SE, Colditz GA, Willett WC (2011) Moderate alcohol consumption during adult life, drinking patterns, and breast cancer risk. JAMA 306:1884–1890

30. Hamajima N, Hirose K, Tajima K, Collaborative Group on Hormonal Factors in Breast Cancer et al (2002) Alcohol, tobacco and breast cancer: collaborative reanalysis of individ-

ual data from 53 epidemiological studies, including 58,515 women with breast cancer and 95,067 women without the disease. Br J Cancer 87:1234–1245

31. Tjonneland A, Christensen J, Olsen A et al (2007) Alcohol intake and breast cancer risk: the European prospective investigation into cancer and nutrition (EPIC). Cancer Causes Control 18:361–373

32. Dong JY, Qin LQ (2011) Soy isoflavones consumption and risk of breast cancer incidence or recurrence: a meta-analysis of prospective studies. Breast Cancer Res Treat 125:315–323

33. Pan SY, Zhou J, Gibbons L, Morrison H, Wen SW (2011) Antioxidants and breast cancer risk—a population-based case-control study in Canada. BMC Cancer 11:372

34. Farvid MS, Cho E, Chen WY, Eliassen AH, Willett WC (2014) Dietary protein sources in early adulthood and breast cancer incidence: prospective cohort study. BMJ 348:g3437

35. Farvid MS, Chen WY, Michels KB, Cho E, Willett WC, Eliassen AH (2016) Fruit and vegetable consumption in adolescence and early adulthood and risk of breast cancer: population based cohort study. BMJ 353:i12343

36. Donaldson MS (2004) Nutrition and cancer: a review of the evidence for an anti-cancer diet. Nutr J 3:19

37. Sieri S, Pala V, Brighenti F, Pellegrini N, Muti P, Micheli A, Evangelista A, Grioni S, Contiero P, Berrino F, Krogh V (2007) Dietary glycemic index, glycemic load, and the risk of breast cancer in an Italian prospective cohort study. Am J Clin Nutr 86:1160–1166

38. Lajous M, Boutron-Ruault MC, Fabre A, Clavel-Chapelon F, Romieu I (2008) Carbohydrate intake, glycemic index, glycemic load, and risk of postmenopausal breast cancer in a prospective study of French women. Am J Clin Nutr 87:1384–1391

39. Shikany JM, Redden DT, Neuhouser ML, Chlebowski RT, Rohan TE, Simon MS, Liu S, Lane DS, Tinker L (2011) Dietary glycemic load, glycemic index, and carbohydrates and risk of breast cancer in the women's health initiative. Nutr Cancer 63:899–907

40. Jonas CR, McCullough ML, Teras LR, Walker-Thurmond KA, Thun MJ, Calle EE (2003) Dietary glycemic index, glycemic load, and risk of incident breast cancer in postmenopausal women. Cancer Epidemiol Biomark Prev 12:573–577

41. Hartman TJ, Gapstur SM, Gaudet MM, Shah R, Flanders WD, Wang Y, McCullough ML (2016) Dietary energy density and postmenopausal breast cancer incidence in the cancer prevention study II nutrition cohort. J Nutr 146:2045–2050

42. Mulholland HG, Murray LJ, Cardwell CR, Cantwell MM (2008) Dietary glycaemic index, glycaemic load and breast cancer risk: a systematic review and meta-analysis. Br J Cancer 99:1170–1175

43. Van Ryswyk K, Villeneuve PJ, Johnson KC, Epidemiology Research Group TC (2016) Dietary patterns and the risk of female breast cancer among participants of the Canadian national enhanced cancer surveillance system. Can J Public Health 107:e49–e55

44. Harris HR, Willett WC, Vaidya RL, Michels KB (2017) An adolescent and early adulthood dietary pattern associated with inflammation and the incidence of breast cancer. Cancer Res 77:1179–1187

45. Buckland G, Travier N, Cottet V et al (2013) Adherence to the Mediterranean diet and risk of breast cancer in the European prospective investigation into cancer and nutrition study. Int J Cancer 132:2918–2927

46. van den Brandt PA, Schulpen M (2017) Mediterranean diet adherence and risk of postmenopausal breast cancer: results of a cohort study and meta-analysis. Int J Cancer 140:2220–2231

47. Kim HJ, Jung S, Eliassen AH, Chen WY, Willett WC, Cho E (2017) Alcohol consumption and breast cancer risk by family history of breast cancer and folate intake in younger women. Am J Epidemiol 186:524–531

48. Neilson HK, Farris MS, Stone CR, Vaska MM, Brenner DR, Friedenreich CM (2017) Moderate-vigorous recreational physical activity and breast cancer risk, stratified by menopause status: a systematic review and meta-analysis. Menopause 24:322–344

49. Friedenreich CM, Neilson HK, Lynch BM (2010) State of the epidemiological evidence on physical activity and cancer prevention. Eur J Cancer 46:2593–2604

50. McTiernan A, Kooperberg C, White E, Wilcox S, Coates R, Adams-Campbell LL, Woods N, Ockene J (2003) Recreational physical activity and the risk of breast cancer in postmenopausal women. The women's health initiative cohort study. JAMA 290:1331–1336
51. Neihoff NM, White AJ, Sandler DP (2017) Childhood and teenage physical activity and breast cancer risk. Breast Cancer Res Treat 164:697–705
52. Kobayashi LC, Janssen I, Richardson H, Lai AS, Spinelli JJ, Aronson KJ (2013) Moderate-to-vigorous intensity physical activity across the life course and risk of pre- and postmenopausal breast cancer. Breast Cancer Res Treat 139:851–861
53. Boeke CE, Eliassen AH, Oh H, Spiegelman D, Willett WC, Tamimi RM (2014) Adolescent physical activity in relation to breast cancer risk. Breast Cancer Res Treat 145:715–724
54. Renehan AG, Tyson M, Egger M, Heller RF, Zwahlen M (2008) Body-mass index and incidence of cancer: a systematic review and meta-analysis of prospective observational studies. Lancet 371:569–578
55. Green J, Cairns BJ, Casabonne D, Wright FL, Reeves G, Beral V (2011) Height and cancer incidence in the million women study: prospective cohort, and meta-analysis of prospective studies of height and total cancer risk. Lancet Oncol 12:785–794
56. McTiernan A, Ulrich C, Slate S, Potter J (1998) Physical activity and cancer etiology: associations and mechanisms. Cancer Causes Control 9:487–509
57. Calle EE, Rodriguez C, Walker-Thurmond K, Thun MJ (2003) Overweight, obesity, and mortality from cancer in a prospectively studied cohort of US adults. N Engl J Med 348:1625–1638
58. Welti LM, Beavers DP, Caan BJ, Sangi-Haghpeykar H, Vitolins MZ, Beavers KM (2017) Weight fluctuation and cancer risk in postmenopausal women: the women's health initiative. Cancer Epidemiol Biomark Prev 26:779–786
59. Feigelson HS, Jonas CR, Teras LR, Thun MJ (2004) Weight gain, body mass index, hormone replacement therapy, and postmenopausal breast cancer in a large prospective study. Cancer Epidemiol Biomark Prev 13:220–224
60. Baer HJ, Tworoger SS, Hankinson SE, Willet WC (2010) Body fatness at young ages and risk of breast cancer throughout life. Am J Epidemiol 171:1183–1194
61. Bruning PF, Bonfrer JM, van Noord PA, Hart AA, de Jong-Bakker M, Nooijen WJ (1992) Insulin resistance and breast cancer risk. Int J Cancer 52:511–516
62. Coughlin SS, Smith SA (2015) The insulin-like growth factor axis, adipokines, physical activity, and obesity in relation to breast cancer incidence and recurrence. Cancer Clin Oncol 4:24–31
63. Talamini R, Franceschi S, Favero A, Negri E, Parazzini F, LaVecchia C (1997) Selected medical conditions and risk of breast cancer. Br J Cancer 75:1699–1703
64. Christopoulos PF, Msaouel P, Koutsilieris M (2015) The role of the insulin-like growth factor-I system in breast cancer. Mol Cancer 14:43
65. Hankinson SE, Willett WC, Colditz GA, Hunter DJ, Michaud DS, Deroo B, Rosner B, Speizer FE, Pollak M (1998) Circulating concentrations of insulin-like growth factor-I and risk of breast cancer. Lancet 351:1393–1396
66. Schernhammer ES, Holly JM, Hunter DJ, Pollak MV, Hankinson SE (2006) Insulin-like growth factor I (IGF-I), its binding proteins (IGFBP-1 and IGFBP-3) and growth hormone and breast cancer risk in the nurses health study II. Endocr Relat Cancer 13:583–592
67. Endogenous Hormones and Breast Cancer Collaborative Group (2010) Insulin-like growth factor 1 (IGF1), IGF binding protein 3 (IGFBP3), and breast cancer risk: pooled individual data analysis of 17 prospective studies. Lancet Oncol 11:530–542
68. Rinaldi S, Toniolo P, Muti P et al (2005) IGF-I, IGFBP-3 and breast cancer in young women: a pooled reanalysis of three prospective studies. Eur J Cancer Prev 14:493–496
69. Harris HR, Tamimi RM, Willett WC, Hankinson SE, Michels KB (2011) Body size across the life course, mammographic density, and risk of breast cancer. Am J Epidemiol 174:909–918
70. Yaghiyan L, Tamimi RM, Bertrand KA, Scott CG, Jensen MR, Pankratz VS, Brandt K, Visscher D, Norman A, Cough F, Shepherd J, Fan B, Chen YY, Ma L, Beck AH, Cummings

SR, Kerlilowske K, Vachon CM (2017) Interaction of mammographic breast density with menopausal status and postmenopausal hormone use in relation to the risk of aggressive breast cancer subyptes. Breast Cancer Res Treat 165:421–431

71. Bertrand KA, Scott CG, Tamimi RM, Jensen MR, Pankratz VS, Norman AD, Visscher DW, Cough FJ, Shepherd J, Chen YY, Fan B, Wu FF, Ma L, Beck AH, Cummings SR, Kerlikowske K, Vachon CM (2015) Dense and nondense mammographic area and risk of breast cancer by age and tumor characteristics. Cancer Epidemiol Biomark Prev 24:798–809

72. Boyd NF, Martin LJ, Yaffe MJ, Minkin S (2011) Mammographic density and breast cancer risk: current understanding and future prospects. Breast Cancer Res 13:223

73. Boyd NF, Melnichouk O, Martin LJ, Hislop G, Chiarelli AM, Yaffe MJ, Minkin S (2011) Mammographic density, response to hormones, and breast cancer risk. J Clin Oncol 29:2985–2929

74. Maskarinec G, Pagano I, Lurie G, Kolonel LN (2006) A longitudinal investigation of mammographic density: the multiethnic cohort. Cancer Epidemiol Biomark Prev 15:732–739

75. Land CE (1995) Studies of cancer and radiation dose among atomic bomb survivors: the example of breast cancer. JAMA 274:402–407

76. Hancock SL, Tucker MA, Hoppe RT (1993) Breast cancer after treatment of Hodgkin's disease. J Natl Cancer Inst 85:25–31

77. Millikan R, DeVoto E, Duell EJ et al (2000) Dichlorodiphenyldichloroethene, polychlorinated biphyenyls, and breast cancer among African-American and white women in North Carolina. Cancer Epidemiol Biomark Prev 9:1233–1240

78. Calle EE, Frumkin H, Henley SJ et al (2002) Organochlorines and breast cancer risk. CA Cancer J Clin 52:301–309

79. Krieger N, Wolff MS, Hiatt RA et al (1994) Breast cancer and serum organochlorines; a prospective study among white, black, and Asian women. J Natl Cancer Inst 86:589–599

80. Institute of Medicine (2012) Breast cancer and the environment: a life course approach. The National Academies Press, Washington, DC

81. Boffetta P, Mundt KA, Adami H-O, Cole P, Mandel JS (2011) TCDD and cancer: a critical review of epidemiologic studies. Crit Rev Toxicol 41:622–636

82. Niehoff N, White AJ, McCullogh LE, Steck SE, Beyea J, Mordukhovich I, Shen J, Neugut AI, Conway K, Santella RM, Gammon MD (2017) Polychyclic aromatic hydrocarbons and postmenopausal breast cancer: an evaluation of effect measure modification by body mass index and weight change. Environ Res 152:17–25

83. Schernhammer ES, Laden F, Speizer FE, Willet WC, Hunter DJ, Kawachi I, Colditz GA (2001) Rotating night shifts and risk of breast cancer in women participating in the nurses' health study. J Natl Cancer Inst 93:1563–1568

84. Blask DE, Hill SM, Dauchy RT, Xiang S, Yuan L, Duplessis T, Mao L, Dauchy E, Sauer LA (2011) Circadian regulation of molecular, dietary, and metabolic signaling mechanisms of human breast cancer growth by the nocturnal melatonin signal and the consequences of its disruption by light at night. J Pineal Res 51:259–269

85. Terry MB, Delgado-Cruzata L, Vin-Raviv N, Wu HC, Santella RM (2011) DNA methylation in white blood cells. Association with risk factors in epidemiologic studies. Epigenetics 6:828–837

86. Phipps AI, Buist DS, Malone KE, Barlow WE, Porter PL, Kerlikowske K, Li CI (2011) Reproductive history and risk of three breast cancer subtypes defined by three biomarkers. Cancer Causes Control 22:399–405

87. de Ruijter TC, Veeck J, de Hoon JPJ, van Engeland M, Tjan-Heijnen VC (2011) Characteristics of triple-negative breast cancer. J Cancer Res Clin Oncol 137:183–192

88. Phipps AI, Chlebowski RT, Prentice R, McTierman A, Wactawski-Wende J, Kuller LH, Adams-Campbell LL, Lane D, Stefanick ML, Vitolins M, Kabat GC, Rohan TE, Li CI (2011) Reproductive history and oral contraceptive use in relation to risk of triple-negative breast cancer. J Natl Cancer Inst 103:470–477

89. Anderson KN, Schwab RB, Martinez ME (2014) Reproductive risk factors and breast cancer subtypes: a review of the literature. Breast Cancer Res Treat 144:1–10

90. Ma H, Ursin G, Xu X, Lee E, Togawa K, Duan L, Lu Y, Malone KE, Marchbanks PA, McDonald JA, Simon MS, Folger SG, Sullivan-Halley J, Deapen DM, Press MF, Bernstein L (2017) Reproductive factors and the risk of triple-negative breast cancer in white women and African-American women: a pooled analysis. Breast Cancer Res 19:6
91. Yang XR, Chang-Claude J, Goode EL et al (2011) Associations of breast cancer risk factors with tumor subtypes: a pooled analysis from the breast cancer association consortium studies. J Natl Cancer Inst 103:250–263
92. Shi J, Kobayashi LC, Grundy A, Richardson H, SenGupta SK, Lohrisch CA, Spinelli JJ, Aronson KJ (2017) Lifetime moderate-to-vigorous physical activity and ER/PR/HER-defined post-menopausal breast cancer risk. Breast Cancer Res Treat 165:201–213
93. Davis AA, Kaklamani VG (2012) Metabolic syndrome and triple-negative breast cancer: a new paradigm. Int J Breast Cancer 2012:809291
94. Mavaddat N, Antoniou AC, Easton DF, Garcia-Closas M (2010) Genetic susceptibility to breast cancer. Mol Oncol 4:174–191
95. Coughlin SS, Khoury MJ, Steinberg KK (1999) BRCA1 and BRCA2 gene mutations and risk of breast cancer. Public health perspectives. Am J Prev Med 16:91–98
96. Newman B, Millikan RC, King M-C (1997) Genetic epidemiology of breast and ovarian cancers. Epidemiol Rev 19:69–79
97. Anderson TI (1996) Genetic heterogeneity in breast cancer susceptibility. Acta Oncol 35:407–410
98. Zhang B, Beeghly-Fadiel A, Long J, Zheng W (2011) Genetic variants associated with breast-cancer risk: comprehensive research synopsis, meta-analysis, and epidemiological evidence. Lancet Oncol 12:477–488
99. Lin WY, Camp NJ, Cannon-Albright LA et al (2011) A role for XRCC2 gene polymorphisms in breast cancer risk and survival. J Med Genet 48:477–484
100. Silva SN, Tomar M, Paulo C, Gomes BC, Azevedo AP, Teixeira V, Pina JE, Rueff J, Gaspar JF (2010) Breast cancer risk and common single nucleotide polymorphisms in homologous recombination DNA repair pathway genes XRCC2, XRCC3, NBS1 and RAD51. Cancer Epidemiol 34:85–92
101. Fulda S (2009) Caspase-8 in cancer biology and therapy. Cancer Lett 281:128–133
102. Turnbull C, Rahman N (2008) Genetic predisposition to breast cancer: past, present, and future. Annu Rev Genomics Hum Genet 9:321–345
103. Antoniou A, Pharoah PD, Narod S et al (2003) Average risks of breast and ovarian cancer associated with BRCA1 or BRCA2 mutations detected in case series unselected for family history: a combined analysis of 22 studies. Am J Hum Genet 72:1117–1113
104. Begg CB, Haile RW, Borg A et al (2008) Variation of breast cancer risk among BRCA1/2 carriers. JAMA 299:194–201
105. Ricks-Santi LJ, Sucheston LE, Yang Y, Freudenheim JL, Isaacs CJ, Schwartz MD, Dumitrescu RG, Marian C, Nie J, Vito D, Edge SB, Shields PG (2011) Association of Rad51 polymorphism with DNA repair in BRCA1 mutation carriers and sporadic breast cancer risk. BMC Cancer 11:278
106. Kuchenbaecker KB, Hopper JL, Barnes DR et al (2017) Risks of breast, ovarian, and contralateral breast cancer for BRCA1 and BRCA2 mutation carriers. JAMA 317:2402–2416
107. Rebbeck TR, Mitra N, Domchek SM et al (2011) Modification of BRCA1-associated breast and ovarian cancer risk by BRCA1-interacting genes. Cancer Res 71:5792–5805
108. Wang X, Pankratz VS, Fredericksen Z et al (2010) Common variants associated with breast cancer in genome-wide association studies are modifiers of breast cancer risk in BRCA1 and BRCA2 mutation carriers. Hum Mol Genet 19:2886–2897
109. Dartois L, Fagherazzi G, Baglietto L et al (2016) Proportion of premenopausal and post-menopausal breast cancers attributable to known risk factors: estimates from the E3N-EPIC cohort. Int J Cancer 138:2415–2427
110. Wilson LF, Page AN, Dunn NA et al (2013) Population attributable risk of modifiable risk factors associated with invasive breast cancer in women aged 45-69 years in Queensland, Australia. Maturitas 76:370–376

111. Taminimi RM, Spiegelman D, Smith-Warner SA, Wang M, Pazaris M, Willett WC, Eliassen AH, Huntr DJ (2016) Population attributable risk of modifiable and nonmodifiable breast cancer risk factors in postmenopausal breast cancer. Am J Epidemiol 184:884–893
112. Coughlin SS, Besenyi GB, Bowen D, De Leo G (2017) Development of a smartphone application for preventing breast cancer in women. mHealth 13(3):288
113. Mokdad AH et al (2017) Trends and patterns of disparities in cancer mortality among US counties, 1980-2014. JAMA 317(4):388–406. https://doi.org/10.1001/jama.2016.20324

Chapter 3
Health and Racial Disparity in Breast Cancer

Clement G. Yedjou, Jennifer N. Sims, Lucio Miele, Felicite Noubissi, Leroy Lowe, Duber D. Fonseca, Richard A. Alo, Marinelle Payton, and Paul B. Tchounwou

Abstract Breast cancer is the most common noncutaneous malignancy and the second most lethal form of cancer among women in the United States. It currently affects more than one in ten women worldwide. The chance for a female to be diagnosed with breast cancer during her lifetime has significantly increased from 1 in 11 women in 1975 to 1 in 8 women (Altekruse, SEER Cancer Statistics Review, 1975–2007. National Cancer Institute, Bethesda, 2010). This chance for a female of being diagnosed with cancer generally increases with age (Howlader et al, SEER Cancer Statistics Review, 1975–2010. National Cancer Institute, Bethesda, 2013). Fortunately, the mortality rate from breast cancer has decreased in recent years due to increased emphasis on early detection and more effective treatments in the White population. Although the mortality rates have declined in some ethnic populations, the overall cancer incidence among African American and Hispanic population has continued to grow. The goal of the work presented in this book chapter is to highlight similarities and differences in breast cancer morbidity and mortality rates

C. G. Yedjou (✉) · F. Noubissi · D. D. Fonseca · R. A. Alo · P. B. Tchounwou
Natural Chemotherapeutics Research Laboratory, NIH/NIMHD RCMI-Center for Environmental Health, College of Science, Engineering and Technology, Jackson State University, Jackson, MS, USA
e-mail: clement.yedjou@jsums.edu; felicite.noubissi_kamdem@jsums.edu; richard.alo@famu.edu; paul.b.tchounwou@jsums.edu

J. N. Sims · M. Payton
Department of Epidemiology and Biostatistics, College of Public Service, Jackson State University, Jackson Medical Mall - Thad Cochran Center, Jackson, MS, USA
e-mail: Jennifer.n.sims@jsums.edu; marinelle.payton@jsums.edu

L. Miele
LSU Health Sciences Center, School of Medicine, Department of Genetics, New Orleans, LA, USA
e-mail: lmiele@lsuhsc.edu

L. Lowe
Getting to Know Cancer (NGO), Truro, NS, Canada
e-mail: leroy.lowe@gettingtoknowcancer.org

© Springer Nature Switzerland AG 2019
A. Ahmad (ed.), *Breast Cancer Metastasis and Drug Resistance*,
Advances in Experimental Medicine and Biology 1152,
https://doi.org/10.1007/978-3-030-20301-6_3

among non-Hispanic white and non-Hispanic black populations. This book chapter also provides an overview of breast cancer, racial/ethnic disparities in breast cancer, breast cancer incidence and mortality rate linked to hereditary, major risk factors of breast cancer among minority population, breast cancer treatment, and health disparity. A considerable amount of breast cancer treatment research have been conducted, but with limited success for African Americans compared to other ethnic groups. Therefore, new strategies and approaches are needed to promote breast cancer prevention, improve survival rates, reduce breast cancer mortality, and ultimately improve the health outcomes of racial/ethnic minorities. In addition, it is vital that leaders and medical professionals from minority population groups be represented in decision-making in research so that racial disparity in breast cancer can be well-studied, fully addressed, and ultimately eliminated in breast cancer.

Keywords Breast cancer · Racial disparity · Black women · White women and other ethnic groups

3.1 Introduction

Apart from skin cancer, breast cancer is the most common form of cancer affecting women in the U.S. It is also the most prevalent cancer affecting women of every ethnic group in the United States. Breast cancer currently affects more than one in ten women worldwide [3]. The rate of getting and dying from breast cancer differs among ethnic groups [4–6]. Recent studies showed that new cases of breast cancer are about the same for Black and White women. However, the incidence rate of breast cancer before age 45 is higher among Black women than White women, whereas between the ages of 60 and 84, breast cancer incidence rates are strikingly higher in White women than in Black women. Yet, Black women are more likely to die from breast cancer at every age [7, 8]. Meanwhile, incidence and death rates for breast cancer are lower among women of other racial and ethnic groups than among non-Hispanic White and Black women. Asian/Pacific Islander women have the lowest incidence and death rates [7, 8].

While racial and ethnic disparities in cancer survival remain, studies have identified potential reasons for this disparity and possible ways of reducing racial disparity in breast cancer outcome in our populations. Different subtypes of breast cancer have been identified; the ER+ and HER2/neu-positive subtype, the ER+ and HER2/neu-negative subtype, and the basal-like breast cancer also known as triple negative tumors which are high-grade tumors and the most aggressive subtype. The incidence of this subtype in Black women especially, younger ones is twice the incidence observed in White women. Studies have now shown that pregnancy and higher parity increase the risk of basal-like breast cancer but reduces the risk of ER+/PR+ breast cancer. However, breastfeeding was found to eliminate that increased risk of triple-negative cancer [9]. It is also observed that Black women have more children especially at a younger age and lower rate of breastfeeding than

White women. These factors could account for the racial disparity in breast cancer. Other studies have identified possible differences in biological properties between Black women and White women, especially in the plasma levels of growth factors and hormones [10], reproductive factors [11, 12], susceptibility loci [13, 14], and primary tumor characteristics, including the presence and expression of steroid and growth factor receptors [12, 15–17], cell cycle proteins [18–20], tumor suppressor genes [21, 22], and chromosomal abnormalities [23]. These possible differences in biological properties between Black women and White women have the potential to influence breast cancer screening and treatment outcomes between the two ethnic groups. Since the early 1990s, several strategies, including early detection and diagnosis, reduction of tobacco smoking, widespread breast cancer screening, and improvement of breast cancer therapies, have been developed to improve the health of patients with breast cancer [24, 25].

Despite medical improvements in early detection, diagnosis and screening, many Black women are less likely to obtain adequate treatment compared with White women [26, 27]. Given all the research work that has been conducted for breast cancer treatment with limited success for African Americans; new strategies and approaches are needed to promote breast cancer prevention, improve survival rates, reduce breast cancer mortality, and improve the health outcomes of racial/ethnic minorities. In addition, it is vital that leaders and medical professionals from minority population groups be represented in decision-making in research studies so that racial disparity in breast cancer can be well-studied, fully addressed, and ultimately eliminated in breast cancer.

3.2   Racial and Ethnic Disparities in Breast Cancer

Racial and ethnicity disparities in breast cancer incidence and mortality rates remain largely unknown, but the possible risk factors include socioeconomic status, late stage of breast cancer at diagnosis, biologic and genetic differences in tumors, differential access to health care, and disease-related molecular mechanistic differences [28]. Traditionally, breast cancer incidence has been lower among Black women compared to White women [29]. Even though the incidence of breast cancer was initially lower in Black women than in White women, breast cancer rates for these two ethnic groups have converged in 2012. This indicated a slow and constant increase in the incidence of breast cancer in Black women while its rate remains stable in White women [30]. Hispanic women show an overall incidence of breast cancer lower than in non-Hispanic white women. However, their breast cancers are often diagnosed at a later stage and they generally present larger tumors than White women. Breast cancer remains the most common cancer (and the leading cause of cancer death) among this ethnic group as well [30]. Meanwhile, the mortality rate of breast cancer remains significantly higher among Black compared to White women and other ethnic groups [30, 31]. Black women tend to be diagnosed with breast cancer at a younger age than White women [32]. For example, the median age at diagnosis for Black women is 59, compared to 63 for White women [32]. Records show an increase in the incidence of breast cancer of 0.4% per year among Black women since 1975 and an increase of 1.5% per year among Asian/Pacific Islanders women since 1992. In contrast, the incidence remained stable among non-Hispanic Whites, Hispanics, or American Indians/Alaska Native women.

Asian-Americans who have recently immigrated to the U.S. show lower rates of breast cancer than those who have lived in the U.S. for many years. However, for Asian American women born in the U.S., the risk is about the same as that of White women [30]. The breast cancer 5-year relative survival rate has increased significantly for both Black and white Women in the last 40 years. Still, substantial racial gap remains. A 5-year survival rate was observed to be 81% for Black women and 92% for White women in recent years [8].

Chinese and Japanese women have the highest breast cancer survival rates whereas Black women have the lowest survival rate of any racial or ethnic group [30]. Overall, breast cancer mortality rate is still higher among Black women compared to White women and other ethnic groups [33]. The gap in breast cancer mortality rate among Black women continues to increase. For example, a report between 2000 and 2010 indicated that breast cancer mortality increased from 30.3% to 41.8% among African American women and that at the advanced stage, 5% of breast cancers are detected among White women compared to 8% of breast cancers among Black women [34].

3.3   Racial and Ethnic Variations in Breast Cancer Incidence and Mortality

Breast cancer does not strike all racial and ethnic groups equally. It varies by race and there is a troubling reality about survival rates for women with breast cancer. White women are more likely to be diagnosed with breast cancer, but Black women are more likely to die from the disease (Table 3.1). Table 3.1 below shows that in 2014, White women had the highest rate of getting breast cancer, followed by Black, Asian/Pacific Islander, Hispanic, and American Indian/Alaska Native (AI/AN) women with the lower incidence rate [29]. It also shows that in 2014, Black women were more likely to die of breast cancer than any other group, followed by White, Hispanic, Asian/Pacific Islander, and American Indian/Alaska Native women with the lower death rate [29].

Table 3.1 Racial or ethnic variations in female breast cancer incidence and mortality per 100,000 people in the United States in 2014 [29]

	White	Black	Asian/Pacific Islander	Hispanic	American Indian/Alaska Native
Incidence rates	127.7	125.1	98.5	93.1	82.2
Death rates	20.6	29.2	11.3	14.4	10.8

As seen on Table 3.1, the gap of breast cancer incidence is quite close between Black women and White women in the United State, but Black women are 42% more likely to die from this disease. Breast cancer also varies between states and different countries. Breast cancer incidence rates around the world vary significantly with approximately 80% in North America, Japan, and Sweden to about 60% in middle-income countries and below 40% in poor countries [35]. In 2012, it was estimated that more than 1.7 million new cases of breast cancer occurred among women worldwide [32].

3.4 Socioeconomic Disparities in Breast Cancer

Breast cancer incidence, survival, mortality rates as well as its risk factors vary not only between race and ethnic groups but also with socioeconomic status [36, 37]. Studies have suggested that racial disparities in breast cancer are reduced compared to the disparity observed when social and economic factors are examined alone. When socioeconomic status is considered, certain studies suggest that racial disparities in breast carcinoma are smaller than when social and economic factors are examined alone, but these disparities still persist [38, 39, 40]. Socioeconomic determinants affecting disparity in breast cancer mortality involve poverty, culture, and social injustice [41].

Poverty is a critical social player driving health disparity [42]. Low income women have significantly lower rates of breast cancer screening, greater probability for late-stage diagnosis, and very often receive inadequate and disparate treatment, resulting in higher mortality from breast cancer [37]. Poverty is associated with poorer breast cancer outcomes for all Americans, regardless of race; however, because a larger proportion of Black than Whites live in poverty [43]. Black are more likely to have the higher mortality rate due to breast cancer [44]. Low income women do not have a regular healthcare provider resulting in lower rates of mammography screening and greater probability for late-stage diagnosis [45, 46]. Living in disadvantaged areas with lack of infrastructures is another challenge that economically deprived women have to face to have access to primary care clinics and physicians for diagnosis, treatment, or follow up [47]. Moreover, health care providers available in underserved communities are not always equipped and trained to provide the adequate information or treatment to the population that they serve [47–50]. Lack or inadequate health insurance is another factor driving breast cancer disparity among women. Studies have shown that Black women are twice as likely to be uninsured and to depend on public insurance as White women [51, 52]. Low income Black women are not always able to take the time off from their job for preventative care due to their very limited financial resources and other competing survival priorities [44, 53]. The prevalence of comorbidity (obesity, diabetes, hypertension, cardiovascular disease, respiratory disease) is higher in low income women and particularly in Black women limiting their treatment options [37, 54, 55].

Poverty is also linked to less education and lack of information on breast cancer prevention and the importance of early detection leading late-stage diagnosis of breast cancer and lower survival rate [47, 56]. Other breast cancer risk factors associated with poverty are tobacco use, poor nutrition, physical inactivity, and obesity. Poor and minority communities are often targets of tobacco companies for marketing. Those populations often have limited access to fresh foods and healthy nutrition, and have fewer opportunities for safe recreational physical activity [45, 57–59]. Those factors result in greater body mass index and abdominal obesity which are associated with poorer breast carcinoma prognosis [60, 61]. Black women are more likely to have a diet high fat diet, low in fruits and vegetables, and are less likely to exercise regularly, and are more likely to be obese than White women [62–64]. Collectively, poverty and its associated factors including lack of primary care physician, geographical location, comorbidity, lack or limited health insurance, poor lifestyle, lack of information and lower education as well as other challenges contribute to breast cancer disparity among women. These conditions are mostly observed in the Black women population [43].

Cultural factors such as spirituality, misconception on the susceptibility of breast cancer, cultural beliefs and views as well as medical mistrust are more prominent in Black women when deciding about breast cancer screening, diagnosis, and treatment options. Spirituality has a strong influence on how many Black women manage their health condition [65, 66]. Black women are more likely than White women to rely on divine intervention alone for treatment rather than seeking appropriate medical treatment which can be detrimental for their survival [67]. However, other studies have suggested that spirituality could be beneficial in the life of some Black women as it can also promote early breast cancer screening and proper treatment [68, 69]. Some Black women tend to believe that they have lower risks of developing breast cancer than White women [67, 70], regardless of their family history of breast cancer [71, 72]. This view contributes to a decrease in mammography screening and inadequate actions to address breast issues [67]. Beliefs and attitudes towards breast cancer differ between White and Black women as well. Some Black women believe that any breast trauma or big breast is risk factors for breast cancer [73, 74]. More likely than White women, Black women would consider any swelling or lump in the breast that is not painful as non-cancerous and would not seek immediate care [75]. Overall, factors such as poverty, culture, and social injustice contribute directly and indirectly to breast cancer disparity among women. Black women are more likely to be affected by those determinants than White women. These factors often lead to lower breast cancer survival rates among Black women as compared to White women.

3.5 Majors Risk Factors in Breast Cancer Affecting Minority Populations

All women are at risk for developing breast cancer; however, there are several factors that alter the degree of risk for individual women. These factors include sex, age, genetic factors, family history, poor diet, personal health history, lack of physical activity and obesity [76]. They may belong to one of the three categories: genetic/family, environmental, and lifestyle.

3.5.1   Age and Sex Risk Factors in Breast Cancer Disparities

Age and sex are considered important risk factors in breast cancer incidence rates and mortality. Breast cancer incidence rates are higher among Blacks than Whites for women under age 45. It is rarely diagnosed in women younger than 25 years of age. The median age a woman is diagnosed with breast cancer is 61 years. The median age of diagnosis for black women is 58 years and 62 years for White women. The median age at breast cancer death is 68 years for all races; 62 years for Black women and 69 years for White women [77]. Approximately 252,710 women and 2470 men are estimated to be diagnosed with breast cancer in 2017. Men have a 1 in 1000 risk of developing breast cancer over his lifetime whereas approximately 1 in 8 women will develop breast cancer in her lifetime. Siegel and colleagues estimated that about 41,070 people (40,610 women and 460 men) will die from breast cancer in 2017 [78].

3.5.2   Family History and Genetic Mutations Risk Factors in Breast Cancer Disparities

One of the most widely recognized breast cancer risk factors is family history. Family history of breast cancer is a heterogeneous risk factor that depends on the number of family members affected, the age at diagnosis, and the number of unaffected women in the pedigree. A woman's breast cancer risk is increased if she has a first-degree relative with breast cancer at a young age or if she has multiple relatives with breast cancer [79–81]. Approximately 5–10% of breast cancers are thought to be hereditary [82]. The BRCA1 (breast cancer gene 1) and BRCA2 (breast cancer gene 2) gene mutations located on chromosomes 17 and 13, respectively, account for most of the autosomal dominant inherited breast cancers. BRCA1 and BRCA2 are human genes that produce tumor suppressor proteins. These proteins help repair damaged DNA and play a role in ensuring the stability of the cell's genetic material. When these genes are mutated, altered, or do not function property, DNA damage is repaired. Thus, cells are more likely to generate additional genetic alterations that can lead to cancer development. Prevalence rates of these mutations vary by ethnicity and race. For instance, BRCA1 mutations, the highest rates occur among Ashkenazi Jewish women (8.3%), followed by Hispanic women (3.5%), non-Hispanic white women (2.2%), Black women (1.3%), and Asian women (0.5%) [83, 84]. Approximately 55–65% of women who inherit a harmful BRCA1 mutation and about 45% of women who inherit a harmful BRCA 2 mutation will develop breast cancer by the age of 70. Moreover, 39% of women who inherit a harmful BRCA1 mutation and 11–17% of women who inherit a harmful BRCA2 mutation will develop ovarian cancer by the age of 70 [85, 86]. Women who have been diagnosed with breast cancer with harmful BRCA1 or BRCA2 mutations are more likely to develop a second cancer in with the ipsilateral breast or the contralateral breast than women who do not carry these mutations. Breast cancers in women with a harmful BRCA1 mutation are also more likely to be triple-negative cancers, which have poorer prognosis than other breast cancers. BRCA2 is a risk factor for male breast cancer [87]. Therefore, doctors recommend that women with early-onset breast cancer and women with a family history consistent with a mutation in BRCA1 and BRCA2 genes have genetic testing when breast cancer is diagnosed.

Although harmful mutations in BRCA 1 and BRCA 2 are responsible for breast cancer in almost 50% of families with multiple cases of breast cancer, a number of mutations in other genes have been associated with increased risks of breast cancer [88, 89]. Rare mutations include PTEN, TP53, MLH1, MLH2, and STK11 genes, as well as ATM, BRIP1, CDH1, CHEK2, MRE11A, NBN, PALB2, RAD50, RAD51C, and SEC23B [90]. The majority of the mutations in these other genes are linked with smaller increases in breast cancer risk than are seen with mutations in BRCA1 and BRCA2. However, mutations in the PALB2 gene are associated with a risk of breast cancer almost as high as the risk associated with inherited BRCA1 and BRCA2 mutations. PALB2 is a tumor suppressor gene. The PALB2 protein interacts with the BRCA1 and BRCA 2 proteins to help repair breaks in DNA. Approximately 33% of women with a harmful mutation in the PALB2 gene will develop breast cancer by age 70. The risk is even higher at 58% for women who have a family history of breast cancer and the harmful PALB2 mutation [91].

The differences in the genetics and biology of breast cancer incidence among Black women compared with White women are well-documented in the literature. A breast cancer study that evaluated 4885 White patients, 1016 Black patients, and 777 Hispanic patients reported significant differences in 5-year survival rates [92]. Findings from this research reported a 5-year survival rate of 75% ± 1% for White patients, 70% ± 2% for Hispanic patients, and 65% ± 2% for Black patients [92]. Despite most of the breast cancers not being of hereditary origin, lifestyle and environmental factors, such as diet, obesity, smoking, alcohol consumption, infectious diseases, and radiation have a profound influence on cancer development [93]. Although the hereditary factors cannot be modified, some lifestyle and environmental factors are modifiable and can be prevented. We recently reviewed and listed possible genes mutations that are associated with breast cancer development (Fig. 3.1) [94]. As seen in Fig. 3.1, BRCA1 and BRCA2 mutations increase breast cancer risk for breast cancer development. Other possible genes mutations that are linked to a smaller increase in breast cancer risk include ATM, CDH1, CHEK2, PALB2, PTEN, TP53, and STK11 genes.

3.5.3 Lack of Physical Activity Risk Factors in Breast Cancer Disparities

Many studies have demonstrated that women who are physically active have a lower risk of breast cancer than inactive women. This reduced risk of breast cancer has been seen in both premenopausal and postmenopausal women; however, the evidence for the association is stronger for postmenopausal breast cancer [95–98].

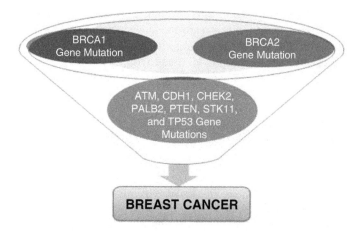

Fig. 3.1 Possible genes mutations associated with breast cancer development

Moreover, postmenopausal women who increase physical activity may result in a lower risk of breast cancer than women who do not exercise after menopause [95, 96]. A retrospective study in 1994 reported that women who were 40 years old and younger who engaged in 4 or more hours of physical activity per week lowered their breast cancer risk by more than 50% when compared with less active women of the same age [99]. In a 2013 meta-analysis study, breast cancer risk was reduced by an average of 12% from physical activity [98]. A report from the International Agency for Research on Cancer estimated that approximately one fourth to one third of cancer cases are associated with elevated body weight and inadequate physical activity [100]. African Americans are often overweight, obese, and have higher BMI and waist-to-hip ratios compared to Caucasians [101, 102]. Scientific data indicated that over 50% of Black women aged 40 years or older are obese and are over 80% overweight [103]. The lack of regular physical exercise among African American may explain why they have higher rates of obesity, a major risk factor of breast cancer [104].

A 2014 study by the Carolina Breast Cancer found racial differences in physical activity among breast cancer survivors revealed that African American women, compared to Caucasian women, are significantly less likely to meet national physical activity guidelines after diagnosis [105]. The lack or limited physical exercises have some implications for breast cancer care. Sisters Network Inc. suggests that only 47% of African American breast cancer survivors may be meeting these physical activity guidelines. Another study by the Northeast Ohio Breast Cancer Survivors found a gradual decline in physical activity levels after high school completion in African American compared to White women and revealed that only 12.3% of African American breast cancer survivors were meeting exercise guidelines [106]. Exercise lowers the levels of estrogen and other growth factors that have been associated with breast cancer development [107]. Exercise also controls blood sugar and regulates blood levels of insulin growth factor, a hormone linked to the growth and function of breast cells. People who are physically active tend to be healthier and are more likely to maintain a healthy body weight compared to people who do not exercise. A proposed breast cancer care model recommended that breast cancer patients should be educated about the importance of physical exercise at the point of breast cancer diagnosis, and provide them with the necessary support to stay active during the stage of breast cancer diagnosis-treatment and beyond [108].

3.5.4 Poor Diet and Obesity Risk Factors in Breast Cancer Disparities

Diet is a major contributor to health disparity in breast cancer and other chronic diseases. A person's diet can increase or decrease his or her risk for cancer. The American Cancer Society recommends eating a diet composed of mostly fruits, vegetables and whole grains. They urge people to consume less red beef, pork, lamb, bacon, sausage, luncheon meats, hot dogs, and fewer sweets. Nutritional factors including, dietary fat, meat, fiber, and vitamin D have been investigated as either promoting or inhibiting breast cancer development and survival [109]. Dietary fat intake is associated with breast cancer outcomes. The Women's Intervention Nutrition Study (WINS) concluded that modest weight loss associated with randomization to a low-fat diet improved relapse-free survival in early-stage breast cancer; however, the significance of these associations was not maintained in the long-term follow-up [110]. Furthermore, the intervention that included fat reduction and a diet high in vegetables, fruits, and fiber but did not lead to weight in the Women's Healthy Eating and Living (WHEL) randomized trial reported no association with recurrence or better prognosis in women with breast cancer [111]. These contradicting results may be a result of weight loss in the WINS and not the WHEL trial [109]. Several studies have demonstrated that a diet rich in vegetables, fruit, poultry, fish, and low-fat dairy products has been associated with a reduced risk of breast cancer. However, it is unclear if specific vegetables, fruits, or other foods can decrease breast cancer risk [109]. For example, the HEAL study recruited African American and Hispanic women from California, Washington, and New Mexico and reported that women with early-stage breast cancer who consumed a diet low in calories, added sugar, alcohol and saturated fat (quality diet) had a 60% reduced risk of all-cause mortality and an 88% lower risk of breast cancer-related mortality [112]. Another report from the HEAL study revealed that a quality diet was correlated with reduced levels of circulating inflammatory markers [113]. The HEAL study is unique since it is one of only a few large studies that is comprised of an ethnically diverse patient population recruited from different geographic locations that investigated an association between diet quality and breast cancer prognosis. Ethnically and racially diverse breast cancer survivors differ in levels of long-term adherence to dietary interventions, levels of physical activity and rates of obesity [114, 115]. Overall, the role of several dietary factors in breast cancer risk is inconclusive; however, there is much evidence from epidemiologic studies that indicate that diet may be linked with promotion or inhibition of the development of breast cancer, which may be due to a woman's food intake. Higher consumption of dietary fiber and vitamin D along with lower intake of saturated fat and red meat may reduce breast cancer risk. Further studies such as, well designed epidemiological and laboratory studies are warranted to investigate the association between diet and breast cancer risk [109].

Obesity has been a significant public health issue. Obesity, cardiovascular disease, and diabetes are more prevalent in Hispanics [116]. Type II diabetes is more prevalent among Native Americans [117]. African Americans have hypertension at an earlier age and tend to develop severe high blood pressure, but they are less likely to receive better treatment [118]. All these disorders are associated with cancer development. Diet-related disparity is a major contributor to differences in breast cancer incidence and treatment outcomes in racial/ethnic minorities compared to Whites. Therefore, in order to address and eliminate breast cancer health disparities, it is important to understand how diet contributes to these disparities. We recently reviewed the impact of poor diet on different types of cancers. We observed that approximately 10–75% of cancer related-deaths are attributed to poor diet (Fig. 3.2) [94]. As seen on Fig. 3.2, if a woman is eating a diet rich in vegetables and fruits, she can reduce her risk of getting breast cancer by 50%. For a man who is eating a diet rich in vegetable and fruit can reduce his risk of getting prostate cancer by 75%.

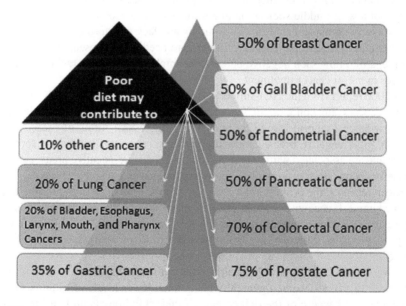

Fig. 3.2 Cancer deaths express in percentage that are associated with poor diet

3.6 Breast Cancer Prevention, Treatment, and Health Disparity

The majority of breast cancer cases are prevented if chemoprevention is applied in appropriate at-risk populations and the major modifiable risk factors such as maintaining a healthy weight, exercising regularly, and reducing alcohol intake are instituted [119]. Lack of insurance, fear of testing, delay in seeking care, barriers to early detection and screening, more advanced stages of disease at diagnosis among minorities, and unequal access to improvements in breast cancer treatment may explain the differences in survival rates between African American and White women [120–122]. Breast cancer tumors among Black and Hispanic women are more likely to be greater than 2 cm in diameter at diagnosis, are more likely to be estrogen-receptor and progesterone-receptor negative, and are more likely to have characteristics of poor differentiation, with nuclear atypia and higher S phase fraction. Furthermore, the prevalence of estrogen receptor-positive breast tumors is lower in African Americans and Hispanics than in Whites [123, 124], which might account for racial/ethnic differences in the use of tamoxifen. Scientific evidence suggests that, because of the increased risk of stroke, pulmonary embolism, and deep vein thrombosis associated with tamoxifen, African Americans, who already have a higher prevalence of risk factors for these conditions, may receive less overall benefit from tamoxifen [125]. Physician behaviors contribute to disparities in breast cancer mortality. For instance, a survey from York State hospitals revealed that physicians have more negative perceptions towards African Americans and people of low or middle socioeconomic status (SES) than of Whites and people of high socioeconomic status [126]. This finding and lack of information on how physician attitudes toward patients affect their care need further research, particularly with regard to how such negative perceptions might contribute to racial/ethnic disparities in breast cancer treatment.

A 2006 report from the NCI-supported research showed that aggressive forms of breast cancers are common in younger African American/Black and Hispanic/Latino women living in low SES areas. These aggressive forms of breast cancer such as triple negative breast cancer are less responsive to standard cancer treatments and are associated with poorer survival [122]. Triple-negative breast cancer is a heterogeneous disease in which tumors are defined by lack of expression of the estrogen receptor, the progesterone receptor, and the human epidermal growth factor receptor 2. It account for about 10–20% of invasive breast cancers and this subtype carries a poorer prognosis than the luminal tumors [22–24]. There are no targeted therapies currently available for the treatment of triple-negative breast cancer.

Low vitamin D levels have been associated with more aggressive triple-negative tumors [127]. Black women generally have much lower levels of vitamin D than White women because of the rich content of their skin in melanin that limits vitamin D absorption from the sun. Collectively, parity at a younger age, multiple parities, low rate of breastfeeding, in addition to lower levels of vitamin D could significantly contribute to the breast cancer disparity between Black women and

White women [128]. Socioeconomic factors are additional determinants of breast cancer disparity among women. Moreover Black women rely more that White women on breast self-examination as effective method for breast cancer detection therefore reducing their rate of mammography screening [129]. Behavior and beliefs also vary between White and Black women in the way they approach screening practices. Black women are more likely to avoid mammography screening by fear of pain, discomfort, embarrassment and radiation [130–132]. In addition, anxiety about the screening outcome is a tangible factor reducing mammography screening in Black women [133].

Misconception about surgery in breast cancer treatment is more prevalent in Black women than in White women [74]. Black women are less likely to seek surgery compared to White women, therefore limiting their treatment options leading to lower breast cancer survival rate [134]. A history of experimentation and abuse endured by Black in general has led to the development of medical mistrust. This factor has been suggested to contribute to the way Black women manage their overall health care and could account for breast cancer disparities between Black and White women [135, 136]. Racial bias may also account for the differences in mammography referrals between Black and White women. Studies have found that found that Black women were more likely than White women to mention lack of recommendation of mammography screening by their physician as a reason for not having undergone breast cancer screening [137]. Another report from the 2000 National Health Interview Study indicated that a 41% of Black women versus 28% of White women stated that their doctor had never suggested mammography [138].

3.7   Conclusions

In this book chapter we sought to describe racial breast cancer disparity primarily in the United State. The mortality rates among breast cancer patients are significantly higher among minority African American women compared to White women and other ethnic group in the United States [139, 140]. There are strong evidences showing that major disparities exist in breast cancer. Scientific data show that breast cancer incidence among Black/non-Hispanic Black women is slightly close to White/non-Hispanic White women [141]. However, Black women have more aggressive breast cancers developing at earlier ages and lower survival rates compared to White women [30, 31]. For example, the percentage of breast cancer mortality among Black women is about 42% higher compared to White women [29]. In addition, breast cancer survival rate has remained lower among White women and has increased over time in Black women [141]. The high mortality and low survival rates in breast cancer among Black women compared to ethnic groups can be attributed to late stage of breast cancer at diagnosis, barriers to health care access, biologic and genetic differences in tumors, and prevalence of risk factors [31, 142]. Other possible reasons for low survival rate among Black women include barriers to early detection and screening, lack of medical coverage, and unequal access to improvements in cancer treatment [121, 122, 124]. The continued growth of the

Black-White breast cancer mortality gap suggests that the current approaches to preventing or eliminating racial/ethnic disparities in breast cancer are not sufficient. Therefore, new strategies and approaches are needed to promote breast cancer prevention, improve survival rates, reduce breast cancer mortality, and improve the health outcomes of racial/ethnic minorities. In addition, it is vital that leaders and medical professionals from minority population groups be represented in decision-making in research studies so that racial disparity in breast cancer can be well-studied, fully addressed, and ultimately eliminated in breast cancer.

Acknowledgments This research was supported in part by the National Institutes of Health (NIH) grant #G12MD007581 through the RCMI-Center for Environmental Health and in part by the NIH grant #P20MD006899 through the Center for Minority Health and Health Disparities at Jackson State University. Research reported in this publication was supported by the National Institute on Minority Health and Health Disparities of the National Institutes of Health under Award Number P20MD006899. The content is solely the responsibility of the authors and does not necessarily represent the official views of the National Institutes of Health.

Author Contributions All authors contributed to the writing of the book chapter.

Conflicts of Interest The authors declare no conflict of interest.

References

1. Altekruse S et al (2010) SEER Cancer statistics review, 1975–2007. National Cancer Institute, Bethesda
2. Howlader et al (2013) SEER Cancer statistics review, 1975–2010. National Cancer Institute, Bethesda
3. Torre LA et al (2015) Global cancer statistics, 2012. CA Cancer J Clin 65(2):87–108
4. Ward E et al (2004) Cancer disparities by race/ethnicity and socioeconomic status. CA Cancer J Clin 54(2):78–93
5. Ries (1998) SEER Cancer statistics review, 1973–1994. National Cancer Institute, Bethesda; 1997 NIH Pub. No. 97–2789
6. Dalaker et al (1999) Bureau of the Census, current population report, series P60–210. Poverty in the United States; 1997. U.S. Government Printing Office, Washington, DC
7. Copeland et al (2015) Cancer in North America: 2008–2012. Volume one: combined Cancer incidence for the United States, Canada and North America. North American Association of Central Cancer Registries, Springfield
8. Howlader et al (2015) SEER Cancer statistics review, 1975–2012. National Cancer Institute, Bethesda
9. Palmer JR et al (2011) Parity and lactation in relation to estrogen receptor negative breast cancer in African American women. Cancer Epidemiol Biomark Prev 20(9):1883–1891
10. Pinheiro SP et al (2005) Racial differences in premenopausal endogenous hormones. Cancer Epidemiol Biomark Prev 14(9):2147–2153
11. Hall IJ et al (2005) Comparative analysis of breast cancer risk factors among African-American women and white women. Am J Epidemiol 161(1):40–51
12. Chlebowski RT et al (2005) Ethnicity and breast cancer: factors influencing differences in incidence and outcome. J Natl Cancer Inst 97(6):439–448
13. Haiman CA et al (2011) A common variant at the TERT-CLPTM1L locus is associated with estrogen receptor-negative breast cancer. Nat Genet 43(12):1210–1214
14. Kato I et al (2009) African American-preponderant single nucleotide polymorphisms (SNPs) and risk of breast cancer. Cancer Epidemiol 33(1):24–30

15. Ray M, Polite BN (2010) Triple-negative breast cancers: a view from 10,000 feet. Cancer J 16(1):17–22
16. Setiawan VW et al (2009) Breast cancer risk factors defined by estrogen and progesterone receptor status: the multiethnic cohort study. Am J Epidemiol 169(10):1251–1259
17. Dunnwald LK, Rossing MA, Li CI (2007) Hormone receptor status, tumor characteristics, and prognosis: a prospective cohort of breast cancer patients. Breast Cancer Res 9(1):R6
18. Porter PL et al (2004) Racial differences in the expression of cell cycle-regulatory proteins in breast carcinoma. Cancer 100(12):2533–2542
19. Martin DN et al (2009) Differences in the tumor microenvironment between African-American and European-American breast cancer patients. PLoS One 4(2):e4531
20. Gukas ID et al (2008) A comparison of clinicopathological features and molecular markers in british and nigerian women with breast cancer. Clin Med Oncol 2:347–351
21. Mehrotra J et al (2004) Estrogen receptor/progesterone receptor-negative breast cancers of young African-American women have a higher frequency of methylation of multiple genes than those of Caucasian women. Clin Cancer Res 10(6):2052–2057
22. Dookeran KA et al (2010) p53 as a marker of prognosis in African-American women with breast cancer. Ann Surg Oncol 17(5):1398–1405
23. Loo LW et al (2011) Genome-wide copy number alterations in subtypes of invasive breast cancers in young white and African American women. Breast Cancer Res Treat 127(1):297–308
24. Yip CH et al (2008) Guideline implementation for breast healthcare in low- and middle-income countries: early detection resource allocation. Cancer 113(8 Suppl):2244–2256
25. Ferlay J et al (2015) Cancer incidence and mortality worldwide: sources, methods and major patterns in GLOBOCAN 2012. Int J Cancer 136(5):E359–E386
26. Tammemagi CM (2007) Racial/ethnic disparities in breast and gynecologic cancer treatment and outcomes. Curr Opin Obstet Gynecol 19(1):31–36
27. Hirschman J, Whitman S, Ansell D (2007) The black:white disparity in breast cancer mortality: the example of Chicago. Cancer Causes Control 18(3):323–333
28. Ademuyiwa FO et al (2011) Impact of body mass index on clinical outcomes in triple-negative breast cancer. Cancer 117(18):4132–4140
29. Howlader et al (2017) SEER Cancer statistics review, 1975–2014. National Cancer Institute, Bethesda
30. ACS, American Cancer Society (2015) Breast cancer facts & figures, 2015–2016. 2015. American Cancer Society, Atlanta
31. ACS, American Cancer Society (2016) Breast cancer facts & figures, 2015–2016. 2016. American Cancer Society, Atlanta
32. Howlader et al (2016) SEER Cancer statistics review, 1975–2013. National Cancer Institute, Bethesda
33. Connor CS et al (2000) Local recurrence following breast conservation therapy in African-American women with invasive breast cancer. Am J Surg 179(1):22–26
34. ACS, American Cancer Society (2013) Cancer facts & figures for African Americans 2013–2014. American Cancer Society, Atlanta, 2013
35. Coleman MP et al (2008) Cancer survival in five continents: a worldwide population-based study (CONCORD). Lancet Oncol 9(8):730–756
36. Newman LA, Martin IK (2007) Disparities in breast cancer. Curr Probl Cancer 31(3):134–156
37. Bigby J, Holmes MD (2005) Disparities across the breast cancer continuum. Cancer Causes Control 16(1):35–44
38. Hunter CP et al (1993) Breast cancer: factors associated with stage at diagnosis in black and white women. Black/white Cancer survival study group. J Natl Cancer Inst 85(14):1129–1137
39. Michalski TA, Nattinger AB (1997) The influence of black race and socioeconomic status on the use of breast-conserving surgery for Medicare beneficiaries. Cancer 79(2):314–319
40. Yood MU et al (1999) Race and differences in breast cancer survival in a managed care population. J Natl Cancer Inst 91(17):1487–1491
41. Freeman HP, Chu KC (2005) Determinants of cancer disparities: barriers to cancer screening, diagnosis, and treatment. Surg Oncol Clin N Am 14(4):655–669, v

42. Freeman HP (2004) Poverty, culture, and social injustice: determinants of cancer disparities. CA Cancer J Clin 54(2):72–77
43. Census (2006) The statistical abstract. 2006, U.S. Census Bureau
44. Gerend MA, Pai M (2008) Social determinants of black-white disparities in breast cancer mortality: a review. Cancer Epidemiol Biomark Prev 17(11):2913–2923
45. Jones BA et al (1997) Severe obesity as an explanatory factor for the black/white difference in stage at diagnosis of breast cancer. Am J Epidemiol 146(5):394–404
46. O'Malley AS, Forrest CB, Mandelblatt J (2002) Adherence of low-income women to cancer screening recommendations. J Gen Intern Med 17(2):144–154
47. Lacey L et al (1993) Referral adherence in an inner city breast and cervical cancer screening program. Cancer 72(3):950–955
48. Williams DR, Jackson PB (2005) Social sources of racial disparities in health. Health Aff (Millwood) 24(2):325–334
49. Tamblyn R et al (2002) Association between licensure examination scores and practice in primary care. JAMA 288(23):3019–3026
50. Bach PB et al (2004) Primary care physicians who treat blacks and whites. N Engl J Med 351(6):575–584
51. Ni et al (2004) Trends in health insurance coverage by race/ethnicity among persons under 65 years of age: United States 1997–2001. National Center for Health Statistics, Hyattsville. 2004
52. Thomasson M (2006) Racial differences in health insurance coverage and medical expenditures in the United States: a historical perspective. Soc Sci Hist 30:529–550
53. Underwood SM et al (1994) Obstacles to cancer care: focus on the economically disadvantaged. Oncol Nurs Forum 21(1):47–52
54. Bickell NA et al (2006) Missed opportunities: racial disparities in adjuvant breast cancer treatment. J Clin Oncol 24(9):1357–1362
55. Tammemagi CM et al (2005) Comorbidity and survival disparities among black and white patients with breast cancer. JAMA 294(14):1765–1772
56. Gazmararian JA et al (1999) Health literacy among Medicare enrollees in a managed care organization. JAMA 281(6):545–551
57. Coates RJ et al (1990) Race, nutritional status, and survival from breast cancer. J Natl Cancer Inst 82(21):1684–1692
58. Forshee RA, Storey ML, Ritenbaugh C (2003) Breast cancer risk and lifestyle differences among premenopausal and postmenopausal African-American women and white women. Cancer 97(1 Suppl):280–288
59. Bernstein L et al (2003) Ethnicity-related variation in breast cancer risk factors. Cancer 97(1 Suppl):222–229
60. Long E (1993) Breast cancer in African-American women. Review of the literature. Cancer Nurs 16(1):1–24
61. Van Loon AJ, Goldbohm RA, Van den Brandt PA (1994) Socioeconomic status and breast cancer incidence: a prospective cohort study. Int J Epidemiol 23(5):899–905
62. Crespo CJ et al (1996) Leisure-time physical activity among US adults. Results from the Third National Health and Nutrition Examination Survey. Arch Intern Med 156(1):93–98
63. Stoll BA (1998) Western diet, early puberty, and breast cancer risk. Breast Cancer Res Treat 49(3):187–193
64. Ogden CL et al (2006) Prevalence of overweight and obesity in the United States, 1999–2004. JAMA 295(13):1549–1555
65. Johnson KS, Elbert-Avila KI, Tulsky JA (2005) The influence of spiritual beliefs and practices on the treatment preferences of African Americans: a review of the literature. J Am Geriatr Soc 53(4):711–719
66. Ellison et al (1996) Turning to prayer: social and situational antecedents of religious coping among African Americans. Rev Relig Res 38:111–130
67. Lannin DR et al (2002) Impacting cultural attitudes in African-American women to decrease breast cancer mortality. Am J Surg 184(5):418–423

68. Mansfield CJ, Mitchell J, King DE (2002) The doctor as God's mechanic? Beliefs in the Southeastern United States. Soc Sci Med 54(3):399–409

69. Potts RG (1996) Spirituality and the experience of cancer in an African American community: implications for psychosocial oncology. J Psychosoc Oncol 14

70. Olsen SJ, Frank-Stromborg M (1994) Cancer prevention and screening activities reported by African-American nurses. Oncol Nurs Forum 21(3):487–494

71. Hughes C, Lerman C, Lustbader E (1996) Ethnic differences in risk perception among women at increased risk for breast cancer. Breast Cancer Res Treat 40(1):25–35

72. Royak-Schaler R et al (1995) Breast cancer in African-American families. Risk perception, cancer worry, and screening practices of first-degree relatives. Ann N Y Acad Sci 768:281–285

73. Carter J et al (2002) Cancer knowledge, attitudes, beliefs, and practices (KABP) of disadvantaged women in the South Bronx. J Cancer Educ 17(3):142–149

74. Skinner CS, Arfken CL, Sykes RK (1998) Knowledge, perceptions, and mammography stage of adoption among older urban women. Am J Prev Med 14(1):54–63

75. Winstead-Fry P et al (1999) The relationship of rural persons' multidimensional health locus of control to knowledge of cancer, cancer myths, and cancer danger signs. Cancer Nurs 22(6):456–462

76. Parkin DM (2011) 1. The fraction of cancer attributable to lifestyle and environmental factors in the UK in 2010. Br J Cancer 105(Suppl 2):S2–S5

77. DeSantis CE et al (2016) Breast cancer statistics, 2015: convergence of incidence rates between black and white women. CA Cancer J Clin 66(1):31–42

78. Siegel RL, Miller KD, Jemal A (2017) Cancer statistics, 2017. CA Cancer J Clin 67(1):7–30

79. Claus EB, Risch NJ, Thompson WD (1990) Age at onset as an indicator of familial risk of breast cancer. Am J Epidemiol 131(6):961–972

80. Collaborative Group on Hormonal Factors in Breast, C (2001) Familial breast cancer: collaborative reanalysis of individual data from 52 epidemiological studies including 58,209 women with breast cancer and 101,986 women without the disease. Lancet 358(9291):1389–1399

81. Metcalfe KA et al (2009) Breast cancer risks in women with a family history of breast or ovarian cancer who have tested negative for a BRCA1 or BRCA2 mutation. Br J Cancer 100(2):421–425

82. Bogdanova N, Helbig S, Dork T (2013) Hereditary breast cancer: ever more pieces to the polygenic puzzle. Hered Cancer Clin Pract 11(1):12

83. John EM et al (2007) Prevalence of pathogenic BRCA1 mutation carriers in 5 US racial/ethnic groups. JAMA 298(24):2869–2876

84. Malone KE et al (2006) Prevalence and predictors of BRCA1 and BRCA2 mutations in a population-based study of breast cancer in white and black American women ages 35 to 64 years. Cancer Res 66(16):8297–8308

85. Antoniou A et al (2003) Average risks of breast and ovarian cancer associated with BRCA1 or BRCA2 mutations detected in case series unselected for family history: a combined analysis of 22 studies. Am J Hum Genet 72(5):1117–1130

86. Chen S, Parmigiani G (2007) Meta-analysis of BRCA1 and BRCA2 penetrance. J Clin Oncol 25(11):1329–1333

87. Breast Cancer Linkage C (1999) Cancer risks in BRCA2 mutation carriers. J Natl Cancer Inst 91(15):1310–1316

88. Campeau PM, Foulkes WD, Tischkowitz MD (2008) Hereditary breast cancer: new genetic developments, new therapeutic avenues. Hum Genet 124(1):31–42

89. Walsh T et al (2006) Spectrum of mutations in BRCA1, BRCA2, CHEK2, and TP53 in families at high risk of breast cancer. JAMA 295(12):1379–1388

90. National Cancer Institute (2016) Genetics of breast and gynecologic cancers (PDQ®) – health professional version. http://www.cancer.gov/types/breast/hp/breast-ovarian-genetics-pdq#section/_88

91. Antoniou AC et al (2014) Breast-cancer risk in families with mutations in PALB2. N Engl J Med 371(6):497–506

92. Genetics of Breast and Gynecologic Cancers (PDQ(R)): Health Professional Version, in PDQ Cancer Information Summaries. 2002: Bethesda
93. Lee IO, Oguma Y (2006) Physical activity. In: Schottenfeld D, Fraumeni JF (eds) Cancer Epidemiology and Prevention, 3rd edn. Oxford University Press, New York
94. Yedjou CG et al (2017) Assessing the racial and ethnic disparities in Breast Cancer mortality in the United States. Int J Environ Res Public Health 14(5)
95. Eliassen AH et al (2010) Physical activity and risk of breast cancer among postmenopausal women. Arch Intern Med 170(19):1758–1764
96. Fournier A et al (2014) Recent recreational physical activity and breast cancer risk in post-menopausal women in the E3N cohort. Cancer Epidemiol Biomark Prev 23(9):1893–1902
97. Hildebrand JS et al (2013) Recreational physical activity and leisure-time sitting in relation to postmenopausal breast cancer risk. Cancer Epidemiol Biomark Prev 22(10):1906–1912
98. Wu Y, Zhang D, Kang S (2013) Physical activity and risk of breast cancer: a meta-analysis of prospective studies. Breast Cancer Res Treat 137(3):869–882
99. Fintor L (1999) Exercise and Breast Cancer risk: lacking consensus. JNCI: J Natl Cancer Inst 91(10):825–827
100. Connolly BS et al (2002) A meta-analysis of published literature on waist-to-hip ratio and risk of breast cancer. Nutr Cancer 44(2):127–138
101. Rose DP, Komninou D, Stephenson GD (2004) Obesity, adipocytokines, and insulin resistance in breast cancer. Obes Rev 5(3):153–165
102. Lamon-Fava S et al (2005) Differences in serum sex hormone and plasma lipid levels in Caucasian and African-American premenopausal women. J Clin Endocrinol Metab 90(8):4516–4520
103. Sephton SE et al (2000) Diurnal cortisol rhythm as a predictor of breast cancer survival. J Natl Cancer Inst 92(12):994–1000
104. Centers for Disease, C. and Prevention (2007) Prevalence of regular physical activity among adults – United States, 2001 and 2005. MMWR Morb Mortal Wkly Rep 56(46):1209–1212
105. Hair BY et al (2014) Racial differences in physical activity among cancer survivors: implications for breast cancer care. Cancer 120(14):2174–2182
106. Thompson CL et al (2014) Race, age, and obesity disparities in adult physical activity levels in breast cancer patients and controls. Front Public Health 2:150
107. Winzer BM et al (2011) Physical activity and cancer prevention: a systematic review of clinical trials. Cancer Causes Control 22(6):811–826
108. Stout NL et al (2012) A prospective surveillance model for rehabilitation for women with breast cancer. Cancer 118(8 Suppl):2191–2200
109. Kotepui M (2016) Diet and risk of breast cancer. Contemp Oncol (Pozn) 20(1):13–19
110. Chlebowski RT et al (2006) Dietary fat reduction and breast cancer outcome: interim efficacy results from the Women's Intervention Nutrition Study. J Natl Cancer Inst 98(24):1767–1776
111. Pierce JP et al (2007) Influence of a diet very high in vegetables, fruit, and fiber and low in fat on prognosis following treatment for breast cancer: the Women's Healthy Eating and Living (WHEL) randomized trial. JAMA 298(3):289–298
112. George SM et al (2011) Postdiagnosis diet quality, the combination of diet quality and recreational physical activity, and prognosis after early-stage breast cancer. Cancer Causes Control 22(4):589–598
113. George SM et al (2010) Postdiagnosis diet quality is inversely related to a biomarker of inflammation among breast cancer survivors. Cancer Epidemiol Biomark Prev 19(9):2220–2228
114. Paxton RJ et al (2011) Was race a factor in the outcomes of the Women's Health Eating and Living Study? Cancer 117(16):3805–3813
115. Paxton RJ et al (2012) Associations among physical activity, body mass index, and health-related quality of life by race/ethnicity in a diverse sample of breast cancer survivors. Cancer 118(16):4024–4031
116. Davidson JA et al (2007) Avoiding the looming Latino/Hispanic cardiovascular health crisis: a call to action. J Cardiometab Syndr 2(4):238–243

117. Egede LE, Dagogo-Jack S (2005) Epidemiology of type 2 diabetes: focus on ethnic minorities. Med Clin North Am 89(5):949–975, viii
118. Hollar D, Agatston AS, Hennekens CH (2004) Hypertension: trends, risks, drug therapies and clinical challenges in African Americans. Ethn Dis 14(4):S2–23-5
119. Colditz GA, Bohlke K (2014) Priorities for the primary prevention of breast cancer. CA Cancer J Clin 64(3):186–194
120. Optenberg SA et al (1995) Race, treatment, and long-term survival from prostate cancer in an equal-access medical care delivery system. JAMA 274(20):1599–1605
121. Eley JW et al (1994) Racial differences in survival from breast cancer. Results of the National Cancer Institute Black/White Cancer Survival Study. JAMA 272(12):947–954
122. Carey LA et al (2006) Race, breast cancer subtypes, and survival in the Carolina Breast Cancer study. JAMA 295(21):2492–2502
123. Elledge RM et al (1994) Tumor biologic factors and breast cancer prognosis among white, Hispanic, and black women in the United States. J Natl Cancer Inst 86(9):705–712
124. Harlan LC et al (1993) Estrogen receptor status and dietary intakes in breast cancer patients. Epidemiology 4(1):25–31
125. ACS, American Cancer Society (2011) Cancer facts and figures for African Americans 2011–2012. American Cancer Society, Atlanta, 2011
126. van Ryn M, Burke J (2000) The effect of patient race and socio-economic status on physicians' perceptions of patients. Soc Sci Med 50(6):813–828
127. Yao S, Ambrosone CB (2013) Associations between vitamin D deficiency and risk of aggressive breast cancer in African-American women. J Steroid Biochem Mol Biol 136:337–341
128. Printz C (2013) Racial and ethnic disparities in breast cancer: experts gain new clues about differences in mortality rates among racial groups. Cancer 119(21):3739–3741
129. Powe BD et al (2005) Perceptions about breast cancer among African American women: do selected educational materials challenge them? Patient Educ Couns 56(2):197–204
130. Friedman LC et al (1995) Breast cancer screening: racial/ethnic differences in behaviors and beliefs. J Cancer Educ 10(4):213–216
131. Phillips JM, Wilbur J (1995) Adherence to breast cancer screening guidelines among African-American women of differing employment status. Cancer Nurs 18(4):258–269
132. Miller AM, Champion VL (1997) Attitudes about breast cancer and mammography: racial, income, and educational differences. Women Health 26(1):41–63
133. Miller LY, Hailey BJ (1994) Cancer anxiety and breast cancer screening in African-American women: a preliminary study. Womens Health Issues 4(3):170–174
134. Lannin DR et al (1998) Influence of socioeconomic and cultural factors on racial differences in late-stage presentation of breast cancer. JAMA 279(22):1801–1807
135. LaVeist TA, Carroll T (2002) Race of physician and satisfaction with care among African-American patients. J Natl Med Assoc 94(11):937–943
136. LaVeist TA et al (2002) Physician referral patterns and race differences in receipt of coronary angiography. Health Serv Res 37(4):949–962
137. Vernon SW et al (1993) Factors associated with perceived risk of breast cancer among women attending a screening program. Breast Cancer Res Treat 28(2):137–144
138. Dawson DA, Thompson GB (1990) Breast cancer risk factors and screening: United States, 1987. Vital Health Stat 10(172):iii–iiv, 1–60
139. Wray CJ et al (2013) The effect of age on race-related breast cancer survival disparities. Ann Surg Oncol 20(8):2541–2547
140. DeSantis C et al (2014) Breast cancer statistics, 2013. CA Cancer J Clin 64(1):52–62
141. ACS, American Cancer Society (2017) Cancer facts and figures 2017. 2017. American Cancer Society, Atlanta
142. Iqbal J et al (2015) Differences in breast cancer stage at diagnosis and cancer-specific survival by race and ethnicity in the United States. JAMA 313(2):165–173

Chapter 4
Breast Cancer: Current Perspectives on the Disease Status

Mohammad Fahad Ullah

Abstract Breast cancer is the most frequently diagnosed cancer in women and ranks second among causes for cancer related death in women. Evidence in literature has shown that the past and ongoing research has an enormous implication in improving the clinical outcome in breast cancer. This has been attributed to the progress made in the realm of screening, diagnosis and therapeutic strategies engaged in breast cancer management. However, poor prognosis in TNBC and drug resistance presents major inhibitions which are also current challenges for containing the disease. Similarly, a focal point of concern is the rising rate of breast cancer incidence and mortality among the population of under developed world. In this chapter, an overview of the current practices for the diagnosis and treatment of breast cancer and associated impediments has been provided.

Keywords Breast carcinoma · Endocrine therapy · Basal like · Metastasis · Drug resistance

4.1 Global Burden: Incidence and Mortality

Cancer is a leading cause of death worldwide in countries across the globe. The existing burden in terms of both the incidence and mortality is expected to grow rapidly due to increased life expectancy and lifestyle issues that increase cancer risk. There were 14.1 million new cancer cases, 8.2 million cancer deaths and 32.6 million people living with cancer (within 5 years of diagnosis) in 2012 worldwide as reported by IARC. Over the years the incidence of cancer disease were more pronounced in the developed world as compared to less developed nations. However, the recent trends show such a disparity being closing in as 57% (8 million) of new

M. Fahad Ullah (✉)
Prince Fahd Research Chair, Department of Medical Laboratory Technology,
Faculty of Applied Medical Science, University of Tabuk, Tabuk-71491, Saudi Arabia
e-mail: m.ullah@ut.edu.sa

© Springer Nature Switzerland AG 2019
A. Ahmad (ed.), *Breast Cancer Metastasis and Drug Resistance*,
Advances in Experimental Medicine and Biology 1152,
https://doi.org/10.1007/978-3-030-20301-6_4

cancer cases, 65% (5.3 million) of the cancer deaths and 48% (15.6 million) of the 5-year prevalent cancer cases occurred in the less developed regions (GLOBACAN 2012) [1]. Consequently, over 20 million new cancer cases are expected annually in less than a decade by 2025 [2]. The burden and patterns in incidence for several common cancers worldwide estimated for more and less developed regions has been shown in Fig. 4.1.

After the lung cancer, breast cancer is estimated to be the second most common cancer overall (1.7 million cases, 11.9%) though it ranks 5th as cause of death (522,000, 6.4%) because of the relatively favorable prognosis. In women, breast cancer is the most common cancer diagnosed in more and less developed regions, with more cases occurring in less developed (883,000 cases) than more developed regions (794,000) as shown in Fig. 4.2 [1, 3].

Earlier the incidence rates of breast cancer increased by about 30% in western countries between 1980 and the late 1990s, primarily due to increased screening, changes in reproductive patterns, and increased use of menopausal hormonal therapy [4, 5]. However, these rapid increases have slowed or plateaued since the early 2000s, probably because of the sensitization of the female population with the associated risk factors. Contrary to the western world, breast cancer incidence rates in many other countries, especially less developed countries, continue to increase due to changing reproductive patterns as well as increased awareness and screening [5, 6].

4.2   Breast Cancer Associated Risk Factors

Considering **age** as a predominant risk factor, compared with lung cancer, the incidence of breast cancer is higher at younger ages with reported incidence doubling about every 10 years until the menopause. Menstrual status also contributes to the age related risk factor with women having menstruation early in life or a late menopause have an increased risk of developing breast cancer. Similarly, the risk of breast cancer in women who have their first child after the age of 30 is about twice that of women who have their first child before the age of 20 and the highest risk groups include women having a first child after the age of 35. Breast cancer susceptibility is generally inherited as an autosomal dominant with limited penetrance (can be transmitted through either sex) and about 10% of breast cancer in Western countries is due to genetic predisposition with higher incidence among close **family** members and first degree relatives. **Lifestyle** issues such as diet (saturated fat), alcohol consumption (excessive intake) and sedentary status leading to abnormal weight (obesity) have also been reported as risk factors. Exposure to **ionizing radiations** at younger age and **hormone replacement therapy** (HRT) also contribute to a higher relative risk. Age adjusted incidence and mortality for breast cancer varies by up to a factor of five between countries with **geographical** variation reporting higher incidence in developed countries (Table 4.1) [7].

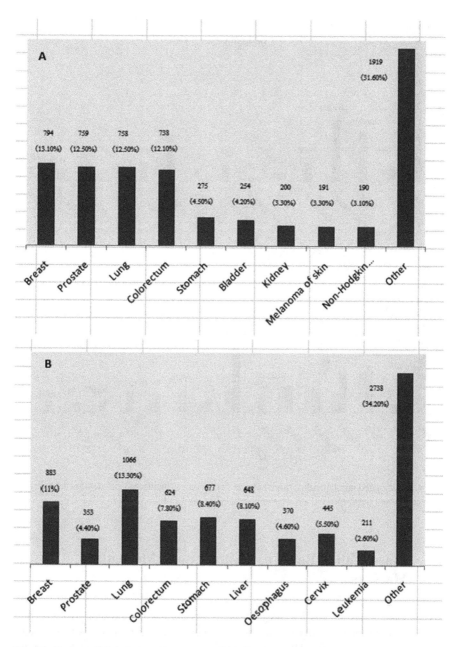

Fig. 4.1 Estimated global numbers of new cases (thousands) of various cancers in populations for (**a**) more developed and (**b**) less developed regions, both sexes combined, 2012

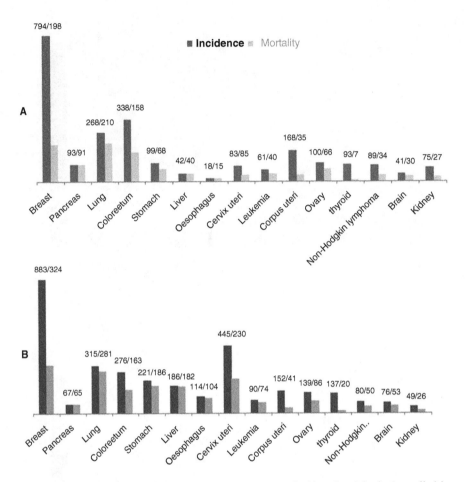

Fig. 4.2 Estimated numbers (thousands) of new cancer cases (incidence) and deaths (mortality) in women in more developed (**a**) and less developed (**b**) regions of the world in 2012

4.3 Classification Based on Histology and Molecular Markers

Breast cancer can be broadly categorized on the basis of histological outcome into in situ carcinoma and *invasive* carcinoma. Breast carcinoma in situ is further sub-classified as either ductal (DCIS; more common) or lobular (LCIS; less common). DCIS has been further sub-classified based on the features of the tumor into five well characterized subtypes: comedo, cribiform, micropapillary, papillary and solid [8, 9]. Similarly, invasive carcinomas are a heterogeneous group of tumors differentiated into histological subtypes that include infiltrating ductal (IDC), invasive

Table 4.1 Common risk factors associated with the incidence of breast cancer

Factors	Relative risk	Exclusive parameters
Age	>10	Beyond 50 years (elderly)
Age at menarche	3	Menarche before age 11
Age at menopause	2	Menopause after age 54
Delayed pregnancy	3	First child in early 40s
Family history	>2	Breast cancer in first degree relative
Diet	1.5	Rich in saturated fat
Alcohol consumption	1.3	Excessive
Body weight:		
(Premenopausal)	0.7	BMI >35
(Postmenopausal)	2	BMI >35
Hormone replacement therapy	1.35	More than 10 years
Ionizing radiations	3	Abnormal exposure in young age
Geographical area	5	Developed nations

lobular, ductal/lobular, mucinous (colloid), tubular, medullary and papillary carcinomas. Among the invasive carcinomas IDC is the most common subtype accounting for 70–80% of all invasive lesions. IDC is further sub-classified as either well-differentiated (grade 1), moderately differentiated (grade 2) or poorly differentiated (grade 3) based on the levels of nuclear pleomorphism, glandular/tubule formation and mitotic index [9–11].

The prognostic value of certain markers such as ER, PR, ErbB2 (Her2/neu) have been utilized to provide a molecular classification of breast cancer subtypes. The classification has been shown to be of high prognostic and predictive significance for IDC (though not utilized for DCIS) and it is recommended that their status be determined on all invasive carcinomas [11, 12]. Immunohistochemical (IHC) techniques are utilized to measure expression of estrogen receptor (ER), progesterone receptor (PR), and overexpression of human epidermal growth factor receptor 2 (HER2/neu). Breast cancers are then classified with respect to the presence or absence of these receptors as Luminal A (ER and/or PR positive, and HER2 negative); Luminal B (ER and/or PR positive, and HER2 positive); HER2-enriched (ER and PR negative, and HER2 positive) and Basal Like (Triple negative breast cancer-ER, PR and HER2 negative) [13]. Triple-negative breast cancers grow and spread faster than most other types of breast cancer. Patients with luminal A and B, and HER2-enriched subtypes are sensitive to targeted treatments, while patients with triple negative characteristic show poor prognosis. The status of these markers helps determine which patients are likely to respond to targeted therapies (i.e., tamoxifen or aromatase inhibitors for ER+/PR+ patients and trastuzumab or lapatinib for HER2/neu patients) while triple negative patients only have chemotherapy as an alternative [14]. Figure 4.3 summarizes the several subtypes of breast cancer based on histological and molecular characterization.

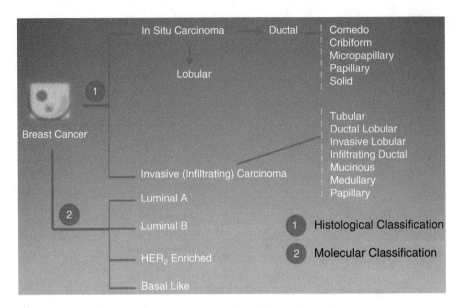

Fig. 4.3 Histological and molecular characterization of breast cancer subtypes

4.4   Tumor Markers in Breast Cancer

Numerous serum tumor markers have been described for breast cancer, including members of the MUC-1family of mucin glycoproteins (e.g., CA 15.3, BR 27.29,MCA, CA 549), carcinoembryonic antigen (CEA), oncoproteins (e.g., HER-2/c-erbB-2) and cytokeratins (e.g. tissue polypeptide antigen and tissue polypeptide-specific antigen). In practice, serum markers in breast cancer are mostly used for monitoring patients with diagnosed disease; tissue based markers are however primarily measured in order to determine prognosis and predict response to therapy. Clinically, the most useful tissue-based markers in breast cancer are estrogen receptor (ER), progesterone receptor (PR) and HER-2 (also known as c-erbB-2 or neu), uPA and PAI-1 [15].

According to the American Society of Clinical Oncology (2007) the following markers showed evidence of clinical utility and were recommended for use in practice: CA 15-3, CA 27.29, carcinoembryonic antigen, estrogen receptor, progesterone receptor, human epidermal growth factor receptor 2, urokinase plasminogen activator, plasminogen activator inhibitor 1, and certain multi-parameter gene expression assays [16].

Breast cancer metastasis accounts for the majority of deaths from breast cancer. Recent method to detect metastasis is the analysis of circulating tumor cells (CTCs). CTCs are tumor cells originating from primary sites or metastases that circulate in the patients' bloodstream and are very rarely found in healthy individuals. CTCs are recognized as critical elements in the metastasis of carcinomas and their analysis enables the prediction of metastatic relapse and progression [17, 18].

4.5 Breast Cancer Metastasis

Breast cancer appears as a disease of mammary epithelial cells which acquire the ability to grow abnormally for years and such a potential remains confined within mammary ducts or lobules (non-invasive breast cancer). This captivity of malignant epithelial cells within the ducto-lobular mesh is an important restraint to breast cancer progression. Since the malignant cells remain contained within the ducts or lobules, the patient survival has been reported to be relatively higher as ~98% of patients diagnosed with localized breast cancer have least probability of cancer recurrence within 5 years. In contrast, breast cancer prognosis markedly deteriorates in the event of cells invading out of the ducto-lobular region into the surrounding stroma (invasive breast cancer). Thus the 5-year survival for regionally invasive breast cancer i.e. breast cancer that has spread to regional lymph nodes, is only 83% (showing a 15% decrease from localized breast cancer). After moving out of the ducts or lobules, cancer cells can metastasize through the blood or lymphatic systems to distant organs such as the lungs, liver, or bones. The presence of distant metastases at the time of diagnosis presents the worst prognosis with only 23% of patients surviving 5 years post-diagnosis [19].

Breast cancer spreads to different distant organs, preferentially to bones, lung, liver and brain. The process of metastasis which includes cell migration and colonization is a multistep cascade of molecular events directed by gene mutations and altered expressions [20]. It is well recognized that metastasis consists of distinct steps in which tumor cells (i) detach and migrate away from the primary tumor site, (ii) invade neighboring tissue and penetrate through basement membrane, (iii) enter the blood or lymphatic vessels, (iv) survive the condition of anoikis while they are detached from the tumor mass and in circulation, (v) exit the blood or lymphatic vessels at a distant organ, (vi) form micrometastatic nodule, (vii) adapt and reprogram the surrounding stroma, and form macrometastases [21]. Metastatic cell migration includes local invasion, intravasation, dissemination and extravasation where as infiltrating distant tissue, evading immune defenses, adapting to supportive niches, surviving as latent tumour-initiating seeds, and eventually breaking out to replace the host tissue, are key steps for metastatic colonization [22].

Changes in cell phenotype between the epithelial and mesenchymal states, defined as the epithelial–mesenchymal transition (EMT; pre-invasion) and mesenchymal–epithelial transition (MET; re-invasion) are recognized as critical events for metastasis of carcinomas. EMT is thought to be critical for the initial transformation from benign to invasive carcinoma, whereas MET (the reverse of EMT) is critical for the later stages of metastasis. In the early stages the cancer cells need to cross its surrounding tissues and also the endothelial cells of the blood vessel in order to get into the blood circulation system. For this a sub-population of cancer cells undergoes EMT. Endothelial-mesenchymal transition is a physiological process characterized by loss of cell-cell adhesion and cytoskeletal alterations, leading to changes in cell morphology and acquisition of invasive and migratory properties [23]. Once accessing into the blood or lymphatic system, these cancer cells migrate to all parts

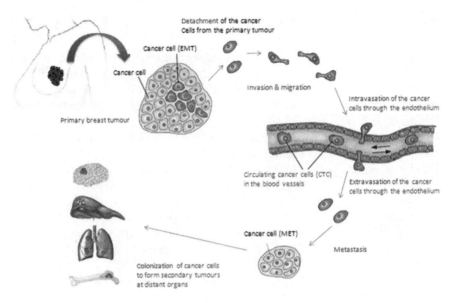

Fig. 4.4 Schematic overview of metastatic cascade

of the body to invade the new tissues by crossing the endothelial cells of the blood vessel. Subsequently, the disseminated mesenchymal tumor cells undergo the reverse transition, MET, at the site of metastases. Figure 4.4 provides a simplistic overview of the metastatic cascade of the breast cancer.

4.6 Therapeutic Strategies

The therapeutic approaches that are employed for breast cancer management include cytoreductive surgery, radiation treatment, targeted endocrine/molecular therapy and chemotherapy [24]. Due to the heterogeneity of the disease the treatment protocol requires rationalized therapy in individual cases according to the characterization and stage of the disease. Traditionally, radical mastectomy and modified radical mastectomy were the mainstream procedures for locoregional management which were eventually replaced by breast conserving surgery with breast radiation as preferred protocols [25]. Subsequently, neoadjuvant (preoperative) chemotherapy for locally advanced and operable breast cancer has been a major development with important implications for locoregional management [26]. Systemic chemotherapy at the time of locoregional recurrence also demonstrated significant improvement in disease-free survival and overall survival for poor-prognosis group [27].

One of the developments that have caused a paradigm shift with global impact in breast cancer prevention is the targeted therapy for estrogen receptor (+ve) and Her2 enriched cancer types [28]. Five years of adjuvant endocrine therapy with the selective estrogen receptor modulator tamoxifen or aromatase inhibitors (AIs, which cause estrogen depletion) reduces breast cancer recurrence and improves overall survival in women with ER-positive early-stage breast cancer [25]. Tamoxifen is a selective estrogen receptor modulator which is antagonist of ER in breast tissue (tamoxifen has agonist actions in other tissues) binds to estrogen receptor and inhibits the proliferative activities of estrogen on mammary epithelium [29], with reports suggesting a decline in the risk of ER+ breast cancer recurrence to 50% and a 28% decrease in morbidity rates [30]. Aromatase (which transforms androstenedione into esterone and testosterone to estrogen) is the chief estrogen source in post-menopausal females and its inhibitors lead to estrogen depletion. As a substitute to tamoxifen in post-menopausal women, (especially in ER+ breast cancer), third generation aromatase inhibitors i.e. letrozole, anastrozole and exemestane, are generally used [31]. It needs a mention that resistance to endocrine therapies that require beyond 5 years of extended therapy remains a clinical challenge. However, gene expression assays on ER expression patterns have implication to identify which patients with ER-positive breast cancers warrant chemotherapy in addition to endocrine therapy and which can be treated adequately with endocrine therapy alone [32].

Trastuzumab is a biologically active, humanized monoclonal antibody which has been reported to improve the survival rates for HER2/neu positive breast cancer patients [33]. It is considered clinically safe and effective in mono-therapy regime of every 3 weeks or in combination with paclitaxel, gemcitabine, vinorelbine or carboplatin [33, 34]. Protein tyrosine kinase inhibitor lapatinib, an orally active, reversible blocker of the HER2 tyrosine kinase is also used for HER2-positive metastatic breast cancer in combination with letrozole as first-line treatment and in patients presenting with trastuzumab resistance [35, 36].

Patients with triple negative breast cancer do not benefit from hormonal or trastuzumab-based therapy because of the loss of target receptors such as ER, PGR, and HER-2. Hence, surgery and chemotherapy, individually or in combination, appear to be the only available modalities [37]. The current highest pathologic complete response (pCR) rates, about 40–45%, are achieved by taxane/anthracycline sequential chemotherapy regimens and inclusion of platinum drugs with the taxane component [38]. Moreover, the addition of platinum agents, under various schedules, to anthracycline/taxane neoadjuvant chemotherapy also demonstrated statistically significantly higher pCR rates (41% vs 54%; 37% vs 53%; 26% vs 51%) [39]. Few novel therapies for TNBC include inhibition of Poly ADP-ribose polymerase enzymes (PARP inhibitor) which are critical for the repair of DNA breaks. Anti-VEGF monoclonal antibody (bevacizumab) targeting angiogensis in tumour region is also under research as tumour VEGF expression is significantly higher in TNBC compared with non TNBC presentations. In patients with metastatic TNBC, a cetuximab (anti-EGFR monoclonal antibody) plus cisplatin combination (BALI-I Trial) has demonstrated an overall better response rate of 20% when compared to a 10% overall better response rate with cisplatin alone. The serine-threonine kinase mammalian target of rapamycin (mTOR) promotes protein translation, angiogenesis,

Table 4.2 Anti-cancer drugs in breast cancer therapy

Natural product	Vinorelbine (vinca alkaloid), paclitaxel (taxane), doxorubicin (antibiotic)
Anti-metabolite analogues	Methotrexate (folic acid analogue), 5-fluorouracil and Capacitabine (pyramidine analogues)
Platinum salts	Carboplatin, cisplatin
Alkylating agent	Cyclophosphamide (nitrogen mustard)
Hormone antagonist	Tamoxifen (anti-estrogen)
Enzyme inhibitors	Letrozole and anastrazole (aromatase inhibitors)
PARP inhibitors	Olaparib
Monoclonal antibody	Trastuzumab (anti-HER2), cetuximab (anti-EGFR). Bevacizumab (anti-VEGF; angiogenesis inhibitor)
Histone deacetylase inhibition (HDAC)	Vorinostat
Protein tyrosine kinase inhibitor	Lapatinib (HER2), Neratinib (EGFR)

proliferation & migration and therapeutic strategies engaging mTOR inhibitors (everolimus) are under investigation. Additional targeted therapies for TNBC include HDAC (histone deacetylase) inhibitors, such as vorinostat which suppress cancer-cell proliferation by inducing cell-cycle arrest and/or apoptosis [40].

Table 4.2 shows anticancer drugs used in treatment regimens for chemotherapy and targeted therapy against breast cancer.

4.7 Drug Resistance in Breast Cancer

Despite numerous drug combinations and regimens, most of the patients with advanced breast cancer inevitably develop resistance to treatment [41]. Drug resistance mechanisms include intracellular drug metabolism/efflux and target modulations as well as extracellular elements of crosstalk between tumor cells and microenvironment [42, 43]. Malignant cells that survive primary treatment continue to evolve, thereby presenting a resistant clone population, which leads to constraint free progression responsible for worst prognosis and death. Estrogen, HER2 signaling, and the PI3K/Akt pathway in drug-resistant breast cancer has been summarized in Fig. 4.5 [44]. It is thus believed that even if ER/HER2 signaling is effectively blocked, cancer proliferation may continue, as downstream pathways may be activated by alternative routes.

Patients with metastatic ER-positive disease develop resistance to endocrine therapy such as against frontline drug tamoxifen. Tamoxifen is a prodrug and to be active against ER it requires bioactivation to the major metabolite, endoxifen [45]. The metabolism involves two members of the cytochrome P450 (CYP) family, CYP2D6 and CYP3A4. The polymorphisms of CYP2D6 is implicated in its catalytic activity and altered drug metabolism as CYP2D6 metabolizer status has been

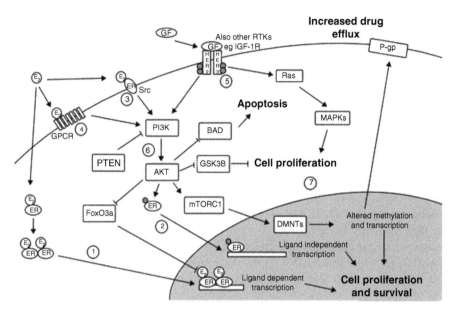

Fig. 4.5 Estrogen, HER2 signalling, and the PI3K/Akt pathway in drug-resistant breast cancer. Notes: ER can activate gene transcription by nuclear translocatin following ligand binding (1) or as a result of receptor phosphorylation in the absence of ligand (2). ERs may also be found associated with the plasma membrane in the presence of SRC and other adaptor proteins. Here, ligand binding triggers nongenomic effects via activation of signaling pathways, including the PI3K/Akt and the Ras/MAPK pathways (not shown) (3). These pathways are also activated by ligand binding to the GPR30 (4) and by growth factor binding to receptor tyrosine kinases, including HER2, inducing autophosphorylation and downstream signalling (5). The PI3K/Akt pathway (6) as indicated is a covergence point in the mechanisms implicated in drug resistance in the three types of breast cancer discussed here, as pathway hyperactivity frequently occurs with multiple downstream effects (7). (Reproduced from the original source [44] under the terms of Creative Common Attribution License)

correlated with response to tamoxifen treatment, with poor metabolizers having greater tumor progression than extensive metabolizers [46]. Moreover, it is known that phosphorylation regulates ERα activity and plays a role in tamoxifen resistance where phosphorylation by protein kinase A or p21-activated kinase-1 modifies the action of tamoxifen from antagonist to agonist. Reports have shown an enhanced activity of these kinases in tamoxifen-resistant breast cancer [47].

Trastuzumab (Herceptin), a monoclonal antibody that binds HER2, has been in use for patients with HER2-positive breast cancer. However, studies have reported de novo resistance to trastuzumab in approximately 65% of cases and induced resistance in approximately 70% of initially sensitive patients [48]. One of the mechanisms of resistance include epitope masking involving mucin 4, a large O-glycosylated membrane-associated protein and CD44/hyaluronan polymer complex which masks the epitope, sterically hindering trastuzumab binding and thereby preventing trastuzumab induced inhibition of HER2 signaling [49]. Trastuzumab resistance has also been reported by activation of downstream signaling *via* alternate routes. For instance trastuzumab treatment also induces upregulation of a number of miRNAs (miR-21) and c-Met leading to the activation of Akt signaling [50, 51]. It has also been reported that in up to 30% of HER2-enriched breast cancers, an amino-terminal truncated form of HER2 is expressed (p95-HER2). The p95-HER2 possesses constitutive kinase activity, triggering downstream signaling, but lacks the trastuzumab binding site, thus generating trastuzumab resistance [44, 52].

Therapeutic options for women presenting with triple negative breast cancer are limited due to the lack of a therapeutic target and as a result, are managed with standard chemotherapy such as paclitaxel (Taxol). Although TNBCs are generally very susceptible to chemotherapy initially, the risk of relapse for TNBC patients in the first 3–5 years is significantly higher than for women presenting with hormone positive breast cancer [53]. ATP-binding cassette (ABC) transporters involved in chemoresistance in TNBC include (a) multidrug-resistant protein-1 (MRP1) which confers resistance to agents such as vinca alkaloids, anthracyclines, and high-dose methotrexate but not paclitaxel or mitoxantrone, (b) breast cancer resistance protein (ABCG2) which is responsible for the efflux of drugs such as doxorubicin, and (c) the P-glycoprotein (MDR1) pump which pumps a wide array of chemotherapeutics out of cancer cells, including paclitaxel [54–56].

References

1. http://globocan.iarc.fr/Pages/fact_sheets_cancer.aspx
2. Bray F (2014) Transitions in human development and the global cancer burden. In: Wild CP, Stewart B (eds) World cancer report 2014. International Agency for Research on Cancer, Lyon
3. Ferlay J, Soerjomataram I, Dikshit R, Eser S, Mathers C, Rebelo M, Parkin DM, Forman D, Bray F (2015) Cancer incidence and mortality worldwide: sources, method sand major patterns in GLOBOCAN 2012. Int J Cancer 136:E359–E386
4. Althuis MD, Dozier JM, Anderson WF, Devesa SS, Brinton LA (2005) Global trends in breast cancer incidence and mortality 1973–1997. Int J Epidemiol 34:405–412
5. Torre LA, Siegel RL, Ward EM, Jemal A (2016) Global cancer incidence and mortality rates and trends—an update. Cancer Epidemiol Biomark Prev 25(1):16–27
6. Colditz GA, Sellers TA, Trapido E (2006) Epidemiology – identifying the causes and preventability of cancer? Nat Rev Cancer 6:75–83
7. McPherson K, Steel CM, Dixon JM (2000) Breast cancer—epidemiology, risk factors, and genetics. BMJ 321:624–628
8. Association of Directors of Anatomic and Surgical Pathology (1995) Recommendations for the Reporting of Breast Carcinoma. Am J Clin Pathol 104:614–619
9. Malhotra GK, Zhao X, Band H, Band V (2010) Histological, molecular and functional subtypes of breast cancers. Cancer Biol Ther 10(10):955–960
10. Li CI, Uribe DJ, Daling JR (2005) Clinical characteristics of different histologic types of breast cancer. Br J Cancer 93:1046–1052
11. Lester SC, Bose S, Chen YY, Connolly JL, de Baca ME, Fitzgibbons PL et al (2009) Protocol for the examination of specimens from patients with invasive carcinoma of the breast. Arch Pathol Lab Med 133:1515–1538
12. Bevers TB, Anderson BO, Bonnacio E et al. (2009) NCCN clinical practice guidelines in oncology:breast cancer screening and diagnosis. J Natl Compr Canc Netw 7:1060–1096

13. Hon JDC, Singh B, Du AysegulSahin G, Wang J, Wang VY, Deng F-M, Zhang DY, Monaco ME, Lee P (2016) Breast cancer molecular subtypes: from TNBC to QNBC. Am J Cancer Res 6(9):1864–1872
14. Payne SJ, Bowen RL, Jones JL, Wells CA (2008) Predictive markers in breast cancer—the present. Histopathology 52:82–90
15. Molina R, Barak V, van Dalen A, Duffy MJ, Einarsson R, Gion M, Goike H, Lamerz R, Nap M, GyörgySölétormos PS (2005) Tumor markers in breast cancer –European Group on Tumor Markers Recommendations. Tumor Biol 26:281–293
16. Harris L, Fritsche H, Mennel R, Norton L, Ravdin P, Taube S, Somerfield MR, Hayes DF, Bast RC Jr (2007) American Society of Clinical Oncology 2007 update of recommendations for the use of tumor markers in breast. Cancer J Clin Oncol 25:5287–5312
17. van de Stolpe A, Pantel K, Sleijfer S, Terstappen LW, den Toonder JM (2011) Circulating tumor cell isolation and diagnostics: toward routine clinical use. Cancer Res 71:5955–5960
18. Pantel K, Alix-Panabieres C, Riethdorf S (2009) Cancer micrometastases. Nat Rev Clin Oncol 6:339–351
19. Howlader NNA, Krapcho M, Neyman N, Aminou R, Waldron W, Altekruse SF, Kosary CL, Ruhl J, Tatalovich Z, Cho H, Mariotto A, Eisner MP, Lewis DR, Chen HS, Feuer EJ, Cronin KA, Edwards BK (2011) SEER cancer statistics review, 1975–2008. National Cancer Institute, Bethesda
20. Weber GF (2008) Molecular mechanisms of metastasis. Cancer Lett 270(2):181–190
21. Steeg PS (2006) Tumor metastasis: mechanistic insights and clinical challenges. Nat Med 12:895–904
22. Massagué J, Obenauf AC (2016) Metastatic colonization. Nature 529(7586):298–306
23. Lin F, Wang N, Zhang TC (2012) The role of endothelial-mesenchymal transition in development and pathological process. IUBMB Life 64(9):717–723
24. Geay JF (2013) Physiopathology, diagnosis and treatment of breast cancer. Soins (776):25–29
25. NIH Consensus Development Conference on the treatment of early-stage breast cancer. Bethesda, June 18–21, 1990. J Natl Cancer Inst Monogr 1–187, 1992
26. Fisher B, Mamounas EP (1995) Preoperative chemotherapy: a model for studying the biology and therapy of primary breast cancer. J Clin Oncol 13:537–540
27. Aebi S, Gelber S, Lang I et al (2012) Chemotherapy prolongs survival for isolated local or regional recurrence of breast cancer: the CALOR trial (Chemotherapy as Adjuvant for Locally Recurrent breast cancer; IBCSG 27-02, NSABP B-37, BIG1-02). Cancer Res 72:96s. (abstr S3-2)
28. Sledge GW, Mamounas EP, Hortobagyi GN, Burstein HJ, Goodwin PJ, Wolff AC (2014) Past, present, and future challenges in breast cancer treatment. J Clin Oncol 32(19):1979–1986
29. Riggs BL, Hartmann LC (2003) Selective estrogen-receptor modulators-mechanisms of action and application to clinical practice. N Engl J Med 348(7):618–629
30. Group EBCTC (1998) Poly chemotherapy for early breast cancer: an overview of the randomized trials. Lancet 352(9132):930–942
31. Bonneterre J, Buzdar A, Nabholtz JM, Robertson JF, Thürlimann B et al (2001) Anastrozole is superior to tamoxifen as first-line therapy in hormone receptor positive advanced breast carcinoma. Cancer 92(9):2247–2258
32. Cancer Genome Atlas Network (2012) Comprehensive molecular portraits of human breast tumours. Nature 490:61–70
33. Baselga J, Carbonell X, Caslaneda Soto N, Clemens M, Green M et al (2004) Phase II study of efficacy, safety, and pharmacokinetics of trastuzumabmonotherapy administered on a 3-weekly schedule. J Clin Oncol 23(10):2162–2171
34. Pegram MD, Konecny GE, O'Callaghan C, Beryt M, Pietras R et al (2004) Rational combinations of trastuzumab with chemotherapeutic drugs used in the treatment of breast cancer. J Natl Cancer Inst 96(10):739–749
35. Toi M, Iwata H, Fujiwara Y, Ito Y, Nakamura S et al (2009) Lapatinib monotherapy in patients with relapsed, advanced, or metastatic breast cancer: efficacy, safety, and biomarker results from Japanese patients phase II studies. Br J Cancer 101(10):1676–1682

36. Blackwell KL, Burstein HJ, Storniolo AM, Rugo H, Sledge G et al (2010) Randomized study of lapatinib alone or in combination with trastuzumab in women with ErbB2-positive, trastuzumab-refractory metastatic breast cancer. J Clin Oncol 28(7):1124–1130
37. Bianchini G, Balko JM, Mayer IA et al (2016) Triple-negative breast cancer: challenges and opportunities of a heterogeneous disease. Nat Rev Clin Oncol 13:674–690
38. Killelea BK, Yang VQ, Mougalian S et al (2015) Neoadjuvant chemotherapy for breast cancer increases the rate of breast conservation: results from the National Cancer Database. J Am Coll Surg 220:1063–1069
39. Sikov WM, Berry DA, Perou CM et al (2015) Impact of the addition of carboplatin and/or bevacizumab to neoadjuvant once-per-week paclitaxel followed by dose-dense doxorubicin and cyclophosphamide on pathologic complete response rates in stage II to III triple-negative breast cancer: CALGB 40603 (Alliance). J Clin Oncol 33:13–21
40. O'Reil EA, Gubbins L, Sharma S et al (2015) The fate of chemoresistance in triple negative breast cancer (TNBC). BBA Clin 3:257–275
41. Gonzalez-Angulo AM, Morales-Vasquez F, Hortobagyi GN (2007) Overview of resistance to systemic therapy in patients with breast cancer. Adv Exp Med Biol 608:1–22
42. Moiseenko F, Volkov N, Bogdanov A, Dubina M, Moiseyenko V (2017) Resistance mechanisms to drug therapy in breast cancer and other solid tumors: an opinion. F1000Res 6:288
43. Ullah MF (2008) Cancer multidrug resistance (MDR): a major impediment to effective chemotherapy. Asian Pac J Cancer Prev 9(1):1–6
44. Martin HL, Smith L, Tomlinson DC (2014) Multidrug-resistant breast cancer: current perspectives. Breast Cancer: Targets Ther 6:1–13
45. Desta Z, Ward BA, Soukhova NV, Flockhart DA (2004) Comprehensive evaluation of tamoxifen sequential biotransformation by the human cytochrome P450 system in vitro: prominent roles for CYP3A and CYP2D6. J Pharmacol Exp Ther 310(3):1062–1075
46. Brauch H, Schwab M (2014) Prediction of tamoxifen outcome by genetic variation of CYP2D6 in postmenopausal women with early breast cancer. Br J Clin Pharmacol 77(4):695–703. Epub August 22, 2013
47. Wang R-A, Mazumdar A, Vadlamudi RK, Kumar R (2002) P21-activated kinase-1 phosphorylates and transactivates estrogen receptor[alpha] and promotes hyperplasia in mammary epithelium. EMBO J 21(20):5437–5447
48. Vu T, Claret FX (2012) Trastuzumab: updated mechanisms of action and resistance in breast cancer. Front Oncol 2:62
49. Palyi-Krekk Z, Barok M, Isola J, Tammi M, Szollosi J, Nagy P (2007) Hyaluronan-induced masking of ErbB2 and CD44-enhanced trastuzumab internalisation in trastuzumab resistant breast cancer. Eur J Cancer 43(16):2423–2433
50. Shattuck DL, Miller JK, Carraway KL 3rd, Sweeney C (2008) Met receptor contributes to trastuzumab resistance of Her2-overexpressing breast cancer cells. Cancer Res 68(5):1471–1477
51. Gong C, Yao Y, Wang Y et al (2011) Up-regulation of miR-21 mediates resistance to trastuzumab therapy for breast cancer. J Biol Chem 286(21):19127–19137
52. Gajria D, Chandarlapaty S (2011) HER2-amplified breast cancer: mechanisms of trastuzumab resistance and novel targeted therapies. Expert Rev Anticancer Ther 11(2):263–275
53. Hudis C, Gianni L (2011) Triple-negative breast cancer: an unmet medical need. Oncologist 16(Suppl 1):1–11
54. Longley DB, Johnston PG (2005) Molecular mechanisms of drug resistance. J Pathol 205:275–292
55. Leonessa F, Clarke R (2003) ATP binding cassette transporters and drug resistance in breast cancer. Endocr Relat Cancer 10:43–73
56. Scharenberg CW, Harkey MA, Torok-Storb B (2002) The ABCG2 transporter is an efficient Hoechst 33342 efflux pump and is preferentially expressed by immature human hematopoietic progenitors. Blood 99:507–512

Chapter 5
Role of Autophagy in Breast Cancer Development and Progression: Opposite Sides of the Same Coin

Mirna Azalea Romero, Oznur Bayraktar Ekmekcigil, Bakiye Goker Bagca, Cigir Biray Avci, Uteuliyev Yerzhan Sabitaliyevich, Tokmurziyeva Gulnara Zhenisovna, Aliye Aras, and Ammad Ahmad Farooqi

Abstract The term "autophagy", which means "self (auto) - eating (phagy)", describes a catabolic process that is evolutionarially conserved among all eukaryotes. Although autophagy is mainly accepted as a cell survival mechanism, it also modulates the process known as "type II cell death". AKT/mTOR pathway is an upstream activator of autophagy and it is tightly regulated by the ATG (autophagy-related genes) signaling cascade. In addition, wide ranging cell signaling pathways and non-coding RNAs played essential roles in the control of autophagy. Autophagy is closely related to pathological processes such as neurodegenerative diseases and cancer as well as physiological conditions. After the Nobel Prize in Physiology or Medicine 2016 was awarded to Yoshinori Ohsumi "for his discoveries of mechanisms for autophagy", there was an explosion in the field of autophagy and molecular biologists started to pay considerable attention to the mechanistic insights related to autophagy in different diseases. Since autophagy behaved dualistically, both as a

M. A. Romero
Facultad de Medicina, Universidad Autónoma de Guerrero, Laboratorio de Investigación Clínica, Av. Solidaridad S/N, Colonia Hornos Insurgentes, Acapulco, Guerrero, Mexico

O. Bayraktar Ekmekcigil
Faculty of Medicine, Department of Medical Biology and Genetics, Okan University, Istanbul, Turkey

B. G. Bagca · C. B. Avci
Medical Faculty, Department of Medical Biology, Ege University, Izmir, Turkey

U. Y. Sabitaliyevich · T. G. Zhenisovna
Kazakhstan Medical University "KSPH", Almaty, Kazakhstan

A. Aras
Department of Botany, Faculty of Science, Istanbul University, Istanbul, Turkey

A. A. Farooqi (✉)
Institute of Biomedical and Genetic Engineering (IBGE), Islamabad, Pakistan
e-mail: ammadfarooqi@rlmclahore.com

© Springer Nature Switzerland AG 2019
A. Ahmad (ed.), *Breast Cancer Metastasis and Drug Resistance*,
Advances in Experimental Medicine and Biology 1152,
https://doi.org/10.1007/978-3-030-20301-6_5

cell death and a cell survival mechanism, it opened new horizons for a deeper analysis of cell type and context dependent behavior of autophagy in different types of cancers. There are numerous studies showing that the induction of autophagy mechanism will promote survival of cancer cells. Since autophagy is mainly a mechanism to keep the cells alive, it may protect breast cancer cells against stress conditions such as starvation and hypoxia. For these reasons, autophagy was noted to be instrumental in metastasis and drug resistance. In this chapter we have emphasized on role of role of autophagy in breast cancer. Additionally we have partitioned this chapter into exciting role of microRNAs in modulation of autophagy in breast cancer. We have also comprehensively summarized how TRAIL-mediated signaling and autophagy operated in breast cancer cells.

Keywords Autophagy · Breast cancer · Apoptosis · Signaling

5.1 Introduction

The link between cell death mechanisms and cancer has become the focus of intensive research. There are two major types of programmed cell death: apoptosis and autophagy. Autophagy, which is defined by formation of double-membraned vesicles in the cytoplasm, has distinct functions during the formation and progression of tumor. The role of autophagy in cancer also depends on tissue type.

Autophagy is one of the main protein degradation routes of the cells. Autophagy also serves as a cellular recycling mechanism since it allows the degradation of long-lived proteins as well as damaged organelles and proteins. Formation of an isolation membrane, also called as 'phagophore', in the cytoplasm around the autophagic target is the hallmark for the onset of autophagy. Isolation membrane is a double-membrane structure and Endoplasmic Reticulum (ER), Golgi or mitochondria might provide the source for isolation membrane [1]. Following elongation and closure of the isolation membrane, double-membrane vesicle containing autophagic cargo is called as 'autophagosome'. Autophagosomes then combine with lysosomes and now called as 'autolysosomes'. The degradation of the autophagic cargo requires hydrolytic activity which is provided by lysosomal hydrolases [1]. Autophagy is induced under several stress factors such as ER stress, accumulation of dysfunctional mitochondria, hypoxia as well as hormone and nutrient deprivation. In addition, autophagy can be induced by certain drugs and proteins [2]. mTOR (mammalian target of Rapamycin) is an important regulator of autophagy. mTORC1 (mTOR complex 1) inhibits ULK1-Atg13-FIP200 complex which is crucial for the beginning of autophagosome formation. mTORC1 is triggered under nutrient-rich conditions. Autophagy might also be triggered in an mTOR-independent manner. The complex of Atg14L, Bif1-UVRAG, Ambra1 and Rab5 induces autophagosome formation [3] (shown in Fig. 5.1).

Autophagic cargo such as damaged or old organelles and misfolded or long-lived proteins are captured in the cytoplasm by a double-membrane structure called phagophore. p62 is the adapter protein that binds to and recruits autophagic cargo

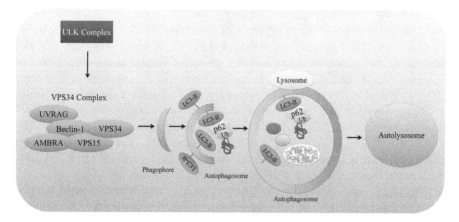

Fig. 5.1 Activation of AMP-activated protein kinase (AMPK) and/or inhibition of mechanistic target of rapamycin complex-1 (mTORC1) by different stress signals triggered activation of the ATG1–ULK1 complex, which promoted the activities of VPS34 complex. Studies have shown that Class III PI3K VPS34 provided PI3P to the phagophores and assisted in positioning of the multi-protein ATG12–ATG5–ATG16L1 signalosome to the membrane. Therefore, after the binding of ATG-complex to the phagophores and LC3 conjugation to PE (LC3-II), the membrane elongated and engulfed cytoplasmic portions that consequently resulted in the formation of the functionally active autophagosomes. Importantly, proteins for example p62, NBR1 and NDP52 established a bridge between LC3-II and specified ubiquitylated cargo through their characteristically unique domains. Finally autophagosomes fused with lysosomes that resultantly induced degradation of the contents of the vesicle

to phagophores and p62 itself is also degraded by the autolysosomes [4]. There are two protein complexes which function in the formation of phagophore. PI3K-III complex is constituted by Atg14L, VPS34, Beclin-1 and VPS15 whereas ULK, ATG13, FIP200 and ATG101 form ULK-complex. Both PI3K-III and ULK complexes promote phagophore formation. Atg12-Atg5-Atg16 complex is responsible for the elongation of phagophore into autophagosome [5] (shown in Fig. 5.1). After closure of the autophagic membrane, fusion with lysosomes is essential for the degradation of autophagic target. Atg5-Atg12 and LC3-phosphatidylethanolamine are two ubiquitin-like conjugation complexes that function in the expansion of the growing autophagosome membrane [6].

Autophagy is a vital mechanism for the most important decision of the cell: to die or to live. It might trigger cell survival or cell death. Therefore, autophagy might facilitate or inhibit tumorigenesis in tissue- and context-dependent manner. At the beginning of tumor formation, autophagy limits tumor growth since it prevents the accumulation of misfolded proteins, organelles and reactive oxygen species [7]. Depletion of autophagy results in an increase in DNA damage response, oxidative stress as well as genomic instability [8].

When autophagy levels are excessively high, inappropriate degradation of organelles and deficiency in caspase activation lead to autophagic cell death. Forty-five percent to 75% of breast tumors do not have caspase three protein and induce autophagic cell death when Bcl-2 is inhibited [9]. Moreover, silencing of Bcl-2 of tumor cells under doxorubicin treatment increased autophagic cell death and limited tumor growth [10]. Stimulation of autophagy might be especially crucial to induce cell death in apoptosis-resistant breast cancer cell lines [9]. Cell lines with high levels of anti-apoptotic proteins such as Bcl-2 and Bcl-xL; or with low levels of Bax and Bak are apoptosis-deficient. Bax and Bak knockout fibroblasts are able to trigger autophagy under chemical treatments such as staurosporine, etoposide and rottlerin [10–14]. Therefore, upregulation of autophagy might alleviate therapeutic response.

Beclin-1 is involved in formation of autophagosomes and lower levels of *beclin-1* increase the risk of HER2-positive breast cancer due to autophagy inhibition [15].

Autophagic and apoptotic cell death can regulate each other and under certain circumstances they might compensate for each other. A reduction in one of the pathways might induce activation of other mechanism of cell death.

The disruption of mitochondria causes mitophagy, a specific subtype of autophagy. Damaged mitochondria are targeted and degraded inside autophagic vesicles during mitophagy. Mitochondria-targeted redox agents (MTAs) were found to trigger mitophagy and autophagic cell death in breast cancer cell lines [16].

5.2   microRNA Regulation of Autophagy in Breast Cancer

Lysosomal protein transmembrane 4 beta (LAPTM4B) and Unc-51 like autophagy activating kinase 1 (ULK1) were found to be directly targeted by miR-489 [21]. There was significant accumulation of LC3B-II in miR-489 overexpressing BCa cells, whereas miR-489 inhibition completely inhibited LC3B-II accumulation. miR-489 inhibited autophagy by blockade of formation of autophagosome and lysosome fusion (Autolysosome). 3-methyladenine (3-MA), an autophagy inhibitor effectively prevented miR-489 mediated autophagosome deposition. 3-MA severely impaired miR-489 induced p62 and LC3B-II deposition [21]. Starvation induced autophagy and miR-489 restoration showed stronger autophagy inhibition under starvation as evidenced by increased accumulation of p62 and LC3B-II in BCa cells. Strategically, miR-489 acted as a drug sensitizer in BCa cells by directly targeting LAPTM4B and consequently inhibiting doxorubicin-triggered cytoprotective autophagy [21]. Data clearly suggested that autophagy inhibition and LAPTM4B downregulation played instrumental role in miR-489-mediated re-sensitization of breast cancer cells to doxorubicin.

Fulvestrant, an FDA-approved "pure anti-estrogen" is useful for treatment of BCa. miR-375 overexpression inhibited growth of fulvestrant-resistant BCa cells, decreased expression of LC3-II and ATG7 and reduced autophagy [20]. Combinatorial inhibition of EGFR and c-ABL elevated expression of miR-375 in BCa cells [20].

Damage-regulated autophagy modulator 1 (DRAM1) played central role in promoting radiation induced autophagy in BCa cells [19]. DRAM1 was negatively regulated by miR-26b and interestingly, DRAM1 was significantly reduced in miR-26b transfected BCa cells. However, on the contrary, miR-26b inhibition resulted in an upregulation of DRAM1 and consequently induced radiation-triggered autophagy in MCF7 cells [19].

Autophagy ensured proper distribution of metabolic substrates to highly demanding breast cancer cells. This mechanism was vital for the survival of BCa cells [23]. Higher LC3-II/LC3-I conversion ratio was observed in miR-23a mimics transfected T47D cells. X-linked inhibitor of apoptosis (XIAP) was directly targeted by miR-23a and intriguingly, enforced expression of XIAP remarkably abolished miR-23a-mediated autophagy in T47D cells. Tumors derived from mice xenografted with miR-23a overexpressing MCF7 were highly invasive [23].

Penetratin, a highly efficient cell-penetrating peptide was used to deliver miR-NAs to BCa cells. Cholesterol-penetratin (Chol-P) conjugates have previously been tested for their ability to deliver payload to target cells [24]. Amphiphilic Chol-P self-assembled into micelles and proficiently delivered obatoclax and miR-124 to BCa cells. Surprisingly, miR-124 was noted to be degraded in the autophagolysosomes. Therefore, obatoclax encapsulated miR-124 was used which strongly inhibited miR-124 degradation in autophagolysosomes. Stability of miR-124 was necessary for maintenance of required concentrations of miR-124 in BCa cells. Moreover, miR-124 induced regression of tumors in mice xenografted with BCa cells [24].

miR-20a inhibited basal and nutrient starvation-triggered lysosomal proteolytic activity and autophagic flux in BCa cells [27]. Additionally, miR-20a overexpression markedly reduced SQSTM1, ATG16L1 or BECN1 in MCF7 and MDA-MB-231 BCa cells. Re-introduction of exogenous SQSTM1, ATG16L1 or BECN1 reversed inhibitory effects exerted by miR-20a on autophagic flux in BCa cells. Tumor growth and development was more pronounced in mice xenografted with the miR-20a-expressing BCa cells [27].

miR-96-5p inhibited autophagy mainly through targeting of FOXO1 and acetylated-FOXO1 in BCa cells [26].

DAPPER antagonist of Beta-Catenin-3 (DACT3) acted as a tumor suppressor in BCa [25]. However, DACT3 was negatively modulated by miR-638. Autophagy was significantly enhanced in DACT3 silenced MCF-7 BCa cells. miR-638 directly targeted DACT3 and induced autophagy in BCa cells [25].

miR-124-3p significantly reduced LC3I and Beclin-1 [29]. miR-124-3p overexpression partially reversed 4-hydroxytamoxifen induced autophagy in BCa cells [29].

miR-18a was found to be considerably enhanced in paclitaxel-resistant triple negative BCa cells (TNBC) [28]. Paclitaxel-resistant MDA-MB-231 BCa cells had significantly higher basal autophagy as compared to MDA-MB-231 cells. More importantly, miR-18a overexpression decreased the expression of phosphorylated mechanistic target of rapamycin (mTOR) and p-p70S6. miR-18a increased autophagy level in MDA-MB-231 cells via inhibition of mTOR signal transduction cascade [28].

Hinokitiol (β-thujaplicin), a tropolone-related natural product efficiently suppressed self-renewing capacity of breast cancer stem cells (BCSCs) [22]. BMI1, an oncogene positively regulated self-renewal capacity of BCSCs. Hinokitiol markedly reduced BMI1 in BT-474 and AS-B145-derived mammospheres. Hinokitiol considerably reduced ALDH+ BCSCs within BT-474 mammospheres, however, Hinokitiol-mediated suppressive effects were impaired in

BMI1-overexpressing BCa cells. miR-494-3p was noted to be upregulated by Hinokitiol in BCSCs [22]. miR-494-3p negatively controlled BMI1 in BCSCs [22]. It will be interesting to see how different natural products modulate oncomiRs and tumor suppressor miRNAs to modulate autophagy in breast cancer.

5.3 Role of TRAIL-Induced Signaling and Autophagy in Breast Cancer

Effective targeting of breast cancer cells has always remained an ultimate goal for pharmacologists and clinicians. Tumor necrosis factor-related apoptosis-inducing ligand (TRAIL) has emerged as a pinnacle molecule because of its ability to selectively target cancer cells.

Quinacrine worked synergistically with TRAIL and increased the levels of ATG5 and LC3-BII in BCa cells [32]. However, levels of ATG5 and LC3-BII were found to be drastically reduced in DR5 silenced MCF-10A BCa cells [32].

Suberoylanilide hydroxamic acid (SAHA), an HDAC inhibitor effectively increased LC3-II and ATG9B in MDA-MB-231 cells, however these effects were impaired in DR5 silenced cells [31]. Additionally, expression levels of Beclin-1, ATG3, ATG7, ATG16, ATG12, ATG4A and ATG5 remained unchanged in MCF-7 cells after SAHA treatment. However, SAHA activated LC3-II, ATG4B and ATG9B and these effects were impaired in DR5 silenced BCa cells [31].

Significantly higher levels of basal autophagosomes were observed in TRAIL-resistant BCa cells (AU565, BT474) under nutrition-rich conditions [30]. Co-localization of DR4 and DR5 with LC3-II was noted in the autophagosomes of TRAIL-resistant BCa cells. Disruption of basal autophagosomes induced efficient restoration of death receptors on surface of BCa cells. MDA-MB-231 BCa cells had higher levels of DR4 and DR5 and negligibly lower level of basal autophagosomes. Inhibition of lysosomal activity triggered autophagosomal accumulation and a reduction in cell surface expression of death receptors [30].

Chronic exposure of BCa cells to TRAIL induced an upregulation of autophagic activity, which highlighted protective role of autophagy and consequently chaperoned BCa cells from TRAIL-driven apoptosis [33].

5.4 Conclusion

Autophagy has emerged as one of the highly studied molecular mechanism in regulation of cancer development and progression. More excitingly, scratching the surface of autophagy-related mechanisms revealed its diametrically opposed roles both as a tumor inducer and tumor suppressor, which urged researchers to drill down deep into the underlying mechanisms. Confluence of information has revolutionized our understanding related to dualistic role of autophagy. Keeping in view the burgeoning evidence about the ability of autophagy to kill cancer cells, the use of autophagy inducing agents cannot be overlooked. However, contemporary and circumstantial evidence also advocates the role of autophagy as a cancer inducer. Because cancer cells utilize autophagy to survive under several stress factors such as nutrient- and oxygen-limited conditions. In RAS-driven tumors, autophagy is increased to trigger the survival and proliferation of cancer cells as well as metastasis [7]. Cancer cells upregulate autophagy also as a response to chemotherapy or radiotherapy [17]. In breast cancer cells, autophagic induction causes a delay in apoptotic cell death resulting from hormone therapy and DNA-damaging agents [11, 18]. Therefore, suppression of autophagy might improve the efficacy of therapeutics in certain cases.

As briefly summarized in this chapter, the results obtained from different studies are contradictory. Induction of autophagy might be either beneficial or harmful depending on cancer-type and the context. In early stages of tumorigenesis, autophagy clears damaged organelles and proteins. Autophagic cell death also limits tumorigenesis. Autophagy and apoptosis are two mechanisms of programmed cell death and they can compensate for each other when one of the mechanisms is inhibited. However, in later stages, cancer cells upregulate autophagy to endure harsh conditions such as limited nutrient, oxygen and hormone. In addition, autophagy is an appropriate way for cancer cells to gain resistance to chemotherapy. Therefore, the link between autophagy and cancer is complex. Consideration should be taken to examine the cancer type in question for the therapeutic approaches.

References

1. Tooze SA, Yoshimori T (2010) The origin of the autophagosomal membrane. Nat Cell Biol 12(9):831–835. https://doi.org/10.1038/ncb0910-831. PubMed PMID: 20811355
2. Gozuacik D, Kimchi A (2007) Autophagy and cell death. Curr Top Dev Biol 78:217–245. https://doi.org/10.1016/S0070-2153(06)78006-1. PubMed PMID: 17338918
3. Das CK, Mandal M, Kogel D (2018) Pro-survival autophagy and cancer cell resistance to therapy. Cancer Metastasis Rev. https://doi.org/10.1007/s10555-018-9727-z. PubMed PMID: 29536228
4. Gozuacik D, Kimchi A (2004) Autophagy as a cell death and tumor suppressor mechanism. Oncogene 23(16):2891–2906. https://doi.org/10.1038/sj.onc.1207521. PubMed PMID: 15077152
5. Dikic I, Elazar Z (2018) Mechanism and medical implications of mammalian autophagy. Nat Rev Mol Cell Biol. https://doi.org/10.1038/s41580-018-0003-4. PubMed PMID: 29618831
6. Jain K, Paranandi KS, Sridharan S, Basu A (2013) Autophagy in breast cancer and its implications for therapy. Am J Cancer Res 3(3):251–265. PubMed PMID: 23841025; PubMed Central PMCID: PMCPMC3696532
7. White E (2015) The role for autophagy in cancer. J Clin Invest 125(1):42–46. https://doi.org/10.1172/JCI73941. PubMed PMID: 25654549; PubMed Central PMCID: PMCPMC4382247
8. Pajares M, Cuadrado A, Engedal N, Jirsova Z, Cahova M (2018) The role of free radicals in autophagy regulation: implications for ageing. Oxidative Med Cell Longev 2018:2450748. https://doi.org/10.1155/2018/2450748. PubMed PMID: 29682156; PubMed Central PMCID: PMCPMC5846360

9. Dalby KN, Tekedereli I, Lopez-Berestein G, Ozpolat B (2010) Targeting the prodeath and prosurvival functions of autophagy as novel therapeutic strategies in cancer. Autophagy 6(3):322–329. PubMed PMID: 20224296; PubMed Central PMCID: PMCPMC2914492

10. Akar U, Chaves-Reyez A, Barria M, Tari A, Sanguino A, Kondo Y et al (2008) Silencing of Bcl-2 expression by small interfering RNA induces autophagic cell death in MCF-7 breast cancer cells. Autophagy 4(5):669–679. PubMed PMID: 18424910

11. Shimizu S, Kanaseki T, Mizushima N, Mizuta T, Arakawa-Kobayashi S, Thompson CB et al (2004) Role of Bcl-2 family proteins in a non-apoptotic programmed cell death dependent on autophagy genes. Nat Cell Biol 6(12):1221–1228. https://doi.org/10.1038/ncb1192. PubMed PMID: 15558033

12. Xue L, Fletcher GC, Tolkovsky AM (1999) Autophagy is activated by apoptotic signalling in sympathetic neurons: an alternative mechanism of death execution. Mol Cell Neurosci 14(3):180–198. https://doi.org/10.1006/mcne.1999.0780. PubMed PMID: 10576889

13. Akar U, Ozpolat B, Mehta K, Fok J, Kondo Y, Lopez-Berestein G (2007) Tissue transglutaminase inhibits autophagy in pancreatic cancer cells. Mol Cancer Res 5(3):241–249. https://doi.org/10.1158/1541-7786.MCR-06-0229. PubMed PMID: 17374730

14. Moretti L, Attia A, Kim KW, Lu B (2007) Crosstalk between Bak/Bax and mTOR signaling regulates radiation-induced autophagy. Autophagy 3(2):142–144. PubMed PMID: 17204849

15. Vega-Rubin-de-Celis S, Zou Z, Fernandez AF, Ci B, Kim M, Xiao G et al (2018) Increased autophagy blocks HER2-mediated breast tumorigenesis. Proc Natl Acad Sci U S A 115(16):4176–4181. https://doi.org/10.1073/pnas.1717800115. PubMed PMID: 29610308; PubMed Central PMCID: PMCPMC5910832

16. Biel TG, Rao VA (2018) Mitochondrial dysfunction activates lysosomal-dependent mitophagy selectively in cancer cells. Oncotarget 9(1):995–1011. https://doi.org/10.18632/oncotarget.23171. PubMed PMID: 29416672; PubMed Central PMCID: PMCPMC5787530

17. Sui X, Chen R, Wang Z, Huang Z, Kong N, Zhang M et al (2013) Autophagy and chemotherapy resistance: a promising therapeutic target for cancer treatment. Cell Death Dis 4:e838. https://doi.org/10.1038/cddis.2013.350. PubMed PMID: 24113172; PubMed Central PMCID: PMCPMC3824660

18. Eisenberg-Lerner A, Bialik S, Simon HU, Kimchi A (2009) Life and death partners: apoptosis, autophagy and the cross-talk between them. Cell Death Differ 16(7):966–975. https://doi.org/10.1038/cdd.2009.33. PubMed PMID: 19325568

19. Meng C, Liu Y, Shen Y, Liu S, Wang Z, Ye Q, Liu H, Liu X, Jia L (2018) MicroRNA-26b suppresses autophagy in breast cancer cells by targeting DRAM1 mRNA, and is downregulated by irradiation. Oncol Lett 15(2):1435–1440. https://doi.org/10.3892/ol.2017.7452.

20. Liu L, Shen W, Zhu Z, Lin J, Fang Q, Ruan Y, Zhao H (2018) Combined inhibition of EGFR and c-ABL suppresses the growth of fulvestrant-resistant breast cancer cells through miR-375-autophagy axis. Biochem Biophys Res Commun 498(3):559–565. https://doi.org/10.1016/j.bbrc.2018.03.019

21. Chen H, Soni M, Patel Y, Markoutsa E, Jie C, Liu S, Xu P (2018). Autophagy Cell viability and chemo-resistance are regulated by miR-489 in breast cancer. Mol Cancer Res. pii: molcanres.0634.2017. https://doi.org/10.1158/1541-7786.MCR-17-0634

22. Chen SM, Wang BY, Lee CH, Lee HT, Li JJ, Hong GC, Hung YC, Chien PJ, Chang CY, Hsu LS, Chang WW (2017). Hinokitiol up-regulates miR-494-3p to suppress BMI1 expression and inhibits self-renewal of breast cancer stem/progenitor cells. Oncotarget 8(44):76057–76068. https://doi.org/10.18632/oncotarget.18648

23. Chen P, He YH, Huang X, Tao SQ, Wang XN, Yan H, Ding KS, Lobie PE, Wu WY, Wu ZS (2017). MiR-23a modulates X-linked inhibitor of apoptosis-mediated autophagy in human luminal breast cancer cell lines. Oncotarget 8(46):80709–80721. https://doi.org/10.18632/oncotarget.21080.

24. Zhang N, Huang Y, Wu F, Zhao Y, Li X, Shen P, Yang L, Luo Y, Yang L, He G (2016). Codelivery of a miR-124 mimic and obatoclax by cholesterol-penetratin micelles simultaneously induces apoptosis and inhibits autophagic flux in breast cancer in vitro and in vivo. Mol Pharm 13(7):2466–2483. https://doi.org/10.1021/acs.molpharmaceut.6b00211

25. Ren Y, Chen Y, Liang X, Lu Y, Pan W, Yang M (2017) MiRNA-638 promotes autophagy and malignant phenotypes of cancer cells via directly suppressing DACT3. Cancer Lett 390:126–136. https://doi.org/10.1016/j.canlet.2017.01.009
26. Shi Y, Zhao Y, Shao N, Ye R, Lin Y, Zhang N, Li W, Zhang Y, Wang S (2017) Overexpression of microRNA-96-5p inhibits autophagy and apoptosis and enhances the proliferation, migration and invasiveness of human breast cancer cells. Oncol Lett 13(6):4402–4412. https://doi.org/10.3892/ol.2017.6025
27. Liu L, He J, Wei X, Wan G, Lao Y, Xu W, Li Z, Hu H, Hu Z, Luo X, Wu J, Xie W, Zhang Y, Xu N (2017) MicroRNA-20a-mediated loss of autophagy contributes to breast tumorigenesis by promoting genomic damage and instability. Oncogene 36(42):5874–5884. https://doi.org/10.1038/onc.2017.193
28. Fan YX, Dai YZ, Wang XL, Ren YQ, Han JJ, Zhang H (2016) MiR-18a upregulation enhances autophagy in triple negative cancer cells via inhibiting mTOR signaling pathway. Eur Rev Med Pharmacol Sci 20(11):2194–2200
29. Zhang F, Wang B, Long H, Yu J, Li F, Hou H, Yang Q (2016). Decreased miR-124-3p expression prompted breast cancer cell progression mainly by targeting Beclin-1. Clin Lab 62(6):1139–1145
30. Di X, Zhang G, Zhang Y, Takeda K, Rivera Rosado LA, Zhang B (2013) Accumulation of autophagosomes in breast cancer cells induces TRAIL resistance through downregulation of surface expression of death receptors 4 and 5. Oncotarget 4(9):1349–1364
31. Han H, Zhou H, Li J, Feng X, Zou D, Zhou W (2017) TRAIL DR5-CTSB crosstalk participates in breast cancer autophagy initiated by SAHA. Cell Death Discov 3:17052. https://doi.org/10.1038/cddiscovery.2017.52. eCollection 2017
32. Das S, Nayak A, Siddharth S, Nayak D, Narayan S, Kundu CN (2017) TRAIL enhances quinacrine-mediated apoptosis in breast cancer cells through induction of autophagy via modulation of p21 and DR5 interactions. Cell Oncol (Dordr) 40(6):593–607. https://doi.org/10.1007/s13402-017-0347-3
33. Lv S, Wang X, Zhang N, Sun M, Qi W, Li, Y, Yang Q (2015) Autophagy facilitates the development of resistance to the tumor necrosis factor superfamily member TRAIL in breast cancer. International Journal of Oncology 46:1286–1294. https://doi.org/10.3892/ijo.2014.2812Pubmed PMID:25572822

Chapter 6
Breast Cancer Heterogeneity in Primary and Metastatic Disease

Lauren Kalinowski, Jodi M. Saunus, Amy E. McCart Reed, and Sunil R. Lakhani

Abstract Breast cancer encompasses a heterogeneous collection of neoplasms with diverse morphologies, molecular phenotypes, responses to therapy, probabilities of relapse and overall survival. Traditional histopathological classification aims to categorise tumours into subgroups to inform clinical management decisions, but the diversity within these subgroups remains considerable. Application of massively parallel sequencing technologies in breast cancer research has revealed the true depth of variability in terms of the genetic, phenotypic, cellular and microenvironmental constitution of individual tumours, with the realisation that each tumour is exquisitely unique. This poses great challenges in predicting the development of drug resistance, and treating metastatic disease. Central to achieving fully personalised clinical management is translating new insights on breast cancer heterogeneity into the clinical setting, to evolve the taxonomy of breast cancer and improve risk stratification.

Keywords Breast cancer classification · Breast cancer molecular subtypes · Clonal evolution · Heterogeneity · Metastasis · Pathology

L. Kalinowski · S. R. Lakhani
Faculty of Medicine, The University of Queensland, Centre for Clinical Research, Royal Brisbane and Women's Hospital, Herston, QLD, Australia

Pathology Queensland, Royal Brisbane and Women's Hospital, Herston, QLD, Australia

J. M. Saunus (✉) · A. E. McCart Reed
Faculty of Medicine, The University of Queensland, Centre for Clinical Research, Royal Brisbane and Women's Hospital, Herston, QLD, Australia
e-mail: j.saunus@uq.edu.au

© Springer Nature Switzerland AG 2019
A. Ahmad (ed.), *Breast Cancer Metastasis and Drug Resistance*,
Advances in Experimental Medicine and Biology 1152,
https://doi.org/10.1007/978-3-030-20301-6_6

6.1   Introduction

Complexity pervades breast tumours at every level – from (epi)genomic, transcriptomic and proteomic landscapes, through to cellular composition and clinical behaviour. This lack of compositional uniformity is referred to as heterogeneity. In breast cancer, this has been historically categorised as intertumoural heterogeneity (diversity between separate tumours) and intratumoural heterogeneity (diversity within a tumour). However, the distinction is becoming increasingly blurred as we understand more about the pathobiology of breast cancer progression. While a single cell acquires the somatic mutations sufficient to launch oncogenic transformation, the cells that eventually comprise clinically detectable deposits arise from clonal selection and expansion as a consequence of a range of different selection pressures, and this has important implications for diagnosis, treatment and drug resistance.

Molecular confirmation of breast cancer heterogeneity has been driven by unparalleled expansion of next generation sequencing technologies over the last decade, with advances in tumour profiling also evolving the traditional taxonomy. Categorising breast tumours into diagnostic and prognostic groups has always been the basis for clinical management, but the *fully* personalised model we are striving for will feature an unprecedented level of precision, matching each patient with the best possible treatments according to specific molecular alterations underpinning their disease. Navigating and rationalising the exponentially growing wealth of new molecular information remains a major challenge to clinical translation.

This chapter will consider the traditional histopathologic classification of breast cancer, broadly examine the molecular basis of genetic, cellular and microenvironment heterogeneity and the ways in which new knowledge is being integrated to complement the existing taxonomy. Finally, we examine the impact of breast cancer heterogeneity on clinical management and translation of emerging research.

6.2   Current Histopathologic Classification of Breast Cancer

6.2.1   Histological Subtypes

Breast carcinoma encompasses a large group of tumours with different morphological, phenotypic and molecular characteristics, and the current classification includes a spectrum of in situ (pre-invasive) to invasive disease. This chapter focuses on invasive disease, where tumour cells breach the basement membrane and invade surrounding tissue, although there is increasing recognition of heterogeneity within in situ carcinoma [1]. The World Health Organisation (WHO) maintains a diagnostic framework that provides practical information to guide tumour diagnosis and patient management (Table 6.1) [2, 3]. Invasive cancers are initially stratified according to

Table 6.1 WHO classification of breast carcinoma (2012)

	Histological type	Frequency
1	Invasive carcinoma of no special type (IC-NST) *Includes: pleomorphic carcinoma, carcinoma with osteoclast-like stromal giant cells, carcinoma with choriocarcinomatous features, carcinoma with melanotic features*	40–75%
2	Invasive lobular carcinoma (ILC) *Includes: classic, solid, alveolar, pleomorphic, tubulolobular, mixed subtypes*	5–15%
3	Tubular carcinoma	2%
4	Cribriform carcinoma	0.3–0.8% (up to 4%)
5	Mucinous carcinoma	2%
6	Carcinoma with medullary features *Includes: medullary carcinoma, atypical medullary carcinoma, IC-NST with medullary features*	<1%
7	Carcinoma with apocrine differentiation	4%
8	Carcinoma with signet ring cell differentiation	<1%
9	Invasive micropapillary carcinoma	0.9–2%
10	Metaplastic carcinoma of no special type *Includes: low-grade adenosquamous carcinoma, fibromatosis-like metasplastic carcinoma, squamous cell carcinoma, spindle cell carcinoma, metasplastic carcinoma with mesenchymal differentiation (chondroid, osseuous, other types), mixed metaplastic carcinoma, myoepithelial carcinoma*	0.2–5%
11	Carcinoma with neuroendocrine features *Includes: well differentiated neuroendocrine tumour, poorly differentiated neuroendocrine tumour (small cell carcinoma), carcinoma with neuroendocrine differentiation*	<1%
12	Secretory carcinoma	<0.15%
13	Invasive papillary carcinoma	<1%
14	Acinic cell carcinoma	<1%
15	Mucoepidermoid carinoma	0.3%
16	Polymorphous carcinoma	<1%
17	Oncocytic carcinoma	<1%
18	Lipid-rich carcinoma	<1–1.6%
19	Glycogen rich clear cell carcinoma	1–3%
20	Sebaceous carcinoma	<1%
21	Adenomyoepithelioma with carcinoma	<1%
22	Adenoid cystic carcinoma	<0.1%
23	Encapsulated papillary carcinoma	<2%
24	Invasive solid papillary carcinoma	<1%

cellular and architectural growth patterns, into histological 'special types' with distinct morphology (25–30% of cases, including 5–15% lobular carcinomas; for examples see Fig. 6.1a, b). As a diagnosis of exclusion, tumours without discriminating morphological features are classified as invasive carcinoma of no special type (IC-NST; 40–75% of cases) [3]. Whilst this distinction appears straightforward,

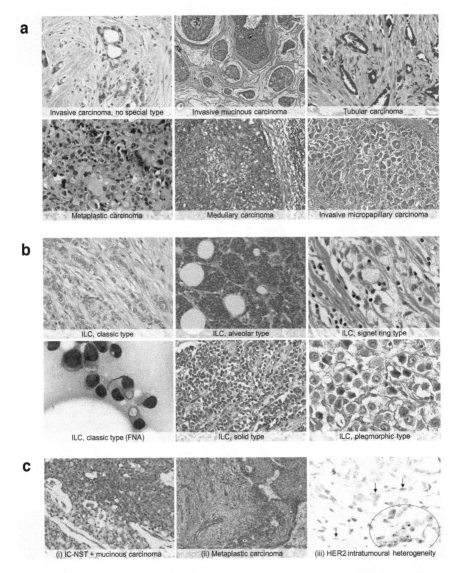

Fig. 6.1 (**a**) Breast cancer heterogeneity exemplified by histological subtypes. Haematoxylin and eosin-stained breast cancer tissues visualised by light microscopy. (**b**) Morphological variation within one histological type, invasive lobular carcinoma (ILC). *FNA, fine needle aspiration cytology.* (**c**) Mixed histological subtypes: (i) Invasive carcinoma (no special type) mixed with invasive mucinous carcinoma; (ii) metaplastic carcinoma exhibiting marked variability in both epithelial and stromal compartments; (iii) intratumoural heterogeneity for HER2 shown by silver *in situ* hybridisation (SISH) – a nest of cells exhibits *ERBB2* gene amplification (circled), while others remain diploid (arrows)

many tumours comprise mixed histology (Fig. 6.1c) – thresholds are used to definitively categorise individual cases, though these are somewhat arbitrary. For example, a pure 'special type' diagnosis is applied if >90% of the tumour area comprises the special morphology, but in 'mixed' cases, separate areas within the same tumour exhibit both 'non-special' and 'special' morphology (10–49% [2]).

In some instances, tumours with distinct morphological features share underlying genetic mutations [4]. Secretory carcinomas are associated with a t(12;15) (p13;q25) translocation and the resulting *ETV6-NTRK3* fusion gene [5]; and, like their counterpart in the salivary gland, adenoid cystic breast carcinomas consistently harbour the t(6;9)(q22–23;p23–24) translocation, leading to *MYB-NFIB* gene fusion and over-expression of the *MYB* oncogene [6]. Genotype-phenotype correlation is epitomised by E-cadherin, which is genomically 'lost' or dysregulated in lobular carcinomas, and tends to occur concomitantly with specific mutations in *PTEN*, *TBX3* and *FOXA1* [7, 8]. However, even subtypes with shared morphological features and mutations exhibit substantial inter-tumoural diversity. For example, within lobular carcinoma, the largest group of special types, genomic and transcriptomic analysis highlighted the existence of distinct prognostic subtypes [8]. Thus overall, histological subtyping alone provides imperfect prognostic information – its value comes from integration with other histopathologic information, namely grade, stage and biomarker status.

6.2.2 Prognostic and Predictive Subgroups

Histopathologic assessment routinely involves quantification of prognostic factors, which predict the natural history of disease irrespective of therapy, and predictive factors, which indicate the likely response to a specific treatment. The disease stage, histological grade and tumour expression of receptors for oestrogen, progesterone and human epidermal growth factor (ER, PR and HER2) are the cornerstones of current prognostic and predictive algorithms. The American Joint Committee on Cancer TNM (tumour/node/metastasis) staging system stratifies broadly based on the burden of the disease by measuring the tumour size, the number of lymph nodes involved, and the extent of distant metastatic disease; stage IV is the most advanced disease, while stage I is the least advanced.

Histological grade is a powerful prognostic indicator [9, 10] and correlates with morphology and molecular features [11]. It is calculated from the degree of nuclear pleomorphism, 'tubule' formation (resemblance to normal ducto-lobular gland structure) and the number of mitoses per ten high power microscope fields [12]. Grading reflects a collective morphological assessment of the biological characteristics of a tumour and therefore encompasses intra-tumoural heterogeneity. It is highly reproducible, and remains a component of widely used prognostic algorithms (e.g. Nottingham and Kalmar Prognostic Indices [13–15]), as well as predictive algorithms used to guide the prescription of chemotherapy [16, 17]. Pathologists have been describing heterogeneity for decades, but given that clinical behaviour is still diverse within these three broad categories, so there is much scope for grading to be complemented by molecular information.

Breast cancers are routinely analysed for ER, PR and HER2 using IHC-based assessment of protein expression levels and frequency. This information is both prognostic and predictive, reflecting critical growth factor signalling dependencies that can be targeted for therapeutic benefit. PR is induced by oestrogen signalling (thus is a surrogate for ER activity), and adds value to the power of ER for predicting response to therapy [18, 19]. ER/PR-positive tumours tend to be lower grade and associated with better outcomes than ER/PR-negative cases, and are candidates for endocrine therapy (*e.g.* tamoxifen, fulvestrant, aromatase inhibitors). The gene encoding HER2 (*ERBB2*) is amplified and/or over-expressed in 15–20% of invasive breast cancers, and correlates with poor prognosis but is also a marker of sensitivity to HER2-targeted therapy (standardly trastuzumab and pertuzumab with chemotherapy) [20–24]. Tumours that are negative for ER/PR and HER2 are currently classified as triple negative breast cancers (TNBC), where there are intensive research efforts ongoing to substratify molecularly distinct subgroups that could be suitable for new therapeutic approaches targeting antitumour host immunity, DNA repair and/or specific signalling pathways [25] (see Sect. 6.4.2).

Importantly, the expression of ER/PR and HER2 is not always uniform, implying that not all tumour cells are dependent on their growth factor ligands. ER/PR-positivity is currently defined by a diagnostic threshold of only 1% [26]. Testing to define HER2 status is based on either protein over-expression as demonstrated by IHC and/or testing for gene amplification. Criteria for gene amplification are based on *ERBB2* copy number or *ERBB2:CEP17* ratio, determined using *in situ* hybridisation (ISH). If the results are equivocal, orthogonal testing is recommended [27]. Whilst conservative cut-offs ensure patients are eligible for treatments that may confer marginal benefit, heterogeneity undoubtedly impacts the clinical response. For example, HER2 heterogeneity is related to low levels of gene amplification, which is more common in ER/PR-positive tumours and associated with shorter disease-free survival [28–30] (Fig. 6.1c).

6.3 Molecular Basis for Heterogeneity in Breast Cancer

The molecular basis for heterogeneity can be divided into tumour cell-intrinsic factors, such as genomic alterations, and their impact on pre-existing differentiation programs in the cell-of-origin; as well as extrinsic factors in the tumour microenvironment. However this division is purely for academic purposes – in reality the tumour and nontumour components are admixed and constantly engaged in feedback signalling [31, 32].

6.3.1 Genetic Heterogeneity

Tumourigenesis occurs by inappropriate expansion of genetically altered clones (groups of isogenic tumour cells derived from a common ancestor; Fig. 6.2, <u>inset</u>) via branching evolution, where the acquisition of a new genetic alteration in a multipotent cell capable of self-renewal represents an evolutionary branching point, and the initiation of a new 'subclone' (Fig. 6.2). Mutations that confer a selective

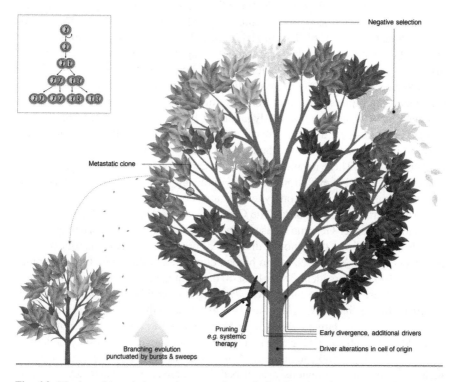

Fig. 6.2 The branching phylogenetic tree analogy of clonal progression, where major branchpoints represent the acquisition of each new driver, and distance from the ground is proportional to divergence from the original founding clone. Coloured bunches of leaves represent major subclones with the same driver combinations, with individual leaves as minor subclones harbouring additional genomic alterations and phenotypic differences (see Fig. 6.3). Evidence suggests that clonal evolution occurs intermittently, with essential fitness advantages acquired at the earliest stages of tumourigenesis in short mutational bursts (often copy-number alterations), followed by stable clonal expansions that form the bulk of the tumour. Selective clonal 'sweeps' may also occur in response to new extrinsic selection pressure (e.g. systemic agents that prune particular subclones). Circulating tumour cell seeds are shed into the blood and lymphatics – those with the requisite capabilities may colonise suitable soil in distant organs, where the branching evolution process continues. (**inset**) Classic clonal expansion, where genetic diversity arises through iterative rounds of somatic mutation (coloured dots) and cell division (arrows), and heritable alterations are passed to daughter cells. *Curved arrow = self-renewal of a cancer stem cell at the top of the clonal hierarchy*

advantage to a clone in its particular microenvironment are referred to as 'drivers', while those that do not immediately confer a selective advantage are 'passengers'. They can be distinguished using algorithms that calculate the rates of non-synonymous *vs* synonymous mutation in each gene, non-random clustering of mutations and/or gene amplification combined with over-expression, which imply positive evolutionary selection [33–35].

Historically, heterogeneity has been considered a byproduct of classical Darwinian evolution, where *de novo* mutations conferring a fitness advantage result in rapid expansion and positive selection of the new clone at the expense of others, resulting in its mutation profile dominating a whole region of the tumour (a so-called 'clonal sweep') [36]. This model implies that tumour cells sustain mutations at a fairly constant tempo, but recent studies suggest that tumourigenesis can be driven by just a few major expansion events followed by long periods of relative evolutionary stasis, challenging gradualistic clonal expansion dogma [37–42]. By sequencing multiple single cells from a tumour, several groups have now found evidence for so-called 'big-bang' dynamics in breast cancer, where critical copy-number alterations are thought to occur as early 'bursts', superimposed with cumulative point mutations that contribute to the genetic diversity observed in tumour biopsies [41, 43]. These detailed studies have given weight to the more progressive 'punctuated' model of evolution – a hybrid of the big-bang and classic clonal expansion paradigms where evolutionary tempos are sporadic.

Large international consortia (The Cancer Genome Atlas (TCGA [44]) and the International Cancer Genome Consortium (ICGC [45, 46])) have made significant inroads characterising the genomic diversity of breast cancer using next-generation sequencing of RNA and DNA from human clinical samples (Table 6.2). An initial survey of 100 tumours identified at least 40 different genes harbouring driver mutations, but these were present in over 70 different combinations [46], with each occurring in less than 10% of tumours [47, 48]. Due to the low overall frequencies of driver mutations, larger cohorts have been required to confirm recurrent alterations. More recently, a landmark whole genome sequencing study using the largest cohort to date (n = 560), identified 93 protein-coding genes as probable drivers, including five with no previously described link to breast cancer (*MED23, FOXP1, MLLT4, XBP1, ZFP36L1*) [49]. Whilst almost all the tumours harboured at least one driver, no two tumours out of 560 shared the same combination. Some of the more frequent changes identified include *ERRB2, CCND1, AKT1* (amplified and over-expressed), *PIK3CA, GATA3* (amplified and overexpressed and/or activating mutation), *TP53, PTEN* and *CDH1* (copy-number loss or inactivating mutation leading to functional insufficiency) [44, 46, 48, 50, 51]. It is thought that breast cancer driver mutations occurring with a frequency of greater than 2% are now known, but it is expected that additional, low frequency drivers are still likely to be found in minor subgroups (e.g. male breast cancer, histological special types) [52]. The particular combination of driver alterations, together with thousands of passenger mutations and structural rearrangements make each breast cancer unique [49, 53, 54]. In general, high levels of genomic heterogeneity tend to be associated with worse clinical outcomes [55].

Table 6.2 Landmark next generation sequencing studies in breast cancer

Study	Year	Cohort size	Approach	Key findings
Shah [156]	2009	1	WGS, RNASeq	First to apply WGS to a matched pair of primary and metastasis 5/32 somatic non-synonymous coding mtuations identified in the metastasis were detected in the primary lobular breast tumour diagnosed 9 years earlier, 6/32 were at low frequency in the primary
Curtis, METABRIC [50]	2012	1992	CNA, GEX	Integration of CNA and GEX data derived 10 molecular subgroups called 'integrative clusters' with distinct clinical outcomes Groups include a high-risk, ER-positive 11q13/14 subgroup and a favourable prognosis subgroup devoid of CNAs Identified *PPP2R2A*, *MTAP* and *MAP2K4* as putative cancer genes
Shah [51]	2012	104	aCGH, WES, WGS, RNASeq,	Basal-like tumours show greater variation in mutations than non-basal TNBC *TP53*, *PIK3CA* and *PTEN* somatic mutations are clonally fominant but in some cases are inconsistent with founder status Mutations in cell shape, cytoskeleton and motitilty genes tend to occur later in tumour progression
TCGA [44]	2012	466	CNA, GEX, methylation, microRNAseq, RPPA, WES	Only *TP53*, *PIK3CA* and *PTEN* somatic mutations occurred in >10% of samples Enrichment of *GATA3*, *PIK3CA* and *MAP3K1* mtuations in luminal tumours Identified two novel protein expression defined subgroups related to microenvironment Molecular commonalities between basal-like tumours and serous ovarian cancers
Stephens [46]	2012	100	CNA, WES	Correlations between number of mutations, age of cancer diagnosis and histological grade Somatic driver point mutations and/or copy number changes were identified in over 40 cancer genes in 73 combinations Maximum of 6 mutated driver genes in a single tumour; 28 tumours showed only 1 driver mutation *TP53*, *PIK3CA*, *ERRB2*, *MYC*, *FGFR1/ZNF703*, *GATA3* and *CCND1* were mutated in >10% of cancers (58% of the driver mutations); remaining 33 mutated cancer genes contributed to the other 42% of driving genetic events 9 new candidate driver genes: *AKT2*, *ARIDIB*, *CASP8*, *CDKN1B*, *MAP3K1*, *MAP3K13*, *NCOR1*, *SMARCD1*, and *TBX3*.

(continued)

Table 6.2 (continued)

Study	Year	Cohort size	Approach	Key findings
Banerji [48]	2012	103 + 22	WES (103), WGS (22)	Confirmed recurrent mutations *PIK3CA, TP53, AKT1, GATA3*, and *MAP3K1* driver mutations Novel mutation *in CBFB* and deletions in *RUNX1* Recurrent *MAGI3-AKT3* fusion enriched in TNBC; leads to activation of AKT kinase
Ellis [172]	2012	77	WES (31), WGS (46)	Biopsies of ER+ tumours from two neo-adjuvant aromatase inhibitor trials were assessed to elucidate biomarkers of response Distinct phenotypes in ER-positive tumours are driven by specific patterns of somatic alteration: *GATA3* – luminal A, low grade, low prolif.; *TP53* – non-luminal A, high grade, high prolif *GATA3* mutations correlated with a treatment-related suppression of proliferation
Wang [41]	2014	2 cases	CNA, nucSeq, WGS, WES	Developed nucSeq approach for single cell sequencing Population and single nuclei sequencing approach in an ER positive tumour and a TNBC No 2 single tumour cells are genetically identical Large numbers of subclonal and de novo mutations
Yates [36]	2015	303 tumours, 50 patients	Targeted sequencing WGS	12 treatment-naive tumours with spatially heterogeneous subclones; all tumours showed at least one clonal driver 4 multi-focal cancers with 2–5 foci; individual foci clonally related but had private mutations suggestive of clonal sweeps Created 'index of heterogeneity', which correlated with age at diagnosis and larger tumour size; no correlation with histology, grade, ER status, intra-tumoral lymphocytes or Ki67 No specific temporal pattern observed – mutations in common breast cancer genes (*PIK3CA, TP53, PTEN, BRACA2* and *MYC*) occurred early in some tumours and late in others
Ciriello [8]	2015	817	CNA, methylation, RPPA, WES	E-cadherin loss and mutations in *PTEN, TBX3* and *FOXA1* in ILC; conversely luminal A IC-NST had mutations in *GATA3* Identified 3 mRNA derived prognostic subgroups of ILC: immune-related, proliferation and reactive-like

Table 6.2 (continued)

Study	Year	Cohort size	Approach	Key findings
Nik-Zainal [49]	2016	560	WGS; mutational signature analysis	Defined 93 protein-coding genes with probable driver mutations (31 dominant, 60 recessive, 2 uncertain) 5 new cancer genes described (*MED23, FOXP1, MLLT4, XBP1, ZFP36L1*) At least 1 driver mutation in >95% of cancers 10 most frequently mutated (62% of drivers): *TP53, PIK3CA, MYC, CCND1, PTEN, ERBB2, ZNF703/FGFR1, GATA3, RB1, MAP3KI* Characterised mutational signatures: 12 base substitutions and 6 rearrangement signatures Specific mutational signatures associated with *BRCA1/2* alterations
Smid [60]	2016	266	RNASeq, meta-analysis of WGS	In luminal tumours, mutation burden correlates directly with adverse outcome Signatures 3 and 13 associated with immune response, increased TILs and better outcomes Specific substitutions more effective in eliciting an immune response than sheer number
Periera [55]	2016	2433	CNA, GEX, targeted sequencing, WES	Assessed intra-tumorual heterogeneity using mutant-allel fractions 40 mutation-driver genes (6/40 oncogenes; 8/40 tumour suppressor genes); most common *PIK3CA* (40.1%) and *TP53* (35.4%) Five genes with coding mutations in >10% samples: *MUC16* (16%), *AHNAK2* (16.2%), *SYNE1* (12%), *KMT2C* (11.4%), *GATA3* (11.1%) *PIK3CA* in lower grade ER+ tumours (associated with reduced survival in 3 subgroups); *TP53* in higher grade tumours, and only associated with worse outcome in ER+ tumours Difference in mutation frequency based on HER status: *TP53* ER-/HER2+ (67.5%) vs ER+/HER2+ (42.6%) 42.5% of tumours had a mutation in the Akt pathway (*PIKC3A, AKT1, PIK3R1, PTEN, FOXO3*) Mutations associated with longer (ER+ *MAP3K1, GATA3*) vs shorter (*SMAD4, USP9X*) survival

aCGH array comparative genomic hybridisation, *CNA* copy number aberration, usually SNP-based, *GEX* gene expression profiling, array-based, *METABRIC* Molecular Taxonomy of Breast Cancer International Consortium, *RNASeq* RNA sequencing, *RPPA* reverse phase protein assays, *SNP* single nucleotide polymorphism, *TCGA* The Cancer Genome Atlas, *WES* whole exome sequencing, *WGS* whole genome sequencing

Focusing on driver mutations has helped to understand the hallmark processes underpinning breast cancer development and define possible drug targets, but there is also increasing interest in passenger mutations – not only in terms of their influence on progression in the context of exposure to extrinsic selection pressures, but as a genomic record of the mutational processes that occurred throughout the development of each tumour. Mutational process signatures are dynamic, varying spatially and temporally depending on both exogenous and endogenous factors (e.g. carcinogen exposure, age-related change or DNA repair defects) [53]. Complex mathematical analysis has identified 21 substitution signatures with different clinicopathologic associations and underlying aetiologies. Like individual mutations, signatures are clonal and coexist at variable frequencies within cancer deposits of each patient. Some are common to different cancers (e.g. age-related), while others are tumour type-specific (e.g. $C \cdot G \rightarrow T \cdot A$ transitions are a feature of signature 7, associated with UV-induced DNA damage in cutaneous cancers) [56, 57].

Breast cancer genomes are characterised by 12 substitution signatures, with six consistently detected in at least 20% of cases [49, 53, 57, 58]. Amongst these, signatures 1 and 5 (which are similar and often classified together as 1B) are associated with age, while signatures 2 and 13 are associated with APOBEC cytidine deaminases, which are normally involved in antiviral immunity and RNA editing, but can also act on long stretches of single-stranded DNA thought to arise during abnormal DNA replication [49]. Signatures 3 and 8 are associated with *BRCA1/BRCA2* deficiency, defective homologous recombination repair, and short (<10 kb) deletions/ tandem duplications [49]. Of the rarer signatures (<20% cases), 6, 20, and 26 are associated with mismatch repair deficiency, while 17, 18, and 30 are of unknown aetiology. The potential implications and clinical applications of mutational signature composition are currently under investigation [58]. For example, they may be useful for characterising cancers with unknown primary origin at diagnosis [59]. Also, signatures 3 and 13 are associated with increased lymphocytic infiltrate and better clinical outcomes, raising the possibility that free DNA and/or mutant peptides associated with this pattern are more immunogenic compared with other mutational processes [60] (see Sect. 6.3.3). Finally, there are possibilities for developing signature-based predictive models, such the 'HRDetect' algorithm that quantifies somatic *BRCA1/2* deficiency, a candidate biomarker of response to polyADP-ribose polymerase (PARP) inhibitors [61, 62].

Sequencing the genomes and transcriptomes of single breast tumour cells is now offering additional insights into heterogeneity. For example, single-cell genome analysis has been applied to understand the dynamics of clonal selection across cohorts of patient-derived tumour xenografts [63]. Also, in an elegant and clinically relevant application of RNA-sequencing, Lee and colleagues compared breast cancer cell subpopulations exhibiting resistance to the microtubule poison paclitaxel in vitro [64]. Residual cells that persisted after treatment expressed variants involved a variety of cellular processes logically connected to drug resistance, including microtubule stabilization and stress. But critically, individual cells expressed different combinations of variant transcripts, suggesting that transcriptional heterogeneity can ultimately generate equivalent phenotypes. The expression profiles of individual cells were not apparent in a pooled analysis of the bulk population, or even as few as five cells. Thus single-cell sequencing has the potential to illuminate aspects of plasticity and clonal evolution that would not be apparent from analysis of tissue homogenates.

6.3.2   Cellular Heterogeneity

Gene expression studies comparing breast tumours with normal breast tissue iden-tified groups of tumours exhibiting transcriptomic similarity to particular mam-mary epithelial compartments. For example, 'luminal-like' tumours are most similar to the specialised luminal epithelia that line ducts and lobules of the breast (Sect. 6.4.1), while the expression profile of 'basal-like' tumours resembles lumi-nal progenitor cells (Sect. 6.4.2) [65]. Functional evidence supporting the idea that global tumour gene expression profiles could reflect the cell type of origin came from transgenic mouse experiments, where oncogenic mutations were introduced into specific compartments of the mouse mammary gland, resulting in formation of tumours that phenocopied metaplastic or *BRCA1*-mutant breast cancer [66, 67]. Thus, heterogeneity reflects the consequences of superimposing the mutational landscape over pre-programmed phenotypic determinants. The cells comprising a tumour exhibit restricted versions of the normal mammary epithelial lineage hier-archy, depending on which cell type sustained the founding oncogenic hits, and how the unique spectrum of alterations impacted lineage differentiation program-ming in its daughters (for example, de-differentiation and phenotypic plasticity). Diversification is also achieved through phenotypic drift (stochastic heterogeneity [31, 68]; Fig. 6.3a). The significance of this is highlighted by the association between stem-like phenotypes and poor outcomes in breast and other cancers [69–71], though it is worth considering that primitive, stem-like cells may be associated with metastasis and treatment resistance simply because they have more potential for generating clonal complexity (*i.e.* better substrates for natural selection) [31], not necessarily because they possess equivalent normal stem cell functions like efficient drug efflux and slow cell cycling.

6.3.3   Microenvironment Heterogeneity

Non-tumour elements contributing to breast cancer heterogeneity include soluble and extracellular matrix proteins, fibroblasts, endothelia, adipocytes, macro-phages and other leukocytes [72] (Fig. 6.3b). A large effort has been directed at investigating clinical implications of the breast cancer microenvironment [73–75]. One area in which there have been key recent developments is in understand-ing how vascular perfusion dynamics impacts tumour progression and treatment

a Effect of the mutational landscape on existing phenotypic programs   **b** Microenvironment heterogeneity

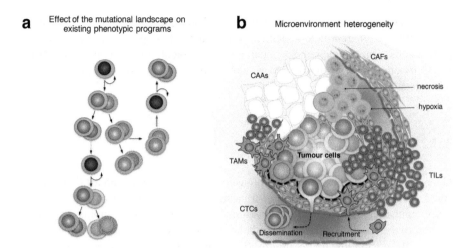

Fig. 6.3 Heterogeneity represents the collective consequences of superimposing the mutational landscape over pre-existing phenotypic programs and interaction with the microenvironment. (**a**) Breast tumour cells exhibit restricted versions of the normal mammary epithelial lineage hierarchy, depending on which cell type sustained the founding oncogenic hits, and how the unique spectrum of alterations impacted lineage differentiation programming in its daughters. The differentiation states (different colours) of stem-like (black nuclei), committed progenitor and daughter cells contribute to phenotypic diversity (deterministic heterogeneity). Phenotypic flux due to cell-specific biochemical processes (patterning in daughter cells) also contributes to phenotypic diversity (stochastic heterogeneity). Daughter cells may acquire stem-cell activity through genetic alteration (dashed arrow) or de-differentiation (blue arrow), acquiring stem cell activity and initiating new clones. (**b**) Stromal elements influence tumour cell phenotypes and clonal selection, and are in turn altered by their interactions with tumour cells, contributing to intratumoural heterogeneity. The figure shows various stromal cell types: cancer-associated adipocytes and fibroblasts (CAAs/CAFs), tumour-infiltrating lymphocytes (TILs), tumour-associated macrophages (TAMs) and circulating tumour cells (CTCs) liberated into surrounding blood vessels. Ongoing tumour cell proliferation fuels pro-tumourigenic cycles of local hypoxia and neoangiogenesis, resulting in chaotic microvascular networks that cannot adequately deliver systemic therapy

efficacy. Ongoing proliferation in solid tumours fuels cycles of hypoxia and neo-angiogenesis, and this in turn creates a chaotic, dysfunctional microvascular bed, with (paradoxically) areas of sluggish blood flow in an otherwise hypervascular environment [76–78]. It is thought that inefficient perfusion directly reduce the delivery of systemic therapeutics, but that drug efficacy is also reduced indirectly in poorly oxygenated tissues. This is because radiotherapy and some chemotherapeutics act by damaging tumour DNA, but breaks are more readily repairable in hypoxic conditions, allowing cells to escape fatal chromosome aberrations, and instead, erroneously repair DNA to increase genetic diversity [79]. Hypoxia is also associated with mesenchymal/stem-cell phenotypes, inflammation, fibrosis, poor drug uptake and immune suppression [80]. This knowledge has driven attempts to improve efficacy and reduce the likelihood of relapse using combination therapies that increase oxygenation by 'normalising' the vascular bed.

Ironically, this strategy uses agents that target vascular endothelial growth factor and its receptor (VEGF/VEGFR), originally intended to starve tumours of nutrients and oxygen (e.g. bevacizumab).

Tumour-infiltrating lymphocytes (TILs) have also been intensively studied in the last 5 years, with evidence rapidly accumulating to support a role in clinical management. A fundamental function of host immunity is to detect and eradicate abnormalities arising from neoplastic transformation (immune-surveillance). Considering that breast tumours are diagnosed once they are detectable by mammography and/or palpation, they are already successfully evading elimination at diagnosis, but chemotherapy and radiotherapy can produce neoantigens that effectively kick-start the immune response, and new therapies that reactivate anticancer immune responses are currently being assessed in clinical trials (e.g. immune-checkpoint inhibitors, personalised cancer vaccines and adoptive T-cell therapy [81, 82]). TILs are most frequent in HER2+ and TN disease, where the overall degree of infiltrate is associated with better outcome, even amongst TNBC patients with residual disease following neoadjuvant chemotherapy, an otherwise poor prognostic group [83].

The breast cancer immune microenvironment is a complex mixture of different functional subsets – mostly T-cells, with smaller proportions of B-cells, dendritic cells, neutrophils, macrophages and natural killer (NK)-cells; with different effects on tumour progression. For example, NK and CD4+ Th1-cells are generally associated with favourable outcomes, whilst myeloid-derived suppressor cells (MDSC) and gamma-delta regulatory T-cells ($\gamma\delta$-T_{reg}) suppress anti-tumour immunity and are associated with poor response to chemotherapy [84–87]. Ultimately, the particular constitution of lymphocytic infiltrate (ratios of different TIL subsets and effectors/modifiers they produce) reaches equilibrium with the tumour compartment, and shapes the microenvironment along a spectrum from an immuno-stimulatory, anti-tumour milieu, to a pro-tumourigenic environment geared toward wound-healing. Despite this complexity, TILs are routinely enumerated *en masse* by examination of haematoxylin and eosin (H&E)-stained tissue sections. Special IHC stains are used occasionally, but at this stage this is purely to help discriminate intratumoural TILs from tumour cells, rather than identify different functional subpopulations [88]. Apart from the fact that the full clinical implications of functional TILs heterogeneity are still being elucidated, there are challenges with standardisation in the diagnostic laboratory, as TILs reside mostly in the stromal compartment, which varies with tumour architecture, and enumeration on two-dimensional tissue sections is difficult because they are heterogeneously distributed in three dimensions. But even without universal standardisation, and somewhat crude histopathologic assessment of overall infiltrate density, there is already strong evidence from multiple prospective clinical trials supporting the prognostic and predictive significance of TILs in HER2+ and TN disease [81]. Thus, improvements in the precision of TIL-based biomarker development and companion therapies will likely play favourably into personalised clinical management models.

6.4   Molecular Classification of Breast Cancer

Molecular profiling has shifted the ways that breast cancer development and heterogeneity are considered. Transcriptomic studies began more than 15 years ago, with the segregation of 38 invasive breast carcinomas by unsupervised hierarchical clustering of gene expression profiles [89, 90]. These 'intrinsic subtypes' have since been extensively confirmed in the field as robust biological entities with distinct mutation profiles and clinical outcomes [70, 91–93] (Table 6.3). In some instances, underlying expression profiles provide a molecular explanation for well-known clinical or morphological features. For example, the clinical behaviour of ER-positive tumours depends largely on histologic grade, and in the intrinsic subtype taxonomy they segregate into luminal-A and -B groups, distinguished by expression of proliferation gene networks [89, 90, 93–95].

Subsequent technological advances have increased the breadth and resolution of the transcriptomic taxonomy (more tumours, more extensive coverage and more accurate RNA quantification), providing a deeper understanding of the underlying biology and potential clinical implications. For example, a subgroup of ER-negative IC-NST that frequently exhibits medullary and metaplastic features is enriched with a 'claudin-low' gene cluster [71, 96]. Another is the 'molecular apocrine' (mApo) group, which is largely triple-negative, yet paradoxically expresses ER-responsive, luminal genes due to expression of the androgen receptor (AR; Table 6.3) [97, 98]. In smaller cohorts with less statistical power, mApo tumours would be classed as basal-like or HER2-enriched [94, 97, 99]. The Molecular Taxonomy of Breast Cancer International Consortium (METABRIC) took expression profile analysis to a different level by integrating expression with copy-number data to stratify 2000 breast tumours on the basis of cancer driver profiles [50]. The ten 'integrative subgroups' overlap variably with intrinsic subtypes and are associated with distinct survival trends.

6.4.1   Heterogeneity in Luminal/ER+ Breast Cancer

The largest subgroup of breast cancers is defined by expression of ER in at least 1% of tumour cells, a conservative cut-off that qualifies around 70% of breast cancer patients for endocrine therapy; though ER+ disease still exhibits marked clinical variability, particularly with respect to late recurrences [50, 100]. While endocrine therapy significantly increases relapse-free survival overall, almost a quarter of patients still relapse within 10 years of diagnosis, with some evidence that mutations in the gene itself (*ESR1*), or ER signalling regulators (e.g. *SMRT*) could contribute [101–103]. In terms of predictive molecular features, luminal-B tumours tend to respond less well to endocrine therapy but better to chemotherapy than luminal-A tumours, with the exception of 'atypical' luminal-A cases, which harbour more *TP53* mutations and copy-number aberrations [101, 104]. Deep molecular analyses have also identified unique differences between luminal-A ILC and IC-NST, with ILCs featuring loss of *CDH1*, AKT signalling activation and *FOXA1*

Table 6.3 Molecular breast cancer subtypes

	Histopath features					
	ER	HER2	Grade	Phenotypic features	Mutations [44]	Differentiation state
Intrinsic subtypes						
Luminal A	+	−	1–2	Expression ER-signalling networks and low molecular-weight cytokeratins (CK8/18)	*PIK3A* (49%), *GATA3* (14%), *MAP3K1* (14%), *TP53* (12%), *CDH1* (9%)	Enriched with the gene expression signature of fully differentiated luminal epithelia
Luminal B	+/−	−/+	2–3	Expression of ER-signalling and proliferation networks	*PIK3A* (32%), *TP53* (32%), *PTEN* (24%)	Enriched with the gene expression signature of fully differentiated luminal epithelia
Her2-enriched	−/+	+	2–3	HER2 overexpressed/amplified, over-expression of genes at 17q22.24	*TP53* (75%), *PIK3CA* (42%) / *PTEN* (19%)	Modest expression of mature luminal and luminal progenitor gene expression signatures
Basal-like	−	−	3	Often triple-negative, high grade, frequent expression of myoepithelial markers (EGRF, CK5/6, CK14), c-kit and FOXC1	*TP53* (84%) / *PIK3CA* (7%)	Most similar to luminal epithelial progenitor cells
Normal-like	−/+	−	1	Expression of adipose and myoepithelium genes; low expression of luminal genes; clusters with fibroadenoma and normal breast samples		Enriched with mammary stem cell and stromal gene expression signatures

(continued)

Table 6.3 (continued)

| | Histopath features | | | | |
	ER	HER2	Grade	Phenotypic features	Mutations [44]	Differentiation state
Additional subtypes						
Claudin-low	–	–	3	Enriched with primitive, CD44$^+$/CD24$^-$, mesenchymal-like cells [71, 96]. Low expression of cell-cell junction proteins, high expression of immune response and epithelial-to-mesenchymal signatures. Overall survival worse than Luminal A [70, 71]	*CDH1, CLDN3/4/7, OCLN*	Primitive, enriched with stem cell and stromal signatures. Epithelial to mesenchymal transition markers
Molecular apocrine	–	+/–	2–3	Frequent apocrine histological features; gene networks associated with AR, calcium and ErbB signalling, lipid and fatty acid synthesis; HER2 over-expression (not associated with 17q22.24 amplification); early recurrence but good response to neoadjuvant therapy [99]	Genes associated with AR, calcium and Her2 signalling, lipid and fatty acid synthesis [97, 99]	Primitive [99]

mutations, while IC-NST showed intact cellular adhesion and *GATA3* mutations [8]. Analysing ILCs as a separate group stratified them into reactive-like, immune-related and proliferative subgroups [8]. It is also worth highlighting that there are two different ligand-activated oestrogen receptors, encoded by separate genes: ERα (*ESR1*) and ERβ *(ESR2)* [105]. ERα is the dominant isoform and the best predictor of response to hormone therapy, but a possible role for ERβ in regulating the immune microenvironment is also now emerging [106], and may provide further insights into luminal breast cancer heterogeneity in the future.

6.4.2 Heterogeneity in Triple-Negative Breast Cancer

TNBC is arguably the most heterogeneous of the major breast cancer subgroups. It is more frequent in individuals with inherited mutations in *BRCA1* and other DNA repair genes and carries a poor prognosis overall, although some patients have complete, durable responses to treatment. TNBCs are usually highly proliferative and of higher histological grade, though there are low-grade variants with a more protracted natural history (namely, adenoid cystic and secretory carcinomas) [70, 90, 91, 107–115]. A defining characteristic of TNBC is its paradoxically impressive initial response to neoadjuvant chemotherapy, yet poor 5-year survival rate. The discrepancy is due to a chemotherapy-resistant subgroup found to have residual disease at the time of breast surgery, which is associated with brain and liver metastasis [116]. TNBC patients who do not relapse within 3 years have a prognosis comparable to ER+ disease [109].

Despite high overall mutation loads, the most common variants are in *TP53* (around 80% of cases, with more frequent nonsense and frameshift mutations than ER/HER2+ disease) and *PI3K* in around 10% of cases [117]. On the other hand, TNBCs harbour characteristic chromosomal alterations, categorised as 'simple', 'amplifier/firestorm' or 'complex/sawtooth' depending on the complexity of causal rearrangements [118]. Integrating CNA with expression data in basal-like TNBC revealed that alterations tend to converge on two major oncogenic signalling pathways: EGFR-ras-MEK and PI3K-mTOR. Common alterations include loss of *PTEN* and *INPP4B* and amplification of *CDK1*, *MYC* and *AKT3*. Interestingly, this profile confers more similarity to serous ovarian cancer than other breast cancers, providing a genomic link between two malignancies associated with germline *BRCA1* mutation [117, 119]. mTOR/MEK inhibitors are promising as combination agents with neoadjuvant chemotherapy, however they are associated with significant toxicity and dosing schedules are still being optimised [120].

Together, these studies have produced critical information on somatic events underpinning TNBC development, however the tumour microenvironment receives little weight in genome-focused approaches. The percentage of 'contaminating' non-tumour cell types is considered a limitation in genomics, but given that immunogenicity is a strong determinant of clinical outcome in TNBC, with TILs at the forefront of personalised therapy for this patient group, there is a valid argument for stratifying TNBCs in a way that encompasses the complexity in tissue homogenates, rather than filtering it out. Two landmark studies attempted to classify TNBC on the basis of unsupervised clustering of gene expression data from large tumour cohorts [121, 122]. They identified four to six major clusters associated with distinct functional gene networks, genomic alterations and clinical outcomes. Independent analyses incorporating laser capture-micro-dissected tumour samples, patient-derived xenografts and cell lines (which lack human non-tumour elements) subsequently showed that tumour cellularity is a critical determinant of clustering [123, 124], and the field is not yet united on a robust classifier that mathematically accounts for this. But overall, the data suggest that basal-like TNBCs (70–80% of cases) can be further segregated according to the degree of active immune infiltrate and tumour-specific immunity, while non-basal TNBCs (20–30%) can be defined by whether they engage ER-independent hormone signalling or exhibit mesenchymal and stem-like features (previously identified as 'claudin-low' as an extension of the intrinsic subtype classifier) [71, 121, 124]. Interest is also gathering around epigenetic dysregulation, and whether differentially methylated regions of the TNBC genome could underpin some of this biological variability [125].

6.5 Clinical Implications of Breast Cancer Heterogeneity

6.5.1 Molecular Diagnostic Tools

As molecular subtypes have emerged, the clinical corollary has been to develop risk stratification signatures. However, many offer no significant benefit beyond current practice standards. In order to be useful, risk stratification signatures must add value to existing histopathological data, accurately classify individual cases (so-called 'single sample predictor') and be readily implemented in the diagnostic laboratory. From a clinical perspective, the most important contribution of molecular subtyping has been the recognition of the luminal A/B subdivision in ER-positive disease, which has informed the development of MammaPrint® [126–130], Oncotype DX® [131–133], EndoPredict® [134] and Prosigna® [94, 131–133]. These tests quantitatively assign the risk of recurrence in ER-positive, node-negative patients, and have implications for sparing a proportion of low-stage patients from receiving chemotherapy. The 'Nottingham Prognostic Index Plus' is another good example of early transitioning to precision medicine – it attempts to blend traditional parameters with a broader IHC panel to better define molecular subtypes and improve stratification [135]. The topic of molecular signatures in breast cancer prognostication has been recently reviewed [136].

Precision medicine is predicated on employing genomics and gene expression profiling to personally tailor a treatment regimen. Theoretically, this is optimal as it allows targeting of appropriate pathways while minimising treatment with agents that may have limited or no benefit. Yet, identifying a targetable mutation does not guarantee that the matching treatment will be effective (for example, one study reported that only 36% of somatic variants were actually expressed [51]). With the exception of *ERRB2*, no single genomic alteration is a clinically useful predictor of therapeutic efficacy [137]. This was exemplified recently in the PALOMA-1 trial where *CDK4/6* amplification was not a reliable predictor of response to a CDK4/6 inhibitor [138]. Predictive tools that incorporate multiple alterations or that complement existing algorithms such as the Nottingham Prognostic Index, are the ideal way to move forward.

It is clear that molecular profiling has a role in breast cancer management, but incorporating the technology and knowledge into routine clinical practice is a major challenge. In the public health setting, there are considerable logistic and economic barriers related to standardization, accreditation and reliable service delivery. The requirements will include infrastructure that is cost-effective and can adapt to evolving technologies; dynamic, curated databases of clinically actionable variants/signatures; major changes to pathology and oncology training programs, and possibly an entirely new precision oncology specialization stream that incorporates genetic counselling, as there are important ethical issues around synthesizing and communicating complex diagnostic results to the clinician and patient in a meaningful way. Finally, how should mutations which are of as-yet-unknown clinical significance be dealt with? Sequencing of close to 1000 breast cancers has identified 128 genes with *putative* targetable alterations [139]. For the vast majority, genotype-drug efficacy relationships are still being elucidated in preclinical and clinical studies, and the cost-effectiveness and overall benefit of matching treatments are unknown [140].

A tumour biopsy is a static representation of a small fraction of a larger mass taken at a single point in time. Given that diagnostic tests used today are still relatively low-resolution with conservative thresholds, tumour under-sampling is not currently a major consideration in clinical practice. However given that precision medicine aims to select rational combinations of targeted agents according to an individual tumour's profile, and yet drug resistant, metastatic clones may represent a minor component of the tumour, the risk of under-sampling will be magnified in a precision oncology context [141, 142]. The potential consequences of basing clinical management on small tumour biopsies has been exemplified by spatial and temporal heterogeneity in amplification and over-expression of HER2 during disease progression [30]. In the case of HER2+ breast cancer, trastuzumab therapy does not preclude later development of metastatic disease; in fact distant recurrence is common and can be HER2-negative [70, 143].

6.5.2   Heterogeneity in Metastatic Breast Cancer

Historically, metastasis was viewed as a complication of end-stage disease with the assumption that distant cancer deposits were virtually the same as the primary tumour from which they arose (linear progression) [144]. However, we have known

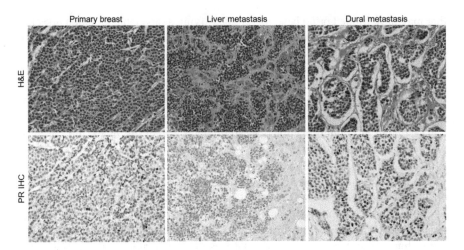

Fig. 6.4 Metastatic breast cancer heterogeneity exemplified by variable expression of progesterone receptor (PR). Approximately 1% of tumour cells in the primary breast tumour are positive for PR, whereas the liver metastasis is negative, and the dural lesion is virually 100% positive. *IHC, immunohistochemistry*

for some time that the expression of clinically relevant biomarkers can differ between primary and metastatic tumours from the same patient (e.g. Fig. 6.4; [145–152]), and American Society of Clinical Oncology (ASCO) practice guidelines now recommend direct biopsy of accessible metastases for repeat HER2/ER/PR testing [153]. More recently, sequencing studies have provided compelling evidence for parallel evolution in regional metastases [154–158]. By applying whole genome sequencing to a large cohort of breast and matching metastatic tumours, Yates and colleagues found that at the time of initial diagnosis, primary tumour genomes are suitable proxies for subclinical metastatic deposits (very encouraging in terms of guiding adjuvant therapy for early breast cancer), but resistant deposits undergo clonal expansion and further diversification, acquiring additional driver alterations before becoming clinically detectable [158] (Fig. 6.2). These findings suggest that early detection of therapeutic resistance will be crucial for optimising therapy, and that re-biopsy will be critical for the success of molecular-targeted therapies in the metastatic setting.

Single-cell genomics can be used to track genomic and transcriptional changes in individual cells, and track clonal evolution over time. There has also been great enthusiasm around applying this technology to circulating tumour cells (CTCs), shed from solid tumours into the circulation or lymphatics and detectable as a source of genetic material [159–161]. CTCs predict survival, disease-related mortality, response to treatment and early disease recurrence [162–164], and it has been argued that the 'liquid biopsy' could represent the entire tumour genome, and provide a means for sensitively monitoring response to treatment over time [165].

However, there are major logistic barriers to realising this goal, not least of which are the low and variable concentrations of CTCs in peripheral blood (1–10 CTC per 10 mL [166]). On the other hand, multiple proof-of-principle studies have underscored the utility of circulating tumour (ct)DNA as an early indicator of therapeutic resistance and the presence of residual disease [165, 167, 168], and suggested value as a collective representation of the tumour genome [169], helping to overcome issues related to tissue sampling bias [170]. As ctDNA profiling is incorporated into more clinical trials, significant developments are expected in the forseeable future [171].

6.6 Concluding Remarks

New knowledge about the extent of heterogeneity in breast cancer and how this relates to clonal evolution is changing the way we think about research, diagnosis and treatment. From a clinical standpoint, the most dire complication of breast cancer heterogeneity is therapeutic resistance. To tackle this, the field has taken a three-pronged approach: (1) reduce the likelihood of relapse in the first place by using more effective agents (and likewise, use agents more effectively) for early breast cancer; (2) detect therapeutic resistance early so that treatment regimens can be optimised; and (3) expand the arsenal of second- and subsequent- line agents so that metastatic disease can be stabilised for as long as possible (though a future goal will be to treat metastatic disease with curative intent).

Achieving these expectations will require continued investment in research and development to identify new therapeutic targets; including druggable alterations, synthetic lethal vulnerabilities, and innovative strategies that combine therapies for maximal efficacy and/or to simultaneously target minor subclones that cause resistance. In parallel, we will need to implement high-resolution companion molecular diagnostic assays that are scalable, adaptive and cost-effective in the public health setting. Implicit in this will be algorithms that accurately predict risk profiles and rank suitable therapeutic regimens according to each tumour's molecular profile, potentially highlighting clinical trial suitability. Clinical training programs will need to evolve to meet precision oncology demands, as oncologists of the future will be expected to synthesise complex diagnostic information, assess optimal therapeutic strategies and deliver complicated diagnostic results and recommendations to their patients. Finally, we need public investment and innovation in clinical trials, including measures to drastically increase access to patients outside major metropolitan centres. Apart from improving equity, conducting trials on a broader scale will be necessary to determine dosing regimens, timing and drug interactions, and to achieve adequate recruitment as the numbers of new targets and agents coming online increases.

References

1. Pinder SE (2010) Ductal carcinoma in situ (DCIS): pathological features, differential diagnosis, prognostic factors and specimen evaluation. Modern Pathol: Off J US Can Acad Pathol 23(Suppl 2):S8–S13
2. Lakhani SR et al (2012) In: Bosman FT (ed) WHO classification of tumours of the breast, World Health Organisation Classification of Tumours. IARC, Lyon
3. Ellis IO et al (2003) Invasive breast carcinomas, WHO Classification of Tumours. Pathology and Genetics of Tumours of the Breast and Female Genital Organs. International Agency for Research on Cancer (IARC), Lyon, France
4. Weigelt B et al (2008) Refinement of breast cancer classification by molecular characterization of histological special types. J Pathol 216(2):141–150
5. Tognon C et al (2002) Expression of the ETV6-NTRK3 gene fusion as a primary event in human secretory breast carcinoma. Cancer Cell 2(5):367–376
6. Persson M et al (2009) Recurrent fusion of MYB and NFIB transcription factor genes in carcinomas of the breast and head and neck. Proc Natl Acad Sci U S A 106(44):18740–18744
7. Rakha EA, Ellis IO (2010) Lobular breast carcinoma and its variants. Semin Diagn Pathol 27(1):49–61
8. Ciriello G et al (2015) Comprehensive molecular portraits of invasive lobular breast cancer. Cell 163(2):506–519
9. Rakha EA et al (2008) Prognostic significance of Nottingham histologic grade in invasive breast carcinoma. J Clin Oncol Off J Am Soc Clin Oncol 26(19):3153–3158
10. Rakha EA et al (2010) Breast cancer prognostic classification in the molecular era: the role of histological grade. Breast Cancer Res: BCR 12(4):207
11. Sotiriou C et al (2006) Gene expression profiling in breast cancer: understanding the molecular basis of histologic grade to improve prognosis. J Natl Cancer Inst 98(4):262–272
12. Elston CW, Ellis IO (1991) Pathological prognostic factors in breast cancer. I. The value of histological grade in breast cancer: experience from a large study with long-term follow-up. Histopathology 19(5):403–410
13. Dalton LW, Page DL, Dupont WD (1994) Histologic grading of breast carcinoma. A reproducibility study. Cancer 73(11):2765–2770
14. Galea MH et al (1992) The Nottingham Prognostic Index in primary breast cancer. Breast Cancer Res Treat 22(3):207–219
15. Sundquist M et al (1999) Applying the Nottingham Prognostic Index to a Swedish breast cancer population. South East Swedish Breast Cancer Study Group. Breast Cancer Res Treat 53(1):1–8
16. Mook S et al (2009) Calibration and discriminatory accuracy of prognosis calculation for breast cancer with the online Adjuvant! program: a hospital-based retrospective cohort study. Lancet Oncol 10(11):1070–1076
17. Goldhirsch A et al (2009) Thresholds for therapies: highlights of the St Gallen International Expert Consensus on the primary therapy of early breast cancer 2009. Ann Oncol: Off J Eur Soc Med Oncol/ESMO 20(8):1319–1329
18. Early Breast Cancer Trialists' Collaborative Group (1998) Tamoxifen for early breast cancer: an overview of the randomised trials. Lancet 351(9114):1451–1467
19. Ravdin PM et al (1992) Prognostic significance of progesterone receptor levels in estrogen receptor-positive patients with metastatic breast cancer treated with tamoxifen: results of a prospective Southwest Oncology Group study. J Clin Oncol Off J Am Soc Clin Oncol 10(8):1284–1291
20. Wolff AC et al (2007) American Society of Clinical Oncology/College of American Pathologists guideline recommendations for human epidermal growth factor receptor 2 testing in breast cancer. Arch Pathol Lab Med 131(1):18–43
21. Slamon DJ et al (1987) Human breast cancer: correlation of relapse and survival with amplification of the HER-2/neu oncogene. Science 235(4785):177–182

22. Tandon AK et al (1989) HER-2/neu oncogene protein and prognosis in breast cancer. J Clin Oncol Off J Am Soc Clin Oncol 7(8):1120–1128
23. Chia S et al (2008) Human epidermal growth factor receptor 2 overexpression as a prognostic factor in a large tissue microarray series of node-negative breast cancers. J Clin Oncol Off J Am Soc Clin Oncol 26(35):5697–5704
24. Madarnas Y et al (2008) Adjuvant/neoadjuvant trastuzumab therapy in women with HER-2/neu-overexpressing breast cancer: a systematic review. Cancer Treat Rev 34(6):539–557
25. Dent R et al (2007) Triple-negative breast cancer: clinical features and patterns of recurrence. Clin Cancer Res 13(15 Pt 1):4429–4434
26. Hammond ME et al (2010) American society of clinical oncology/college of american pathologists guideline recommendations for immunohistochemical testing of estrogen and progesterone receptors in breast cancer. J Oncolo Prac/Am Soc Clin Oncol 6(4):195–197
27. Wolff AC et al (2013) Recommendations for human epidermal growth factor receptor 2 testing in breast cancer: American Society of Clinical Oncology/College of American Pathologists clinical practice guideline update. J Clin Oncol 31(31):3997–4013
28. Lee HJ et al (2014) Two histopathologically different diseases: hormone receptor-positive and hormone receptor-negative tumors in HER2-positive breast cancer. Breast Cancer Res Treat 145(3):615–623
29. Lee HJ et al (2015) Clinicopathologic significance of the intratumoral heterogeneity of HER2 gene amplification in HER2-positive breast cancer patients treated with adjuvant trastuzumab. Am J Clin Pathol 144(4):570–578
30. Seol H et al (2012) Intratumoral heterogeneity of HER2 gene amplification in breast cancer: its clinicopathological significance. Mod Pathol: Off J US Can Acad Pathol 25:938
31. Marusyk A, Almendro V, Polyak K (2012) Intra-tumour heterogeneity: a looking glass for cancer? Nat Rev Cancer 12(5):323–334
32. Marusyk A, Polyak K (2010) Tumor heterogeneity: causes and consequences. Biochim Biophys Acta 1805(1):105–117
33. Carter H et al (2009) Cancer-specific high-throughput annotation of somatic mutations: computational prediction of driver missense mutations. Cancer Res 69(16):6660–6667
34. Wood LD et al (2007) The genomic landscapes of human breast and colorectal cancers. Science 318(5853):108–113
35. Torkamani A, Schork NJ (2008) Prediction of cancer driver mutations in protein kinases. Cancer Res 68(6):1675–1682
36. Yates LR et al (2015) Subclonal diversification of primary breast cancer revealed by multiregion sequencing. Nat Med 21(7):751–759
37. Greaves M, Maley CC (2012) Clonal evolution in cancer. Nature 481(7381):306–313
38. Nowell PC (1976) The clonal evolution of tumor cell populations. Science 194(4260):23–28
39. Navin N et al (2011) Tumour evolution inferred by single-cell sequencing. Nature 472(7341):90–94
40. Stephens PJ et al (2011) Massive genomic rearrangement acquired in a single catastrophic event during cancer development. Cell 144(1):27–40
41. Wang Y et al (2014) Clonal evolution in breast cancer revealed by single nucleus genome sequencing. Nature 512(7513):155–160
42. Gao Y et al (2017) Single-cell sequencing deciphers a convergent evolution of copy number alterations from primary to circulating tumour cells. Genome Res 27:1312
43. Gao R et al (2016) Punctuated copy number evolution and clonal stasis in triple-negative breast cancer. Nat Genet 48(10):1119–1130
44. Cancer Genome Atlas, N (2012) Comprehensive molecular portraits of human breast tumours. Nature 490(7418):61–70
45. Zhang J et al (2011) International Cancer Genome Consortium Data Portal – a one-stop shop for cancer genomics data. Database (Oxford) 2011:bar026
46. Stephens PJ et al (2012) The landscape of cancer genes and mutational processes in breast cancer. Nature 486(7403):400
47. Polyak K, Metzger Filho O (2012) SnapShot: breast cancer. Cancer Cell 22(4):562–562 e1

48. Banerji S et al (2012) Sequence analysis of mutations and translocations across breast cancer subtypes. Nature 486(7403):405–409
49. Nik-Zainal S et al (2016) Landscape of somatic mutations in 560 breast cancer whole-genome sequences. Nature 534(7605):47–54
50. Curtis C et al (2012) The genomic and transcriptomic architecture of 2,000 breast tumours reveals novel subgroups. Nature 486:346
51. Shah SP et al (2012) The clonal and mutational evolution spectrum of primary triple-negative breast cancers. Nature 486(7403):395–399
52. Yates LR, Desmedt C (2017) Translational genomics: practical applications of the genomic revolution in breast cancer. Clin Cancer Res 23(11):2630–2639
53. Nik-Zainal S et al (2012) Mutational processes molding the genomes of 21 breast cancers. Cell 149(5):979–993
54. Nik-Zainal S et al (2012) The life history of 21 breast cancers. Cell 149(5):994–1007
55. Pereira B et al (2016) The somatic mutation profiles of 2,433 breast cancers refines their genomic and transcriptomic landscapes. Nat Commun 7:11479
56. Alexandrov LB, Stratton MR (2014) Mutational signatures: the patterns of somatic mutations hidden in cancer genomes. Curr Opin Genet Dev 24:52–60
57. Alexandrov LB et al (2013) Signatures of mutational processes in human cancer. Nature 500(7463):415–421
58. Nik-Zainal S, Morganella S (2017) Mutational signatures in breast cancer: the problem at the DNA level. Clin Cancer Res 23(11):2617–2629
59. Saunus JM et al (2015) Integrated genomic and transcriptomic analysis of human brain metastases identifies alterations of potential clinical significance. J Pathol 237(3):363–378
60. Smid M et al (2016) Breast cancer genome and transcriptome integration implicates specific mutational signatures with immune cell infiltration. Nat Commun 7:12910
61. Davies H et al (2017) HRDetect is a predictor of BRCA1 and BRCA2 deficiency based on mutational signatures. Nat Med 23(4):517–525
62. Lord CJ, Ashworth A (2016) BRCAness revisited. Nat Rev Cancer 16(2):110–120
63. Eirew P et al (2015) Dynamics of genomic clones in breast cancer patient xenografts at single-cell resolution. Nature 518(7539):422–426
64. Lee MC et al (2014) Single-cell analyses of transcriptional heterogeneity during drug tolerance transition in cancer cells by RNA sequencing. Proc Natl Acad Sci U S A 111(44):E4726–E4735
65. Lim E et al (2009) Aberrant luminal progenitors as the candidate target population for basal tumor development in BRCA1 mutation carriers. Nat Med 15(8):907–913
66. Keller PJ et al (2012) Defining the cellular precursors to human breast cancer. Proc Natl Acad Sci U S A 109(8):2772–2777
67. Molyneux G et al (2010) BRCA1 basal-like breast cancers originate from luminal epithelial progenitors and not from basal stem cells. Cell Stem Cell 7(3):403–417
68. Chaffer CL et al (2011) Normal and neoplastic nonstem cells can spontaneously convert to a stem-like state. Proc Natl Acad Sci U S A 108(19):7950–7955
69. Clevers H (2011) The cancer stem cell: premises, promises and challenges. Nat Med 17(3):313–319
70. Harrell JC et al (2011) Genomic analysis identifies unique signatures predictive of brain, lung, and liver relapse. Breast Cancer Res Treat 132:523
71. Prat A et al (2010) Phenotypic and molecular characterization of the claudin-low intrinsic subtype of breast cancer. Breast Cancer Res: BCR 12(5):R68
72. Korkaya H, Liu S, Wicha MS (2011) Breast cancer stem cells, cytokine networks, and the tumor microenvironment. J Clin Invest 121(10):3804–3809
73. Finak G et al (2008) Stromal gene expression predicts clinical outcome in breast cancer. Nat Med 14(5):518–527
74. Allinen M et al (2004) Molecular characterization of the tumor microenvironment in breast cancer. Cancer Cell 6(1):17–32

75. Ma XJ et al (2009) Gene expression profiling of the tumor microenvironment during breast cancer progression. Breast Cancer Res: BCR 11(1):R7
76. Kienast Y et al (2010) Real-time imaging reveals the single steps of brain metastasis formation. Nat Med 16(1):116–122
77. Carmeliet P, Jain RK (2011) Principles and mechanisms of vessel normalization for cancer and other angiogenic diseases. Nat Rev Drug Discov 10(6):417–427
78. Monsky WL et al (2002) Role of host microenvironment in angiogenesis and microvascular functions in human breast cancer xenografts: mammary fat pad versus cranial tumors. Clin Cancer Res 8(4):1008–1013
79. Moeller BJ, Richardson RA, Dewhirst MW (2007) Hypoxia and radiotherapy: opportunities for improved outcomes in cancer treatment. Cancer Metastasis Rev 26(2):241–248
80. Jain RK (2014) Antiangiogenesis strategies revisited: from starving tumors to alleviating hypoxia. Cancer Cell 26(5):605–622
81. Savas P et al (2016) Clinical relevance of host immunity in breast cancer: from TILs to the clinic. Nat Rev Clin Oncol 13(4):228–241
82. US National Institutes of Health (n.d.). www.clinicaltrials.gov. 7th Aug 2017
83. Dieci MV et al (2014) Prognostic value of tumor-infiltrating lymphocytes on residual disease after primary chemotherapy for triple-negative breast cancer: a retrospective multicenter study. Ann Oncol 25(3):611–618
84. Mahmoud SM et al (2011) Tumor-infiltrating CD8+ lymphocytes predict clinical outcome in breast cancer. J Clin Oncol Off J Am Soc Clin Oncol 29(15):1949–1955
85. Rody A et al (2011) A clinically relevant gene signature in triple negative and basal-like breast cancer. Breast Cancer Res: BCR 13(5):R97
86. Ye J et al (2013) Specific recruitment of gammadelta regulatory T cells in human breast cancer. Cancer Res 73(20):6137–6148
87. Ladoire S et al (2008) Pathologic complete response to neoadjuvant chemotherapy of breast carcinoma is associated with the disappearance of tumor-infiltrating foxp3+ regulatory T cells. Clin Cancer Res 14(8):2413–2420
88. Salgado R et al (2015) The evaluation of tumor-infiltrating lymphocytes (TILs) in breast cancer: recommendations by an international TILs working group 2014. Ann Oncol 26(2):259–271
89. Perou CM et al (2000) Molecular portraits of human breast tumours. Nature 406(6797):747–752
90. Sorlie T et al (2001) Gene expression patterns of breast carcinomas distinguish tumor subclasses with clinical implications. Proc Natl Acad Sci U S A 98(19):10869–10874
91. Kennecke H et al (2010) Metastatic behavior of breast cancer subtypes. J Clin Oncol Off J Am Soc Clin Oncol 28(20):3271–3277
92. Korde LA et al (2010) Gene expression pathway analysis to predict response to neoadjuvant docetaxel and capecitabine for breast cancer. Breast Cancer Res Treat 119(3):685–699
93. Rouzier R et al (2005) Breast cancer molecular subtypes respond differently to preoperative chemotherapy. Clin Cancer Res 11(16):5678–5685
94. Parker JS et al (2009) Supervised risk predictor of breast cancer based on intrinsic subtypes. J Clin Oncol 27(8):1160–1167
95. Sorlie T et al (2003) Repeated observation of breast tumor subtypes in independent gene expression data sets. Proc Natl Acad Sci U S A 100(14):8418–8423
96. Hennessy BT et al (2009) Characterization of a naturally occurring breast cancer subset enriched in epithelial-to-mesenchymal transition and stem cell characteristics. Cancer Res 69(10):4116–4124
97. Farmer P et al (2005) Identification of molecular apocrine breast tumours by microarray analysis. Oncogene 24(29):4660–4671
98. Doane AS et al (2006) An estrogen receptor-negative breast cancer subset characterized by a hormonally regulated transcriptional program and response to androgen. Oncogene 25(28):3994–4008

 99. Guedj M et al (2011) A refined molecular taxonomy of breast cancer. Oncogene 31:1196
100. Haque R et al (2012) Impact of breast cancer subtypes and treatment on survival: an analysis spanning two decades. Cancer Epidemiol Biomark Prev 21(10):1848–1855
101. Ciriello G et al (2013) The molecular diversity of Luminal A breast tumors. Breast Cancer Res Treat 141(3):409–420
102. (EBCTCG), E.B.C.T.C.G (2005) Effects of chemotherapy and hormonal therapy for early breast cancer on recurrence and 15-year survival: an overview of the randomised trials. Lancet 365(9472):1687–1717
103. Jeselsohn R et al (2015) ESR1 mutations-a mechanism for acquired endocrine resistance in breast cancer. Nat Rev Clin Oncol 12(10):573–583
104. Creighton CJ (2012) The molecular profile of luminal B breast cancer. Biologics 6:289–297
105. Huang B, Warner M, Gustafsson JA (2015) Estrogen receptors in breast carcinogenesis and endocrine therapy. Mol Cell Endocrinol 418(Pt 3):240–244
106. Huang B et al (2014) Differential expression of estrogen receptor alpha, beta1, and beta2 in lobular and ductal breast cancer. Proc Natl Acad Sci U S A 111(5):1933–1938
107. Badve S et al (2011) Basal-like and triple-negative breast cancers: a critical review with an emphasis on the implications for pathologists and oncologists. Mod Pathol: Off J US Can Acade Pathol 24(2):157–167
108. Turner NC et al (2007) BRCA1 dysfunction in sporadic basal-like breast cancer. Oncogene 26(14):2126–2132
109. Lehmann BD, Pietenpol JA (2015) Clinical implications of molecular heterogeneity in triple negative breast cancer. Breast 24(Suppl 2):S36–S40
110. Fulford LG et al (2006) Specific morphological features predictive for the basal phenotype in grade 3 invasive ductal carcinoma of breast. Histopathology 49(1):22–34
111. Livasy CA et al (2006) Phenotypic evaluation of the basal-like subtype of invasive breast carcinoma. Mod Pathol 19(2):264–271
112. Banerjee S et al (2006) Basal-like breast carcinomas: clinical outcome and response to chemotherapy. J Clin Pathol 59(7):729–735
113. Bergamaschi A et al (2006) Distinct patterns of DNA copy number alteration are associated with different clinicopathological features and gene-expression subtypes of breast cancer. Genes Chromosomes Cancer 45(11):1033–1040
114. Chin K et al (2006) Genomic and transcriptional aberrations linked to breast cancer pathophysiologies. Cancer Cell 10(6):529–541
115. Hu Z et al (2006) The molecular portraits of breast tumors are conserved across microarray platforms. BMC Genomics 7:96
116. Fulford LG et al (2007) Basal-like grade III invasive ductal carcinoma of the breast: patterns of metastasis and long-term survival. Breast Cancer Res 9(1):R4
117. TCGA, Cancer Genome Atlas Network (2012) Comprehensive molecular portraits of human breast tumours. Nature 490(7418):61–70
118. Kwei KA et al (2010) Genomic instability in breast cancer: pathogenesis and clinical implications. Mol Oncol 4(3):255–266
119. Encinas G et al (2015) Somatic mutations in breast and serous ovarian cancer young patients: a systematic review and meta-analysis. Rev Assoc Med Bras (1992) 61(5):474–483
120. Jokinen E, Koivunen JP (2015) MEK and PI3K inhibition in solid tumors: rationale and evidence to date. Ther Adv Med Oncol 7(3):170–180
121. Burstein MD et al (2015) Comprehensive genomic analysis identifies novel subtypes and targets of triple-negative breast cancer. Clin Cancer Res 21(7):1688–1698
122. Lehmann BD et al (2011) Identification of human triple-negative breast cancer subtypes and preclinical models for selection of targeted therapies. J Clin Invest 121(7):2750–2767
123. Lehmann BD et al (2016) Refinement of triple-negative breast cancer molecular subtypes: implications for neoadjuvant chemotherapy selection. PLoS One 11(6):e0157368
124. Prat A et al (2013) Molecular characterization of basal-like and non-basal-like triple-negative breast cancer. Oncologist 18(2):123–133

125. Stirzaker C et al (2015) Methylome sequencing in triple-negative breast cancer reveals distinct methylation clusters with prognostic value. Nat Commun 6:5899
126. van 't Veer LJ et al (2002) Gene expression profiling predicts clinical outcome of breast cancer. Nature 415(6871):530–536
127. van de Vijver MJ et al (2002) A gene-expression signature as a predictor of survival in breast cancer. N Engl J Med 347(25):1999–2009
128. Buyse M et al (2006) Validation and clinical utility of a 70-gene prognostic signature for women with node-negative breast cancer. J Natl Cancer Inst 98(17):1183–1192
129. Bueno-de-Mesquita JM et al (2009) Validation of 70-gene prognosis signature in node-negative breast cancer. Breast Cancer Res Treat 117(3):483–495
130. Cardoso F et al (2008) Clinical application of the 70-gene profile: the MINDACT trial. J Clin Oncol Off J Am Soc Clin Oncol 26(5):729–735
131. Goldstein LJ et al (2008) Prognostic utility of the 21-gene assay in hormone receptor-positive operable breast cancer compared with classical clinicopathologic features. J Clin Oncol Off J Am Soc Clin Oncol 26(25):4063–4071
132. Paik S (2007) Development and clinical utility of a 21-gene recurrence score prognostic assay in patients with early breast cancer treated with tamoxifen. Oncologist 12(6):631–635
133. Paik S et al (2004) A multigene assay to predict recurrence of tamoxifen-treated, node-negative breast cancer. N Engl J Med 351(27):2817–2826
134. Filipits M et al (2011) A new molecular predictor of distant recurrence in ER-positive, HER2-negative breast cancer adds independent information to conventional clinical risk factors. Clin Cancer Res 17(18):6012–6020
135. Rakha EA et al (2014) Nottingham Prognostic Index Plus (NPI+): a modern clinical decision making tool in breast cancer. Br J Cancer 110(7):1688–1697
136. Lal S et al (2017) Molecular signatures in breast cancer. Methods 131:135
137. Santarpia L et al (2016) Deciphering and targeting oncogenic mutations and pathways in breast cancer. Oncologist 21(9):1063–1078
138. Finn RS et al (2015) The cyclin-dependent kinase 4/6 inhibitor palbociclib in combination with letrozole versus letrozole alone as first-line treatment of oestrogen receptor-positive, HER2-negative, advanced breast cancer (PALOMA-1/TRIO-18): a randomised phase 2 study. Lancet Oncol 16(1):25–35
139. Van Allen EM et al (2014) Whole-exome sequencing and clinical interpretation of formalin-fixed, paraffin-embedded tumor samples to guide precision cancer medicine. Nat Med 20(6):682–688
140. Kalita-de Croft P et al (2016) Omics approaches in breast cancer research and clinical practice. Adv Anat Pathol 23(6):356–367
141. Ding L et al (2012) Clonal evolution in relapsed acute myeloid leukaemia revealed by whole-genome sequencing. Nature 481(7382):506–510
142. Gerlinger M et al (2012) Intratumor heterogeneity and branched evolution revealed by multiregion sequencing. N Engl J Med 366(10):883–892
143. Wu JM, Halushka MK, Argani P (2010) Intratumoral heterogeneity of HER-2 gene amplification and protein overexpression in breast cancer. Hum Pathol 41(6):914–917
144. Weigelt B et al (2003) Gene expression profiles of primary breast tumors maintained in distant metastases. Proc Natl Acad Sci U S A 100(26):15901–15905
145. Da Silva L et al (2010) HER3 and downstream pathways are involved in colonization of brain metastases from breast cancer. Breast Cancer Res 12(4):R46
146. Wu JM et al (2008) Heterogeneity of breast cancer metastases: comparison of therapeutic target expression and promoter methylation between primary tumors and their multifocal metastases. Clin Cancer Res: Off J Am Assoc Cancer Res 14(7):1938–1946
147. Arslan C et al (2011) Variation in hormone receptor and HER-2 status between primary and metastatic breast cancer: review of the literature. Expert Opin Ther Targets 15(1):21–30
148. St Romain P et al (2012) Organotropism and prognostic marker discordance in distant metastases of breast carcinoma: fact or fiction? A clinicopathologic analysis. Hum Pathol 43(3):398–404

149. Houssami N et al (2011) HER2 discordance between primary breast cancer and its paired metastasis: tumor biology or test artefact? Insights through meta-analysis. Breast Cancer Res Treat 129(3):659–674
150. Cummings MC et al (2014) Metastatic progression of breast cancer: insights from 50 years of autopsies. J Pathol 232(1):23–31
151. Cejalvo JM et al (2017) Intrinsic subtypes and gene expression profiles in primary and metastatic breast cancer. Cancer Res 77(9):2213–2221
152. Amir E et al (2012) Prospective study evaluating the impact of tissue confirmation of metastatic disease in patients with breast cancer. J Clin Oncol Off J Am Soc Clin Oncol 30(6):587–592
153. Van Poznak C et al (2015) Use of biomarkers to guide decisions on systemic therapy for women with metastatic breast cancer: American Society of Clinical Oncology Clinical Practice Guideline. J Clin Oncol 33(24):2695–U174
154. Almendro V et al (2014) Genetic and phenotypic diversity in breast tumor metastases. Cancer Res 74(5):1338–1348
155. Ding L et al (2010) Genome remodelling in a basal-like breast cancer metastasis and xenograft. Nature 464(7291):999–1005
156. Shah SP et al (2009) Mutational evolution in a lobular breast tumour profiled at single nucleotide resolution. Nature 461(7265):809–813
157. Klein CA (2009) Parallel progression of primary tumours and metastases. Nat Rev Cancer 9(4):302–312
158. Yates LR et al (2017) Genomic evolution of breast cancer metastasis and relapse. Cancer Cell 32(2):169–184 e7
159. Shaw JA et al (2017) Mutation analysis of cell-free DNA and single circulating tumor cells in metastatic breast cancer patients with high circulating tumor cell counts. Clin Cancer Res 23(1):88–96
160. Sieuwerts AM et al (2011) mRNA and microRNA expression profiles in circulating tumor cells and primary tumors of metastatic breast cancer patients. Clin Cancer Res 17(11):3600–3618
161. Babayan A et al (2013) Heterogeneity of estrogen receptor expression in circulating tumor cells from metastatic breast cancer patients. PLoS One 8(9):e75038
162. Smerage JB et al (2014) Circulating tumor cells and response to chemotherapy in metastatic breast cancer: SWOG S0500. J Clin Oncol 32(31):3483–3489
163. Janni WJ et al (2016) Pooled analysis of the prognostic relevance of circulating tumor cells in primary breast cancer. Clin Cancer Res 22(10):2583–2593
164. Lv Q et al (2016) Prognostic value of circulating tumor cells in metastatic breast cancer: a systemic review and meta-analysis. Clin Transl Oncol 18(3):322–330
165. Dawson SJ et al (2013) Analysis of circulating tumor DNA to monitor metastatic breast cancer. N Engl J Med 368(13):1199–1209
166. Alix-Panabieres C, Pantel K (2014) Challenges in circulating tumour cell research. Nat Rev Cancer 14(9):623–631
167. Murtaza M et al (2013) Non-invasive analysis of acquired resistance to cancer therapy by sequencing of plasma DNA. Nature 497(7447):108–112
168. Garcia-Murillas I et al (2015) Mutation tracking in circulating tumor DNA predicts relapse in early breast cancer. Sci Transl Med 7(302):302ra133
169. Murtaza M et al (2015) Multifocal clonal evolution characterized using circulating tumour DNA in a case of metastatic breast cancer. Nat Commun 6:8760
170. Chan KC et al (2013) Cancer genome scanning in plasma: detection of tumor-associated copy number aberrations, single-nucleotide variants, and tumoral heterogeneity by massively parallel sequencing. Clin Chem 59(1):211–224
171. Openshaw MR et al (2016) The role of ctDNA detection and the potential of the liquid biopsy for breast cancer monitoring. Expert Rev Mol Diagn 16(7):751–755
172. Ellis MJ et al (2012) Whole-genome analysis informs breast cancer response to aromatase inhibition. Nature 486(7403):353–360

Chapter 7
Bone Metastasis of Breast Cancer

Rie K. Tahara, Takae M. Brewer, Richard L. Theriault, and Naoto T. Ueno

Abstract Bone is the most common site of metastasis for breast cancer. Bone metastasis significantly affects both quality of life and survival of the breast cancer patient. Clinically, complications secondary to bone metastasis include pain, pathologic fractures, spinal cord compression, and hypercalcemia of malignancy. Because bone metastasis is extremely common in patients with metastatic breast cancer, clinical management of bone metastases is an important and challenging aspect of treatment in the metastatic setting.

The skeleton is a metabolically active organ system that undergoes continuous remodeling throughout life. A delicate balance of the bone-forming osteoblasts and bone-resorbing osteoclasts in the dynamic microenvironment of the skeleton maintains normal bone remodeling and integrity. The presence of metastatic lesions in bone disrupts the normal bone microenvironment and upsets the fine balance between the key components. The changes in the bone microenvironment then create a vicious cycle that further promotes bone destruction and tumor progression.

Various therapeutic options are available for bone metastases of breast cancer. Treatment can be tailored for each patient and, often requires multiple therapeutic interventions. Commonly used modalities include local therapies such as surgery, radiation therapy and radiofrequency ablation (RFA) together with systemic therapies such as endocrine therapy, chemotherapy, monoclonal antibody-based therapy, bone-enhancing therapy and radioisotope therapy. Despite the use of various therapeutic modalities, bone metastases eventually become resistant to therapy, and disease progresses.

In this chapter, we describe the clinical picture and biological mechanism of bone metastases in breast cancer. We also discuss known risk factors as well as detection and assessment of bone metastases. We present therapeutic options for

R. K. Tahara · R. L. Theriault · N. T. Ueno (✉)
Department of Breast Medical Oncology, The University of Texas MD Anderson Cancer Center, Houston, TX, USA
e-mail: nueno@mdanderson.org

T. M. Brewer
Genomic Medicine Institute, Cleveland Clinic, Cleveland, OH, USA

© Springer Nature Switzerland AG 2019
A. Ahmad (ed.), *Breast Cancer Metastasis and Drug Resistance*,
Advances in Experimental Medicine and Biology 1152,
https://doi.org/10.1007/978-3-030-20301-6_7

bone metastasis using a multidisciplinary approach. Further, we describe future directions for bone metastasis management, focusing on novel bone-specific targeted therapies.

Keywords Bone · Metastasis · Mechanism of bone metastases · Bone-targeted therapy · Therapy · Detection · Assessment

7.1   Clinical Picture of Bone Metastasis in Breast Cancer

Bone metastasis develops in approximately 70% of patients with advanced breast cancer and contributes to significant morbidity due to pain and skeletal related events (SREs) [1]. Among patients with bone metastases, two thirds will eventually develop skeletal related events [2]. Bone-only metastasis has been reported to develop in 17–37% of women with metastatic disease [3–5]. SREs are often defined as a pathologic fracture, a requirement for surgical intervention for the bone metastases and need for palliative radiotherapy, hypercalcemia of malignancy, and spinal cord compression. Having pain alone, immobility and analgesic use do not define SREs. Table 7.1 summarizes the definition of skeletal-related events [2].

Bone metastasis not only adversely affects quality of life of the patient but also reduces overall survival. Sathiakumar et al. studied 98,260 women with breast cancer who were U.S. Medicare beneficiaries between 1999 and 2005, among which 7189 (7.3%) had bone metastases either at the time of diagnosis or during the follow-up period. They found that the presence of bone metastases was strongly associated with a higher mortality rate among these women, and the association was stronger for bone metastasis complicated by SREs (HR of 1.5: 95% CI 1.4–1.6) [6]. It is important to note, however, that several studies have shown that patients with bone-only metastatic disease tend to survive longer than those with visceral metastases, with

Table 7.1 Definition of skeletal related events

Generally definition includes
Pathological fractures
Spinal cord compression
Surgery for bone complications
Radiotherapy for bone complications
Hypercalcemia of malignancy (HCM)
Change of antineoplastic therapy for bone pain
Definition does not include
Pain only
Immobility
Analgesic use
Non-hospital costs (physiotherapy)

median survival times of 26 months to 4.3 years for those with bone-only metastases whereas median survival was 13–18 months for visceral-only metastases [4, 5].

Low-grade and ER-positive tumors are more likely to be associated with the development of bone metastases [7]. Colleoni et al. found that ER-negative tumors had a higher early incidence of bone metastasis while ER-positive tumors had a greater frequency of long-term incidence of bone recurrence, probably due to good recurrence control with endocrine therapy [8]. Other factors associated with increased risk of bone metastasis include lymph node status at presentation of breast cancer (number of positive lymph nodes greater than 4), large tumor size (>2 cm), and younger age (<35 years) [8]. Lousquy et al. reviewed 4175 patients with non-metastatic disease and developed a nomogram to predict subsequent bone metastasis [9].

In summary, the skeleton is the most common site of systemic metastasis in breast cancer and it is important for clinicians to recognize the clinical problems associated with metastases in breast cancer. Also, in the future, it would be useful to develop reliable tools to predict who may be at higher risk for bone metastases so that both patients and clinicians have a more realistic understanding of the behavior of the disease.

7.2   Biological Mechanism of Bone Metastasis in Breast Cancer

In order to discuss therapeutic approaches to bone metastasis in breast cancer, it is important to review the biological mechanism of bone metastases. Remodeling occurs constantly in the healthy skeleton to regulate calcium homeostasis, to repair damage to the bone and to withstand new external stresses to the skeleton. In addition, remodeling is important to replace damaged and aging bone in order to preserve function of the skeletal system.

In adults, normal bone turnover mainly occurs through bone remodeling, which involves a well-coordinated activity of and interaction among osteocytes, osteoblasts, osteoclasts and chondrocytes. The basic multicellular unit (BMU), composed of osteoclasts and osteoblasts, is a temporary anatomic unit which moves through the bone during remodeling. The leading group of osteoclasts in the BMU destroys the preexisting bone, a process called *resorption*, while the osteoblasts behind them rebuild and replace the matrix and minerals lost by resorption [10]. Recent studies suggest osteocytes, rather than osteoblasts, are the major source of cytokine receptor activator of Nuckear Factor-κB ligand (RANKL) and thus function as the chief driving component in bone remodeling [11]. RANKL is essential for differentiation and proper function of osteoclasts. Interestingly, the osteoclasts arising at different sites require different supporting cells. Although osteoblasts have long been recognized as the major source of RANKL, recent experimental data suggest hypertrophic chondrocytes are the major source of RANKL in endochondral bone formation whereas osteocytes are the major source of RANKL in cancellous bone remodeling [11]. Researchers speculate that osteocytes and hypertrophic chondrocytes, embedded within mineralized matrix, detect the need for bone resorption and send signals to stimulate osteoclast differentiation and activity [11].

Hormones, cytokines and growth factors modulate the proliferation of osteoclast and osteoblast progenitor cells, mainly through up regulating RANKL expression by osteocytes. Parathyroid hormone (PTH) promotes osteoclastogenesis by stimulation of RANKL in osteocytes [12]. When osteocytes undergo apoptosis, RANKL production increases from undetermined sources, promoting resorption of the bone [13]. Sex steroids suppress osteoclastogenesis, and loss of sex hormones may promote bone resorption by increasing osteocyte apoptosis [11].

When the normal balance among these key components is disrupted, it can result in bone destruction as observed in osteolytic metastases, which appear as "less dense than normal" areas on X-ray, or excessive bone deposition as observed in osteoblastic lesions, which appear "more dense than normal". In the healthy human, bone density declines after reaching a peak between age 25 and 30 years [14]. In women, the bone loss accelerates after menopause around age 50, due to declining levels of estrogens, which have inhibitory effects on the bone-resorbing osteoclast [7]. Breast cancer survivors, after going through chemotherapy and adjuvant hormonal therapy including tamoxifen and aromatase inhibitors, are at an increased risk for low bone density and osteoporosis [15, 16].

Once breast cancer cells metastasize to the bone, they disrupt the normal bone homeostasis and this starts a vicious cycle. It is still unclear why certain types of breast cancer cells have a tendency to metastasize to bone. It was postulated that the phenomenon of metastasis is not a random event but rather tumor cells growing selectively in the specific microenvironment of selected organs [17]. This model is named the "Seed and Soil" hypothesis. Multiple studies have demonstrated that neoplasms are biologically heterogeneous and that metastasis is an extremely selective process, involving a series of alterations during the course of the disease [18]. The cancer cells that succeed in the multiple steps leading to metastasis, including invasion, embolization, survival in the circulation, arrest in a distant capillary bed, and extravasation into and multiplication within the organ parenchyma, can then establish metastatic lesions in the microenvironment that promote tumor-cell growth, survival, angiogenesis, invasion and metastasis [18]. The trabecular bone is highly vascular and appears to be the preferred site to which breast cancer cells metastasize once breast cancer cells succeed in hematogenous spread [19].

Studies have shown that RANK is expressed on the surface of breast cancer cells and RANKL is overexpressed in bone [20, 21]. Furthermore, CXCR4, a chemokine receptor, is highly expressed in breast cancer tissue and its ligand, CXCL12, is overexpressed in common metastatic sites in breast cancer, including bone marrow [22]. Cadherin-11 also promotes breast cancer cells to metastasize to bone [19]. These findings may explain the homing of breast cancer cells to the bone, in support of Paget's seed and soil hypothesis.

Bone metastases in breast cancer often have evidence of both osteolytic and osteoblastic features. Although osteolytic lesions usually predominate [23], 12–50%

of patients with bone metastases have predominantly osteoblastic disease [24]. Moreover, bone destruction in osteolytic lesions induces secondary new bone formation, leading to osteoblastic changes [25, 26], which may explain the presence of mixed lesions in bone metastases in breast cancer.

The process of metastatic lesion development in the bone is complex and involves various proteins and cytokines produced by metastatic breast cancer cells, which in turn stimulate the osteoblast to initiate a *vicious cycle* (Fig. 7.1) [27], leading to initiation of destructive bone lesions and tumor progression [28]. The initial step involves cancer cells in the bone, which produce several factors that promote differentiation of the osteoblast. These factors include parathyroid hormone-related peptide (PTHrP), interleukin-1 (IL-1), IL-6, IL-11, prostaglandin E2 (PGE2), tumor necrosis factor (TNF), and macrophage colony-stimulating factor (M-CSF) [29]. Furthermore, breast cancer cells produce Receptor Activator of Nuclear Factor-κB (RANK) and upregulate RANK ligand (RANKL) expression on the surface of the osteoblast [29]. RANKL then binds to RANK on the surfaces of monocytes, and under the stimulation of macrophage colony-stimulating factor (M-CSF), several monocytes fuse to form a multinucleated osteoclast [19]. RANKL also enhances the activity of preexisting osteoclasts by binding to RANK on their surface [29]. In turn, the osteoblast secretes osteoprotegerin (OPG), a member of the TNF receptor

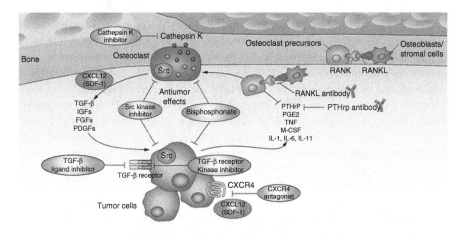

Fig. 7.1 A 'vicious cycle' accelerates both bone destruction and tumor growth as tumor cells secrete osteoclast-stimulating factors, and the bone marrow stromal cells secrete tumor growth factors. A 'vicious cycle' accelerates both bone destruction and tumor growth as tumor cells secrete osteoclast-stimulating factors, and the bone marrow stromal cells secrete tumor growth factors. Various drugs targeting these factors, which include RANKL, Src kinase, cathepsin K, and TGF-β are under development. *Abbreviations*: *CXCL12* C-X-C motif chemokine 12, *CXCR4* C-X-C chemokine receptor type 4, *FGF* fibroblast growth factor, *IGF* insulin-like growth factor, *IL* interleukin, *M-CSF* macrophage colony-stimulating factor, *PDGF* platelet-derived growth factor, *PGE2* prostaglandin E2, *PTHrP* parathyroid hormone-related peptide, *RANK* receptor activator of nuclear factor κB, *RANKL* RANK ligand, *SDF-1* stromal cell-derived factor 1, *Src* proto-oncogene tyrosine-protein kinase, *TGF-β* transforming growth factor β, *TNF* tumor necrosis factor [27]

superfamily, which competitively binds RANKL and suppresses the osteoclast activity [30]. PTHrP from cancer cells, however, suppresses the OPG activity [30]. Other factors which stimulate osteoclast differentiation include interleukin 6 (IL-6), IL-1, prostaglandins, and CSFs (colony stimulating factors) [19]. Once activated, the osteoclast reabsorbs bone by removing mineralized matrix as well as breaking up the organic bone [29]. Activated osteoclasts do so by first binding to the bone matrix via integrin proteins and then secreting acid and lysosomal enzymes to degrade bone [19].

The bone matrix stores several important growth factors including insulin-growth factor (IGF-1), transforming growth factor β (TGF-β), fibroblast growth factor (FGFs), and platelet-derived growth factor (PDGF) as well as bone morphogenetic proteins (BMPs) [29]. These factors are released upon bone resorption. IGF-1 stimulates breast cancer cell growth and directs the cancer cells to migrate into bone by activating signaling molecules, such as PI-3 kinase, Akt, and NF-κB [19].

The enhanced bone resorption alters the calcium concentration in the affected bone, further weakening the bone. The various factors mentioned above as well as the environment high in calcium further enhance proliferation of the cancer cell as well as PTHrP secretion, which promotes the activity of the osteoclasts [31]. The interaction between tumor cells and other key components of the bone metastasis are shown in Fig. 7.1. The vicious cycle is summarized and divided into four major steps in Table 7.2 [27, 29].

The Wnt signaling cascade, an important pathway in embryogenesis, promotes osteoblast differentiation and induces osteoblast activity [32]. Dickkopf-1 (DKK-1) is a gene in embryo development and is known to inhibit Wnt signaling [33], thus preventing osteoblast differentiation. Voorzanger-Rousselot et al. showed DDK-1 was produced by osteolytic breast cancer cells and increased circulating levels were found in patients with breast cancer and bone metastases [33]. In other words, DKK-1 blocks Wnt-signaling and, as a consequence, inhibits osteoblast differentiation [34]. Along with DDK-1, breast cancer cells secrete actin A (a member of TGF β superfamily) and noggin (bone morphogenetic protein [BMP] antagonist), all of which inhibit osteoblast differentiation [35], which favors osteoclastic activities and promotes osteolysis.

The mechanism of development of osteoblastic lesions is less well-understood but accumulating evidence suggests it also is a complex mechanism involving various factors. Core binding factor alpha 1 (Cbfα1), also known as Runx-2, is a

Table 7.2 Four major steps of progression of lytic bone lesions in breast cancer [27]

Step 1: Breast cancer cells secrete parathyroid hormone-related peptide (PTHrP) and other factors, which stimulate the osteoblasts to produce RANKL
Step 2: RANKL stimulates the osteoclast, causing bone resorption
Step 3: Bone resorption stimulates production of growth factors, such as TGF-β which are released into the microenvironment
Step 4: Released growth factors promote cancer cell proliferation, which in turn further stimulates osteoclast activity

Created from text in Onishi [27]

transcription factor linked to osteoblast differentiation [36]. Other factors which enhance the growth, differentiation and activity of the osteoblast include platelet derived growth factor (PDGF) [37], fibroblast growth factor (FGF) [38], TGF-beta [39], bone morphogenic proteins (BMPs) [40], and Endothelin-1 [41].

Endothelin-1 is known to mediate the development of osteoblastic metastases [41] by increasing osteoblast proliferation and activity through inhibition of expression of Dickkopf-1 (DKK-1) gene by marrow stroma cells [42]. As previously mentioned, DKK-1 blocks Wnt signaling and inhibits osteoblastic differentiation. When this inhibition is reversed, there will be more mature osteoblasts, favoring the development of osteoblastic lesions. Thus, the mechanism of bone metastases appears to involve an intricate interplay between osteoblasts and osteoclasts as well as multiple factors in the bone microenvironment. Some breast cancer cell lines which cause osteoblastic metastases secrete endothelin-1, stimulating new bone formation [43]. As mentioned previously, PTHrP and TGF-β are important mediators in metastatic bone lesions and can be therapeutic targets. Important molecules and signaling pathways involved in bone metastasis are summarized by Theriault as shown in Table 7.3 [19].

Table 7.3 Molecules and signaling pathways involved in bone metastasis of breast cancer [12]

Cytokines	Role	Result
Parathyroid hormone-related peptide (PTHrP)	Interacts with PTHR1 to cause expression of RANKL	Stimulates osteoclast-mediated bone resorption
Receptor activator of nuclear factor κB ligand (RANKL)	Binds to RANK receptor on precursor osteoclasts	Stimulates osteoclast development and activation, leading to bone resorption
Osteoprotegerin (OPG)	Acts as a decoy RANK receptor	Blocks RANK/RANKL interaction, inhibits osteoclast development
Insulin-like growth factor 1 (IGF-1)	Stimulates chemotaxis of cancer cells and directs migration	Causes proliferation of cancer cells in bone
Transforming growth factor beta (TGF-β)	Enhances production of PTHrP	Stimulates osteoclast-mediated bone resorption
Interleukin 6 (IL-6)	Induces osteoclastogenesis and suppresses osteblasts	Leads to bone resorption, decreased bone production
Interleukin 11 (IL-11)	Induces osteoclastogenesis and suppresses osteoblasts	Leads to bone resorption, decreased bone production
Prostaglandin E2	Increases expression of RANKL leading to enhanced osteoclast formation	Stimulates bone resorption
Macrophage colony-stimulating factor (M-CSF)	Induces osteoclastogenesis and suppresses osteoblasts	Leads to bone resorption
Tumor necrosis factor alpha (TNF-α)	Induces osteoclastogenesis and suppresses osteoblasts	Leads to bone resorption
Integrins	Allows cancer cells to arrest in target organs	Allows proliferation of cancer cells in bone
Cadherins	Unknown mechanism	Involved in migration and invasion
Osteopontin (OPN)/bone sialoprotein (BSP)	Stimulates osteoblast proliferation	Leads to bone resorption

In summary, bone metastasis is a complicated biological phenomenon, involving multiple cellular and biochemical components interacting with each other. The complicated nature of bone metastasis makes it a challenge to develop targeted therapy and to stop completely or to reverse the metastatic events. Regardless, multiple treatment modalities are currently available for combating bone metastasis in breast cancer. These are discussed next.

7.3 Current Therapeutic Options

A multidisciplinary team, consisting of a medical oncologist, a diagnostic imaging physician, a radiation oncologist, and a surgeon, is often necessary for optimally treating patients with bone metastases. Currently, the mainstay of treatment for bone metastases includes external beam radiation therapy, osteoclast inhibitors, systemic endocrine and chemotherapy, radioisotopes, and supportive interventions including analgesics. In addition, surgery can be utilized for patients with localized disease, with a single or few detectable metastatic lesions. The treatment plan should be tailored for each patient, since the number, locations and biological features of tumors dictate the course of treatment most suitable for the patient. In most cases the goal is not curative but palliative. Surgery, radiation therapy, and radiofrequency ablation (RFA) are effective for pain control and for preventing pathological fractures.

A small percentage of stage IV bone disease (1–10%) is potentially curable, especially when the metastasis is limited to an isolated loco-regional or distant site [44]. However, resection with curative intent for bone metastases has limited utility except for selected cases such as isolated spine or sternal legions [45, 46]. Surgical correction is useful in order to prevent impeding fractures in weight-bearing bones [47]. Surgery is especially indicated for locations such as the femur, humerus, pelvis, and vertebrae because pathological fractures at these sites may lead to significant disability. Several surgical techniques including plate osteosynthesis, nailing, and insertion of a prosthesis are often employed for effective management [48]. External beam radiation is effective for alleviating pain and preventing fractures in weight-bearing bones and may be used in combination with surgical fixation [49]. For more emergent cases such as those involving spinal cord or cauda equina compression, high-dose corticosteroids in combination with external beam radiation or surgical decompression is needed to preserve neurologic function [50].

Once the patient develops bone metastasis, the disease is considered systemic and thus requires systemic treatments. Compared to patients with visceral metastases, those with bone only metastases have a more indolent course [4, 5, 51, 52]. Bone-only metastases are more common in hormone receptor positive patients and hormonal therapy is an important key treatment for them [53]. However the optimal treatment algorithms for bone metastases are difficult to determine at the present time and it is not yet clear which treatment modality or combination of treatments is most effective in prolonging survival for patients with bone-only metastasis [54].

Among several molecularly targeted agents, osteoclast inhibitors such as bisphosphonates and denosumab target the osteolysis associated with bone lesions and deserve special attention here. Bisphosphonates reduce pain and the incidence of SREs [55, 56]. Patients with stage IV disease confined to the skeleton at the time of diagnosis are most likely to develop SREs and may benefit the most from bisphosphonate treatment [4]. The mechanism of action of this class of drugs is inhibition of bone resorption by suppression of osteoclast activity. Early generation bisphosphonates (clodronate and etidronate) are taken up and metabolized by osteoclasts and induce apoptosis by their metabolites, cytotoxic ATP analogs. On the other hand, later-generation bisphosphonates (pamidronate, ibandronate and zoledronate) are internalized but not metabolized by osteoclasts [20]. They inhibit the function of farnesyl diphosphonate (FPP) synthase, which is necessary for prenylation of GTPase such as Ras, Rho, and Rac, as part of post-translational modification. Without proper GTPase function, osteoclasts fail to form ruffled borders, which are necessary for adhesion to the bone surface [20].

Bisphosphonates reduce the SRE risk, delay the time to SREs, reduce bone pain and improve patients' quality of life [56]. Furthermore, bisphosphonates rapidly normalize calcium levels in tumor-induced hypercalcemia (TIH); therefore they are the current standard of care in patients with TIH. Bisphosphonates, however, do not appear to improve overall survival of breast cancer patients with bone metastases [56]. It is also important to note that bisphosphonates are associated with potentially serious side effects including renal failure, gastrointestinal side effects and osteonecrosis of the jaw, necessitating close monitoring during their use [57]. There also has been reported to be an increased risk of atypical femoral fracture among those treated with bisphosphonates [58].

Denosumab is another effective osteoclast inhibitor which is useful in management of bone metastasis in breast cancer. Denosumab is a monoclonal antibody, targeting the receptor activator of nuclear factor kappa B ligand (RANKL) [59]. As mentioned previously, up regulation of RANKL contributes to the vicious cycle of bone destruction in metastatic bone disease. Tumor cells in bone secrete cytokines, which in turn induce osteoblasts to secrete RANKL. RANKL then stimulates osteoclasts to resorb bone. Denosumab inhibits the function of RANKL, thus inhibiting bone destruction [60].

Denosumab has been shown to be superior to the bisphosphonate zoledronic acid in several trials involving patients with bone metastases. Compared to bisphosphonates, denosumab is more effective in reducing the risk of developing SREs as well as delaying the time to SREs in breast cancer [61–65]. Patients receiving denosumab demonstrated a greater level of clinical improvement regarding health-related quality of life than patients receiving bisphosphonates [66]. Compared with bisphosphonates, denosumab reduced the incidence of certain indicators of adverse events, including pyrexia, bone pain, edema and renal failure while hypocalcemia and toothache, not associated with osteonecrosis of the jaw (ONJ), were more frequent in the denosumab group [61, 66]. Rates of severe (defined as Common Terminology Criteria of Adverse Events grade ≥3) and serious adverse events (e.g. life threatening or requiring hospitalization) were similar between zoledronic acid and denosumab [61]. Denosumab has much less renal toxicity, and thus it may be beneficial for patients being treated with nephrotoxic compounds and for those with decreased creatinine clearance [66]. However, like bisphosphonates, denosumab does not make a significant difference in overall patient survival [56].

ONJ is the most severe adverse event of osteoclast inhibitor. The majority of ONJ cases have been associated with known risk factors involving invasive dental procedures and poor oral hygiene. The incidence rate is 1.4–2.9% in patients with breast cancer [61, 67, 68] and increased with the duration of anti-resorptive therapy [67, 68]. Before starting an osteoclast inhibitor, patients should receive a dental checkup. Also it is preferable to avoid surgical procedures for dental problems during treatment with an osteoclast inhibitor. A statistically significant difference in the incidence of ONJ has not been observed between denosumab-treated and zoledronic acid-treated groups [61, 68]. ONJ resolved in over one-third of the patients [68].

The long-term safety of osteoclast inhibitors in bone metastasis has not been adequately studied in controlled trials, and concerns regarding long-term complications including renal toxicity, ONJ, and atypical femoral fractures remain a primary rationale for the current practice of withholding therapy or implementing a less intensive schedule of therapy. The ZOOM trial [69] and the OPTIMIZE-2 trial [70] compared zoledronic acid standard every 4 weeks vs. 12 weeks after 10–15 months of previous bisphosphonate therapy. The every 12 weeks regimen was not inferior to the every 4 weeks regimen for SRE. This outcome supports decreasing the frequency of administration of zoledronic acid to a 12-weekly regimen to reduce zoledronic acid exposure from the 2nd year. On the other hand, the use of zoledronic acid every 12 weeks did not result in an increased risk of SRE compared with every 4 weeks for patients with no previous zoledronic acid therapy [71]. The safety profiles did not differ significantly between the treatment groups in these trials. But there may be a possibility to decrease adverse events with longer treatment duration. This 12 week interval regimen of bisphosphonate may be an acceptable treatment option. At present there are insufficient data supporting the longer interval administration of denosumab yet.

Another systemic treatment modality, which targets bone more specifically, are radioisotopes with affinity for bone. Isotopes such as strontium-89 and samarium-153, are given systemically but localized in sites of active bone turnover, treating all sites of bone metastases simultaneously. These isotopes release beta-particles (electrons), which are cytotoxic to cancer cells in the metastatic bone lesions, providing effective pain relief with response rates ranging from 40% to 95% [72].

Although clinical management of bone metastases is challenging, multiple treatment modalities are currently available to alleviate pain and minimize the risk for SREs for breast cancer patients with bone metastases. The current therapeutic options for bone metastatic breast cancer are summarized in Table 7.4. These treatments, however, are only beneficial if given following good detection and under appropriate assessment of bone metastases. Further, bone specific therapies which specifically target the tumors need to be developed. In the next section, we discuss the current techniques used to detect bone metastases and to assess the response to treatment.

Table 7.4 Current therapeutic options for bone metastatic breast cancer

Therapeutic options	Main indications
External beam radiation therapy	Pain control
	Prevention of pathological fractures
Surgery	Curative intent for localized disease (rare)
	Correction of pathological fractures
	Prevention of pathological fractures
Systemic endocrine therapy	Intent to control disease
Systemic chemotherapy	Intent to control disease
Systemic targeted therapy	Intent to control disease
Bone-targeted therapy (bisphosphonates, denosumab)	Pain control
	Reduction of SRE risks
	Delaying time to SREs
Radioisotopes (strontium-89, samarium-153)	Pain control
Supportive interventions (analgesics)	Pain control

7.4 Detection and Assessments

To assess bone involvement from breast cancer, multiple imaging studies are currently available including plain x-ray films, bone scintigraphy, computed tomography (CT) scan, magnetic resonance imaging (MRI), positron emission tomography (PET) scan, and PET/CT [73]. PET-CT has higher sensitivity and accuracy for detection of bone metastases in breast cancer patients compared with bone scintigraphy [74]. Although PET-magnetic resonance (PET-MR) imaging is an innovative technique still under investigation, PET-MR detected a higher number of osseous metastases than did same-day PET-CT and was positive for 12% of the patients deemed osseous metastasis-negative by PET-CT [75]. According to the National Comprehensive Cancer Network, use of these imaging studies for evaluation of patients with primary breast cancers are optional unless directed by symptoms or abnormal laboratory results [76]. Excessive imaging by radiographs and CT is not only extremely expensive but also puts the patient at risk for unnecessary radiation exposure and/or invasive procedures undertaken because of false positive findings. When necessary, treatment response for bone metastases is assessed by a combination of methods, including imaging, blood analyses and symptomologies [73, 77–79].

The most widely used criteria for assessing tumor response are based on the anatomic measurement of solid tumors. Because bone metastases are typically located in irregularly shaped bones and are difficult to measure with rulers, they have been previously considered as unmeasurable disease. New developments in cancer response criteria have increased awareness of the importance of the response of bone metastases to therapy. Three well-established organizations, namely Union International Against Cancer [UICC], World Health Organization [WHO] and MD Anderson Cancer Center [MDA], have established criteria to assess the bone response to treatment [77]. UICC recommends plain films only; WHO, plain films and bone scan and MDA, plain films, bone scan, CT and MRI. The MDA criteria updated the UICC and WHO bone response criteria by expanding radiographic assessment and incorporating both CT and MRI in order to classify the response into four distinctive types: complete response, partial response, no change or stable disease, and progressive disease. On plain film, osteolytic lesions are recognized as a hole in the bone cortex while osteoblastic lesions appear dense and "whiter" than the surrounding bone. The lesions in the cortex are best demonstrated on CT with bone windows, whereas trabecular lesions are best demonstrated on MRI [19]. Since CT and MRI are able to detect detailed anatomic changes, MDA criteria appear to be superior to UICC and WHO's to assess the response of bone metastasis lesions to treatment and to interpret the clinical behavior of bone metastasis [77].

The updated Response Evaluation Criteria in Solid Tumors (RECIST 1.1) now consider bone metastases with soft tissue masses >10 mm to be measurable disease. Functional imaging criteria, such as the Positron Emission Tomography Response Criteria in Solid Tumors (PERCIST) using PET-CT allow response to be measured in the absence of anatomic change through assessment of metabolic activity [80, 81]. A decrease in FDG uptake of PET-CT has proved to indicate treatment response in patients with breast cancer [82, 83]. FDG uptake of PET-CT has also been shown to provide more rapid response data than anatomic measurements [83, 84]. Therefore, PERCIST appears to be superior to RECIST and more suitable for assessing tumor response than RECIST criteria [80, 85].

At present, biochemical tests by blood analysis are not very specific for assessment of bone metastases. However, bone resorption and osteoblastic markers may be useful in identifying patients at increased risks of SREs as well as monitoring progression of the disease and evaluating treatment response [86]. Since the bone matrix contains type I collagen as its major organic component, byproducts of collagen breakdown are released during bone resorption [86]. These collagen-related biomarkers of bone resorption include: pyridinoline (PYD), deoxypyridinoline (DPD), urinary collagen cross-linked nitrogen-terminal N-telopeptide (NTX) and collagen I carboxyl-terminal C-telopeptide (CTX). These urinary waste products of the collagen crosslinks are very accurate predictors of the response to bisphosphonate therapy, compared to other markers such as bone alkaline phosphatase, urinary calcium and hydroxyproline [87]. Elevated levels of bone-specific alkaline phosphatase indicates the state of increased bone turnover and new bone formation, alerting the physician that new bone metastases may now be present or, if the presence of bone metastases is already known, that the disease is progressing [86].

Other biomarkers used to predict presence and response of bone metastasis are circulating tumor cells (CTCs) and disseminated tumor cells in the bone marrow. The number of CTCs and the presence of micro-metastasis in the bone marrow before first-line treatment is associated with a poor prognosis in patients with metastatic breast cancer [88–91]. This prognostic value has also been observed during treatment [92]. The presence of extensive bone metastases detected by FDG-PET/CT is associated with increased CTC numbers in metastatic breast cancer [93].

It has also been suggested that CTC count could provide additional prognostic information beyond Tumor Markers for metastatic breast cancer [94, 95]. A recent study suggested that the identification of CTCs in epithelial-to-mesenchymal transition is associated with a poor prognosis [96]. CTC status can also serve as an indicator to monitor the effectiveness of treatments and guide subsequent therapies in breast cancer [97, 98]. CTC can potentially evaluate patient prognosis with CTC clusters during treatment and provide a noninvasive and inexpensive assessment that can guide drug discovery development or therapeutic choices for personalized treatment [99].

Both circulating tumor cells and disseminated tumor cells could, therefore, be potential surrogates for the presence of bone lesions, and could be used to stratify high-risk patients and monitor treatment response.

As described in this section, various imaging studies and blood tests are available for detection and assessment of bone metastases. Since sophisticated imaging studies are expensive and false results can be problematic, surrogate biomarkers would be extremely useful. Thus, along with developing new therapeutic strategies, novel and effective biomarkers of bone disease and response are needed.

7.5   Future Directions for Bone Metastasis Management: Novel Treatments

As described previously, bone metastasis is a complex phenomenon, which involves multiple genes, signaling pathways, and cellular and biochemical components. Despite various types of treatment and a thorough multidisciplinary approach, the metastatic disease eventually becomes resistant to therapies and the disease progresses. The mechanism of resistance to bone-targeted therapies is not well-understood. Some researchers postulate that cancer stem cells, which are insensitive to currently available therapies, are the culprit for therapy resistance in metastatic diseases including bone [100]. Epithelial-mesenchymal transition (EMT), which is viewed as the generation of cancer stem cell phenotypes, is another concept which might explain the mechanism of bone metastasis development and resistance to therapy [101].

Laboratory studies and clinical trials are being undertaken in order to develop new, more effective therapies. Recent advances in understanding the mechanism of bone metastases in breast cancer have led to several promising bone-specific, molecular targets under investigation, which target osteoclast activities, osteoblasts and the bone microenvironment favoring metastatic lesions. The emerging therapeutic targets bring much hope and deserve special attention in this chapter. Recent developments in new therapeutic targets and modalities for bone metastases in breast cancer are discussed here (Table 7.5).

Table 7.5 Ongoing clinical trials of targeted agents and Ra-223 in breast cancer or solid tumor

Target	Compound (agent)	Phase	NCT	Cancer type	Combination	Bone-specific endpoint	Status
c-Src	BMS-354825 (dasatinib)	I, II	NCT00820170	Breast	Paclitaxel	None	Ongoing
	AZD0530 (saracatinib)	II	NCT02085603	Cancer with bone metastasis		Pain/analgesic drug usage/bone markers	Recruiting
TGFβ	GC1008 (fresolimumab)	II	NCT01401062	Breast	Radiation	None	Ongoing
	Y2157299 (galunisertib)	I	NCT02672475	Breast	Paclitaxel	None	Recruiting
		II	NCT02538471	Breast	Radiation	None	Recruiting
CXCR4	LY2510924	I	NCT02737072	Solid tumors		None	Recruiting
	USL311	I	NCT02765165	Solid tumors		None	Recruiting
Radium-223		II	NCT02258464	Breast with bone metastasis	Hormonal therapy	Symptomatic skeletal event free survival/pain	Recruiting
		II	NCT02258451	Breast with bone metastasis	Exemestane/everolimus	Symptomatic skeletal event free survival/pain	Recruiting
		II	NCT02366130	Breast with bone metastasis	Hormonal therapy	Efficacy evaluation of bone	Recruiting

7.5.1   *c-Src*

c-Src is a proto-oncogene, encoding a non-receptor tyrosine kinase, which controls various signaling pathways in tumorigenesis. It is often overexpressed in human cancer cells and is activated by RANKL/RANK interaction and plays a central role in osteoclast function [102]. The c-Src expression is a potential independent predictor of poor prognosis in breast cancer patients with bone metastasis [103]. It was shown that c-Src inhibitors effectively inhibit invasion of cancer cells and growth of breast cancer bone metastases in mice [104]. Dasatinib, one of the Src-targeting agents, was studied as monotherapy in several Phase 2 studies and did not exhibit significant antitumor activity in metastatic breast cancer [105–107]. But some Phase 1 studies showed tolerability of dasatinib in combination with chemotherapy, such as paclitaxel and capecitabine [108–110]. A Phase 2 study of dasatinib plus paclitaxel for metastatic breast cancer is now ongoing (Table 7.5). For treatment of breast cancer bone metastasis, there has been a Phase 1/2 study of dasatinib combined with zoledronic acid which was well tolerated and produced responses [111]. Saracatinib is other Src inhibitor that is now being studied in Phase 2 placebo controlled study for cancer-induced bone pain (Table 7.5).

7.5.2   *TGFβ*

Transforming growth factor β (TGFβ) is known for having multiple effects on development and progression of bone metastasis. TGFβ regulates various cellular functions such as cell growth and differentiation, extra cellular matrix production, cell motility and immunosuppression [112]. Interestingly, TGFβ switches roles in cancer, exerting tumor suppressor effects in early stage metastases and promoter effects as the tumor progresses [112]. It is known that extracellular TGFβ is associated with advancing disease stage [113] and TGFβ receptor is a prognostic indicator [114]. Moreover, blocking TGFβ in breast cancer might prevent tumor cells from metastasizing and growing [115–118]. In bone metastases, TGFβ inhibition interrupts the vicious cycle driven by TGFβ and other key components, halting tumor growth [119, 120]. A cytokine belonging to the TGF β superfamily, the dual nature of TGF β may pose a challenge upon developing therapies targeting TGFβ. It is worth noting that serious side effects might arise from targeting TGFβ due to its pleotropic effects. It is possible that chronic inflammation and autoimmune reactions as well as the development of premalignant lesions might occur upon suppressing the immunosuppressive effect of TGFβ. Several strategies targeting the TGFβ signaling system are under investigation, including monoclonal antibodies against TGFβ ligands, TGF receptor inhibitors, and antisense oligonucleotides which inhibit TGFβ production. These have proven to be effective in preclinical studies, some of which are now in clinical development [121].

7.5.3   CXCR4/CXCL12

CXCR4 is a chemokine receptor which exclusively binds to stromal cell-derived factor 1 (known as SDF-1 or CXCL12) [22]. CXCR4 is highly expressed in breast cancer tissue and CXCL12 is overexpressed in common metastatic sites in breast cancer, such as bone marrow, lymph node, lung and liver [22]. CXCR4 is more likely to be expressed in bone metastases than visceral metastasis and may contribute to the homing of breast cancer cells to the bone [122]. CXCL12 is produced by multiple types of bone marrow cells, including osteoblasts [122]. Thus, the CXCR4/CXCL12 interaction is important in the homing of breast cancer cells to distant sites and is another attractive therapeutic target in bone metastasis [122]. Several CXCR4/CXCL12 antagonists have been tested in preclinical studies and demonstrated an ability to reduce metastasis as well as primary tumor growth in animal breast cancer models [123–129]. Several CXCR4 antagonists, such as LY2510924, USL311, are in Phase 1 clinical trials (Table 7.5).

7.5.4   Radium-223

Radium-223 dichloride (Ra-223) is a radioisotope which emits alpha-particles, and is under investigation for management of bone metastases in breast cancer. It delivers an intense and highly localized radiation to the affected bone surface while delivering substantially less irradiation to healthy bone marrow compared with standard bone-seeking beta-emitting radioisotopes (strontium-89) [130]. This is due to alpha-particles having a lower penetration depth than beta-particles, thus sparing surrounding healthy bone and bone marrow tissues. In a Phase 2 study for patients with prostate cancer, Ra-233 reduced pain secondary to bone metastases, decreased the incidence of SREs, and reduced bone-specific ALP concentrations [131]. Furthermore, data from a Phase III trial (ALSYMPCA trial) have shown significant improvement in overall survival among patients with castration-resistant prostate cancer, with the treatment group having a median overall survival of 14.9 months compared with 11.3 months for the placebo group (p < 0.001) [132]. The U.S.FDA approved Ra-223 for treatment of patients with castration-resistant prostate cancer with bone metastases in 2013. Ra-223 has also shown promising preliminary results in a Phase II trial in breast cancer. This trial recruited breast cancer patients with bone metastases no longer responsive to endocrine therapy. These results showed that Ra-223 was well-tolerated and reduced the levels of bone alkaline phosphatase as well as urine N-telopeptide, both of which are important bone turnover markers associated with bone metastases. This study also showed metabolic decrease in FDG PET/CT of bone lesions [133]. Some clinical trials of Ra-223 for breast cancer patients with bone metastasis are now ongoing to determine the clinical benefit (Table 7.5).

7.6   Conclusion

In summary, there are multiple potential therapeutic targets under investigation for bone metastases in breast cancer. Until definitive control of disease is possible, bone metastases in breast cancer remain difficult to cure and their resistance to pre-existing therapies continues to pose challenges. However, new discoveries elucidating the molecular mechanism of bone metastases and new emerging targets under study provide hope for patients. Since bone metastasis in breast cancer is a complicated process, a multidisciplinary approach should continue to be employed in order to provide the best available care for breast cancer patients with bone metastases.

References

1. Coleman RE (2006) Clinical features of metastatic bone disease and risk of skeletal morbidity. Clin Cancer Res 12(20):6243s–6249s
2. Gainford MC, Dranitsaris G, Clemons M (2005) Recent developments in bisphosphonates for patients with metastatic breast cancer. BMJ 330(7494):769–773
3. Scheid V, Buzdar AU, Smith TL, Hortobagyi GN (1986) Clinical course of breast cancer patients with osseous metastasis treated with combination chemotherapy. Cancer 58(12):2589–2593
4. Plunkett TA, Smith P, Rubens RD (2000) Risk of complications from bone metastases in breast cancer. Implications for management. Eur J Cancer 36(4):476–482
5. Domchek SM, Younger J, Finkelstein DM, Seiden MV (2000) Predictors of skeletal complications in patients with metastatic breast carcinoma. Cancer 89(2):363–368
6. Sathiakumar N, Delzell E, Morrisey MA, Falkson C, Yong M, Chia V, Blackburn J, Arora T, Brill I, Kilgore ML (2012) Mortality following bone metastasis and skeletal-related events among women with breast cancer: a population-based analysis of U.S. Medicare beneficiaries, 1999–2006. Breast Cancer Res Treat 131(1):231–238
7. James JJ, Evans AJ, Pinder SE, Gutteridge E, Cheung KL, Chan S, Robertson JFR (2003) Bone metastases from breast carcinoma: histopathological – radiological correlations and prognostic features. Br J Cancer 89(4):660–665
8. Colleoni M, O'Neill A, Goldhirsch A, Gelber RD, Bonetti M, Thürlimann B, Price KN, Castiglione-Gertsch M, Coates AS, Lindtner J, Collins J, Senn H-J, Cavalli F, Forbes J, Gudgeon A, Simoncini E, Cortes-Funes H, Veronesi A, Fey M, Rudenstam C-M (2000) Identifying breast cancer patients at high risk for bone metastases. J Clin Oncol 18(23):3925–3935
9. Delpech Y, Bashour SI, Lousquy R, Rouzier R, Hess K, Coutant C, Barranger E, Esteva FJ, Ueno NT, Pusztai L, Ibrahim NK (2015) Clinical nomogram to predict bone-only metastasis in patients with early breast carcinoma. Br J Cancer 113(7):1003–1009
10. Parfitt AM (2002) Targeted and nontargeted bone remodeling: relationship to basic multicellular unit origination and progression. Bone 30(1):5–7
11. Xiong J, O'Brien CA (2012) Osteocyte RANKL: new insights into the control of bone remodeling. J Bone Miner Res 27(3):499–505
12. Fu Q, Manolagas SC, O'Brien CA (2006) Parathyroid hormone controls receptor activator of NF- B ligand gene expression via a distant transcriptional enhancer. Mol Cell Biol 26(17):6453–6468
13. Tatsumi S, Ishii K, Amizuka N, Li M, Kobayashi T, Kohno K, Ito M, Takeshita S, Ikeda K (2007) Targeted ablation of osteocytes induces osteoporosis with defective mechanotransduction. Cell Metab 5(6):464–475

122   R. K. Tahara et al.

14. O'Flaherty EJ (2000) Modeling normal aging bone loss, with consideration of bone loss in osteoporosis. Toxicol Sci 55(1):171–188
15. Chen Z, Maricic M, Pettinger M, Ritenbaugh C, Lopez AM, Barad DH, Gass M, LeBoff MS, Bassford TL (2005) Osteoporosis and rate of bone loss among postmenopausal survivors of breast cancer. Cancer 104(7):1520–1530
16. Van Poznak C, Sauter NP (2005) Clinical management of osteoporosis in women with a history of breast carcinoma. Cancer 104(3):443–456
17. Mathot L, Stenninger J (2012) Behavior of seeds and soil in the mechanism of metastasis: a deeper understanding. Cancer Sci 103(4):626–631
18. Fidler IJ (2003) Timeline: the pathogenesis of cancer metastasis: the 'seed and soil' hypothesis revisited. Nat Rev Cancer 3(6):453–458
19. Theriault RL, Theriault RL (2012) Biology of bone metastases. Cancer Control 19(2):92–101
20. Rose AA, Siegel PM (2010) Emerging therapeutic targets in breast cancer bone metastasis. Future Oncol 6(1):55–74
21. Jones DH, Nakashima T, Sanchez OH, Kozieradzki I, Komarova SV, Sarosi I, Morony S, Rubin E, Sarao R, Hojilla CV, Komnenovic V, Kong Y-Y, Schreiber M, Dixon SJ, Sims SM, Khokha R, Wada T, Penninger JM (2006) Regulation of cancer cell migration and bone metastasis by RANKL. Nature 440(7084):692–696
22. Müller A, Homey B, Soto H, Ge N, Catron D, Buchanan ME, McClanahan T, Murphy E, Yuan W, Wagner SN, Barrera JL, Mohar A, Verástegui E, Zlotnik A (2001) Involvement of chemokine receptors in breast cancer metastasis. Nature 410(6824):50–56
23. Kozlow W, Guise TA (2005) Breast cancer metastasis to bone: mechanisms of osteolysis and implications for therapy. J Mammary Gland Biol Neoplasia 10(2):169–180
24. Coleman RE, Seaman JJ (2001) The role of zoledronic acid in cancer: clinical studies in the treatment and prevention of bone metastases. Semin Oncol 28(2 Suppl 6):11–16
25. Chirgwin JM, Guise TA (2000) Molecular mechanisms of tumor-bone interactions in osteolytic metastases. Crit Rev Eukaryot Gene Expr 10(2):159–178
26. Chiang AC, Massagué J (2008) Molecular basis of metastasis. N Engl J Med 359(26):2814–2823
27. Onishi T, Hayashi N, Theriault RL, Hortobagyi GN, Ueno NT (2010) Future directions of bone-targeted therapy for metastatic breast cancer. Nat Rev Clin Oncol 7(11):641–651
28. Guise TA (2002) The vicious cycle of bone metastases. J Musculoskelet Neuronal Interact 2(6):570–572
29. Roodman GD (2004) Mechanisms of bone metastasis. N Engl J Med 350(16):1655–1664
30. Simonet WS, Lacey DL, Dunstan CR, Kelley M, Chang MS, Lüthy R, Nguyen HQ, Wooden S, Bennett L, Boone T, Shimamoto G, DeRose M, Elliott R, Colombero A, Tan HL, Trail G, Sullivan J, Davy E, Bucay N, Renshaw-Gegg L, Hughes TM, Hill D, Pattison W, Campbell P, Sander S, Van G, Tarpley J, Derby P, Lee R, Boyle WJ (1997) Osteoprotegerin: a novel secreted protein involved in the regulation of bone density. Cell 89(2):309–319
31. Clines GA, Guise TA (2005) Hypercalcaemia of malignancy and basic research on mechanisms responsible for osteolytic and osteoblastic metastasis to bone. Endocr Relat Cancer 12(3):549–583
32. Clevers H (2006) Wnt/β-catenin signaling in development and disease. Cell 127(3):469–480
33. Voorzanger-Rousselot N, Goehrig D, Journe F, Doriath V, Body JJ, Clézardin P, Garnero P (2007) Increased Dickkopf-1 expression in breast cancer bone metastases. Br J Cancer 97(7):964–970
34. Tian E, Zhan F, Walker R, Rasmussen E, Ma Y, Barlogie B, Shaughnessy JD (2003) The role of the Wnt-signaling antagonist DKK1 in the development of osteolytic lesions in multiple myeloma. N Engl J Med 349(26):2483–2494
35. Clézardin P (2011) Therapeutic targets for bone metastases in breast cancer. Breast Cancer Res 13(2):207
36. Yang X, Karsenty G (2002) Transcription factors in bone: developmental and pathological aspects. Trends Mol Med 8(7):340–345

37. Yi B, Williams PJ, Niewolna M, Wang Y, Yoneda T (2002) Tumor-derived platelet-derived growth factor-BB plays a critical role in osteosclerotic bone metastasis in an animal model of human breast cancer. Cancer Res 62(3):917–923

38. Valta MP, Hentunen T, Qu Q, Valve EM, Harjula A, Seppänen JA, Väänänen HK, Härkönen PL (2006) Regulation of osteoblast differentiation: a novel function for fibroblast growth factor 8. Endocrinology 147(5):2171–2182

39. Dunn LK, Mohammad KS, Fournier PGJ, McKenna CR, Davis HW, Niewolna M, Peng XH, Chirgwin JM, Guise TA (2009) Hypoxia and TGF-β drive breast cancer bone metastases through parallel signaling pathways in tumor cells and the bone microenvironment. PLoS One 4(9):e6896

40. Dai J, Keller J, Zhang J, Lu Y, Yao Z, Keller ET (2005) Bone morphogenetic protein-6 promotes osteoblastic prostate cancer bone metastases through a dual mechanism. Cancer Res 65(18):8274–8285

41. Guise TA, Yin JJ, Mohammad KS (2003) Role of endothelin-1 in osteoblastic bone metastases. Cancer 97(S3):779–784

42. Clines GA, Mohammad KS, Bao Y, Stephens OW, Suva LJ, Shaughnessy JD, Fox JW, Chirgwin JM, Guise TA (2007) Dickkopf homolog 1 mediates endothelin-1-stimulated new bone formation. Mol Endocrinol 21(2):486–498

43. Yin JJ, Mohammad KS, Kakonen SM, Harris S, Wu-Wong JR, Wessale JL, Padley RJ, Garrett IR, Chirgwin JM, Guise TA (2003) A causal role for endothelin-1 in the pathogenesis of osteoblastic bone metastases. Proc Natl Acad Sci 100(19):10954–10959

44. Hanrahan EO, Broglio KR, Buzdar AU, Theriault RL, Valero V, Cristofanilli M, Yin G, Kau S-WC, Hortobagyi GN, Rivera E (2005) Combined-modality treatment for isolated recurrences of breast carcinoma: update on 30 years of experience at the University of Texas M.D. Anderson Cancer Center and assessment of prognostic factors. Cancer 104(6):1158–1171

45. Incarbone M, Nava M, Lequaglie C, Ravasi G, Pastorino U (1997) Sternal resection for primary or secondary tumors. J Thorac Cardiovasc Surg 114(1):93–99

46. Dürr HR, Müller PE, Lenz T, Baur A, Jansson V, Refior HJ (2002) Surgical treatment of bone metastases in patients with breast cancer. Clin Orthop Relat Res 396:191–196

47. Thompson RC (1992) Impending fracture associated with bone destruction. Orthopedics 15(5):547–550

48. Harrington KD (1997) Orthopedic surgical management of skeletal complications of malignancy. Cancer 80(8 Suppl):1614–1627

49. Tong D, Gillick L, Hendrickson FR (1982) The palliation of symptomatic osseous metastases: final results of the study by the Radiation Therapy Oncology Group. Cancer 50(5):893–899

50. Maranzano E, Latini P (1995) Effectiveness of radiation therapy without surgery in metastatic spinal cord compression: final results from a prospective trial. Int J Radiat Oncol Biol Phys 32(4):959–967

51. Perez JE, Machiavelli M, Leone BA, Romero A, Rabinovich MG, Vallejo CT, Bianco A, Rodriguez R, Cuevas MA, Alvarez LA (1990) Bone-only versus visceral-only metastatic pattern in breast cancer: analysis of 150 patients. A GOCS study. Grupo Oncológico Cooperativo del Sur. Am J Clin Oncol 13(4):294–298

52. Leone BA, Vallejo CT, Romero AO, Machiavelli MR, Pérez JE, Leone J, Leone JP (2017) Prognostic impact of metastatic pattern in stage IV breast cancer at initial diagnosis. Breast Cancer Res Treat 161(3):537–548

53. Lee SJ, Park S, Ahn HK, Yi JH, Cho EY, Sun JM, Lee JE, Nam SJ, Yang J-H, Park YH, Ahn JS, Im Y-H (2011) Implications of bone-only metastases in breast cancer: favorable preference with excellent outcomes of hormone receptor positive breast cancer. Cancer Res Treat 43(2):89–95

54. Niikura N, Liu J, Hayashi N, Palla SL, Tokuda Y, Hortobagyi GN, Ueno NT, Theriault RL (2011) Treatment outcome and prognostic factors for patients with bone-only metastases of breast cancer: a single-institution retrospective analysis. Oncologist 16(2):155–164

55. Diel IJ (2007) Effectiveness of bisphosphonates on bone pain and quality of life in breast cancer patients with metastatic bone disease: a review. Support Care Cancer 15(11):1243–1249

56. Wong MH, Stockler MR, Pavlakis N (2012) Bisphosphonates and other bone agents for breast cancer. In: Pavlakis N (ed) Cochrane database of systematic reviews, no. 2. Wiley, Chichester, p CD003474

57. Petrut B, Trinkaus M, Simmons C, Clemons M (2008) A primer of bone metastases management in breast cancer patients. Curr Oncol 15(Suppl 1):S50–S57

58. Gedmintas L, Solomon DH, Kim SC (2013) Bisphosphonates and risk of subtrochanteric, femoral shaft, and atypical femur fracture: a systematic review and meta-analysis. J Bone Miner Res 28(8):1729–1737

59. Lipton A, Steger GG, Figueroa J, Alvarado C, Solal-Celigny P, Body J-J, de Boer R, Berardi R, Gascon P, Tonkin KS, Coleman R, Paterson AHG, Peterson MC, Fan M, Kinsey A, Jun S (2007) Randomized active-controlled phase II study of denosumab efficacy and safety in patients with breast cancer-related bone metastases. J Clin Oncol 25(28):4431–4437

60. Canon JR, Roudier M, Bryant R, Morony S, Stolina M, Kostenuik PJ, Dougall WC (2008) Inhibition of RANKL blocks skeletal tumor progression and improves survival in a mouse model of breast cancer bone metastasis. Clin Exp Metastasis 25(2):119–129

61. Stopeck AT, Lipton A, Body J-J, Steger GG, Tonkin K, de Boer RH, Lichinitser M, Fujiwara Y, Yardley DA, Viniegra M, Fan M, Jiang Q, Dansey R, Jun S, Braun A (2010) Denosumab compared with zoledronic acid for the treatment of bone metastases in patients with advanced breast cancer: a randomized, double-blind study. J Clin Oncol 28(35):5132–5139

62. Fizazi K, Carducci M, Smith M, Damião R, Brown J, Karsh L, Milecki P, Shore N, Rader M, Wang H, Jiang Q, Tadros S, Dansey R, Goessl C (2011) Denosumab versus zoledronic acid for treatment of bone metastases in men with castration-resistant prostate cancer: a randomised, double-blind study. Lancet 377(9768):813–822

63. Henry DH, Costa L, Goldwasser F, Hirsh V, Hungria V, Prausova J, Scagliotti GV, Sleeboom H, Spencer A, Vadhan-Raj S, von Moos R, Willenbacher W, Woll PJ, Wang J, Jiang Q, Jun S, Dansey R, Yeh H (2011) Randomized, double-blind study of denosumab versus zoledronic acid in the treatment of bone metastases in patients with advanced cancer (excluding breast and prostate cancer) or multiple myeloma. J Clin Oncol 29(9):1125–1132

64. Lipton A, Fizazi K, Stopeck AT, Henry DH, Brown JE, Yardley DA, Richardson GE, Siena S, Maroto P, Clemens M, Bilynskyy B, Charu V, Beuzeboc P, Rader M, Viniegra M, Saad F, Ke C, Braun A, Jun S (2012) Superiority of denosumab to zoledronic acid for prevention of skeletal-related events: a combined analysis of 3 pivotal, randomised, phase 3 trials. Eur J Cancer 48(16):3082–3092

65. Henry D, Vadhan-Raj S, Hirsh V, von Moos R, Hungria V, Costa L, Woll PJ, Scagliotti G, Smith G, Feng A, Jun S, Dansey R, Yeh H (2014) Delaying skeletal-related events in a randomized phase 3 study of denosumab versus zoledronic acid in patients with advanced cancer: an analysis of data from patients with solid tumors. Support Care Cancer 22(3):679–687

66. Wang X, Yang KH, Wanyan P, Tian JH (2014) Comparison of the efficacy and safety of denosumab versus bisphosphonates in breast cancer and bone metastases treatment: a meta-analysis of randomized controlled trials. Oncol Lett 7(6):1997–2002

67. Bamias A, Kastritis E, Bamia C, Moulopoulos LA, Melakopoulos I, Bozas G, Koutsoukou V, Gika D, Anagnostopoulos A, Papadimitriou C, Terpos E, Dimopoulos MA (2005) Osteonecrosis of the jaw in cancer after treatment with bisphosphonates: incidence and risk factors. J Clin Oncol 23(34):8580–8587

68. Saad F, Brown JE, Van Poznak C, Ibrahim T, Stemmer SM, Stopeck AT, Diel IJ, Takahashi S, Shore N, Henry DH, Barrios CH, Facon T, Senecal F, Fizazi K, Zhou L, Daniels A, Carrière P, Dansey R (2012) Incidence, risk factors, and outcomes of osteonecrosis of the jaw: integrated analysis from three blinded active-controlled phase III trials in cancer patients with bone metastases. Ann Oncol 23(5):1341–1347

69. Amadori D, Aglietta M, Alessi B, Gianni L, Ibrahim T, Farina G, Gaion F, Bertoldo F, Santini D, Rondena R, Bogani P, Ripamonti CI (2013) Efficacy and safety of 12-weekly

versus 4-weekly zoledronic acid for prolonged treatment of patients with bone metastases from breast cancer (ZOOM): a phase 3, open-label, randomised, non-inferiority trial. Lancet Oncol 14(7):663–670

70. Hortobagyi GN, Van Poznak C, Harker WG, Gradishar WJ, Chew H, Dakhil SR, Haley BB, Sauter N, Mohanlal R, Zheng M, Lipton A (2017) Continued treatment effect of zoledronic acid dosing every 12 vs 4 weeks in women with breast cancer metastatic to bone: The OPTIMIZE-2 randomized clinical trial. JAMA Oncol 3(7):906–912

71. Himelstein AL, Foster JC, Khatcheressian JL, Roberts JD, Seisler DK, Novotny PJ, Qin R, Go RS, Grubbs SS, O'Connor T, Velasco MR, Weckstein D, O'Mara A, Loprinzi CL, Shapiro CL (2017) Effect of longer-interval vs standard dosing of zoledronic acid on skeletal events in patients with bone metastases. JAMA 317(1):48

72. Finlay IG, Mason MD, Shelley M (2005) Radioisotopes for the palliation of metastatic bone cancer: a systematic review. Lancet Oncol 6(6):392–400

73. Hamaoka T, Madewell JE, Podoloff DA, Hortobagyi GN, Ueno NT (2004) Bone imaging in metastatic breast cancer. J Clin Oncol 22(14):2942–2953

74. Rong J, Wang S, Ding Q, Yun M, Zheng Z, Ye S (2013) Comparison of 18FDG PET-CT and bone scintigraphy for detection of bone metastases in breast cancer patients. A meta-analysis. Surg Oncol 22(2):86–91

75. Catalano OA, Nicolai E, Rosen BR, Luongo A, Catalano M, Iannace C, Guimaraes A, Vangel MG, Mahmood U, Soricelli A, Salvatore M (2015) Comparison of CE-FDG-PET/CT with CE-FDG-PET/MR in the evaluation of osseous metastases in breast cancer patients. Br J Cancer 112(9):1452–1460

76. Carlson RW, Allred DC, Anderson BO, Burstein HJ, Carter WB, Edge SB, Erban JK, Farrar WB, Forero A, Giordano SH, Goldstein LJ, Gradishar WJ, Hayes DF, Hudis CA, Ljung B-M, Mankoff DA, Marcom PK, Mayer IA, McCormick B, Pierce LJ, Reed EC, Sachdev J, Lou Smith M, Somlo G, Ward JH, Wolff AC, Zellars R, National Comprehensive Cancer Network (2011) Invasive breast cancer. J Natl Compr Cancer Netw 9(2):136–222

77. Hamaoka T, Costelloe CM, Madewell JE, Liu P, Berry DA, Islam R, Theriault RL, Hortobagyi GN, Ueno NT (2010) Tumour response interpretation with new tumour response criteria vs the World Health Organisation criteria in patients with bone-only metastatic breast cancer. Br J Cancer 102(4):651–657

78. De Giorgi U, Mego M, Rohren EM, Liu P, Handy BC, Reuben JM, Macapinlac HA, Hortobagyi GN, Cristofanilli M, Ueno NT (2010) 18F-FDG PET/CT findings and circulating tumor cell counts in the monitoring of systemic therapies for bone metastases from breast cancer. J Nucl Med 51(8):1213–1218

79. Avril S, Muzic RF, Plecha D, Traughber BJ, Vinayak S, Avril N (2016) 18F-FDG PET/CT for monitoring of treatment response in breast cancer. J Nucl Med 57(Suppl_1):34S–39S

80. Riedl CC, Pinker K, Ulaner GA, Ong LT, Baltzer P, Jochelson MS, McArthur HL, Gönen M, Dickler M, Weber WA (2017) Comparison of FDG-PET/CT and contrast-enhanced CT for monitoring therapy response in patients with metastatic breast cancer. Eur J Nucl Med Mol Imaging 44(9):1428–1437

81. Costelloe CM, Chuang HH, Madewell JE, Ueno NT (2010) Cancer response criteria and bone metastases: RECIST 1.1, MDA and PERCIST. J Cancer 1:80–92

82. Smith IC, Welch AE, Hutcheon AW, Miller ID, Payne S, Chilcott F, Waikar S, Whitaker T, Ah-See AK, Eremin O, Heys SD, Gilbert FJ, Sharp PF (2000) Positron emission tomography using [18F]-fluorodeoxy-d-glucose to predict the pathologic response of breast cancer to primary chemotherapy. J Clin Oncol 18(8):1676–1688

83. Brücher BL, Weber W, Bauer M, Fink U, Avril N, Stein HJ, Werner M, Zimmerman F, Siewert JR, Schwaiger M (2001) Neoadjuvant therapy of esophageal squamous cell carcinoma: response evaluation by positron emission tomography. Ann Surg 233(3):300–309

84. Dose Schwarz J, Bader M, Jenicke L, Hemminger G, Jänicke F, Avril N (2005) Early prediction of response to chemotherapy in metastatic breast cancer using sequential 18F-FDG PET. J Nucl Med 46(7):1144–1150

85. Min SJ, Jang HJ, Kim JH (2016) Comparison of the RECIST and PERCIST criteria in solid tumors: a pooled analysis and review. Oncotarget 7(19):27848–27854
86. Clines GA, Guise TA (2004) Mechanisms and treatment for bone metastases. Clin Adv Hematol Oncol 2(5):295–302
87. Pickering LM, Mansi JL (2002) The role of bisphosphonates in breast cancer management: review article. Curr Med Res Opin 18(5):284–295
88. Cristofanilli M, Budd GT, Ellis MJ, Stopeck A, Matera J, Miller MC, Reuben JM, Doyle GV, Allard WJ, Terstappen LWMM, Hayes DF (2004) Circulating tumor cells, disease progression, and survival in metastatic breast cancer. N Engl J Med 351(8):781–791
89. Cristofanilli M, Hayes DF, Budd GT, Ellis MJ, Stopeck A, Reuben JM, Doyle GV, Matera J, Allard WJ, Miller MC, Fritsche HA, Hortobagyi GN, Terstappen LWMM (2005) Circulating tumor cells: a novel prognostic factor for newly diagnosed metastatic breast cancer. J Clin Oncol 23(7):1420–1430
90. Braun S, Vogl FD, Naume B, Janni W, Osborne MP, Coombes RC, Schlimok G, Diel IJ, Gerber B, Gebauer G, Pierga J-Y, Marth C, Oruzio D, Wiedswang G, Solomayer E-F, Kundt G, Strobl B, Fehm T, Wong GYC, Bliss J, Vincent-Salomon A, Pantel K (2005) A pooled analysis of bone marrow micrometastasis in breast cancer. N Engl J Med 353(8):793–802
91. Mu Z, Wang C, Ye Z, Austin L, Civan J, Hyslop T, Palazzo JP, Jaslow R, Li B, Myers RE, Jiang J, Xing J, Yang H, Cristofanilli M (2015) Prospective assessment of the prognostic value of circulating tumor cells and their clusters in patients with advanced-stage breast cancer. Breast Cancer Res Treat 154(3):563–571
92. Hayes DF, Cristofanilli M, Budd GT, Ellis MJ, Stopeck A, Miller MC, Matera J, Allard WJ, Doyle GV, Terstappen LWWM (2006) Circulating tumor cells at each follow-up time point during therapy of metastatic breast cancer patients predict progression-free and overall survival. Clin Cancer Res 12(14):4218–4224
93. De Giorgi U, Valero V, Rohren E, Mego M, Doyle GV, Miller MC, Ueno NT, Handy BC, Reuben JM, Macapinlac HA, Hortobagyi GN, Cristofanilli M (2010) Circulating tumor cells and bone metastases as detected by FDG-PET/CT in patients with metastatic breast cancer. Ann Oncol 21(1):33–39
94. Bidard F-C, Peeters DJ, Fehm T, Nolé F, Gisbert-Criado R, Mavroudis D, Grisanti S, Generali D, Garcia-Saenz JA, Stebbing J, Caldas C, Gazzaniga P, Manso L, Zamarchi R, de Lascoiti AF, De Mattos-Arruda L, Ignatiadis M, Lebofsky R, van Laere SJ, Meier-Stiegen F, Sandri M-T, Vidal-Martinez J, Politaki E, Consoli F, Bottini A, Diaz-Rubio E, Krell J, Dawson S-J, Raimondi C, Rutten A, Janni W, Munzone E, Carañana V, Agelaki S, Almici C, Dirix L, Solomayer E-F, Zorzino L, Johannes H, Reis-Filho JS, Pantel K, Pierga J-Y, Michiels S (2014) Clinical validity of circulating tumour cells in patients with metastatic breast cancer: a pooled analysis of individual patient data. Lancet Oncol 15(4):406–414
95. Shiomi-Mouri Y, Kousaka J, Ando T, Tetsuka R, Nakano S, Yoshida M, Fujii K, Akizuki M, Imai T, Fukutomi T, Kobayashi K (2016) Clinical significance of circulating tumor cells (CTCs) with respect to optimal cut-off value and tumor markers in advanced/metastatic breast cancer. Breast Cancer 23(1):120–127
96. Bulfoni M, Gerratana L, Del Ben F, Marzinotto S, Sorrentino M, Turetta M, Scoles G, Toffoletto B, Isola M, Beltrami CA, Di Loreto C, Beltrami AP, Puglisi F, Cesselli D (2016) In patients with metastatic breast cancer the identification of circulating tumor cells in epithelial-to-mesenchymal transition is associated with a poor prognosis. Breast Cancer Res 18(1):30
97. Yan W-T, Cui X, Chen Q, Li Y-F, Cui Y-H, Wang Y, Jiang J (2017) Circulating tumor cell status monitors the treatment responses in breast cancer patients: a meta-analysis. Sci Rep 7:43464
98. Pierga J-Y, Hajage D, Bachelot T, Delaloge S, Brain E, Campone M, Dieras V, Rolland E, Mignot L, Mathiot C, Bidard F-C (2012) High independent prognostic and predictive value of circulating tumor cells compared with serum tumor markers in a large prospective trial in first-line chemotherapy for metastatic breast cancer patients. Ann Oncol 23(3):618–624

99. Khoo BL, Grenci G, Jing T, Lim YB, Lee SC, Thiery JP, Han J, Lim CT (2016) Liquid biopsy and therapeutic response: circulating tumor cell cultures for evaluation of anticancer treatment. Sci Adv 2(7):e1600274
100. Britton KM, Kirby JA, Lennard TWJ, Meeson AP (2011) Cancer stem cells and side population cells in breast cancer and metastasis. Cancer (Basel) 3(4):2106–2130
101. Marchini C, Montani M, Konstantinidou G, Orrù R, Mannucci S, Ramadori G, Gabrielli F, Baruzzi A, Berton G, Merigo F, Fin S, Iezzi M, Bisaro B, Sbarbati A, Zerani M, Galiè M, Amici A (2010) Mesenchymal/stromal gene expression signature relates to basal-like breast cancers, identifies bone metastasis and predicts resistance to therapies. PLoS One 5(11):e14131
102. Saad F, Lipton A (2010) SRC kinase inhibition: targeting bone metastases and tumor growth in prostate and breast cancer. Cancer Treat Rev 36(2):177–184
103. Zhang L, Teng Y, Zhang Y, Liu J, Xu L, Qu J, Hou K, Yang X, Liu Y, Qu X (2012) c-Src expression is predictive of poor prognosis in breast cancer patients with bone metastasis, but not in patients with visceral metastasis. APMIS 120(7):549–557
104. Rucci N, Recchia I, Angelucci A, Alamanou M, Del Fattore A, Fortunati D, Susa M, Fabbro D, Bologna M, Teti A (2006) Inhibition of protein kinase c-Src reduces the incidence of breast cancer metastases and increases survival in mice: implications for therapy. J Pharmacol Exp Ther 318(1):161–172
105. Mayer EL, Baurain J-F, Sparano J, Strauss L, Campone M, Fumoleau P, Rugo H, Awada A, Sy O, Llombart-Cussac A (2011) A phase 2 trial of dasatinib in patients with advanced HER2-positive and/or hormone receptor-positive breast cancer. Clin Cancer Res 17(21):6897–6904
106. Herold CI, Chadaram V, Peterson BL, Marcom PK, Hopkins J, Kimmick GG, Favaro J, Hamilton E, Welch RA, Bacus S, Blackwell KL (2011) Phase II trial of dasatinib in patients with metastatic breast cancer using real-time pharmacodynamic tissue biomarkers of Src inhibition to escalate dosing. Clin Cancer Res 17(18):6061–6070
107. Schott AF, Barlow WE, Van Poznak CH, Hayes DF, Moinpour CM, Lew DL, Dy PA, Keller ET, Keller JM, Hortobagyi GN (2016) Phase II studies of two different schedules of dasatinib in bone metastasis predominant metastatic breast cancer: SWOG S0622. Breast Cancer Res Treat 159(1):87–95
108. Fornier MN, Morris PG, Abbruzzi A, D'Andrea G, Gilewski T, Bromberg J, Dang C, Dickler M, Modi S, Seidman AD, Sklarin N, Chang J, Norton L, Hudis CA (2011) A phase I study of dasatinib and weekly paclitaxel for metastatic breast cancer. Ann Oncol 22(12):2575–2581
109. Somlo G, Atzori F, Strauss LC, Geese WJ, Specht JM, Gradishar WJ, Rybicki A, Sy O, Vahdat LT, Cortes J (2013) Dasatinib plus capecitabine for advanced breast cancer: safety and efficacy in phase I study CA180004. Clin Cancer Res 19(7):1884–1893
110. Ocana A, Gil-Martin M, Martín M, Rojo F, Antolín S, Guerrero Á, Trigo JM, Muñoz M, Carrasco E, Urruticoechea A, Bezares S, Caballero R, Carrasco E, Urruticoechea A (2015) A phase I study of the SRC kinase inhibitor dasatinib with trastuzumab and paclitaxel as first line therapy for patients with HER2-overexpressing advanced breast cancer. GEICAM/2010-04 study. Oncotarget 8:73144–73153
111. Mitri Z, Nanda R, Blackwell K, Costelloe CM, Hood I, Wei C, Brewster AM, Ibrahim NK, Koenig KB, Hortobagyi GN, Van Poznak C, Rimawi MF, Moulder-Thompson S, Translational Breast Cancer Research Consortium (2016) TBCRC-010: phase I/II study of dasatinib in combination with zoledronic acid for the treatment of breast cancer bone metastasis. Clin Cancer Res 22(23):5706–5712
112. Iyer S, Wang Z-G, Akhtari M, Zhao W, Seth P (2005) Targeting TGFbeta signaling for cancer therapy. Cancer Biol Ther 4(3):261–266
113. Dalal BI, Keown PA, Greenberg AH (1993) Immunocytochemical localization of secreted transforming growth factor-beta 1 to the advancing edges of primary tumors and to lymph node metastases of human mammary carcinoma. Am J Pathol 143(2):381–389
114. Buck MB, Fritz P, Dippon J, Zugmaier G, Knabbe C (2004) Prognostic significance of transforming growth factor beta receptor II in estrogen receptor-negative breast cancer patients. Clin Cancer Res 10(2):491–498

115. Rausch MP, Hahn T, Ramanathapuram L, Bradley-Dunlop D, Mahadevan D, Mercado-Pimentel ME, Runyan RB, Besselsen DG, Zhang X, Cheung H-K, Lee W-C, Ling LE, Akporiaye ET (2009) An orally active small molecule TGF-beta receptor I antagonist inhibits the growth of metastatic murine breast cancer. Anticancer Res 29(6):2099–2109

116. Garrison K, Hahn T, Lee W-C, Ling LE, Weinberg AD, Akporiaye ET (2012) The small molecule TGF-β signaling inhibitor SM16 synergizes with agonistic OX40 antibody to suppress established mammary tumors and reduce spontaneous metastasis. Cancer Immunol Immunother 61(4):511–521

117. Ganapathy V, Ge R, Grazioli A, Xie W, Banach-Petrosky W, Kang Y, Lonning S, McPherson J, Yingling JM, Biswas S, Mundy GR, Reiss M (2010) Targeting the transforming growth factor-β pathway inhibits human basal-like breast cancer metastasis. Mol Cancer 9(1):122

118. Fang Y, Chen Y, Yu L, Zheng C, Qi Y, Li Z, Yang Z, Zhang Y, Shi T, Luo J, Liu M (2013) Inhibition of breast cancer metastases by a novel inhibitor of TGF receptor 1. J Natl Cancer Inst 105(1):47–58

119. Yin JJ, Selander K, Chirgwin JM, Dallas M, Grubbs BG, Wieser R, Massagué J, Mundy GR, Guise TA (1999) TGF-β signaling blockade inhibits PTHrP secretion by breast cancer cells and bone metastases development. J Clin Invest 103(2):197–206

120. Wright LE, Frye JB, Lukefahr AL, Timmermann BN, Mohammad KS, Guise TA, Funk JL (2013) Curcuminoids block TGF-β signaling in human breast cancer cells and limit osteolysis in a murine model of breast cancer bone metastasis. J Nat Prod 76(3):316–321

121. Neuzillet C, Tijeras-Raballand A, Cohen R, Cros J, Faivre S, Raymond E, de Gramont A (2015) Targeting the TGFβ pathway for cancer therapy. Pharmacol Ther 147:22–31

122. Cabioglu N, Sahin AA, Morandi P, Meric-Bernstam F, Islam R, Lin HY, Bucana CD, Gonzalez-Angulo AM, Hortobagyi GN, Cristofanilli M (2009) Chemokine receptors in advanced breast cancer: differential expression in metastatic disease sites with diagnostic and therapeutic implications. Ann Oncol 20(6):1013–1019

123. Richert MM, Vaidya KS, Mills CN, Wong D, Korz W, Hurst DR, Welch DR (2009) Inhibition of CXCR4 by CTCE-9908 inhibits breast cancer metastasis to lung and bone. Oncol Rep 21(3):761–767

124. Wong D, Korz W (2008) Translating an antagonist of chemokine receptor CXCR4: from bench to bedside. Clin Cancer Res 14(24):7975–7980

125. Huang EH, Singh B, Cristofanilli M, Gelovani J, Wei C, Vincent L, Cook KR, Lucci A (2009) A CXCR4 antagonist CTCE-9908 inhibits primary tumor growth and metastasis of breast cancer. J Surg Res 155(2):231–236

126. Hassan S, Buchanan M, Jahan K, Aguilar-Mahecha A, Gaboury L, Muller WJ, Alsawafi Y, Mourskaia AA, Siegel PM, Salvucci O, Basik M (2011) CXCR4 peptide antagonist inhibits primary breast tumor growth, metastasis and enhances the efficacy of anti-VEGF treatment or docetaxel in a transgenic mouse model. Int J Cancer 129(1):225–232

127. Williams SA, Harata-Lee Y, Comerford I, Anderson RL, Smyth MJ, McColl SR (2010) Multiple functions of CXCL12 in a syngeneic model of breast cancer. Mol Cancer 9(1):250

128. Gil M, Seshadri M, Komorowski MP, Abrams SI, Kozbor D (2013) Targeting CXCL12/CXCR4 signaling with oncolytic virotherapy disrupts tumor vasculature and inhibits breast cancer metastases. Proc Natl Acad Sci 110(14):E1291–E1300

129. Peng S-B, Zhang X, Paul D, Kays LM, Gough W, Stewart J, Uhlik MT, Chen Q, Hui Y-H, Zamek-Gliszczynski MJ, Wijsman JA, Credille KM, Yan LZ (2015) Targeting CXCL12/CXCR4 signaling with oncolytic virotherapy disrupts tumor vasculature and inhibits breast cancer metastases. Mol Cancer Ther 14(2):480–490

130. Henriksen G, Fisher DR, Roeske JC, Bruland ØS, Larsen RH (2003) Targeting of osseous sites with alpha-emitting 223Ra: comparison with the beta-emitter 89Sr in mice. J Nucl Med 44(2):252–259

131. Nilsson S, Franzén L, Parker C, Tyrrell C, Blom R, Tennvall J, Lennernäs B, Petersson U, Johannessen DC, Sokal M, Pigott K, Yachnin J, Garkavij M, Strang P, Harmenberg J, Bolstad B, Bruland OS (2007) Bone-targeted radium-223 in symptomatic, hormone-refractory

prostate cancer: a randomised, multicentre, placebo-controlled phase II study. Lancet Oncol 8(7):587–594

132. Parker C, Nilsson S, Heinrich D, Helle SI, O'Sullivan JM, Fosså SD, Chodacki A, Wiechno P, Logue J, Seke M, Widmark A, Johannessen DC, Hoskin P, Bottomley D, James ND, Solberg A, Syndikus I, Kliment J, Wedel S, Boehmer S, Dall'Oglio M, Franzén L, Coleman R, Vogelzang NJ, O'Bryan-Tear CG, Staudacher K, Garcia-Vargas J, Shan M, Bruland ØS, Sartor O, ALSYMPCA Investigators (2013) Alpha emitter radium-223 and survival in metastatic prostate cancer. N Engl J Med 369(3):213–223

133. Coleman R, Aksnes A-K, Naume B, Garcia C, Jerusalem G, Piccart M, Vobecky N, Thuresson M, Flamen P (2014) A phase IIa, nonrandomized study of radium-223 dichloride in advanced breast cancer patients with bone-dominant disease. Breast Cancer Res Treat 145(2):411–418

Chapter 8
Therapeutic Options for Metastatic Breast Cancer

Manpreet Sambi, Bessi Qorri, William Harless, and Myron R. Szewczuk

Abstract Metastatic breast cancer is the most common cancer in women after skin cancer, with a 5-year survival rate of 26%. Due to its high prevalence, it is important to develop therapies that go beyond those that just provide palliation of symptoms. Currently, there are several types of therapies available to help treat breast cancer including: hormone therapy, immunotherapy, and chemotherapy, with each one depending on both the location of metastases and morphological characteristics. Although technological and scientific advancements continue to pave the way for improved therapies that adopt a targeted and personalized approach, the fact remains that the outcomes of current first-line therapies have not significantly improved over the last decade. In this chapter, we review the current understanding of the pathology of metastatic breast cancer before thoroughly discussing local and systemic therapies that are administered to patients diagnosed with metastatic breast cancer. In addition, our review will also elaborate on the genetic profile that is characteristic of breast cancer as well as the local tumor microenvironment that shapes and promotes tumor growth and cancer progression. Lastly, we will present promising novel therapies being developed for the treatment of this disease.

Keywords Metastatic breast cancer · Targeted therapies · Tumor microenvironment · Nanoparticles · Drug delivery systems · Immunotherapy · Oseltamivir phosphate

Manpreet Sambi and Bessi Qorri contributed equally as first authors.

M. Sambi · B. Qorri · M. R. Szewczuk (✉)
Department of Biomedical and Molecular Sciences, Queen's University,
Kingston, ON, Canada
e-mail: 13ms84@queensu.ca; szewczuk@queensu.ca

W. Harless
Encyt Technologies Inc., Membertou, NS, Canada

© Springer Nature Switzerland AG 2019
A. Ahmad (ed.), *Breast Cancer Metastasis and Drug Resistance*,
Advances in Experimental Medicine and Biology 1152,
https://doi.org/10.1007/978-3-030-20301-6_8

8.1   Introduction

With cancer rates projected to rise up to 30–40% within the next decade and a half [1], developing a treatment protocol that is effective at prolonging progression-free survival (PFS), or perhaps even a cure for metastatic breast cancer is an important and difficult task. This task may be particularly challenging for metastatic breast cancer as it has a unique pathophysiology that separates it from other forms of cancer. Clinical manifestation of metastatic disease may not appear until decades after it is first diagnosed – at which point metastases may take over the rest of the body. Following establishment of metastases, resection is often not possible and disease progression becomes inevitable. Metastatic disease prognoses have slowly improved over the last 30 years but survival rates remain low with only 2–5% of patients diagnosed with metastatic breast cancer surviving at least 10 years [2]. Novel approaches are now emerging that may improve our ability to treat this disease more effectively. An understanding of the most recent advancements and their potential to improve the clinical treatment of patients with metastatic breast cancer is of great importance.

This chapter will provide an overview of the pathology of metastatic breast cancer, including the genetic profile of the disease, as well as current therapeutic options available to patients who present with this disease. We will also be placing an emphasis on the unique microenvironment of metastatic breast cancer and the relevant targets that are currently being explored as candidates for targeted therapy as well as novel therapeutic options for the treatment of this malignancy.

8.2   Overview of Metastatic Breast Cancer Pathology

Metastasis is a complex process that ultimately permits malignant cells to establish secondary tumors at distant sites. This process is divided into three main components – local invasion, intravasation, and extravasation [3]. As depicted in Fig. 8.1, following formation and establishment of the primary tumor, the malignant cells begin the first phase of the metastatic cascade: initiating invasion of the local tumor microenvironment (TME) and tumor stroma. At this stage, malignant cells begin to disaggregate as a result of a disruption in their cell-cell adhesion. This is marked by the loss of epithelial cell adhesion marker E-cadherin, which forms the core of the epithelial adherens junction. Additionally, loss of E-cadherin expression has also been associated with the diffused cytoplasmic and nuclear localization of β-catenin, which would otherwise be associated with cell-cell junctions. The liberated and unphosphorylated β-catenin then promotes the expression of mesenchymal proteins such as N-cadherin, vimentin and fibronectin [4]. Thus, loss of E-cadherin expression and its associated downstream events mediate the process of epithelial-to-mesenchymal transition (EMT) during which malignant cells undergo morphological changes acquiring a more invasive and highly motile phenotype [5]. During

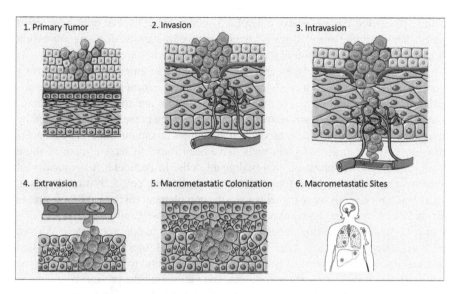

Fig. 8.1 General schematic of the metastatic cascade. Following formation of the primary tumor (1), malignant cells invade the local TME and stroma (2), intravasate into the blood and/or lymphatic vessels (3) extravasate to a distant secondary site (4), and establish macrometastatic colonies (5) resulting in the development of metastatic tumor clusters at specific parts of the body, particular the brain, lungs, liver and bones

intravasation, malignant cells invade the basal membrane and enter blood and lymphatic vessels. This is a critical step of metastatic progression as only those malignant cells that are capable of detaching from the primary tumor and surviving in circulation are then able to exit the bloodstream at some predetermined sites [6]. Once disseminated cells reach their destination, the next stage of the metastatic cascade is initiated – extravasation. This process is highly dynamic and involves the modulation of invading tumor cells and the endothelial cells comprising the vessel wall to induce vessel remodeling and simultaneously inhibiting vascular leakage. At the molecular level, this particular process is mediated by the pro-metastatic gene expression of Twist, which targets cell adhesion and intravascular migration of malignant cells [7]. Upon exiting the vasculature, malignant cells are then able to establish micro- and macrometastatic colonies at distant sites thereby contributing to metastatic disease as each metastatic colony contributes to the overall progression of metastatic disease.

Each type of cancer that develops metastases has certain organs in which metastases are prevalent, with the most common across all cancer types being the brain, lungs, and bones [8, 9]. To explain this seemingly preferential spread of metastatic clusters, Stephen Paget proposed the 'seed and soil' hypothesis stating that tumor metastasis is the result of favorable interactions amid metastatic tumor cells (the 'seed'), and their organ microenvironment ('the soil') [10]. As such, the cross-talk between the tumor cells and the tumor microenvironment (TME) plays a critical role in regulating the metastatic potential of malignant cells. For breast cancer in particular, a defining morphological characteristic of metastatic disease progression is the architectural disruption of the glandular microenvironment [11].

As an extension of the 'seed and soil' hypothesis, an emerging field in further understanding the advent of predetermined sites where cancer cells in systemic circulation of metastatic therapy is the study of exosomes and their role in 'priming' secondary sites for metastasis. Exosomes are small membrane vesicles secreted by many cell types that provide a mode of intercellular communication [12]. Rapidly growing cells, such as malignant cells, have been found to secrete more of these vesicles than slower-growing, non-malignant cells. In particular, the quantity of secreted exosomes has been found to increase following cell activation, hypoxia, oxidative injury, exposure to proteins from the complement cascade and exposure to stress [13]. Due to increased exosome secretion in these conditions that are hallmarks of cancer progression, it has been postulated that tumor- and platelet-derived exosomes are components of the TME that play pivotal roles in tumor progression and metastasis. Tumor-derived exosomes have been found to play roles in altering the local and systemic microenvironment, and facilitating the pre-metastatic niche allowing for metastases to establish in specific areas [14]. The critical roles of the TME and exosomes as they pertain to cancer progression will be covered in detail in the sections below.

8.3   Current Therapeutic Options for Metastatic Breast Cancer

8.3.1   Local Treatments

8.3.1.1   Surgery

Presently, metastatic breast cancer is considered an incurable disease and treatment is focused on therapies designed to prolong a patient's life and to palliate symptoms associated with the disease process. Exceptions to this general principle include a small subset of patients who present with oligometastatic disease characterized by solitary or very few metastatic deposits. However, it is estimated that less than 10% of patients presenting with metastatic breast cancer are amenable to surgical removal [15]. The efficacy of surgical resection of metastatic breast cancer has been documented in patients with only liver metastases. An aggressive hepatic surgical approach has been associated with favorable long term survival, with 2- and 5-year survival rates of 86% and 61%, respectively [16]. In addition, hepatic surgery for breast cancer that has metastasized to the liver has allowed for the discontinuation of chemotherapy in 46% of cases of patients with breast cancer presenting liver metastases, ultimately prolonging overall survival [17]. In contrast to oligometastatic disease in colorectal cancer, where an aggressive surgical approach to oligometastases remains a standard of care, this has not become standard practice in treating metastatic breast cancer and remains highly individualized. However, distinct patients may benefit from an aggressive surgical approach in an attempt to cure the disease, thereby making clinical judgement and multidisciplinary collaborations essential when determining the optimal approach for these patients owing to the fact that a cure currently remains a theoretical possibility.

Surgical removal of the primary breast tumor in patients with metastatic breast cancer remains an area of controversy with no consensus on a standard of care. A review of ten retrospective studies in women with metastatic breast cancer undergoing surgical removal of the primary tumor revealed an improved PFS compared to the women not undergoing surgery. The pooled hazard ratio for overall mortality in these studies was 0.65 (95% confidence interval (CI) 0.59–0.72) in favor of patients undergoing surgery [18]. In a population-based study of women with metastatic breast cancer, it was found that women with excision of the primary breast tumor with negative surgical margins had a marked 40% reduced risk of death from the disease when compared to women who did not undergo surgery. Reduced mortality risk was noted amongst patients with different metastatic sites, but was particularly evident in women with metastases in the bone. Women with positive surgical margins did not have a statistically significant difference in survival from those who did not undergo surgery [19, 20]. Following control for factors such as age, comorbidities, tumor grade, histology, and sites of metastases, primary tumor resection was associated with a median survival of 31.9 months compared to only 15.4 months for those who did not undergo surgery [21].

Contrary to these results, a recent prospective study revealed that there was no survival benefit following surgical removal of the breast and lymph nodes in women with metastatic breast cancer [22]. It is evident from these conflicting findings that further research is necessary to establish the role of surgical removal of the breast in patients with metastatic breast cancer.

8.3.1.2 Radiation

Radiotherapy is treatment with high-energy rays or particles that target and destroy cancer cell DNA, resulting in necrosis, apoptosis, or accelerated cell senescence [23]. There are two main forms of radiotherapy: external beam radiation, which occurs from outside of the body, and internal radiation, also referred to as brachytherapy, in which the radioactive source is delivered inside the body for a short period of time [24]. Radiation is most efficacious in cases where there are relatively few malignant cells that are well vascularized; therefore, radiation has been shown to be best suited for tumor cells that are located at the periphery as opposed to those in the center where there is a large volume of malignant cells typically found in hypoxic conditions [23]. However, radiation therapy in metastatic disease is almost entirely reserved for the palliation of symptoms associated with metastases at various sites in the body, especially bone metastases.

An area in which radiotherapy potentially plays a curative role is in the treatment of CNS metastases. Brain metastases as a result of breast cancer occur in approximately 10–16% of cases, typically among women with larger tumors and more aggressive histological subtypes. Whole brain radiation therapy and sterotactic radiation are currently the standard of care for CNS metastases; however, it is not yet clear whether these methods are as efficacious in breast cancer compared with other solid tumors [25, 26]. Though sterotactic radiation may be a treatment option for those patients with isolated lesions, this represents only a small subset of patients where disease spread is confined to an isolated lesion in the CNS, and thus is mainly used for palliation of symptoms.

8.3.2 Systemic Therapies

8.3.2.1 Hormone Therapy

Following surgery, hormone therapy can be used as an additional treatment option if it proves efficacious for the patient; however, it is highly dependent on the cell type(s) present in the cancer. While local therapies are ideal for targeting primary tumor masses or large metastases, systemic therapies allow for the effective treatment of cancer that has already metastasized. Cancer cells are referred to as hormone positive if they express the estrogen receptor (ER) and/or the progesterone receptor (PR). For hormone receptor positive metastatic breast cancer, hormone therapy is generally the first treatment option provided that the patient is not suffering metastatic disease that is threatening visceral organ function [27]. Randomized studies have demonstrated that the initiation of hormone therapy yields comparable long-term results to chemotherapy while avoiding the associated negative side effects [28]. Hormone therapy works to arrest or delay the progression of hormone-sensitive tumors by either blocking the body's ability to produce hormones or by interfering with the effect of those hormones on breast cancer cells. There are several classes of drugs with distinct mechanisms of action.

Gonadotropin-releasing hormone (GnRH) agonists, for example, also known as luteinizing hormone-releasing hormone (LH-RH) agonists block ovarian function by interfering with signals from the pituitary gland that stimulate the ovaries to produce estrogen [29]. Alternatively, estrogen production can be blocked through aromatase inhibitors (AIs). Aromatase is the enzyme used by the body's peripheral tissues to make estrogen. Anastrozole and letrozole are two nonsteroidal AIs that temporarily inactivate aromatase; however, letrozole has been found to be a more potent suppressor of body aromatization and estrogen levels [30]. Exemestane is an orally active steroidal AI that permanently inactivates the enzyme [31]. It has been shown that exemestane demonstrates activity following prior failure of other AIs. In addition, patients are also able to receive exemestane as their first AI and still have therapeutic effects from anastrozole or letrozole if their disease progresses, suggesting that partial resistance between the steroidal and non-steroidal AIs is independent of the sequence in which they are administered [32]. Selective estrogen receptor modulators (SERMs) are synthetic molecules that bind to ER, preventing estrogen from binding and blocking its effects. Tamoxifen is the typical SERM for ER+ breast cancer, exerting its effects by blocking the effects of estrogen in breast tissue (acting as an estrogen antagonist) but acts similar to estrogen in the uterus and bone (acting as an estrogen agonist) [33]. Alternatively, fulvestrant has a higher affinity for the ER compared to tamoxifen, but has no agonistic effects, functioning only as an estrogen antagonist. Following fulvestrant binding to the ER, both the receptor and the cell are targeted for destruction [34]. However, it is important to consider the menopausal status of women when prescribing hormonal therapies.

Premenopausal women Premenopausal women with functioning ovaries and ER+/PR+ breast cancer, have a large amount of aromatase in their ovaries. General treatment options include ovarian ablation using surgical oophorectomy, suppression of estrogen through LH-RH agonists, or SERMs like tamoxifen [35]. All of these treatment options work to limit estrogen levels. Following the decrease in estrogen levels, gonadotrophin levels increase, and the ovarian aromatase promoter is highly sensitive to them. As such, AIs are contraindicated in premenopausal women for breast cancer treatment without administration in combination with LH-RH agonists [36].

Postmenopausal women Postmenopausal women have a decline and complete arrest in estrogen production from the ovaries; thus, it is understandable that their hormonal therapy would differ from that of premenopausal women. Studies have documented that postmenopausal women with ER+/PR+ metastatic breast cancer benefit more from treatment with AI rather than treatment with tamoxifen [32].

In general, the aforementioned hormone therapies are well-tolerated by the body. Although women who respond to one hormonal intervention may eventually become less sensitive to it effects, it was found that they could still respond to a second type of hormone therapy. As a result, some patients benefit from three or four hormonal therapies in sequence, such as switching between AIs and estrogen agonists, which have demonstrated good quality of life outcomes [37]. However, even sequential treatment with various hormone therapies results in metastatic breast cancer eventually becoming refractory to hormonal treatment. At this point, refractory breast cancer as well as ER- breast cancer is typically treated with chemotherapy.

8.3.2.2 Chemotherapy

Advanced breast cancer is not considered curative and the disease is aggressive in its spread throughout the body; as such, the goal of chemotherapy treatment is to prolong survival, alleviate or prevent tumor-associated symptoms, and improve overall quality of life. Paradoxically, chemotherapy causes a variety of toxicities to the body. Although endocrine therapy yields comparable long-term results to chemotherapy, patients that are refractive to endocrine therapy are started on chemotherapy so as to induce a rapid tumor response. The duration and dosage of chemotherapeutic drugs play a major role in patient outcomes, with patients more likely to respond to and have extended periods of tumor control with first-line chemotherapy [28]. With each subsequent line of treatment, there is a decrease in response rate and time for tumor progression. Although therapies of various chemo drugs are used to treat earlier stage breast cancer, advanced metastatic breast cancer is typically treated with single chemotherapy drugs as combination chemotherapy has not been shown to be clearly superior to single agent chemotherapy drugs used sequentially.

Chemotherapy works by targeting cell division. This is critical as malignant cells are characterized by uncontrolled cell growth – and thus are appropriate targets for this kind of therapy. However, there are other non-malignant cells such as those found in hair follicles, nails, mouth, digestive tract, and bone marrow that also exhibit a proliferation profile similar to that of cancer cell growth which ultimately leads to the adverse effects associated with chemotherapy treatment [28]. Chemotherapy is given either as a neoadjuvant, prior to surgery, so that less tissue needs to be removed, or as an adjuvant following recovery after surgery. Classes of chemo drugs for metastatic breast cancer include taxanes, anthracyclines and antimetabolities [38].

Taxanes, such as docetaxel and paclitaxel, are microtubule inhibitors that are the most commonly used agents for metastatic breast cancer [38]. Over the last few years, there have been a growing number of clinical trials demonstrating progression free survival advantages in metastatic disease using taxanes. Taxane-based therapy is currently the primary treatment option for patients previously treated with anthracyclines that faced disease progression or recurrence [39].

Alternatively, anthracyclines such as doxorubicin, epirubicin, and pegylated lipodoxorubicin (PLD) target cancer cells by damaging their genetic material [38]. Anthracyclines were one of the first chemotherapeutic agents discovered; however, cardiac toxicity and secondary hematological malignancy concerns still remain [40]. Of these, doxorubicin is the most widely used anthracycline; however, its efficacy is limited by its high toxicity, which may lead to drug resistance. PLD, which is doxorubicin confined in liposomes, has comparable results for progression free survival to doxorubicin while avoiding toxicities such as cardiotoxicity, vomiting and alopecia [41].

Capecitabine is a pyrimidine antimetabolite that is a 5-fluorouracil (5-FU) prodrug that acts as an oral chemotherapy agent [38]. Capecitabine has been efficacious in paclitaxel-refractory metastatic breast cancer patients who had been previously administered an anthracycline. In addition to its efficacy in taxane-refractory breast cancer, being an oral drug that can be administered at home renders, it is more advantageous over other chemotherapeutic drugs [42].

8.3.2.3   Targeted Therapies

Biological Agents as Cancer Immunotherapy

Human epidermal growth factor receptor (HER2) is overexpressed in approximately 30% of breast cancers. When HER2 is amplified, the encoded protein, a transmembrane glycoprotein receptor ($P185^{HER2}$), is expressed at abnormally high levels in malignant cells, acting as a HER2 receptor [43]. Cells with HER2 gene amplification and protein overexpression are referred to as HER2+ cells and are associated with a clinically aggressive disease phenotype and a poorer prognosis due to shorter disease-free and overall survival [44]. HER2 overexpression has been found to confer resistance to endocrine therapies resulting in a need for additional therapies required for treatment. In a randomized study of patients with ER+, PR+ or both ER+ and PR+ metastatic breast cancer, patients were divided into three independent clinical trials to receive second-line hormone therapy and were subsequently analyzed for HER2 serum levels. Patients with ER+ breast cancer with serum HER2 were less likely to respond to hormone treatment (23%) compared to those with non-elevated HER2 levels (45%) [45]. These findings suggest that HER2 expression can decrease sensitivity to hormone therapy in patients with hormone receptor positive breast cancer. Models have also demonstrated that even ER+ breast cancer cells that originally lack HER2 acquire resistance over time with enhanced expression of receptors involved in cross-talk with ER [46].

HER2+ cancers are typically treated with anti-HER2 drugs such as trastuzumab (Herceptin). Trastuzumab is a recombinant monoclonal antibody that recognizes and targets an extracellular domain of $P185^{HER2}$. Trastuzumab is active and well tolerated as a first-line treatment for women with metastatic breast cancer with HER2 overexpression [44]. As a safety precaution, the occurrence of cardiac events is monitored while patients are treated with trastuzumab or other anti-HER2 drugs such as pertuzumab. Reports of the risk of cardiac toxicity was shown to be moderate and reversible in the majority of the patients [47].

Another monoclonal antibody used for targeted therapies of metastatic breast cancer is bevacizumab, which recognizes vascular endothelial growth factor (VEGF). VEGF is known to promote angiogenesis and has been implicated in the growth and metastasis of breast cancer. In previously treated metastatic breast cancer, bevacizumab was evaluated in a dose-escalated trial with the 10 mg/kg every other week, which was the optimal dose with acceptable toxicity [48, 49]. Additional details of the role of VEGF and angiogenesis in metastatic breast cancer progression will be covered in detail in upcoming sections.

Nanoparticles as a Targeted Delivery System

In recent years, advancements in polymer science have allowed for the development of polymeric nanoparticles capable of encapsulating therapeutic drugs, with a particular focus on cancer therapy [50]. This targeted therapy is unique in that it can utilize any of the previously mentioned therapies, both local and systemic, and deliver them in a way to target specifically malignant cell types. By doing so they typically offer improved pharmacokinetics, controlled and sustained drug release, and most importantly, lower systemic toxicity, which is a limitation of the many of the current therapies [51]. This form of targeted therapy allows for the utilization of the tumor microenvironment to direct therapy specifically to malignant cells in hopes of avoiding potentially toxic treatment to normal healthy cells. This method is currently in use for the delivery of taxanes such as paclitaxel, demonstrating efficacy in taxane-resistant cancer [52]; however, it has the potential to be expanded to delivering other therapies including hormone and biological agents without having their associated widespread effects and related toxicities. The increased efficacy of this type of therapy relies on the functionalization of these polymers in order to specifically target malignant cells. This is accomplished through the use of pH responsive [53], conjugated [54], functionalized [55], amphiphilic polymers capable of self-assembly [56]. Additional details on the development of nanoparticles and their applications are discussed in further detail in sections below.

8.3.2.4   Combination Therapies

Each of the aforementioned therapies comes with its own benefits and drawbacks. In an attempt to avoid potential adverse effects, combination therapies have been increasingly studied with the intention of maximizing the efficacy of treatment. These combination therapies are particularly focused on utilizing a therapy as an adjuvant or neoadjuvant to chemotherapy to improve survival outcomes and disease-free progression. For example, individuals with HER2- tumors do not receive additional benefits when their chemotherapy treatment is supplemented with trastuzumab; however, administering trastuzumab in addition to chemotherapy has demonstrated favorable outcomes for individuals with HER2+ tumors [28]. Trastuzumab and other biological agents that are active against metastatic breast cancer have also demonstrated great potential for enhancing the effects of chemotherapy to improve survival outcomes. Synergistic activity has been observed between trastuzumab and chemotherapies such as docetaxel and carboplatin and additive activity has been observed with paclitaxel, doxorubicin and epirubicin. However, there is a substantially increased risk of cardiotoxicity employing anthracyclines with trastuzumab and this combination is generally avoided [39]. When combined with docetaxel, trastuzumab was demonstrated to be superior to docetaxel monotherapy as first-line treatment of patients with HER2+ metastatic breast cancer in terms of overall survival, response rate, response duration, time to progression, and time to treatment failure, with generally little to no additional toxicity. However, neutropenia was seen more commonly with combination therapy than with docetaxel alone [57].

Trastuzumab in combination with anastrozole has been found to improve outcomes for patients with HER2+/ER+ metastatic breast cancer; however, adverse and serious adverse events were observed more frequently with the combination therapy. This was the first study (TAnDEM trial) to combine a hormonal agent, trastuzumab and chemotherapy for HER2/ER co-positive breast cancer [58]. Although potentially more effective as a short-term treatment, these combination therapies appear to be associated with increased risk of adverse effects. As such, dosages that are more effective within the therapeutic windows need to be elucidated for combination therapies to exert their effects while minimizing negative side effects. In a study evaluating the efficacy of trastuzumab, patients with HER2+ metastatic breast cancer were assigned to receive either standard chemotherapy alone, or standard chemotherapy in addition to trastuzumab. Those patients who had not previously received adjuvant therapy with an anthracycline were treated with doxorubicin and cyclophosphamide with or without trastuzumab. Patients who had been previously treated with adjuvant anthracycline were treated with paclitaxel alone or with trastuzumab. In both chemotherapy options, combination with trastuzumab was associated with a significantly higher rate of overall response and a significantly lower rate of death at 1 year [43].

Bevacizumab, another targeted therapy has also been studied for efficacy and safety when combined with other standard chemotherapy regimens versus chemotherapy alone for first-line treatment of patients with HER2- metastatic breast cancer. The combination of bevacizumab with capecitabine, taxane-based paclitaxel, or anthracycline-based chemotherapies results in increased progression free survival with a safety profile that is comparable to prior phase III studies [59]. The efficacy of bevacizumab is noted as treatment of 15 mg/kg every 3 weeks resulted in a significant increase in progression-free survival when combined with docetaxel as first-line therapy for metastatic breast cancer when compared with docetaxel with a placebo. Furthermore, it is important to note that the addition of bevacizumab to docetaxel did not significantly impact the safety profile of docetaxel [60].

In summary, treatments for cancer are generally divided into local and systemic therapies. Metastatic breast cancer is largely a systemic disease that requires systemic options; however, an important caveat remains that non-specific treatment is often toxic to non-malignant cells in the body and results in numerous adverse effects. The efficacy of systemic therapies is highly dependent upon the expression of ER/PR and EGFR. A graphic representation of the various treatment options discussed above is provided below and is based on the expression of the three candidate hormone receptors (Fig. 8.2).

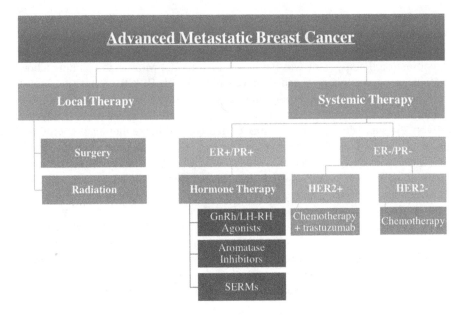

Fig. 8.2 Overview of the treatment options for metastatic breast cancer. Depending on the location and size of metastases, local or systemic therapy may be chosen. Therapy will also depend on the cancer cell subtypes present in the patient, as well as the patient's menopausal status

8.4 Genetic Profile of Metastatic Breast Cancer: Implications, Current and Potential Therapeutic Targets

8.4.1 Currently Identified Driver Mutations of Metastatic Breast Cancer

A key area of research interest is to determine the underlying genetic events that drive metastatic breast cancer in order to develop more efficient treatment methods. There are several candidate driver genes that have been uncovered that will be discussed in detail below. Firstly, driver mutations either directly or indirectly "drive" or facilitate the alteration of normal cells to cancer cells by activating oncogenes (mutations that act through gain-of-function) or inactivating tumor suppressor genes (mutations that act through loss of function) [61]. Passenger mutations, on the other hand, are random mutations that accumulate over time and do not influence tumorigenesis [62]. Through computational analysis, Lee et al. [62] were able to elucidate five candidate driver mutations that may be involved in breast cancer metastasis: SLC22A5, NUP93, PCGF6, PKP2 and lastly, ADPGK. Mutations in these genes are known to induce EMT and increase migratory capability. Specifically, PKP2 is an activator of cancer metastasis and therefore, a mutation in this driver gene has been proposed to lead to hyperactivity of this gene. The roles that SLC22A5, NUP93, PCGF6 and ADPGK play in breast cancer have not yet been elucidated; however, both SLC22A5 and NUP93 have been confirmed as being one of ten breast cancer driver genes [63–65].

In contrast, Lefebvre et al. [66] identified 12 additional driver genes that have been implicated in the progression of metastatic breast cancers including TP53, PIK3CA, GATA3, MAP3K1, CDH1, AKT1, MAP2K4, PTEN, CBFB, and CDKN2A. A genomic analysis study done on 105 breast cancer patients revealed that TP53 mutations were identified in 15.2% of breast tumors, whereas PIK3CA accounts for 35.2% of mutations in breast tumors [67]. The above have been previously identified as drivers of breast cancer; however, two new driver genes were identified through computational analysis of the genetic profiles of 216 metastatic breast cancers: ESR1 (EStrogen Receptor 1) and RB1 (retinoblastoma tumor suppressor gene) [66]. Both have been shown to mediate resistance to endocrine therapy as patients with ESR1 mutations did not respond well to endocrine therapy. ESR1 was the most frequently observed mutation in metastatic cells. RB1 is a tumor suppressor protein that regulates the cell cycle and is normally phosphorylated by CDK4. In metastatic breast cancers, a mutation in RB1 presents as a loss of function of the protein. Palbociclib[1] is a potent small molecule inhibitor of CDK4 and requires the presence of RB1 in order to exhibit therapeutic effects, thus, metastatic breast cancers with a mutation in this gene would not be positively affected by this inhibitor, resulting in RB1 mutations being able to potentially predict the efficacy of this inhibitor.

From these separate studies alone, there has yet to be a consensus on which driver genes are involved in the progression of metastatic breast cancer. Furthermore, genetic variations between cells of the primary tumor and those of the metastatic sites of kidney cancer reveal a 30% genetic match of cancer cells [66]. Therefore, not only are there potential driver mutations that can act as screening tools, but mutations that take place at secondary sites have an even more unique genetic profile that may be exploited when developing therapies.

8.4.2 Epigenetic Changes of Metastatic Breast Cancer and Potential Therapeutic Targets

Epigenetic changes present an additional facet of metastatic breast cancer biology to consider when determining how to proceed with treatment options as genetic alterations go beyond mutations. For example, demethylation at one locus and hypermethylation at another can lead to cancer development and progression. Oncogenes, for example, are a subset of genes that are normally under tight regulation and activation of these genes leads to tumor progression [70]. HER2, which

---

[1] Palbociclib is a selective inhibitor applied to HER2-negative and ER-positive metastatic breast cancer patients. It was recently approved to be administered as a treatment option when given alongside aromatase inhibitors, such as letrozole, and has shown to be efficacious, particularly for patients who had previously received endocrine therapy [68, 69].

was discussed in detail above, is an example of an oncogene that is activated in about 20% of breast cancer and amplification of this gene has been associated with a more aggressive phenotype [70]. In contrast, tumor suppressor genes, as the name suggests, act to prevent tumorigenesis and a loss of function in these genes leads to tumor development. Tumor suppressor genes have been shown to be abnormally silenced, while oncogenes increase their expression in a number of cancers [70]. Examples of silenced tumor suppressor genes include PTEN, TP53, BRCA1, ATM and others.

DNA methyltransferases (DNMTs) are required to facilitate genetic alterations and thus are continuously active and are critical to the growth and development of cancer. DNMTs are particularly important when altering the genetic profile of cancer cells in response to the changes in the surrounding environment [71]. For example, DNMTs can be involved in upregulating proliferative pathways to compensate for the effects of cytotoxic therapy. Therefore, because the activity level of DNMTs is higher in cancer cells when compared with normal cells, DNMTs could be a potential therapeutic target and a change in their activity could severely limit the ability of cancer cells to upregulate or downregulate various pathways that are crucial to their growth and response to the TME.

A knockout study conducted on DNMT, Dmnt-1 of leukemic stem cells, was able to successfully impede leukemogeneis and leukemic stem cell renewal without affecting normal hematopoiesis [72]. Inhibitors that are capable of targeting specific DNMTs that are critical to the epigenetic events that take place to promote breast cancer progression and metastasis are an area that should be further explored. In particular, the events that mediate hypermeythation and hypomethylation are proposed to be independent events that may be controlled by different processes [73]. For example, methylation of the p16 gene, a tumor suppressor gene that normally controls cell growth, was shown to be silenced and has been implicated in metastasis [74]. Szyf et al., eloquently outline aberrantly methylated genes in breast cancer in their review [73]. In brief, they present 33 hypermethylated genes that are implicated in breast cancer progression and metastasis including the BRAC-1 oncogene, ER, and p16, to name a few. Similar to the knockout study on Dmnt-1, inhibition of this gene through the use of the nucleoside analog 5-aza-Cd and an antisense oligonucleotide have different effects, but have shown some promising results that ultimately led to the induction of tumor suppressor genes and inhibition of DNA replication.

The caveat of using DNMT inhibitors as potential therapeutic agents is their negative effects on the normal methylation events that take place in cells. For example, one potent, yet unstable methylation inhibitor that was applied to inhibit the metastatic ability of MDA-MB-231 cells is SAM (S-adenosyl-L-methionine). SAM acts to inhibit active demethylation of cells and in turn, results in in inhibition of the invasiveness of MDA-MB-231 cells [73]. Therefore, while there are a large number of candidate genes whose methylation patterns are changed and lead to the progression of metastasis, determining which methyltransferase to target without negatively affecting normal cells is an important distinction to consider.

8.4.3 CRISPR-Cas9 Technology and Its Applications for Metastatic Breast Cancer

CRISPR-Cas9 (clustered, regularly interspaced, short palindromic repeats with its CRISPR-associated protein 9) has been proposed as a therapeutic option for editing genetic mutations including, but not limited to, those that confer resistance to therapy and those that allow cancer to grow uncontrollably. CRISPR is a component of the bacterial immune system and its mode of action is described in detail in several papers [75, 76]. In brief, it is a gene-editing tool that has the capacity to seek out a gene of interest and "cut" it out and replace the removed portion with a new genetic code i.e., the correct sequence when editing a mutation.

The technological relevance of CRISPR to cancer comes in many forms, with one such avenue being the generation of more accurate study models in order to map disease progression as a function of genetic mutations. Recently, Xue et al. [77], generated a liver cancer mouse model through CRISPR-mediated gene alterations of two very critical tumor suppressor genes: PTEN and p53. This method of generating mouse models that are capable of mimicking the genetic events that may drive the progression of other malignancies provides a more accurate modeling system that is organ specific and can lead to more efficient drug development.

Specifically in relation to metastatic breast cancer, while there are several candidate models that allow scientists to understand disease progression and design therapeutic targets that are able to reduce tumor growth and metastasis [78], the fact remains that these models come with their limitations when accurately modelling human disease progression. This is particularly important when considering the manner in which carcinogenesis is facilitated in these mouse models. Currently, development of breast cancer mouse models includes spontaneous or chemical induction of breast cancer, knockout mice and tumor transplants [78]. While some of these models may represent a small portion of breast cancer patients, CRISPR technology is capable of providing a more accurate model of induction and genetic alternations that may be far more accurate in mimicking the progression of cancer as it presents in humans.

Although CRISPR has yet to be applied as a therapeutic tool, its possibilities extend beyond generating better cancer models. Potential applications of CRISPR technology on cancer are reviewed in detailed elsewhere [61]. However, determining exactly how to apply this particular technology to cancer remains controversial. Targeting a specific subset of mutated genes, such as tumor suppressor genes or oncogenes, might prove futile as CRISPR would have to locate every single cell with this mutation and edit each one. CRISPR might prove most effective by targeting the cancer stem cell subpopulation and self-renewal. Genetically altering a subset of T cells that are capable of seeking out malignant cancer cells is an application that might be possible. As CRISPR technology is currently in a state of infancy, its application to cancer as a therapeutic option has yet to be realized but the possibilities seem to be very promising.

8.5 Components of the Tumor Microenvironment and Their Respective Therapeutic Targets

8.5.1 Inflammation and Potential Anti-inflammatory Drugs

Inflammation plays both an anti- and pro-tumorigenic role in the progression and induction of cancer. Chronic inflammation in particular, is a potent inducer of tumors. The infiltration of the TME with bioactive molecules such as cytokines, growth factors, chemokines, cell survival signals, pro-angiogenic factors, and extracellular matrix-modifying enzymes such as metalloproteinases that promote EMT potentiate the risk of cancer as a result of disrupting tissue architecture as well as protein and DNA alterations [79]. Depending on the TME, and the cytokines present, these can be targeted in therapies in order to prevent cell transformation and malignancy.

Tumor necrosis factor alpha (TNF-α) has been implicated in carcinogenesis due to its involvement in chronic inflammatory diseases. This pro-inflammatory cytokine is recognized by ubiquitously expressed TNF-α receptor-1 (TNF-αR-1) and TNF-αR-2 expressed primarily on immune cells. TNF-α binding to its receptor results in the activation of signaling pathways ultimately resulting in the induction of nuclear factor kappa-light-chain-enhancer of activated B cells (NF-κB). Low, sustained TNF-α production can induce a tumor phenotype which is based on reactive oxygen species (ROS) and reactive nitrogen species (RNS) generation that can induce DNA damage resulting in tumorigenesis [80]. Furthermore, TNF-α enhances tumor angiogenesis through angiogenic factors such as IL-8, and VEGF through both a JNK- and an AP-1-dependent pathway [81].

Targeting this pro-inflammatory cytokine and preventing its chronic activation, presents as a potential therapy for the regulation of tumorigenesis. Since TNF-α activates NF-κB and subsequently activates transcription factor cyclooxygenase-2 (COX-2), non-steroidal anti-inflammatory drugs (NSAIDs) have been investigated as potential therapies to limit cancer-associated inflammation. Patients with NSAID use at both pre- and post-diagnosis have demonstrated a significantly reduced risk of distant metastasis [82]. Additionally, elevated prostaglandin (PG) levels have been observed in human tumors and contribute to carcinogenesis as they influence cell proliferation, tumor promotion and metastasis. As such, common NSAIDs acetylsalicylic acid (ASA), and celecoxib have been used to inhibit and regulate PG levels [83]. ASA and other COX-2 specific drugs have also been studied in terms of reducing risk of breast cancer; however, their use as a potential therapy is yet to be elucidated [84].

8.5.2 Hypoxic Tumor Microenvironment and Its Targets

Another hallmark of solid tumors is hypoxic regions where oxygen levels are significantly lower than in healthy tissues. Hypoxia has been previously found to contribute to and increase angiogenesis, cancer cell survival and metastasis and plays a critical role in regulating each step of the metastatic cascade [85]. Hypoxia induces the transcription of genes involved in biological processes important for tumor growth and metastatic disease such as cell proliferation, migration, invasion, and ECM remodeling. A wide range of genes associated with breast cancer metastasis have been reported to be upregulated under hypoxic conditions, that are then associated with poorer outcomes in breast cancer [86, 87]. Hypoxia-inducible factor 1-alpha (HIF-1α) expression has been linked to metastatic disease. Breast cancer studies have shown overexpression of HIF-1α in approximately 70% of breast cancer metastases. This HIF-α overexpression results from an imbalance in the supply and consumption of oxygen by tumor cells, contributing to their more aggressive phenotypes [88].

HIF expression plays an important role in metastatic breast cancer as it has been linked to influencing metastatic seeding at distant organs prior to cancer cell arrival, regulating pre-metastatic niche formation [86]. This is accomplished through the induction of members of the lysyl oxidase (LOX) family, which catalyze collagen cross-linking in the lungs prior to bone marrow-derived cell (BMDC) recruitment, as well as CXCR4. Only a small subset of LOX family members have been found to be expressed in any breast cancer; however, HIF-1 was required for their expression in every case. The requirement of HIF-1 was confirmed when knock-out of HIF-1 resulted in the reduction of collagen cross-linking CD11b+ BMDC recruitment as well as metastasis formation in the lungs of mice following orthotopic transplantation of human breast cancer cells [89]. These HIF-inducible genes also function in secondary tumor growth, as a result of angiogenesis [86].

In hypoxic conditions, malignant cells secrete additional molecules that modulate the TME to facilitate angiogenesis and metastasis. Hypoxia results in the loss of cell-cell adhesion in squamous carcinoma cells [90]. This is due to HIFs inducing the expression of SNAIL1, SNAIL2 and TWIST1, all of which work to suppress E-cadherin [89]. Under hypoxic conditions, E-cadherin, which is necessary for cell-cell adhesion, was found clustered in the plasma membrane and cytoplasm. This cell adhesion loss was confirmed with real time PCR for Snail, a negative E-cadherin transcription regulator. Additionally, conditioned media from hypoxia-treated cells resulted in the induction of angiogenesis in vivo. Hypoxia enhanced the angiogenic potential of this malignant cell secretion and provided a mechanism to facilitate tumor angiogenesis in a growing tumor with a hypoxic core. Immunoblotting against hypoxia-induced factor-1 alpha (HIF-1α), demonstrated elevation under hypoxic conditions [90]. HIFs promote motility by increasing mesenchymal-to-epithelial transition (MET), and increase invasion through the increase of MMP2 and MMP9. HIFs increase intravasation by increasing VEGFA and ANGFT2, and increase extravasation by increasing L1CAM and ANGPTL4 [89].

Due to the countless implications of HIFs in all aspects of metastasis, they are important targets for therapies to target. HIFs are targeted by HIF inhibitors which block primary tumor growth and metastasis, and have already been efficacious as demonstrated in orthotopic mouse models of breast cancer metastasis [89]. However, a reason for the lack of efficacious use of HIF inhibitors as a part of cancer therapy lies in their lack of specificity, resulting in the inhibition of multiple targets.

A potential therapy that may increase specificity to HIF-1α is targeting its mRNA expression. EZN-2968 is highly specific, binding HIF-1α with high affinity, causing down-regulation and ultimately reduction of HIF-1α protein levels [91]. A caveat to HIF expression is that it functions as a transcription factor for VEGF, which is a crucial growth factor in angiogenesis and vascularization. HIF-1 binds to the hypoxic response element (HRE) on VEGF, activating VEGF transcription, with VEGF synthesis increasing angiogenesis [92]. Angiogenesis as another component of the TME that presents as a target for cancer therapies and is discussed below as a separate subsection.

8.5.3   Angiogenesis and Neovascularization of the Tumor

8.5.3.1   Preventing Metastasis Through the Normalization of Tumor Vasculature

Tumor vasculature is abnormal when compared with the vessels feeding into healthy organs because tumors neovascularize existing vessels [93]. The abnormality of tumor vasculature stems from the fact that these new blood vessels are leaky, dilated and have a disorganized arrangement leading to compromised structural and functional integrity. For example, pericytes that normally provide support to endothelial cells, are few or absent and are disorganized; endothelial cells have an abnormal phenotype and the basement membrane is not present or unnaturally thick in some areas. These abnormalities in tumor vasculature all contribute to the unique tumor microenvironment that allows tumor cells to grow in hypoxic conditions and in turn become resistant to therapies. Furthermore, a hypoxic environment also selects for cells with a more aggressive and malignant phenotype, increasing their ability to metastasize to distant organs. Therefore, the architecture of the network of vessels surrounding the tumor plays an important role in facilitating metastasis.

The concept of vessel normalization consequently involves establishing a balance between proangigogenic and antiangiogenic processes so that a normal network of vessels can be established without causing the existing vessels from regressing. The short window of time during the normalization process (1–6 days) is quite limited as the tumor eventually acquires resistance to the angiogenic therapies that are administered and is able to find alternative ways to facilitate blood vessel formation Reports by Jain [94] and Goel et al. [95] have proposed that the application of antiangiogenic therapy should also take place at a critical time point during which time the vessels have begun to normalize and are delivering oxygen to the tumor. During this window of normalization (which lasts about 6 days), cancer cells are rendered sensitive to radiation therapy because the level of reactive oxygen species is increased due to the overall increase in oxygen (Fig. 8.3).

As a treatment option, antiangiogenic therapies have been proposed to be given in conjunction with cytotoxic drugs in order to provide an effective method to kill cancer cells but to also deprive them of nutrients they require to survive. Candidate

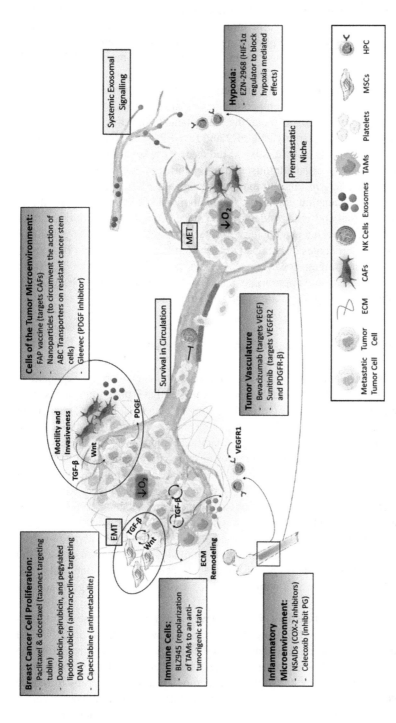

Fig. 8.3 Components of the tumor microenvironment and their respective therapeutic targets key features of the TME as well as malignant and non-malignant cells associated with tumor progression and the development of the premetastatic niche are depicted above in detail. The legend in the bottom right corner shows a few candidate cells and additional component involved in tumorigenesis as discussed in the body of this chapter and provides a brief overview of the TME. Tumor development is a multistage process with multiple therapeutic targets. These targets are shown in boxes with currently approved drugs and inhibitors that have shown some efficacy when administered in combination with chemotherapies (shown in "Breast Cancer Proliferation")

targets include blocking VEGF [93] as it is crucial to the normal development of vasculature in mice. For example, the monoclonal antibody bevacizumab has been shown to bind to VEGF thereby preventing its subsequent binding to its receptors. Unfortunately, the patient response to this therapy has been modest [96]. Similar results were observed when it was administered in conjunction with chemotherapeutic agent such as docetaxel [96]. Furthermore, a number of small inhibitor molecules have been proposed as therapeutic agents that are tyrosine kinase inhibitors with angiogenic pathway targets including: Vandetanib (which targets VEGFR2 and EGFR), Sunitinib (which targets VEGFR2 and PDGFR-β) and others described by Nielsen et al. [96]. However, results from studies on these small molecule inhibitors as well as their effects when administered in combination with therapeutic agents have yielded conflicting results and thus additional studies are required.

One possible explanation could be that the application of antiangiogenic therapies is multifactorial and is dependent on the stage of angiogenesis during tumor development and thus other candidate growth factors might need to be targeted. For example, in the early stages of breast tumor development, VEGF would be considered an appropriate target; however, in later stages, FGF1, FGF2 and TGFB, to name a few, would be more appropriate than VEGF as the tumor would have developed vasculature at this point of antiangiogenic treatment.

8.5.3.2 Implications of Vascular Leakiness on Metastasis

While the abnormality of the tumor vasculature is well understood, its implications on efficacy of drug treatments and therapies are an area that is under intense research for several important reasons as outlined in detail by Jain [94]. In brief, changes in interstitial fluid pressure cause fluids containing cancer cells and growth factors to spill into surrounding tissues and thereby facilitate tumor progression. Secondly, hypoxia is established due to the differences in vessel architecture. This means that while one region of the tumor receives adequate blood flow, another region might not receive this same type of blood. This creates a heterogeneous vessel network that can generate a hypoxic tumor microenvironment that is known to select for an aggressive phenotype and mediate metastasis. This change in oxygenation also generates a lower than normal pH in the extracellular components. Thirdly, many drug treatments (i.e. chemotherapy, radiation, and immunotherapy) require oxygen and sustained blood flow in order to be effective. Thus, because of the abnormal architecture of the tumor, there is a reduced level of access for these drugs, rendering them less effective.

Currently, only ten antiangiogenic drugs have been approved for use in conjunction with chemotherapies [94]. However, determining whether these drugs will be effective depends on the stage of cancer and the vascular network surrounding the tumor. This is because depending on the stage of tumor growth, blood vessel formation may not be affected by antiangiogenic therapy. Anti-VEGF therapy to reduce formation of new blood vessels as well as to normalize existing tumor vessels; however, it is not always effective and therefore it is important to determine which cancer types would benefit from this type of therapy. This therapy is proposed to be ineffective for triple negative breast cancer (among others) and is related to the higher expression levels of soluble VEGFR1. VEGFA inhibition is only effective on newly formed or forming vessels because mature vessels are surrounded by the ECM and pericytes that are unaffected by the inhibition of VEGFA [97]. PDGF is another candidate that can be inhibited to prevent vascularization of the tumor because it has been shown to recruit angiogenic stromal cells that can secrete VEGFA and other factors involved in angiogenesis [97]. For example, Gleevec, a tyrosine kinase inhibitor, acts directly on PDGF by inhibiting PDGF receptor function on non-small cell lung cancers [98].

As discussed in earlier sections, VEGF is an important growth factor that is required in the development of tumor vessels; therefore, its inhibition is an important therapeutic target in order to reduce the formation of blood vessels to the tumor [95]. Although this form of therapy has not "starved" the tumor, it does however, appear to make cytotoxic therapies more effective when used as a concomitant treatment strategy. In a phase III trial of patients with HER negative metastatic breast cancer, patients were divided into two groups: those that were given chemotherapy alone or chemotherapy in conjunction with bevacizumab [99]. It was found that there was an increase in PFS in patients receiving the additional treatment; unfortunately, the increase was only 2 months compares to patients who only received chemotherapy. However, as with any targeted therapy, the efficacy of normalizing tumor vasculature and inhibiting growth factors involved in blood vessel formation is highly dependent on the stage, progression and type of malignancy and requires further studies in order to apply it to metastatic breast cancer.

8.5.4 Cells Found in the Tumor Microenvironment and Their Targets

8.5.4.1 Tumor-Associated Macrophages

Tumor-associated macrophages (TAMs) are abundant in metastases of multiple cancer types, and enhance tumor progression through supporting growth, angiogenesis and invasion from the secretion of pro-tumorigenic proteases, cytokines and growth factors [100]. These cells are educated by the TME so they adopt a trophic role that facilitates matrix breakdown and tumor cell motility, contributing to the metastatic process. Macrophages also produce mutagenic oxygen and nitrogen radicals as well as angiogenic factors [101]. These cells create an inflammatory environment that is mutagenic. In this way, macrophages prepare target tissues for the arrival of tumor cells [102]. In addition, primary tumors have been found to induce the expression of matrix metalloproteinase MMP9 in macrophages at the sites of lung metastasis, causing the release of bound VEGF, which promotes angiogenesis [102]. These TAMs are preprogrammed to inhibit lymphocyte function through the release of inhibitory cytokines such as IL-10, prostaglandins, or reactive oxygen species [103]. Thus, it is evident that various components of the TME are interrelated. Figure 8.4 highlights the role that TAMs play in facilitating the changes that occur in the TME to promote and foster tumor progression and survival.

High TAM density has been correlated with poor patient prognosis and poor survival outcomes in over 8% of cancer studies published [102]. TAMs are composed of multiple subtypes that share features of both M1 and M2 type macrophages, but have an overall greater similarity to those macrophages involved in developmental processes. The differentiation and chemotaxis of macrophages is regulated by macrophage growth factor colony-stimulating-factor-1 (CSF-1). The overexpression of CSF-1 has been implicated with poor prognoses in breast,

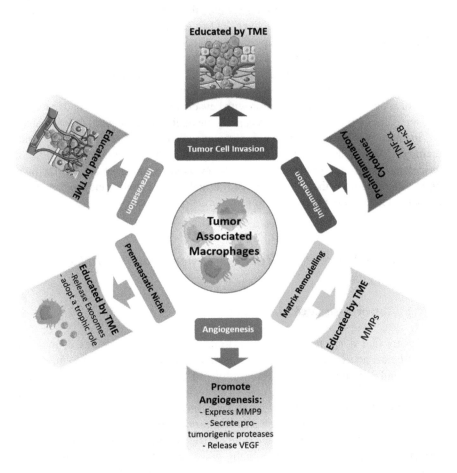

Fig. 8.4 Role of TAMs in facilitating tumor growth and cancer progression. TAMs play crucial roles in the metastatic process, including invasion and extravasation, as well as in facilitating the metastatic niche through exosome release. Through recruitment of pro-inflammatory cytokines, and MMP9, TAMs promote inflammation and angiogenesis, with matrix remodeling taking place as a result of establishment of new metastases

ovarian, and endometrial cancer [100]. The role of macrophages in tumor progression was further observed when they were removed in mice via null mutation of CSF-1, and a reduced rate of tumor progression almost complete metastasis ablation was observed in a tumor mouse model of breast cancer. Epidermal growth factor (EGF) is one of the growth factors secreted by TAMs, which acts in a paracrine signaling loop through CSF-1 [102]. The repolarization of macrophages from an anti-tumorigenic state to a pro-tumorigenic state promotes along with EGFR signaling promote the exit of tumor cells from a state of dormancy. As such, CSF-1R inhibitors such as BLZ945 present as potential therapies by targeting CSF-1 [104].

8.5.4.2 Cancer-Associated Fibroblasts

Cancer-associated fibroblasts (CAFs) comprise the bulk of the cancer stroma, moderating the TME by promoting cancer initiation, angiogenesis, invasion and metastasis. In breast cancer, CAFs have been found to promote tumor progression as well as induce resistance to therapy. Removal of fibroblast activation protein (FAP)-expressing tumor stromal cells resulted in stunted tumor growth [105]. Due to the presence of these tumor stromal cells, targeting FAP-tumor stromal cells presents as a potential therapeutic target in controlling the TME in metastatic disease. The origins of CAFs have been narrowed to activated resident fibroblasts, bone-marrow-derived MSCs, and cancer cells that undergo EMT. CAFs induce mammary carcinogenesis, but also promote invasion and metastasis. CAFs induce invasion through increasing matrix metalloproteinase expression and activity (MMP14, and MMP9). CAFs also induce EMT changes in breast epithelial cells, and secreted CXCL12/SDF-1 to promote angiogenesis in the primary site by recruiting endothelial progenitor cells. Cancer cells secrete growth factors and chemokines, such as CCL2 to activate CAFs and recruit macrophages. CCL2 secreted from CAFs also increases breast cancer stem cells, which promotes metastasis [105]. Through their role as key modulators of immune polarization in the TME, CAFs are strong candidates for targeted therapy in metastatic breast cancer treatment. Elimination of CAFs results in a Th2 to Th1 polarization, which is characterized by suppressed recruitment of TAMs, myeloid-derived suppressor cells, regulatory T cells, as well as degreased angiogenesis and lymphangiogenesis [106].

Therapies targeting CAFs include a DNA vaccine for FAP that resulted in improved anti-metastatic effects of doxorubicin chemotherapy. In addition, the use of the vaccine enhanced IL-6 and Il-4 suppression while increasing dendritic cell and CD8+ T cell recruitment. This combined DNA vaccine with chemotherapy was also found to reduce tumor-associated VEGF, PDGFC, and CSF mRNA and protein expression [106]. Targeting CAFs present in the tumor stroma allows for regulation of many components of metastasis and angiogenesis. As cancer therapies targeting CAFs have demonstrated to improve chemotherapy efficacy, this proposes a potentially efficacious combination therapy that may be used in the multi-modal treatment of metastatic breast cancer. Including these drugs that target CAFs is of utmost importance as CAFs are also a key source of VEGF, which would otherwise continue to support angiogenesis during tumor growth.

8.5.4.3 Mesenchymal Stem Cells

Mesenchymal stem cells (MSCs) are pluripotent progenitor cells that contribute to the maintenance and regeneration of connective tissue. These cells are highly prevalent in the TME, and it is postulated that the TME facilitates metastatic spread due to a reversible change in the phenotype of malignant cells [8]. Mesenchymal cells are highly motile and invasive in nature. To determine if the presence of MSCs alters the phenotype of malignant cells to promote metastatic spread, MSCs bone-marrow-derived human MSCs mixed with human breast carcinoma cells were analyzed, and resulted in an increase in metastatic potency. This is thought to be due to the malignant cells stimulating de novo secretion of CCL5 chemokine from MSCs, which ultimately enhances motility, invasion, and metastasis [8]. Through the repeated cross-talk between malignant cells and cells in the TME, metastasis and tumor growth are moderated.

Human breast cancer cells were investigated to see if they attracted human MSCs. Bone-marrow-derived MSCs were allowed to migrate towards media from breast cancer cell cultures. MSCs migrated more avidly towards media from the breast cancer cell cultures, than the controls. MSCs also accelerated the growth of breast cancer cells (BCC) without effecting tumor kinetics. MSCs promote metastasis, as mice xenografts with just BCCs exhibited few micrometastases, whereas those implanted with BCCs and MSCs displayed an up to sevenfold increase in micro- and macroscopic metastasis. Implantation of MSCs contralateral to the tumor or in a separate site didn't affect metastatic potential [8]. This suggests that MSC-induced metastasis occurs only when in proximity to the primary tumor, and do not migrate to the metastatic site.

However, due to the ability of MSCs to migrate towards tumor sites, they have been increasingly studied as efficient targeted-delivery vehicles for cancer gene therapy [107]. This has been tested for the administration of interferon beta (IFN-β) in vivo as although at high concentrations has been found to inhibit malignant cell growth in vitro, has limited effects in vivo due to excessive toxicity when systemically administered at high doses. Human MSCs transduced with an adenoviral expression vector carrying IFN-β gene (MSC-IFNβ cells) were injected in immunodeficient mouse xenograft models. The co-culture of MSC-IFN-β cells with A375SM or MDA 231 cells significantly inhibited tumor cell growth when compared to tumor cells cultured alone. The injected MSC-IFN-β cells resulted in suppression of pulmonary metastases – likely due to local production of IFN-β in the TME [108].

8.5.4.4 Exosomes

Exosomes, as previously mentioned, are extracellular vesicles released by cells that are found to be upregulated in metastatic cells. Locally, they promote cell proliferation and increase chemoresistance through the transfer of oncogenic proteins and multidrug transporters, ultimately promoting the proliferation of more aggressive and malignant cells. Furthermore, fibroblasts are activated to myofibroblasts which work within the TME to participate and facilitate angiogenesis. Systemically, exosome-mediated signaling results in the recruitment of bone marrow-derived hematopoietic cells to form a pre-metastatic niche in distant organs. These exosomes also interact with myeloid-derived cells to suppress the anti-tumor immune response [14]. These actions of exosomes are summarized in Fig. 8.5.

Stromal and breast cancer cells have been shown to use both paracrine and juxtacrine signaling to facilitate chemoresistance. The non-coding RNA transcripts within these exosomes stimulate pattern recognition receptor (PRR) RIG-1 to activate STAT1-dependent antiviral signaling [109]. Tumor-derived exosomes have also been demonstrated to contribute to forming a pre-metastatic niche that promotes tumor growth [110]. Exosome release is regulated by a calcium-dependent mechanism [111]. As such, utilizing therapies that alter intracellular Ca^{2+} levels will further modulate exosome secretion.

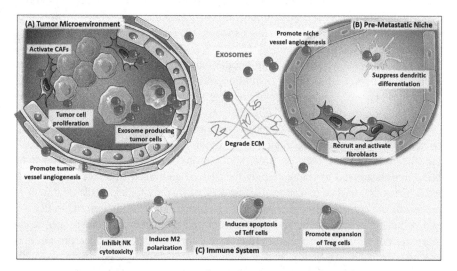

Fig. 8.5 Mechanisms of action of exosomes. Exosomes are vesicles containing proteins and nucleic acids produced by specific tumor cells that have the capacity to act on components of the local tumor microenvironment (**a**) as well as components of the premetastatic niche (**b**) and immune system (**c**). Local exosomal targets include CAFs which are activated to differentiate, and endothelial cells of the local vasculature and neighboring tumor cells, which are signaled to proliferate. At the premetastatic niche, several processes take place that prime the site for colonization by disseminated tumor cells including suppression of dendritic cell differentiation, promotion of angiogenesis and recruitment of fibroblasts. Further protective events also take place to inhibit the action of the immune system as outlined in (**c**)

MSCs have been found to release exosomes, and exosome-mediated signaling promotes tumor progression due to communication between the tumor and the tumor stroma, resulting in the activation of proliferative and angiogenic pathways because of immune suppression, and the initiation of pre-metastatic sites. Due to evidence of both exosome-mediated, and hypoxia-mediated metastasis, King and colleagues set out to determine if there is a role for hypoxic tumor cell-derived exosomes in promoting angiogenic signaling. MCF7 breast cancer cells exposed to moderate hypoxia (1% O_2) demonstrated exosomes with significantly higher nanoparticle concentrations when compared with exosome fractions from normoxic controls. MDA-MB-231 and SKBR3 breast cancer cell lines displayed similar results. Exposure to more severe hypoxic conditions (0.1% O_2) resulted in significantly higher nanoparticle concentrations per cell count compared to normoxic control exosome fractions for all three cell lines. Hypoxic tumor-derived exosomes contain pro-angiogenic factors, promoting angiogenesis and endothelial activation [112].

8.5.4.5   Cancer Stem Cells, Chemoresistance and Overcoming Resistance to Therapy

The existence of the cancer stem cell population was proposed over 40 years ago [113] and has only recently been characterized in multiple malignancies [114–116]. Since then, this cancer stem cell/tumor initiating population has been identified in several malignancies including breast cancer [114, 117]. This population is characterized as being $CD44^+CD24^{-/low}$ Lineage$^-$ [117]. Not only is this population postulated to be the core tumor renewing population, this cell population has also been proposed to be the main culprit behind chemoresistance in patients receiving chemotherapy. The mechanisms behind this chemoresistance is eloquently outlined by Zhao [118] and by Abdullah and Chow [119].

In brief, resistance to chemotherapy can present itself in two forms: intrinsic resistance, where cancer cells are inherently resistant to chemotherapy in patients receiving chemotherapy for the first time, and acquired resistance, where cancer cells become desensitized to chemotherapy because of continued exposure to this treatment. Chemoresistance is responsible for 90% of therapy failure in the treatment of metastatic cancer, including metastatic breast cancer [120]. Although the molecular and cellular mechanisms behind cancer stem cell mediated chemoresistance resistance are not well understood, there are several theories that have been proposed as potential explanations. Firstly, similar to their normal counterparts, cancer stem cells are proposed to establish a protective niche that allows them to self-renew and differentiate without exposure to therapeutics such as cytotoxic drugs. Although the specific cells and proteins involved in establishing this niche have not been determined, the establishment of a hypoxic niche has been shown to be an important facilitator of cancer stem cell proliferation and expansion in several cancer types including breast cancer [121]. Secondly, stromal components including CAFs, the ECM and immune cells have all been implicated in establishing a protective niche that is able to facilitate chemoresistance in cancer stem cells. This is achieved by secreting growth factors and cytokines such as HGF (hepatocyte growth factor), FGF (fibroblast growth factor) and IL6 (interleukin-6), which upregulate stemness and survival pathways that allow cancer stem cells to counteract the effects of anti-cancer drugs such as RAF inhibitors [122]. In the event that cytotoxic drugs are able to penetrate the above external defense, cancer stem cells are also capable of activating drug efflux mechanisms that are able to transport drugs out of the cytoplasm through the action of the ABCT (adenosine triphosphate binding cassette transporter) family of drug transporters. In addition, cancer stem cells are also able to enter the quiescent phase of the cell cycle thereby reducing their proliferation and effectively avoiding the action of cytotoxic therapies that are traditionally designed to target rapidly proliferating cells.

The cancer stem cell population presents as a challenge when developing targeted therapies as there are multiple mechanisms in place that serve to protect these cells. As stated earlier, this cellular population is present in many different malignancies and is the likely cause for cancer relapse because of its resilience during treatment [119]. Particularly in the case of breast cancer, the NF-κB pathway, which plays a dual role in preventing and promoting tumorigenesis, has been shown to confer resistance to paclitaxcel therapy; however, upon administration of disulfram and copper, whose mode of action is via inhibition of the NF-κB pathway, this resistance can be reversed [119]. Inhibition of the NF-κB pathway through the action of parthenolide has also been shown to reduce its protective effects on metastatic breast cancer cells and renders cancer cells more sensitive to the cytotoxic effects of paclitaxel [123].

Additional mechanisms that have been proposed to reverse this resistance include overcoming the action of drug efflux by resistant cells with a more effective drug delivery system that can circumvent the action of ABC transporter proteins. For example, nanodiamond based delivery systems have shown promising results in in vivo studies [124]. The mode of action for this particular delivery system was prolonged retention of the chemotherapeutic, doxycycline, in the 4T1 metastatic breast tumor model thereby overriding the efflux of the drug and increasing the cytotoxic effects of doxycycline as observed through reduced tumor sizes. In addition, the toxicity and the immune response normally mediated by doxycycline treatment was also reduced in normal tissues when administered through the nanodiamond drug delivery system. Other drug delivery systems that could be efficacious include those that target specific receptors that are overexpressed on the surface of cancer cells and can be internalized thereby bypassing pumps that are able to remove chemotherapeutic drugs from the cytoplasm of cancer cells. One such example of a nanoparticle capable of such an action is a folic acid functionalized amphiphilic alternating copolymer poly(styrene-*alt*-maleic anhydride) (FA-DABA-SMA) [53, 125]. FA-DABA-SMA is not only capable of binding to overexpressed folate receptors on cancer cells, it is also pH sensitive and is capable of being internalized by the cancer cells and can release its payload directly inside the cell. While this particular drug delivery system has only been administered to pancreatic cancer cells, its mode of action is applicable to breast cancer cells because overexpression of folate acid receptors is a hallmark of poor prognosis of breast cancer patients [126] and can therefore be exploited by nanoparticles that are designed to target this receptor (Fig. 8.6).

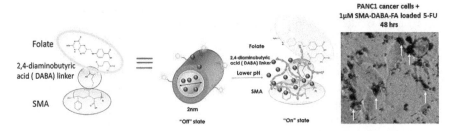

Fig. 8.6 Graphical representation of SMA-DABA-FA The panel on the far left depicts the chemical structure of the polymer SMA linked to Folate via the DABA linker. The "off" state (middle panel) of the polymer occurs at a neutral pH, specifically when the hydrophobic interior has encapsulated the compound of interest, in this particular image the chemotherapeutic agent 5-fluorouracil has been encapsulated. Upon exposure to an acidic environment, the polymer switches to an "on" state at which point it releases its payload. The functionalization of the polymer allows it to dock on the folate receptors on cancer cells and be internalized and localized to the nucleus, where the acid environment allows for the payload's release in the interior of the cell, effectively bypassing the action of efflux transporter pumps that would normally prevent cytotoxic drugs from having an effect. (Reproduced with permission from Sambi et al. [50]. https://doi.org/10.15406/mojps.2017.01.000)

8.6 Novel Therapies for the Treatment of Metastatic Breast Cancer

8.6.1 Applications of Cancer Immunotherapy in the Treatment of Metastatic Breast Cancer

Immunotherapy is a therapeutic approach that involves the stimulation of the immune system. This form of therapy has several mechanisms of action including: targeting specific antigens found on the surface of tumor cells and enhancing the antitumor effects of the immune system. As discussed in Sect. 8.5 the TME is composed of a mosaic of cells with a diverse range of functions and that could be targeted by the immune system. An alternative area of interest is enhancing the effects of the immune system by blocking or stimulating the immune checkpoints that have been hijacked by the tumor. Both areas of immunotherapy are currently being studied and applied to the treatment of metastatic breast cancer and will be discussed below.

8.6.1.1 Current Progress on Immune Checkpoints and Targeting Metastatic Breast Cancer

Immune checkpoints are important regulatory pathways that can have an inhibitory or stimulatory effect on immune function [127]. With regard to tumor progression, cancer cells are able to hijack these immune checkpoints and are able to inhibit the antitumor action of T-cells in their favor [128]. While there are several immune checkpoints, there are currently two candidate checkpoints that are being extensively studied with respect to cancer immunotherapy: blockade of cytotoxic T-lymphocyte-associated antigen 4 (CTLA-4) and programmed cell death protein-1 (PD-1) inhibitors.

CTLA-4 is an important immune checkpoint located on T-cells and modulates the amplitude of T-cell activation in its early stages thereby preventing an excessively intensified response from being initiated [128]. During tumor progression, the inhibition of T-cell activity by CTLA-4 can prevent the anticancer effects of cytotoxic T-cells. Blocking this receptor as a means to enhance the antitumor response of activated T-cells has been proposed as a potential therapy [128]. Initial CTLA4-knockout mice models suggested that a blockade of this receptor could potentially be lethal and lead to immune toxicities [127]. However, subsequent preclinical animal studies reported that there was a critical therapeutic window when CTLA-4 should be inhibited in order to elicit a favorable antitumor response [129]. As such, two CTLA-4 antibodies have been approved for clinical trials: tremelimumab and ipilimumab, both of which were initially tested on patients presenting with melanoma [127]. In relation to metastatic breast cancer, in preclinical animal studies, mice bearing 4T1 metastatic mammary carcinoma tumors were given radiation therapy in conjunction with CTLA-4 blockade with a monoclonal antibody [128]. Results of this studied revealed that lung metastases were reduced when CTLA-4 was inhibited and given in combination with radiation therapy. However, additional studies are required on the applications of CTLA-4 inhibition for the treatment of metastatic breast cancer.

A second emerging immune checkpoint of interest is the PD-1 receptor. In healthy tissues, this particular immune checkpoint is involved in reducing the activation of T-cells during an inflammatory response to prevent autoimmunity [130, 131]. The mechanism of action involves the binding of the PD-1 ligand 1 (PDL-1), which is located on the cell surface, to the PD-1 receptor, which is located on T-cells. PDL-1 overexpression has been observed on several tumor types, specifically triple negative breast cancer [132]. Additionally, overexpression of PDL-1 has been shown to be regulated by the loss of PTEN, an effect that is mediated through the P13K pathway [132]. Furthermore, increased PDL-1 expression reduced the activation and proliferation of T-cells and allowed triple negative breast cancer cells to evade an immune response. Thus far, PDL-1/PD-1 inhibition has only been applied to malignancies other than metastatic breast cancer; however, additional preclinical studies are required in order to determine the efficacy of this form of immunotherapy in the treatment of metastatic breast cancer.

8.6.2   Selective Inhibition as a Targeted Therapeutic Approach for Metastatic Breast Cancer

The administration of small inhibitor molecules as a mode of targeted therapy has shifted the focus of cytotoxic only treatments for patients with cancer, to that of a more personalized and targeted approach. Small inhibitor molecules are designed to inhibit pathways that are involved in tumor development and progression as a whole. For the purpose of this chapter, we will focus on the pathways as they pertain to the progression of metastatic breast cancer.

8.6.2.1 PLD-2 Inhibition

Macrophages and their effects on the establishment of the tumor microenvironment (as discussed earlier in Sect. 8.4), have been well established. In brief, macrophages that are associated with tumors are identified as TAMs and have been shown to be key drivers of the inflammatory environment that aids tumor growth through a number of processes including providing a protective niche for cancer stem cells, promoting metastasis and allowing for genetic instability [133]. Phospholipase D-2, an enzyme that is regulated by protein kinase C, has an important role in macrophage and neutrophil signaling as well as cell migration and is therefore an important molecular target in order to mitigate the action of macrophages in tumor development [134].

Recently, Henkels et al. [135] reported that mice injected MCF-7 cells with overly expressed PLD-2 were able to form tumors more efficiently when compared with mice injected with MDAMB231 cells with silenced PLD-2 expression. Furthermore, cohorts with overexpressed PLD-2 also had a faster tumor onset as well as increased lung metastases. The inhibitors used for this study were FIPI and VU0155072-2 PLD inhibitors. The key findings of this study were that upon inhibition of PLD-2, there was reduced TAM and tumor associated neutrophil recruitment to the tumor and a reduction in metastatic burden and tumor volume. A novel and surprising finding of this study was that upon inhibition of PLD-2, there appeared to be an increase in M1 macrophages, which are less invasive and more anti-tumoral growth when compared with the M2 population that is normally present in the tumor microenvironment owing to their supportive effect on tumorigenesis.

8.6.2.2 EGFR/ERBB-2 Pathway Inhibition

The EGFR (epidermal growth factor receptor) transmembrane glycoprotein and its overexpression in cancer cells has been implicated in a number of cellular progresses that are required for the progression of cancer [136]. The EGFR family is made up of four receptors: EGFR, ErbB2, ErbB3 and ErbB4, of these four, only ErbB2 does not have a ligand associated with its action. In breast cancer specifically, ErbB2, also known as HER2, has been shown to be overexpressed in 25–30% of invasive breast cancers [137, 138] and has been associated with poor survival [139]. ErbB2 has also been implicated in a number of signaling cascades mediating cancer progression including metastasis. It has also been proposed as a mediator of chemoresistance [136].

The small molecule inhibitor lapatinib is an EGFR/ERBB2 inhibitor that has been administered to ErbB2-positive breast cancer patients [140]. In a recent report by Li and Marchenko [141], this inhibitor was also shown to suppress tumor growth by inactivating HSF1, a transcription factor whose target is the Hsp90 (heat shock protein 90), and ultimately leads to the downregulation of the mutated p53 tumor suppressor gene. Mutations in the p53 tumor suppressor gene play a critical role in tumor progression and by downregulating its action with lapatinib, the therapeutic potential of this inhibitor molecule could lead to a more positive prognosis for ErbB2 positive breast cancer patients.

8.6.2.3   PARP1 Inhibition

There are five important modes through which DNA repair occurs in human cells including: mismatch repair (MMB), base excision repair (BER), nucleotide excision repair (NER) and double-strand break (DSB) recombinational repair [142]. The tumor suppressor genes BRCA1 and BRCA2 have been implicated in playing an important role in DNA repair processes and are regulators of transcription. Specifically, BRCA1 has been shown to complex and activate p53, another tumor suppressor gene [143]. In normal cells, p53 is involved in locating DNA damage and stopping the cell cycle in order to repair the error or initiate cell death.

In addition, poly-ADP-ribose polymerases (PARPs) are another family of enzymes that are also activated by DNA damage and are crucial in the repairing of single-strand breaks in DNA to prevent apoptosis in cells with these breaks [144]. PARP1 specifically is activated in repair pathways involving single strand breaks or BER [143]. Its mode of action involves binding to the damaged region of the DNA, where it recruits proteins and forms a repair complex. Because DNA repair and replication are pivotal in cancer survival, inhibiting the action of PARP in cells with a mutation in the BRCA1 and BRCA2 genes is particularly detrimental to cancer cell survival because these genes cannot repair these breaks [145]. With additional breaks in DNA, the genomic instability can lead to apoptosis.

This is the rationale of employing the use of PARP inhibitors to prevent repair mechanisms from mending double stranded breaks in tumors with BRCA1, BRCA2 mutations that are incapable of repairing the breaks and thus require PARP1 [145]. Therefore, by allowing these double stranded breaks to accumulate cell death can result. PARP1 inhibitors, such as the commercially known Iniparib, have been put forward as potential anti-cancer agents for the treatment of metastatic breast cancer [146]. When administered in conjunction with platinum-based chemotherapy, a phase II study showed that patients with metastatic triple negative breast cancer showed a 52% response rate with minimal toxicity when compared with the 32% response rate seen in patients receiving only chemotherapy [146].

Recent studies have shown that PARP inhibitors may have two modes of action: (a) inhibitors that prevent the enzymatic activity of PARP in repair mechanisms and (b) PARP inhibitors that are able to block this activity as well as help to localize PARP proteins to sites of damage in regions associated with anti-tumor activity thereby blocking DNA replication [147]. This particular study revealed the therapeutic range of PARP inhibitors currently being studied in clinical trials and their respective potency based on their mechanism of action. Olaparib was found to be more potent than veliparib and MK-4817, which was the least potent in relation to its inhibitory action; however, it was the more toxic agent [147].

However, while this type of therapy has been revealed to be efficacious when administered in conjunction with chemotherapy, it is important to note that its action is very specific and has been shown to be efficacious for patients that have mutations in the BRCA1 gene [145] and its potency varies based on its mode of action as well (Fig. 8.7).

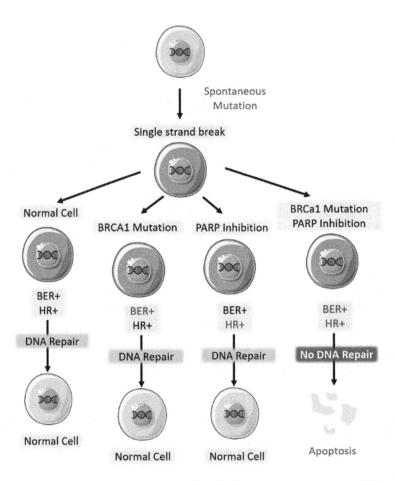

Fig. 8.7 Genetic mutations and the efficacy of PARP Inhibition The occurrence of a SSB in DNA leads to a number of repair processes in normal cells. Normal cells have BER and HR repair mechanisms that are able to repair the SSB and return the cell to its viable and stable state. In the event of a BRCA1 mutation, it is possible for other the DNA repair mechanisms to repair SSB and return the cells to its functional state as long as HR remains unaffected by BRCA1 mutations. Therefore, PARP inhibitors are only able to have an effect on cells that have a BRCA-1 mutation and have impaired HR function

8.6.2.4 Neuraminidase Inhibition as a Multi-faceted Therapy

Our group recently published a series of reports outlining the importance of the enzyme neuraminidase-1 (Neu-1) and the subsequent effects on its inhibition through the application of oseltamivir phosphate (OP) in regulating the downstream signaling of several receptors including the epidermal growth factor receptor (EGFR) [148], Toll-like receptors [149–152] as well as insulin receptor [153–155]. Activation of these receptors mediates several key processes involved in tumor progression that are outlined in detail elsewhere [156]. In brief, these receptors are involved in chemoresistance, immune-mediated tumorigenesis, tumorigenesis, and the upregulation of survival pathways and cell proliferation. Normally, Neu-1 cleaves α-2,3 sialic acid and facilitates crosstalk between matrix metalloproteinase-9 (MMP9) and G protein-coupled receptor(s) (GPCR). This signaling paradigm is regulates a number of downstream signaling events involved in multistage tumorigenesis through the action of receptor tyrosine kinases (RTKs) and TOLL-like (TLR) receptors [156].

We have previously reported that OP is a potent inhibitor of this signaling cascade by preventing the cleavage of α-2,3 sialic acid and has anti-tumor effects on pancreatic [148,157,158], ovarian [159] and metastatic breast [160] cancer mouse models. Specifically, PANC-1 and MiaPaCa-2 pancreatic tumor mouse models treated with OP showed an overall improvement in animal health and survival as well as reduced neovascularization of the developing tumor, reduced tumor size (as measured by tumor volume) and metastasis to the lungs and liver [148, 157, 158]. Similar results were observed in the therapeutic effects of OP in not only regulating multistage tumorigenesis [156], but O'Shea et al. was also able to show the chemotherapeutic sensitizing effects of OP of pancreatic cancer cells that were resistant to gemcitabine, tamoxifen, cisplatin and other chemotherapeutic agents [158] (Fig. 8.8).

In mouse models of metastatic breast cancer, Haxho et al. [160] showed long term survival for 180 days in addition to reduced tumor volume and reduced tumor vasculature when cohorts were treated with 50 mg/kg of OP. Additional characterization of the tissues harvested from untreated and OP treated cohorts revealed a reduction in N-cadherin expression as well as reduced CD31+ endothelial cells, which are normally expressed when blood vessel formation is occurring. Most surprising was that OP treated cohorts did not show any sign of relapse once they were taken off treatment for 56 days suggesting an irreversible effect of OP on cell proliferation and tumor volume reduction. Consistent observations across multiple malignancies of varying origins suggest that OP is capable of targeting a signaling pathway that is conserved across multiple cancer types and provides a promising addition that can be given in conjunction with chemotherapy. This is particularly important for metastatic breast cancer as OP was able to significantly reduce metastatic burden, which was localized to liver and lungs in untreated cohorts. Further study is required in its treatment enhancing potential when administered with chemotherapy as a multimodal-targeted strategy.

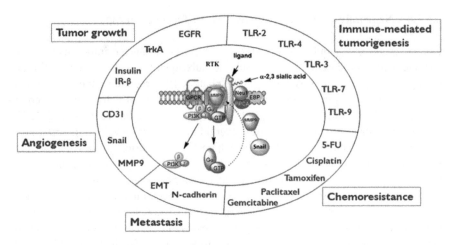

Fig. 8.8 Graphical representation of the proposed downstream effects of Neuraminidase inhibition. Neuraminadase (Neu-1) cleavage of α-2,3 sialic acid allows for crosstalk between matrixmetalloproteiase 9 (MMP9), and the G-protein coupled receptor, GPCR, in order to regulate the action of receptor tyrosine kinases (RTKs) and Toll-like (TLR) receptors of cancer cells. Oseltamivir phosphate acts to inhibit Neu-1 from cleaving α-2,3 sialic acid thereby indirectly inhibiting the mechanisms involved in multistagte tumorigenesis including metastasis and chemoresistance. (Reproduced in part with permission from in part from: ©Abdulkhalek et al. [159, 161]. Publisher and licensee Dove Medical Press Ltd. This is an Open Access article which permits unrestricted non-commercial use, provided the original work is properly cited)

8.7 Conclusion

Current therapeutic options for patients with metastatic breast cancer range from treating this malignancy at the molecular/genetic level to treatment of the tumor microenvironment. One key aspect of the disease progression of metastatic breast cancer is abundantly clear: designing a treatment protocol cannot be approached with a "one size fits all" lens, instead, a personalized approach is required. This is particularly true when considering that the unique genetic profile of this malignancy varies from patient to patient, from stage to stage and from cell to cell. While there has been an increase in our understanding of what drives this disease process at the molecular level, with a number of possible therapeutic targets/treatments emerging from that understanding, chemotherapy is still the main treatment option. Unfortunately, chemotherapy was initially designed with the outdated understanding that all cancer cells are created equal and hence equally susceptible to therapies targeting cellular proliferation. In light of research characterizing the heterogeneity of breast and other cancers, particularly the paradigm shift that has occurred with the cancer stem cell hypothesis, cytotoxic therapies need to be delivered in conjunction with additional therapies for a multimodal approach that targets multiple pathways that are critical to the development and progression of these malignancies. As outlined in this chapter, many candidate pathways can be exploited in breast cancer patients depending on their unique tumor microenvironment and genetic profile. While these candidate drugs may all have promising benefits to extend survivorship, realistically, the efficacy of these additional inhibitors depends on the unique profile of the disease and whether the cells express the molecular targets upon which candidate inhibitors can act. Furthermore, it has been well established that the tumor microenvironment or the tumor itself has mechanisms to compensate for the inhibition of one pathway by upregulating others. Therefore, designing multimodal therapies must not only target a particular molecular pathway facilitating tumor growth and survival, but target the compensating pathways upregulated by the initial targeted approach.

Acknowledgements This work was supported in part by grants to MR Szewczuk from the Natural Sciences and Engineering Research Council of Canada (NSERC), a private sector cancer funding from the Josefowitz Family and Encyt Technologies, Inc. to MR Szewczuk.

M Sambi is a recipient of the Queen's Graduate Award (QGA). B Qorri is a recipient of the QGA and the 2017 Terry Fox Research Institute Transdisciplinary Training Program in Cancer Research. The authors report no other conflicts of interest in this work.

Author Contributions All authors contributed equally toward drafting and critically revising the paper and agree to be equally accountable for all aspects of the work.

References

1. Canadian Cancer Society's Advisory Committee on Cancer Statistics (2017)
2. Cheng YC, Ueno NT (2012) Improvement of survival and prospect of cure in patients with metastatic breast cancer. Breast Cancer 19(3):191–199
3. Chaffer CL, Weinberg RA (2011) A perspective on cancer cell metastasis. Science 331(6024):1559
4. Onder TT, Gupta PB, Mani SA, Yang J, Lander ES, Weinberg RA (2008) Loss of E-cadherin promotes metastasis via multiple downstream transcriptional pathways. Cancer Res 68(10):3645
5. Taube JH, Herschkowitz JI, Komurov K et al (2010) Core epithelial-to-mesenchymal transition interactome gene-expression signature is associated with claudin-low and metaplastic breast cancer subtypes. Proc Natl Acad Sci 107(35):15449–15454
6. Patel LR, Camacho DF, Shiozawa Y, Pienta KJ, Taichman RS (2011) Mechanisms of cancer cell metastasis to the bone: a multistep process. Future Oncol 7(11):1285–1297
7. Stoletov K, Kato H, Zardouzian E et al (2010) Visualizing extravasation dynamics of metastatic tumor cells. J Cell Sci 123(13):2332–2341
8. Karnoub AE, Dash AB, Vo AP et al (2007) Mesenchymal stem cells within tumour stroma promote breast cancer metastasis. Nature 449:557–563
9. Yang J, Weinberg RA (2008) Epithelial-mesenchymal transition: at the crossroads of development and tumor metastasis. Dev Cell 14(6):818–829
10. Langley RR, Fidler IJ (2011) The seed and soil hypothesis revisited—the role of tumor-stroma interactions in metastasis to different organs. Int J Cancer 128(11):2527–2535
11. Roskelley CD, Bissell MJ (2002) The dominance of the microenvironment in breast and ovarian cancer. Semin Cancer Biol 12(2):97–104
12. Luga V, Zhang L, Viloria-Petit Alicia M et al (2012) Exosomes mediate stromal mobilization of autocrine Wnt-PCP signaling in breast cancer cell migration. Cell 151(7):1542–1556

13. Ratajczak J, Wysoczynski M, Hayek F, Janowska-Wieczorek A, Ratajczak MZ (2006) Membrane-derived microvesicles: important and underappreciated mediators of cell-to-cell communication. Leukemia 20(9):1487–1495
14. Kahlert C, Kalluri R (2013) Exosomes in tumor microenvironment influence cancer progression and metastasis. J Mol Med 91(4):431–437
15. Pagani O, Senkus E, Wood W et al (2010) International guidelines for management of metastatic breast cancer: can metastatic breast cancer be cured? JNCI J Natl Cancer Inst 102(7):456–463
16. Vlastos G, Smith DL, Singletary SE et al (2004) Long-term survival after an aggressive surgical approach in patients with breast cancer hepatic metastases. Ann Surg Oncol 11(9):869–874
17. Pocard M, Pouillart P, Asselain B, Salmon RJ (2000) Hepatic resection in metastatic breast cancer: results and prognostic factors. Eur J Surg Oncol (EJSO) 26(2):155–159
18. Jetske Ruiterkamp ACV, Bosscha K, Vivianne CG, Tjan-Heijnen MFE (2009) Impact of breast surgery on survival in patients with distant metastases at initial presentation: a systematic review of the literature. Breast Cancer Res Treat 120(1):9–16
19. Rapiti E, Verkooijen HM, Vlastos G et al (2006) Complete excision of primary breast tumor improves survival of patients with metastatic breast cancer at diagnosis. J Clin Oncol 24(18):2743–2749
20. Gnerlich J, Jeffe DB, Deshpande AD, Beers C, Zander C, Margenthaler JA (2007) Surgical removal of the primary tumor increases overall survival in patients with metastatic breast cancer: analysis of the 1988–2003 SEER data. Ann Surg Oncol 14(8):2187–2194
21. Fields RC, Jeffe DB, Trinkaus K et al (2007) Surgical resection of the primary tumor is associated with increased long-term survival in patients with stage IV breast cancer after controlling for site of metastasis. Ann Surg Oncol 14(12):3345–3351
22. Badwe R, Parmar B (2013) Surgical removal of primary breast tumor and axillary lymph nodes at first presentation in women with metastatic breast cancer; a prospective randomized controlled trial. Breast Cancer Symposium. San Antonio
23. Morrow M, Burstein H, Harris JR (2015) Malignant tumors of the breast. In: Cancer: principles and practice of oncology, 10th edn. Philadelphia, Pa, Lippincott Williams & Wilkins
24. Smith GL, Xu Y, Buchholz TA et al (2012) Association between treatment with brachytherapy vs whole-breast irradiation and subsequent mastectomy, complications, and survival among older women with invasive breast cancer. JAMA 307(17):1827–1837
25. Dawood S, Gonzalez-Angulo AM (2013) Progress in the biological understanding and management of breast cancer-associated central nervous system metastases. Oncologist 18(6):675–684
26. Dellas K (2011) Does radiotherapy have curative potential in metastatic patients? The concept of local therapy in oligometastatic breast cancer. Breast Care 6(5):363–368
27. Paridaens R, Dirix L, Lohrisch C et al (2003) Mature results of a randomized phase II multicenter study of exemestane versus tamoxifen as first-line hormone therapy for postmenopausal women with metastatic breast cancer. Ann Oncol 14(9):1391–1398
28. Mayer EL, Burstein HJ (2007) Chemotherapy for metastatic breast cancer. Hematol Oncol Clin N Am 21(2):257–272
29. Del Mastro L, Catzeddu T, Boni L et al (2006) Prevention of chemotherapy-induced menopause by temporary ovarian suppression with goserelin in young, early breast cancer patients. Ann Oncol 17(1):74–78
30. Geisler J, Haynes B, Anker G, Dowsett M, Lønning PE (2002) Influence of letrozole and anastrozole on total body aromatization and plasma estrogen levels in postmenopausal breast cancer patients evaluated in a randomized, cross-over study. J Clin Oncol 20(3):751–757
31. Buzdar A (2000) Exemestane in advanced breast cancer. Anti-Cancer Drugs 11(8):609–616
32. Bertelli G, Garrone O, Merlano M et al (2005) Sequential treatment with exemestane and non-steroidal aromatase inhibitors in advanced breast cancer. Oncology 69(6):471–477

33. Peng J, Sengupta S, Jordan VC (2009) Potential of selective estrogen receptor modulators as treatments and preventives of breast cancer. Anti-Cancer Agents Med Chem 9(5):481–499
34. Howell SJ, Johnston SRD, Howell A (2004) The use of selective estrogen receptor modulators and selective estrogen receptor down-regulators in breast cancer. Best Pract Res Clin Endocrinol Metab 18(1):47–66
35. Francis PA, Regan MM, Fleming GF et al (2014) Adjuvant ovarian suppression in premenopausal breast cancer. N Engl J Med 372(5):436–446
36. Mathew A, Davidson NE (2015) Adjuvant endocrine therapy for premenopausal women with hormone-responsive breast cancer. Breast 24:S120–S125
37. Hortobagyi GN (1998) Treatment of breast cancer. N Engl J Med 339(14):974–984
38. Zeichner SB, Terawaki H, Gogineni K (2016) A review of systemic treatment in metastatic triple-negative breast cancer. Breast Cancer Basic Clin Res 10:25–36
39. O'Shaughnessy J (2005) Extending survival with chemotherapy in metastatic breast cancer. Oncologist 10(3):20–29
40. Crozier JA, Swaika A, Moreno-Aspitia A (2014) Adjuvant chemotherapy in breast cancer: to use or not to use, the anthracyclines. World J Clin Oncol 5(3):529–538
41. O'Brien MER, Wigler N, Inbar M et al (2004) Reduced cardiotoxicity and comparable efficacy in a phase III trial of pegylated liposomal doxorubicin HCl (CAELYX™/Doxil®) versus conventional doxorubicin for first-line treatment of metastatic breast cancer. Ann Oncol 15(3):440–449
42. Blum JL, Jones SE, Buzdar AU et al (1999) Multicenter phase II study of capecitabine in paclitaxel-refractory metastatic breast cancer. J Clin Oncol 17(2):485–485
43. Slamon DJ, Leyland-Jones B, Shak S et al (2001) Use of chemotherapy plus a monoclonal antibody against HER2 for metastatic breast cancer that overexpresses HER2. N Engl J Med 344(11):783–792
44. Vogel CL, Cobleigh MA, Tripathy D et al (2002) Efficacy and safety of trastuzumab as a single agent in first-line treatment of HER2-overexpressing metastatic breast cancer. J Clin Oncol 20(3):719–726
45. Lipton A, Ali SM, Leitzel K et al (2002) Elevated serum HER-2/neu level predicts decreased response to hormone therapy in metastatic breast cancer. J Clin Oncol 20(6):1467–1472
46. Johnston S, Pippen J, Pivot X et al (2009) Lapatinib combined with letrozole versus letrozole and placebo as first-line therapy for postmenopausal hormone receptor–positive metastatic breast cancer. J Clin Oncol 27(33):5538–5546
47. Guarneri V, Lenihan DJ, Valero V et al (2006) Long-term cardiac tolerability of trastuzumab in metastatic breast cancer: the M.D. Anderson cancer center experience. J Clin Oncol 24(25):4107–4115
48. Cobleigh MA, Langmuir VK, Sledge GW et al (2003) A phase I/II dose-escalation trial of bevacizumab in previously treated metastatic breast cancer. Semin Oncol 30:117–124
49. Valachis A, Polyzos NP, Patsopoulos NA, Georgoulias V, Mavroudis D, Mauri D (2010) Bevacizumab in metastatic breast cancer: a meta-analysis of randomized controlled trials. Breast Cancer Res Treat 122(1):1–7
50. Sambi M, Qorri B, Malardier-Jugroot C, Szewczuk M (2017) Advancements in polymer science: 'Smart' drug delivery systems for the treatment of cancer. MOJ Polym Sci 1(3):00016
51. Malam Y, Loizidou M, Seifalian AM (2009) Liposomes and nanoparticles: nanosized vehicles for drug delivery in cancer. Trends Pharmacol Sci 30(11):592–599
52. Haley B, Frenkel E (2008) Nanoparticles for drug delivery in cancer treatment. Urol Oncol Semin Original Inv 26(1):57–64
53. Li X, McTaggart M, Malardier-Jugroot C (2016) Synthesis and characterization of a pH responsive folic acid functionalized polymeric drug delivery system. Biophys Chem 214–215:17–26
54. Li X, Szewczuk MR, Malardier-Jugroot C (2016) Folic acid-conjugated amphiphilic alternating copolymer as a new active tumor targeting drug delivery platform. Drug Des Devel Ther 10:4101–4110

55. Heo DN, Yang DH, Moon H-J et al (2012) Gold nanoparticles surface-functionalized with paclitaxel drug and biotin receptor as theranostic agents for cancer therapy. Biomaterials 33(3):856–866
56. Lal S, Clare SE, Halas NJ (2008) Nanoshell-enabled photothermal cancer therapy: impending clinical impact. Acc Chem Res 41(12):1842–1851
57. Marty M, Cognetti F, Maraninchi D et al (2005) Randomized phase II trial of the efficacy and safety of trastuzumab combined with docetaxel in patients with human epidermal growth factor receptor 2–positive metastatic breast cancer administered as first-line treatment: the M77001 study group. J Clin Oncol 23(19):4265–4274
58. Kaufman B, Mackey JR, Clemens MR et al (2009) Trastuzumab plus anastrozole aersus anastrozole alone for the treatment of postmenopausal women with human epidermal growth factor receptor 2–positive, hormone receptor–positive metastatic breast cancer: results from the randomized phase III TAnDEM study. J Clin Oncol 27(33):5529–5537
59. Robert NJ, Diéras V, Glaspy J et al (2011) RIBBON-1: randomized, double-blind, placebo-controlled, phase III trial of chemotherapy with or without bevacizumab for first-line treatment of human epidermal growth factor receptor 2–negative, locally recurrent or metastatic breast cancer. J Clin Oncol 29(10):1252–1260
60. Miles DW, Chan A, Dirix LY et al (2010) Phase III study of bevacizumab plus docetaxel compared with placebo plus docetaxel for the first-line treatment of human epidermal growth factor receptor 2–negative metastatic breast cancer. J Clin Oncol 28(20):3239–3247
61. Sanchez-Rivera FJ, Jacks T (2015) Applications of the CRISPR-Cas9 system in cancer biology. Nat Rev Cancer 15(7):387–395
62. Lee JH, Zhao XM, Yoon I et al (2016) Integrative analysis of mutational and transcriptional profiles reveals driver mutations of metastatic breast cancers. Cell Discov 2:16025
63. Wang CY, Uray IP, Mazumdar A, Mayer JA, Brown PH (2012) SLC22A5/OCTN2 expression in breast cancer is induced by estrogen via a novel intronic estrogen-response element (ERE). Breast Cancer Res Treat 134(1):101–115
64. Tran LM, Zhang B, Zhang Z et al (2011) Inferring causal genomic alterations in breast cancer using gene expression data. BMC Syst Biol 5:121
65. Zhang NG, Ge GQ, Meyer R et al (2008) Overexpression of Separase induces aneuploidy and mammary tumorigenesis. Proc Natl Acad Sci U S A 105(35):13033–13038
66. Lefebvre C, Bachelot T, Filleron T et al (2016) Mutational profile of metastatic breast cancers: a retrospective analysis. PLoS Med 13(12):e1002201
67. Bai X, Zhang E, Ye H et al (2014) PIK3CA and TP53 gene mutations in human breast cancer tumors frequently detected by ion torrent DNA sequencing. PLoS One 9(6):e99306
68. Finn RS, Martin M, Rugo HS et al (2016) Palbociclib and letrozole in advanced breast cancer. N Engl J Med 375(20):1925–1936
69. Chirila C, Mitra D, Colosia A et al (2017) Comparison of palbociclib in combination with letrozole or fulvestrant with endocrine therapies for advanced/metastatic breast cancer: network meta-analysis. Curr Med Res Opin 33(8):1457–1466
70. Osborne C, Wilson P, Tripathy D (2004) Oncogenes and tumor suppressor genes in breast cancer: potential diagnostic and therapeutic applications. Oncologist 9(4):361–377
71. Yao SH, He ZY, Chen C (2015) CRISPR/Cas9-mediated genome editing of epigenetic factors for cancer therapy. Hum Gene Ther 26(7):463–471
72. Trowbridge JJ, Sinha AU, Zhu N, Li M, Armstrong SA, Orkin SH (2012) Haploinsufficiency of Dnmt1 impairs leukemia stem cell function through derepression of bivalent chromatin domains. Genes Dev 26(4):344–349
73. Szyf M, Pakneshan P, Rabbani SA (2004) DNA methylation and breast cancer. Biochem Pharmacol 68(6):1187–1197
74. Hu XC, Wong IH, Chow LW (2003) Tumor-derived aberrant methylation in plasma of invasive ductal breast cancer patients: clinical implications. Oncol Rep 10(6):1811–1815
75. Sander JD, Joung JK (2014) CRISPR-Cas systems for editing, regulating and targeting genomes. Nat Biotechnol 32(4):347–355

76. Horvath P, Barrangou R (2010) CRISPR/Cas, the immune system of bacteria and archaea. Science 327(5962):167–170
77. Xue W, Chen S, Yin H et al (2014) CRISPR-mediated direct mutation of cancer genes in the mouse liver. Nature 514(7522):380–384
78. Fantozzi A, Christofori G (2006) Mouse models of breast cancer metastasis. Breast Cancer Res BCR 8(4):212
79. de Visser KE, Eichten A, Coussens LM (2006) Paradoxical roles of the immune system during cancer development. Nat Rev Cancer 6(1):24–37
80. Landskron G, De la Fuente M, Thuwajit P, Thuwajit C, Hermoso MA (2014) Chronic inflammation and cytokines in the tumor microenvironment. J Immunol Res 2014:19
81. Wu Y, Zhou BP (2010) TNF-α/NF-κB/Snail pathway in cancer cell migration and invasion. Br J Cancer 102(4):639–644
82. Zhao X, Xu Z, Li H (2017) NSAIDs use and reduced metastasis in cancer patients: results from a meta-analysis. Sci Rep 7(1):1875
83. Kumar N, Drabu S, Mondal SC (2013) NSAID's and selectively COX-2 inhibitors as potential chemoprotective agents against cancer: 1st Cancer Update. Arab J Chem 6(1):1–23
84. Dierssen-Sotos T, Gómez-Acebo I, de Pedro M et al (2016) Use of non-steroidal anti-inflammatory drugs and risk of breast cancer: the Spanish Multi-Case-control (MCC) study. BMC Cancer 16(1):660
85. Rankin EB, Giaccia AJ (2016) Hypoxic control of metastasis. Science (New York, NY) 352(6282):175–180
86. Gilkes DM, Semenza GL (2013) Role of hypoxia-inducible factors in breast cancer metastasis. Future Oncol (London, England) 9(11):1623–1636
87. Favaro E, Lord S, Harris AL, Buffa FM (2011) Gene expression and hypoxia in breast cancer. Genome Med 3(8):55–55
88. Muz B, de la Puente P, Azab F, Azab AK (2015) The role of hypoxia in cancer progression, angiogenesis, metastasis, and resistance to therapy. Hypoxia 3:83–92
89. Wong CC-L, Gilkes DM, Zhang H et al (2011) Hypoxia-inducible factor 1 is a master regulator of breast cancer metastatic niche formation. Proc Natl Acad Sci 108(39):16369–16374
90. Park JE, Tan HS, Datta A et al (2010) Hypoxic tumor cell modulates its microenvironment to enhance angiogenic and metastatic potential by secretion of proteins and exosomes. Mol Cell Proteomics 9(6):1085–1099
91. Onnis B, Rapisarda A, Melillo G (2009) Development of HIF-1 inhibitors for cancer therapy. J Cell Mol Med 13(9a):2780–2786
92. Burroughs SK, Kaluz S, Wang D, Wang K, Van Meir EG, Wang B (2013) Hypoxia inducible factor pathway inhibitors as anticancer therapeutics. Future Med Chem 5(5):553–572. https://doi.org/10.4155/fmc.4113.4117
93. Jain RK (2005) Normalization of tumor vasculature: an emerging concept in antiangiogenic therapy. Science 307(5706):58–62
94. Jain RK (2013) Normalizing tumor microenvironment to treat cancer: bench to bedside to biomarkers. J Clin Oncol 31(17):2205–2218
95. Goel S, Wong AH, Jain RK (2012) Vascular normalization as a therapeutic strategy for malignant and nonmalignant disease. Cold Spring Harb Perspect Med 2(3):a006486
96. Nielsen DL, Andersson M, Andersen JL, Kamby C (2010) Antiangiogenic therapy for breast cancer. Breast Cancer Res BCR 12(5):209
97. Ferrara N, Kerbel RS (2005) Angiogenesis as a therapeutic target. Nature 438(7070):967–974
98. Zhang P, Gao WY, Turner S, Ducatman BS (2003) Gleevec (STI-571) inhibits lung cancer cell growth (A549) and potentiates the cisplatin effect in vitro. Mol Cancer 2:1
99. Brufsky A, Rivera RR, Hurvitz SA et al (2010) Progression-free survival. (PFS) in patient subgroups in RIBBON-2, a phase III trial of chemotherapy (chemo) plus or minus bevacizumab (BV) for second-line treatment of HER2-negative, locally recurrent or metastatic breast cancer (MBC). J Clin Oncol 28:15_suppl, 1021

100. Qian B-Z, Pollard JW (2010) Macrophage diversity enhances tumor progression and metastasis. Cell 141(1):39–51
101. Pollard JW (2004) Tumour-educated macrophages promote tumour progression and metastasis. Nat Rev Cancer 4(1):71–78
102. Condeelis J, Pollard JW (2006) Macrophages: obligate partners for tumor cell migration, invasion, and metastasis. Cell 124(2):263–266
103. Whiteside TL (2008) The tumor microenvironment and its role in promoting tumor growth. Oncogene 27(45):5904–5912
104. Pyonteck SM, Akkari L, Schuhmacher AJ et al (2013) CSF-1R inhibition alters macrophage polarization and blocks glioma progression. Nat Med 19(10):1264–1272
105. Mao Y, Keller ET, Garfield DH, Shen K, Wang J (2013) Stromal cells in tumor microenvironment and breast cancer. Cancer Metastasis Rev 32(1–2):303–315
106. Liao D, Luo Y, Markowitz D, Xiang R, Reisfeld RA (2009) Cancer associated fibroblasts promote tumor growth and metastasis by modulating the tumor immune microenvironment in a 4T1 murine breast cancer model. PLoS One 4(11):e7965
107. Hu Y-L, Fu Y-H, Tabata Y, Gao J-Q (2010) Mesenchymal stem cells: a promising targeted-delivery vehicle in cancer gene therapy. J Control Release 147(2):154–162
108. Studeny M, Marini FC, Dembinski JL et al (2004) Mesenchymal stem cells: potential precursors for tumor stroma and targeted-delivery vehicles for anticancer agents. JNCI J Natl Cancer Inst 96(21):1593–1603
109. Boelens Mirjam C, Wu Tony J, Nabet Barzin Y et al (2014) Exosome transfer from stromal to breast cancer cells regulates therapy resistance pathways. Cell 159(3):499–513
110. Suetsugu A, Honma K, Saji S, Moriwaki H, Ochiya T, Hoffman RM (2013) Imaging exosome transfer from breast cancer cells to stroma at metastatic sites in orthotopic nude-mouse models. Adv Drug Deliv Rev 65(3):383–390
111. Savina A, Furlán M, Vidal M, Colombo MI (2003) Exosome release is regulated by a calcium-dependent mechanism in K562 cells. J Biol Chem 278(22):20083–20090
112. King HW, Michael MZ, Gleadle JM (2012) Hypoxic enhancement of exosome release by breast cancer cells. BMC Cancer 12(1):421
113. Bruce WR, Van Der Gaag H (1963) A quantitative assay for the number of murine lymphoma cells capable of proliferation in vivo. Nature 199:79–80
114. Dick JE (2003) Breast cancer stem cells revealed. Proc Natl Acad Sci U S A 100(7):3547–3549
115. Li C, Heidt DG, Dalerba P et al (2007) Identification of pancreatic cancer stem cells. Cancer Res 67(3):1030–1037
116. Dalerba P, Dylla SJ, Park IK et al (2007) Phenotypic characterization of human colorectal cancer stem cells. Proc Natl Acad Sci U S A 104(24):10158–10163
117. Al-Hajj M, Wicha MS, Benito-Hernandez A, Morrison SJ, Clarke MF (2003) Prospective identification of tumorigenic breast cancer cells. Proc Natl Acad Sci U S A 100(7):3983–3988
118. Zhao J (2016) Cancer stem cells and chemoresistance: the smartest survives the raid. Pharmacol Ther 160:145–158
119. Abdullah LN, Chow EK (2013) Mechanisms of chemoresistance in cancer stem cells. Clin Transl Med 2(1):3
120. Longley DB, Johnston PG (2005) Molecular mechanisms of drug resistance. J Pathol 205(2):275–292
121. Schwab LP, Peacock DL, Majumdar D et al (2012) Hypoxia-inducible factor 1alpha promotes primary tumor growth and tumor-initiating cell activity in breast cancer. Breast Cancer Res BCR 14(1):R6
122. Wilson TR, Fridlyand J, Yan Y et al (2012) Widespread potential for growth-factor-driven resistance to anticancer kinase inhibitors. Nature 487(7408):505–509
123. Patel NM, Nozaki S, Shortle NH et al (2000) Paclitaxel sensitivity of breast cancer cells with constitutively active NF-kappaB is enhanced by IkappaBalpha super-repressor and parthenolide. Oncogene 19(36):4159–4169
124. Chow EK, Zhang XQ, Chen M et al (2011) Nanodiamond therapeutic delivery agents mediate enhanced chemoresistant tumor treatment. Sci Transl Med 3(73):73ra21

125. Li X, Sambi M, DeCarlo A et al (2018) Functionalized folic acid-conjugated amphiphilic alternating copolymer actively targets 3D multicellular tumour spheroids and delivers the hydrophobic drug to the inner core. Nanomaterials 8: 588–608

126. Hartmann LC, Keeney GL, Lingle WL et al (2007) Folate receptor overexpression is associated with poor outcome in breast cancer. Int J Cancer 121(5):938–942

127. Pardoll DM (2012) The blockade of immune checkpoints in cancer immunotherapy. Nat Rev Cancer 12(4):252–264

128. Demaria S, Kawashima N, Yang AM et al (2005) Immune-mediated inhibition of metastases after treatment with local radiation and CTLA-4 blockade in a mouse model of breast cancer. Clin Cancer Res Off J Am Assoc Cancer Res 11(2 Pt 1):728–734

129. van Elsas A, Hurwitz AA, Allison JP (1999) Combination immunotherapy of B16 melanoma using anti-cytotoxic T lymphocyte-associated antigen 4 (CTLA-4) and granulocyte/macrophage colony-stimulating factor (GM-CSF)-producing vaccines induces rejection of subcutaneous and metastatic tumors accompanied by autoimmune depigmentation. J Exp Med 190(3):355–366

130. Freeman GJ, Long AJ, Iwai Y et al (2000) Engagement of the PD-1 immunoinhibitory receptor by a novel B7 family member leads to negative regulation of lymphocyte activation. J Exp Med 192(7):1027–1034

131. Nishimura H, Nose M, Hiai H, Minato N, Honjo T (1999) Development of lupus-like autoimmune diseases by disruption of the PD-1 gene encoding an ITIM motif-carrying immunoreceptor. Immunity 11(2):141–151

132. Mittendorf EA, Philips AV, Meric-Bernstam F et al (2014) PD-L1 expression in triple-negative breast cancer. Cancer Immunol Res 2(4):361–370

133. Mantovani A, Marchesi F, Malesci A, Laghi L, Allavena P (2017) Tumour-associated macrophages as treatment targets in oncology. Nat Rev Clin Oncol 14(7):399–416

134. Meats JE, Steele L, Bowen JG (1993) Identification of phospholipase D (PLD) activity in mouse peritoneal macrophages. Agents Actions 39 Spec No:C14–C16

135. Henkels KM, Muppani NR, Gomez-Cambronero J (2016) PLD-specific small-molecule inhibitors decrease tumor-associated macrophages and neutrophils infiltration in breast tumors and lung and liver metastases. PLoS One 11(11):e0166553

136. Tan M, Yu D (2007) Molecular mechanisms of erbB2-mediated breast cancer chemoresistance. Adv Exp Med Biol 608:119–129

137. Slamon DJ, Godolphin W, Jones LA et al (1989) Studies of the HER-2/neu proto-oncogene in human breast and ovarian cancer. Science 244(4905):707–712

138. Wang Y (2010) Breast cancer metastasis driven by ErbB2 and 14-3-3zeta: a division of labor. Cell Adhes Migr 4(1):7–9

139. Eccles SA (2011) The epidermal growth factor receptor/Erb-B/HER family in normal and malignant breast biology. Int J Dev Biol 55(7–9):685–696

140. Hoelder S, Clarke PA, Workman P (2012) Discovery of small molecule cancer drugs: successes, challenges and opportunities. Mol Oncol 6(2):155–176

141. Li D, Marchenko ND (2017) ErbB2 inhibition by lapatinib promotes degradation of mutant p53 protein in cancer cells. Oncotarget 8(4):5823–5833

142. Dziadkowiec KN, Gasiorowska E, Nowak-Markwitz E, Jankowska A (2016) PARP inhibitors: review of mechanisms of action and BRCA1/2 mutation targeting. Prz Menopauzalny 15(4):215–219

143. Ouchi T, Monteiro AN, August A, Aaronson SA, Hanafusa H (1998) BRCA1 regulates p53-dependent gene expression. Proc Natl Acad Sci U S A 95(5):2302–2306

144. Morales J, Li L, Fattah FJ et al (2014) Review of poly (ADP-ribose) polymerase (PARP) mechanisms of action and rationale for targeting in cancer and other diseases. Crit Rev Eukaryot Gene Expr 24(1):15–28

145. Chalmers AJ (2009) The potential role and application of PARP inhibitors in cancer treatment. Br Med Bull 89:23–40

146. O'Shaughnessy J, Osborne C, Pippen JE et al (2011) Iniparib plus chemotherapy in metastatic triple-negative breast cancer. N Engl J Med 364(3):205–214

147. Murai J, Huang SY, Das BB et al (2012) Trapping of PARP1 and PARP2 by clinical PARP inhibitors. Cancer Res 72(21):5588–5599
148. Gilmour AM, Abdulkhalek S, Cheng TS et al (2013) A novel epidermal growth factor receptor-signaling platform and its targeted translation in pancreatic cancer. Cell Signal25(12):2587–2603
149. Amith SR, Jayanth P, Franchuk S et al (2010) Neu1 desialylation of sialyl α-2,3-linked β-galactosyl residues of TOLL-like is essential for receptor activation and cellular signaling. Cellular Signalling 22: 314–324
150. Abdulkhalek S, Amith SR, Franchuk SL et al (2011) Neu1 sialidase and matrix metalloproteinase-9 cross-talk Is essential for Toll-like receptor activation and cellular signaling. J Biol Chem 286 (42): 36532–36549
151. Abdulkhalek S, Guo M, Amith SR et al (2012) G-protein coupled receptor agonists mediate Neu1 sialidase and matrix metalloproteinase-9 cross-talk to induce transactivation of TOLL-like receptors and cellular signaling. Cellular Signalling 24: 2035–2042
152. Abdulkhalek S, Szewczuk MR (2013) Neu1 sialidase and matrix metalloproteinase-9 cross-talk regulates nucleic acid-induced endosomal TOLL-like receptor-7 and -9 activation, cellular signaling and pro-inflammatory responses. Cellular Signalling 25: 2093–2105
153. Alghamdi F, Guo M, Abdulkhalek S et al (2014) A novel insulin receptor-signaling platform and its link to insulin resistance and type 2 diabetes. Cellular Signalling 26: 1355–1368
154. Haxho F, Alghamdi F, Neufeld RJ et al (2014) Novel Insulin Receptor-Signaling Platform. Int J Diabetes Clin Res 1:1-10
155. Haxho F, Haq S, Szewczuk MR (2018) Biased G protein-coupled receptor agonism mediates Neu1 sialidase and matrix metalloproteinase-9 crosstalk to induce transactivation of insulin receptor signaling. Cellular Signalling 43: 71–84
156. Haxho F, Neufeld RJ, Szewczuk MR (2016) Neuraminidase-1: A novel therapeutic target in multistage tumorigenesis. Oncotarget 7: 40860–40881
157. Hrynyk M, Ellis JP, Haxho F et al (2015) Therapeutic designed poly (lactic-co-glycolic acid) cylindrical oseltamivir phosphate-loaded implants impede tumor neovascularization, growth and metastasis in mouse model of human pancreatic carcinoma. Drug Des Devel Ther 9:4573–4586
158. O'Shea LK, Abdulkhalek S, Allison S, Neufeld RJ, Szewczuk MR (2014) Therapeutic targeting of Neu1 sialidase with oseltamivir phosphate (Tamiflu(R)) disables cancer cell survival in human pancreatic cancer with acquired chemoresistance. Oncotarget Ther 7:117– 134
159. Abdulkhalek S, Geen OD, Brodhagenn L, Haxho F et al (2014) Transcriptional factor snail controls tumor neovascularization, growth and metastasis in mouse model of human ovarian carcinoma. Clinical and Translational Medicine 3: 1-28
160. Haxho F, Allison S, Alghamdi F et al (2014) Oseltamivir phosphate monotherapy ablates tumor neovascularization, growth, and metastasis in mouse model of human triple-negative breast adenocarcinoma. Breast Cancer Targets Ther 6:191–203
161. Abdulkhalek S, Hrynyk M, Szewczuk MR (2013) A novel G-protein-coupled receptorsignaling platform and its targeted translation in human disease. Res Rep Biochem 3:17–30

Chapter 9
Chemotherapy and Inflammatory Cytokine Signalling in Cancer Cells and the Tumour Microenvironment

Derek W. Edwardson, Amadeo M. Parissenti, and A. Thomas Kovala

Abstract Cancer is the result of a cell's acquisition of a variety of biological capabilities or 'hallmarks' as outlined by Hanahan and Weinberg. These include sustained proliferative signalling, the ability to evade growth suppressors, resisting cell death, enabling replicative immortality, inducing angiogenesis, and the ability to invade other tissue and metastasize. More recently, the ability to escape immune destruction has been recognized as another important hallmark of tumours. It is suggested that genome instability and *inflammation* accelerates the acquisition of a variety of the above hallmarks. Inflammation, is a product of the body's response to tissue damage or pathogen invasion. It is required for tissue repair and host defense, but prolonged inflammation can often be the cause for disease. In a cancer patient, it is often unclear whether inflammation plays a protective or deleterious role in disease progression. Chemotherapy drugs can suppress tumour growth but also induce pathways in tumour cells that have been shown experimentally to support tumour progression or, in other cases, encourage an anti-tumour immune response.

D. W. Edwardson
Graduate Program in Biomolecular Sciences, Laurentian University, Sudbury, ON, Canada

A. M. Parissenti (✉)
Graduate Program in Biomolecular Sciences, Laurentian University, Sudbury, ON, Canada

Department of Chemistry and Biochemistry, Laurentian University, Sudbury, ON, Canada

Division of Medical Sciences, Northern Ontario School of Medicine, Sudbury, ON, Canada

Health Sciences North Research Institute, Sudbury, ON, Canada

Division of Oncology, Faculty of Medicine, University of Ottawa, Ottawa, ON, Canada
e-mail: aparissenti@hsnsudbury.ca

A. T. Kovala
Graduate Program in Biomolecular Sciences, Laurentian University, Sudbury, ON, Canada

Department of Chemistry and Biochemistry, Laurentian University, Sudbury, ON, Canada

Division of Medical Sciences, Northern Ontario School of Medicine, Sudbury, ON, Canada

Department of Biology, Laurentian University, Sudbury, ON, Canada
e-mail: tkovala@nosm.ca

© Springer Nature Switzerland AG 2019
A. Ahmad (ed.), *Breast Cancer Metastasis and Drug Resistance*,
Advances in Experimental Medicine and Biology 1152,
https://doi.org/10.1007/978-3-030-20301-6_9

Thus, with the goal of better understanding the context under which each of these possible outcomes occurs, recent progress exploring chemotherapy-induced inflammatory cytokine production and the effects of cytokines on drug efficacy in the tumour microenvironment will be reviewed. The implications of chemotherapy on host and tumour cytokine pathways and their effect on the treatment of cancer patients will also be discussed.

Keywords Chemotherapy response · Induction · Cytokines · Tumour microenvironment · Response biomarkers · Drug resistance

9.1 Introduction

The intersection between tumour development and progression, inflammation, and the immune system is now well recognized but not completely understood. The key role of the tumour microenvironment has become an increasingly important topic for both basic and clinical cancer research. Mediators of inflammatory reactions, produced by the tumour cells themselves, associated stroma and vascular cells, or the immune cells infiltrating the tumour, and their influence on all aspects of tumourigenesis, are under extensive investigation. An enormous number of cytokines, growth factors, lipids, and other signalling molecules are produced by different cell types, which impact both negatively and positively on tumour progression. Much of this is highly dependent upon the tumour microenvironment. There is currently an extensive literature on the influence of inflammatory pathways and the immune system on tumour development, with many excellent general reviews in this area [1–5].

Cytokines are the major regulators of inflammatory processes, and drive many of the interactions between immune cells. Cytokines are a very diverse group of small (generally 2–20 kDa) proteins, including such different families as the chemokines, interleukins (IL), adipokines, interferons (IFN), transforming growth factors (TGF) and tumour necrosis factors (TNF). Chemokines are chemotactic cytokines, while interleukins were originally believed to mediate communication between leukocytes. The latter are now known to be produced by numerous cell types. Adipokines are cytokines produced by adipocytes. An individual cytokine can belong to several of these groupings. The nomenclature of cytokines has historically been confusing, where multiple names for individual cytokines coexist as different groups identified functional activities in different systems. More rational, systematic classifications based on functional and/or structural characteristics have been developed, but historical names are often deeply ingrained and still commonly used. In this review we will try to provide both the systematic name and the most common name where possible.

Functionally, cytokines can be divided into groups involved in adaptive immunity, pro-inflammatory processes, and anti-inflammatory processes. Many cytokines also exhibit other activities, some of which are context dependent [6].Structurally, the majority of chemokines belong to either the CCL family with two adjacent cysteine residues (31 family members), as compared to the CXCL family, where the cysteines are separated by a variable amino acid residue (18 family members). Smaller families of chemokines include those with a single cysteine (XCL1 and XCL2) and the CX3CL family, with a single member, fractalkine. The interleukin family currently has 38 identified members [7, 8], while to date ten interferons (IFN) have been identified, of which seven are expressed in humans [9]. The TNF superfamily has 19 members [10] and the TGFβ superfamily contains over 30 members [11]. The prototypical members of each family have been thoroughly studied, but much less is often known about many of the more newly identified members.

For decades, inflammatory cytokines have been the topic of extensive study in oncology, implicated as promoters, or in some cases, inhibitors of tumour cell proliferation. They also are known to have effects on tumour angiogenesis, metastasis, and other malignant cell behaviour [2, 12]. Prior studies have shown that several therapeutic agents used in the treatment of cancer can stimulate the production of several inflammatory cytokines from both cells of the immune system as well as the tumour, as we will discuss in this review. The extracellular space proximal to a tumour contains a repertoire of recruited, apparently normal cells, collectively referred to as the tumour microenvironment, which can contribute to progression of disease. Originating from either the tumour or other cells within its microenvironment, the presence of inflammatory cytokines in the tumour microenvironment plays a major role in cancer behaviour in general [13], and in breast cancer specifically (reviewed in [14–18]).

The taxane class of chemotherapy drugs, including docetaxel and paclitaxel, are commonly used in the treatment of breast and other cancers. Taxanes bind to β-tubulin where they exert their cytotoxic effects on tumour cells through the stabilization of microtubules and the resulting arrest in mitosis [19]. The development of resistance to these drugs by a variety of mechanisms poses serious limitations in the successful treatment of patients [20, 21]. Among the first documented studies of inflammatory cytokine production in response to treatment with chemotherapeutic drugs were reports of murine macrophages that increased their production of TNF-α and IL-1 after exposure to paclitaxel [22]. It was later suggested that this action of paclitaxel is distinct from its cytotoxic activity [23]. Since then, the ability of taxanes, along with other drug families, to induce inflammatory cytokine production has been observed, in some cases from immune cells, and in other cases from tumour cell lines. A variety of studies have reported chemotherapy-induced cytokine release (Table 9.1) in vitro and in vivo and the effects of stromal- or tumour-derived cytokines on drug sensitivity (Table 9.2).

Cellular modulation of activity by cytokines can be either autocrine or paracrine, and a role for numerous cytokines has been identified in multiple aspects of tumour development. A far less understood area concerns the impact of chemotherapeutic drugs on the tumour microenvironment, and the impact of the tumour microenvironment on drug sensitivity in the tumour. This review will concentrate on two key aspects: (a) the ability of chemotherapy drugs to induce the expression of cytokines by tumour cells or associated stromal cells, and (b) the ability of

Table 9.1 Chemotherapy-induced release of a variety of inflammatory cytokines from various tumour and immune cell lines

Chemotherapy drug	Cytokine(s) induced	Cell type	Reference
Camptothecin	IL-6	Lung cancer cell lines	[72]
Carboplatin	MIC1	Prostate cancer	[156]
Cisplatin	IL-6	Lung cancer cell lines	[72]
Cisplatin	CCL2	Ovarian stromal fibroblasts	[132]
Cisplatin	CCL5	CAF – ovarian cancer	[132]
Cisplatin	MIC1	Lung cancer, A2780	[159]
Cisplatin	IL-6, CXCL8, CCL2, CCL5, BFGF, G-CSF, VEGF	Various cancer cell lines	[210]
Dacarbazine	CXCL8, VEGF	Melanoma	[211, 212]
Docetaxel	C5/C5a, I-309, IFNγ, IL-1α, IL-1rα, RANTES	Prostate cancer cells PC3	[213]
Docetaxel	IL-10	Docetaxel-resistant PC3 (prostate)	[213]
Docetaxel	CXCL1, RANTES	PC3 (prostate)/U937 (monocyte) mixed culture	[213]
Docetaxel	GCSF, IL-27	Docetaxel-resistant PC3 (prostate)/U937 (monocyte) mixed	[214]
Docetaxel	TNF-α	MCF-7 (breast), A2780 (ovarian) tumour cells	[26]
Docetaxel	CCL2	Prostate cancer	[128]
Docetaxel	CXCL10, MIC-1, IL1β	Prostate cancer cells (PC3, DU145) LuCaP 35V xenografts	[156]
Doxorubicin	CCL2, IL-6, CXCL8	MCF-7	[59]
Doxorubicin	TNF-α	Breast epithelial cells (in vivo mouse)	[33]
Doxorubicin	IFNγ	Various cancer cell lines	[172]
Doxorubicin	IL-6, CXCL8, CCL2, CCL5, BFGF, G-CSF, VEGF	Various cancer cell lines	[210]
Genistein	MIC1	Lung cancer cell, A2780	[159]
Mitoxantrone	CXCL10, MIC-1	Prostate cancer cells PC3, DU145	[156]
Mitoxantrone	IFNγ	Various cancer cell lines	[172]
Oxaliplatin	CXCL8, CXCL1	Prostate cancer cell lines PC3, DU145	[63]
Paclitaxel	TNF-α, IL-1α/β	Murine macrophages	[22]
Paclitaxel	CXCL8	Ovarian tumour cells	[54]
Paclitaxel	CXCL8	Primary ovarian tumour cells	[55]
Paclitaxel	CXCL8	Human lung carcinoma	[56]

(continued)

Table 9.1 (continued)

Chemotherapy drug	Cytokine(s) induced	Cell type	Reference
PLX4032	CCL2	Melanoma cell lines	[127]
Trastuzumab	EGF, IL-6	Breast cancer (BT-474) and gastric cancer (NCI-N87)	[75]
Cytarabine, Daunorubicin, Etoposide, Methotrexate, Vincristine	CXCR4	Leukemia cell lines; up-regulation (697, MOLM-14, and MV4-11) or down-regulation (HB-1119, Nalm-6, SEM-K2)	[106]

Table 9.2 Cytokines identified as playing a role in resistance to cytotoxic agents via autocrine/paracrine signalling

Cytokine(s)	Cytotoxic agent	Cell types involved	Tumour cell targets	Reference
Chemoresistance-inducing				
IL-6	Gemcitabine	Pancreatic cancer cells	FAK and ERK1/2	[215]
IL-6	Trastuzumab	MCF-7 and SUM-159 HER2+ cells	IL-6R/STAT3/AKT/ NF-κB	[212]
IL-6	Trastuzumab	NCI-N87 gastric cancer cells	STAT3/Jagged-1/ Notch	[76]
IL-6, EGF	Trastuzumab	BT-474 (breast) and NCI-N87 (gastric)	STAT3	[75]
IL-6	Dexamethasone	Various myeloma cell lines		[86]
IL-6	Cisplatin	Non-small cell lung cancer cells (A549 and H157)	IL-6 gene transcription	[78]
IL-6	Paclitaxel	SKOV3 and SKOV3/TR	IL-6 gene transcription/STAT3	[216]
IL-6	Various anti-HER2 agents	ER-/HER2+ Breast cancer cells	IL-6/JAK/STAT3/ Calprotectin	[77]
IL-6	Camptothecin, cisplatin	Various lung cancer cell lines	Ataxia telangiectasia mutated/NF-κB	[72]
IL-6	Doxorubicin, vincristine, paclitaxel	MCF-7	C/EBPβ, C/EBP, MDR-1	[71]
IL-6	Tamoxifen	CAOV-3, SKOV-2, ES-2, A2780	ER-α activity through MEK/ERK and PI3K/Akt	[217]
IL-6	Cisplatin, paclitaxel	A2780, SKOV-3, CAOV-3	MEK/ERK and PI3K/Akt	[58]
IL-6	Paclitaxel, doxorubicin	MCF-7	P-gp	[59]
IL-6	Cisplatin, paclitaxel	A2780, SKOV-3, CAOV-3	MEK/ERK and PI3K/Akt	[58]
IL-7	Cisplatin	Glioma		[141]
IL-10	Paclitaxel	Breast cancer		[148]

(continued)

Table 9.2 (continued)

Cytokine(s)	Cytotoxic agent	Cell types involved	Tumour cell targets	Reference
IL-10	Paclitaxel	Dendritic		[218]
IL-10, IL-4	Cisplatin, doxorubicin, taxol	Thyroid carcinoma	Bcl2, Bcl-X$_L$	[219]
IL-18	Doxorubicin	MCF-7		[150]
IL18	Pemetrexed, vorinostat	Mesothelioma cell lines		[151]
IL-34	Doxorubicin	Adenocarcinoma A459	PI3K/Akt	[153]
CXCL12	Doxorubicin, Ara-C	AML		[220]
CXCL12	Doxorubicin, cytarabine	AML		[221]
CXCL12	Docetaxel	Prostate cancer		[152]
CXCL12	Docetaxel	Prostate cancer		[105]
CXCL12	Temsirolimus	Pancreatic cancer		[102]
CXCL12	Gemcitabine	Pancreatic cancer	IL-6	[215]
CXCL8	Paclitaxel, doxorubicin	MCF-7	P-gp	[59]
CXCL8	Oxaliplatin	Prostate cancer cell lines PC3, DU145	NF-κB	[63]
CCL2	Docetaxel	Prostate cancer	ERK/PI3K	[128]
CCL2	5-FU, gentamycin	Breast cancer	Smad3/ERK	[121]
CCL2	Paclitaxel, cisplatin	Ovarian cancer		[222]
CCL2	PLX4032	Melanoma		[127]
CCL5	Tamoxifen	Breast cancer	STAT3	[131]
CCL5	Cisplatin	Ovarian cancer	STAT3/Akt	[132]
CCL25	Cisplatin	Breast cancer	Akt/PI3K/FAK	[139]
CCL25	Cisplatin	Ovarian cancer	Akt/GSK3b/FKHR	[135]
CCL25	Etoposide	Prostate cancer	PI3K/Akt	[136]
CCL25	TNF-α	Leukemia	JNK, Livin	[138]
MIC1	Docetaxel	Prostate PC-3		[157]
MIC1	Docetaxel	Prostate PC-3, LNCaP		[158]
MIC1	Docetaxel, mitoxantrone	Prostate cancer, PC3, DU145		[156]
MIC1	Mitoxantrone	AML		[162]
MIC1	Cisplatin	Ovarian cancer A2780		[159]
MIC1	Trastuzumab	Breast cancer		[160]
MIC1	Trastuzumab	Breast cancer		[161]
TGF-β	Docetaxel	Prostate cancer, PC3, DU145		[223]
TGF-β	Docetaxel	Prostate cancer		[96]
TGF-β	Erlotinib	NSCLC	IL-6	[97]
TGF-β	Cisplatin, radiation	Oral cancer, SCC4, SCC25	IL-6	[99]
TGF-β	Gemcitabine	Biliary tract cancer cell lines	IL-6, SMAD4	[98]

(continued)

Table 9.2 (continued)

Cytokine(s)	Cytotoxic agent	Cell types involved	Tumour cell targets	Reference
TNF-α	Docetaxel	Docetaxel-resistant MCF-7	TNFR2/NF-κB	[26]
Chemosensitizing				
IFN/ CXCL10	Doxorubicin	Fibrosarcomas, melanomas	TLR3, IFNAR	[172]
IL-24	Adriamycin	MCF-7/ADM	STAT3, P-gp	[170]
IL-24	Paclitaxel	MDA-M-231, Bcap-37		[169]
IL-24	Doxorubicin	Osteosarcoma	P-gp, BCRP1	[166]
IL-24	Cisplatin, epirubicin, vinblastine	B cell lymphoma	RhoA, ERK	[165]
IL-24	Radiation	Primary glioma	Bcl-2, Bad	[167, 171]
IL-24	Temozolomide	Glioma (U87, U251)	PKR, Bcl-2	[168]

cytokines to influence the efficacy of chemotherapy drug treatment on tumour cells. Some of the potential clinical implications of chemotherapy-induced cytokine expression and cytokine modulation of physiological processes will also discussed. These interactions are vital to the development of drug resistance in many tumours and an understanding of the mechanisms behind these interactions will be important for the development of more effective treatment options for cancer patients, with reduced host toxicities [24].

9.2 Chemotherapy, Cytokines and Drug Resistance

9.2.1 Tumour Necrosis Factor-α (TNF-α)

TNF-α is perhaps the most widely studied inflammatory cytokine, playing important roles in regulating both the innate and adaptive immune response pathways through its ability to affect a variety of cell types. It has been dubbed "a master regulator of leukocyte movement" [25], and recently has been shown to affect tumour cells directly through autocrine action.

We have shown that TNF-α is released from breast and ovarian tumour cells in response to treatment with various classes of chemotherapy drugs, including the taxanes [26], anthracyclines, platinating agents, and nucleoside analogs [26, 27]. We further observed that treatment of MCF-7 breast tumour cells with a neutralizing antibody specific for TNF-α receptor 1 (TNFR1) resulted in less cellular sensitivity to the growth inhibitory effects of docetaxel [26]. An explanation for this is that docetaxel-induced autocrine TNF-α signalling, through TNFR1, contributed to the drug's cytotoxic action on MCF-7 cells [26]. Another study reported that addition of TNF-α, in recombinant form, potentiated the cytotoxic effect of paclitaxel in human SKOV3 ovarian cancer cells [28].

We also found that breast cancer cells, which were selected for survival in increasing concentrations of docetaxel, increased their production of TNF-α at intermediate selection doses [26]. An investigation into the expression of TNF-α receptors revealed that concomitant with the acquisition of docetaxel resistance, there was a significant decrease in the level of TNFR1 protein levels, with no change in TNFR2 levels [26]. Thus, it is possible that while TNF-α signalling through TNFR1 activates a death pathway in the presence of docetaxel, abrogation of this pathway during acquisition of drug resistance shifts the effective balance of TNF-α signalling to the TNFR2 pathway, promoting survival. In support of this view, it was demonstrated that inhibition of TNFR2 signalling using a TNFR2-neutralizing antibody caused a sensitization of docetaxel-resistant breast tumour cells to docetaxel [26]. Thus, it appears that depending on the relative levels of the two TNF-α receptors, TNF-α signalling can either increase or decrease the sensitivity of breast tumour cells to docetaxel. The above findings suggest that the autocrine role of TNF-α on tumour cells is context-dependent, depending upon the relative levels of TNF-α receptors present on target cells [26]. As discussed later, the effects of drug-induced TNF-α release was found to also be dependent upon the level of TNF-α [29], and whether it is in the membrane-bound or soluble form [30].

As with all inflammatory cytokines, TNF-α does not act in isolation. Clinical research has demonstrated what appears to be an intricate link between chemoresistance and metastasis in cancer [31, 32]. A potential explanation for this is highlighted in a recent study describing a paracrine signalling network involving endothelial, myeloid, and breast tumour cells, whereby the alarmin S100A8/9 (calprotectin), as well as inflammatory cytokines CXCL1 and TNF-α, play key roles in the interactions between tumour and healthy host cells [33]. These studies used a mouse model to show that chemotherapy agents such as doxorubicin, paclitaxel, and cyclophosphamide, although toxic to tumour cells, are capable of inducing TNF-α production in endothelial cells. This in turn, causes increased expression and release of chemokines CXCL1 and CXCL2 from tumour cells, which recruit CXCR2-expressing (CD11b+Gr1+) myeloid cells to the tumour [33]. Recruited myeloid cells, in turn, release the alarmin heterodimer S100A8/S100A9, which promotes lung metastasis as well as breast cancer cell survival [33]. The tumour-promoting effect of this heterodimer was shown to be mediated by ERK1/2 and p70S6K activation in tumour cells, as inhibition of these kinases was found to increase tumour sensitivity to doxorubicin [33].

While TNF-α is an important factor in cancer progression, its role appears to be quite dependent on the nature of the tumour and on the tumour microenvironment. Along with its well established effects on endothelial cells [34], more recent studies have shown a role for tumour TNF-α production on tumour behaviour via its effect on tumour-associated myeloid cells. One study showed that "although high doses of TNF-α have antitumour activity" [29], TNF-α expressed endogenously by tumours can cause differentiation of tumour-associated myeloid cells, resulting in a sub-population that expresses the vascular endothelial growth factor receptor 2 (VEGFR2). Furthermore, this myeloid-endothelial subpopulation can support tumour progression in a variety of ways. In nude mice, significant increases in microvessel density (as measured by PECAM-1/CD31 immunoreactivity) were observed in the microenvironment of murine melanoma (B-16), murine lung (LLC) and murine breast (Py-mT) tumour cells upon transfection with an expression plasmid housing TNF-α cDNA. Plasmids lacking the TNF-α cDNA were without effect. Consistent with this view, overexpression of TNF-α prevented necrosis in B16 and LLC tumour cells [29]. Moreover, increased tumour cell proliferation was observed in TNF-α-overexpressing B-16 (melanoma) and Py-mT (mammary) tumours, as quantified by Ki-67 immunoreactivity [29]. Similar to the results in CXCL8 studies [35], these tumour-supporting effects of TNF-α were not likely due to autocrine action, since overexpression of TNF-α did not significantly affect growth or survival of tumour cells in culture [29]. While TNF-α overexpression from tumours gave rise to significantly larger CD11b+/F4-80+ myeloid cell populations expressing either VEGFR2 or VE-cadherin, these trends were not observed in TNFR1/2 double-knockout mice, thus confirming that TNF-α signalling through at least one TNF-α receptor was required for recruitment of the tumour-supporting myeloid cell population [29].

It has been suggested that TNF-α "orchestrates the interplay" between tumours and myeloid cell tissue, and that this interplay is important for tumour growth and metastasis [30]. This cytokine is first produced as a membrane-bound protein (mTNF-α) before it is cleaved by matrix metalloproteases and released from the cell membrane [36]. Studies have strongly supported a role for TNF-α that is distinct from its soluble form (sTNF-α). An in vivo study using mice with implanted lung or melanoma tumour cell lines revealed that the expression of mTNF-α in these cells caused a significant *reduction* in the tumour-associated myeloid-monocyte lineage (anti-ER-HR3, CD11b, F4/80), among tumour-associated T cells (anti-CD3), B cells (anti-B220b), and neutrophils (anti-Ly6G), while tumour-associated T cells (anti-CD3), B cells (anti-B220b), and neutrophils (anti-Ly6G) were unaffected. More specifically, the study concluded that mTNF-α imposes a cytotoxic effect on myeloid cells, via the generation of intracellular reactive oxygen species. This in turn *prevents* the tumour-supporting behaviour of myeloid cells and results in reduced tumour growth [30]. Similarly, a distinction between the effects of mTNF-α and sTNF-α is highlighted in an in vivo study that examined the potential association between relative levels of TNF-α isoforms and patient outcome [37]. Using gene expression data from 442 lung adenocarcinoma patients, these investigators found that higher tumour expression of TNF-α converting enzyme (TACE/ADAM-17) was associated with lower overall survival [37]. Also, tumours with high TNF-α expression and low TACE levels (indicating a high mTNF-α:sTNF-α ratio) had longer survival times than patients with high TNF-α expression and high TACE (indicating a low mTNF-α:sTNF-α ratio) [37].

Certain chemotherapy agents have been reported to induce *immunogenic* cell death in tumour cells and growing evidence supports the idea that successful treatment of solid tumours in vivo with specific chemotherapy agents involves drug-induced signals originating from tumour cells that promote tumour destruction by the host immune system [38–41]. During chemotherapy administration a certain portion of the tumour cell population will succumb to treatment, thereby releasing molecules called damage-associated molecular patterns (DAMPs) that provoke a response in nearby antigen-presenting cells. For example, one study [39] reported that HMGB1, released from tumours, activates a receptor on nearby dendritic cells that activates a dendritic cell pathway. This pathway delays the degradation of tumour-specific antigens, permitting more frequent presentation of tumour-specific antigens to lymphocytes. This, in turn, facilitates the tumour-targeted adaptive immune response [39]. Other DAMPs released from tumour cells, such as ATP, recruit myeloid cells to tumours, stimulating myeloid cell differentiation, and the phagocytosis of tumour antigens [42]. Likely the cancer treatment regimen, whether ionizing radiation or chemotherapy, dictates the immune response to dying cells, and this response determines the clinical outcome [43]. Given the above observations, there is little doubt that inflammatory cytokines, along with DAMPs, play major roles within the tumour microenvironment that, in turn, affect anti-tumour immune responses.

TNF-α can increase tumour vascularization, through its ability to induce an endothelial phenotype in tumour-associated myeloid cells [29]. Although increased vascularization reportedly increases tumour proliferation and progression in mouse tumour studies [29, 35], it is likely that increased blood flow to tumours would result in increased chemotherapy drug cytotoxicity through improved drug delivery to the tumour. Consistent with all in vivo studies reviewed here, production of the inflammatory cytokines CXCL8, CXCL1 or TNF-α by tumour cells seems to affect tumour-associated myeloid cell behaviour. Whether these effects are in support of tumour progression (or protective against it) depends upon one or more confounding factors.

9.2.2   CXCL8 (IL-8)

Another inflammatory cytokine, CXCL8, commonly known as interleukin-8 (IL-8), has been studied for its potential role in cancer progression [44, 45], metastasis [46], and drug resistance [35, 47]. CXCL8 plays many roles in immune responses and is released by a variety of immune cells, including monocytes, neutrophils, endothelial cells, mesothelial cells, and tumour cells [47]. It possesses chemotactic activity and the ability to recruit neutrophils, basophils and T-cells to a site of immune activation [48–51]. CXCL8 elicits its effects through two known cell-surface G protein-coupled receptors, CXCR1 and CXCR2 (IL-8RA and IL-8RB), which are expressed by most tumour cells [47, 52] as well as endothelial cells [53].

Along with TNF-α, CXCL8 was found to be released from ovarian cancer cell lines in response to paclitaxel [54]. Approximately 50% of human ovarian cancer cell lines responded to paclitaxel with increased CXCL8 production, a trend that extended to freshly explanted primary ovarian cancer cells [55]. In responding cells, paclitaxel-induced CXCL8 expression required accumulation of drug within tumour cells and involved increased gene transcription [54]. Also, paclitaxel-responsive elements located within the CXCL8 gene promoter are necessary and sufficient for paclitaxel-induced CXCL8 production in responsive ovarian cancer cell lines [54].

Consistently, paclitaxel has been shown to upregulate CXCL8 synthesis in a subset of human lung carcinoma cell lines [56] and an independent study later showed that CXCL8 is a growth factor for both non-small and small cell lung carcinoma [57], specifically through the CXCL8 receptor CXCR1, but not through CXCR2 [57].

Another study found that the level of basal CXCL8 production in A2780, SKOV-3, and CAOV-3 ovarian cancer cells was negatively correlated with sensitivity to either paclitaxel or cisplatin, suggesting that CXCL8 expression promotes drug resistance. In experiments where CXCL8 was over-expressed in poorly-expressing A2780 cells, cells exhibited increased resistance to both paclitaxel and cisplatin [47]. In these studies, the authors suggested that CXCL8-induced drug resistance may be due to increased expression of the gene for the ABCB1 drug transporter *MDR-1*, which expresses P-glycoprotein (P-gp), as well as other genes. Similar findings from the same research group concluded that tumour IL-6 production, and subsequent autocrine signalling, resulted in increased resistance to paclitaxel and cisplatin in ovarian cancer cells, through increased expression of multidrug resistance genes and apoptosis inhibitory proteins, as well as the activation of survival pathways [58].

In another study, the expression levels of IL-6 and CXCL8 were found to increase in the MCF-7 breast cancer cells selected for resistance to paclitaxel. These cells were not only resistant to paclitaxel, but also to doxorubicin and 5-fluorouracil (5-FU), and exhibited increased expression of the ABC transporter P-gp [59]. Furthermore, treatment with neutralizing antibodies or transfection with siRNAs targeting IL-6 and CXCL8 expression increased sensitivity of the drug-resistant cells to both paclitaxel and doxorubicin. In support of a role for IL-6 and CXCL8 in drug resistance, the over-expression of both cytokines resulted in increased resistance to both paclitaxel and doxorubicin in drug-naive MCF-7 cells [59]. The authors of these studies suggest that P-gp activity limits the accumulation of drug within cells, but that there are other factors contributing to drug resistance, since inhibition of the transporter with verapamil only partially restored sensitivity to drug [59]. Critically speaking, without evidence that verapamil treatments completely restored accumulation of drug in the drug-resistant cells, it is possible that only partial inhibition of P-gp was achieved and this accounted for residual drug resistance. Thus, the drug-resistant phenotype could be mediated by P-gp and cellular export of drug, entirely. Nevertheless, these cytokines could indeed be drivers of P-gp expression or activity, and/or may activate survival pathways in tumour cells.

It is worth noting that CXCL8 transcript expression is consistently elevated upon acquisition of taxane-resistance in a number of cancer cell lines [59, 60], consistent with observations in breast cancer cell lines selected for resistance to docetaxel [27]. It is unclear whether CXCL8 plays a role in tumour drug resistance in a clinical setting. However, consistent with a role in drug resistance, elevated levels of CXCL8 in the tumours of patients with ovarian carcinoma were associated with poor prognosis in some studies [61, 62].

CXCL8 also appears to mediate resistance to oxaliplatin in androgen-independent prostate cancer cells [63], since the drug induced activation of NF-κB and increased transcription of genes for CXCL8, CXCL1 and the related receptors, CXCR1and CXCR2. Inhibition of CXCR2 signalling resulted in abrogation of drug-induced NF-κB activation and increased oxaliplatin cytotoxicity [63]. Table 9.2 lists studies where chemotherapy agents promote drug resistance through their ability to promote the expression of inflammatory cytokines via autocrine signalling.

As mentioned, CXCL8 production in ovarian tumour cell lines was found to be triggered by paclitaxel [54], a frontline therapy used in the treatment of ovarian carcinoma. The biological significance of this phenomenon was assessed by the same group using an in vivo mouse model, whereby human ovarian cancer cells transfected with a CXCL8 expression vector were injected into nude mice and the number of resulting tumours quantified [64]. Interestingly, while CXCL8 expression did not affect the growth of tumour cells in vitro, the tumours of CXCL8-expressing cells were significantly smaller than those of control cells [64]. Consistently, injection of a neutralizing antibody for CXCL8 resulted in increased tumour growth in mice injected with CXCL8-overexpressing tumour cells. Examination of mouse tissue near the injection site revealed dramatically elevated levels of neutrophils and macrophages in mice that were injected with CXCL8-expressing tumour cells. This led to the hypothesis that the elevation of immune cells within the tumour microenvironment may be due to CXCL8-dependent chemotaxis [64].

On the other hand, other studies have found that over-expression of CXCL8 in ovarian carcinomas was found to be directly associated with increased tumour growth and vascularity [52], as well as metastasis in melanomas [65]. In a clinical setting, immunohistochemical analysis of human ovarian tumours revealed a positive correlation between CXCL8 levels and disease-specific mortality [35]. This particular finding prompted a study involving orthotopically-implanted human ovarian tumour cell lines in mice, which demonstrated that silencing of CXCL8 by administration of liposome-encapsulated CXCL8 siRNA molecules suppressed multiple tumourigenic properties, including angiogenesis and tumour cell invasiveness [35]. The authors further provided data suggesting the production of CXCL8 by tumour cells promotes angiogenesis in vivo, as measured by elevated tumour levels of the blood vessel endothelial cell marker CD31 [35]. In addition, the study showed that CXCL8 also induced MMP expression, which was associated with increased invasiveness of tumour cells [35]. CXCL8 had no effect on the proliferation of HeyA8 and SKOV3ip cells in the study [35]. This suggested that although CXCL8 autocrine signalling may promote invasiveness via MMP induction, its effect on tumour cell proliferation in vivo may be through effects on the endothelial cells of blood vessels. Immunohistochemical analysis of implanted tumours in the study also revealed elevated CXCL8 expression from mice treated with docetaxel and a CXCL8 siRNA, relative to those treated with the CXCL8 siRNA alone [35]. Docetaxel treatment, however, did not result in changes in serum CXCL8 levels, thus suggesting that chemotherapy-induced CXCL8 production was somewhat specific to the tumour in this case.

In a clinical setting, it remains unclear whether chemotherapy treatment induces cytokine release from tumours. Among several cytokines examined, blood levels of IL-6, CXCL8, and CCL2 were found to decrease in patients with epithelial ovarian cancer following administration of steroids, but then significantly increased 24 h after the administration of paclitaxel [66]. The levels of these cytokines were also found to be constitutively elevated in peritoneal fluid, at concentrations two to three logs greater than those found in serum [66]. Higher serum levels of IL-6 and CXCL8 were found in patients with ovarian cancer relative to healthy controls, and high levels of these cytokines were found to be associated with a poor immediate response to paclitaxel [66]. In another study, IL-6 and CXCL8, among six cytokines tested, increased slightly in the blood serum of patients given paclitaxel for the treatment of non-metastatic breast cancer [67]. However, the source of systemic inflammatory cytokines could be a variety of tissues, including peripheral blood leukocytes, tumour stroma, or tumour cells, and it is unclear whether increased cytokine production in a tumour would be detected in patient sera.

It should be noted that mice do not normally produce CXCL8. However, they are arguably relevant models for such studies, since cells expressing both known CXCL8 receptors (CXCR1 and 2) are present in murine tissues and can thus be stimulated by CXCL8 produced and secreted by implanted human or murine tumours. In vivo mouse studies have demonstrated that tumour production of CXCL8 can promote a variety of important changes to the tumour microenvironment, including recruitment of myeloid cells, and changes in the behaviour of tumour-associated stromal cells. Taken together, the above studies suggest that the biological effect of CXCL8 release from tumours appears to be dependent upon the tumour context, either inhibiting tumour progression [64] or, in many cases, supporting a variety of malignant phenotypes, including increased tumour vascularization through its effects on endothelial cell function [35].

9.2.3   Interleukin-6 (IL-6)

IL-6 has both pro- and anti-inflammatory properties [68]. It has been widely studied for its contribution to chemotherapy drug resistance (reviewed in [69, 70]). Resistance to multiple chemotherapy drugs (multidrug resistance) has been correlated with IL-6 overexpression in breast cancer [71] and lung cancer [72] cells. Multidrug resistance in lung cancers results from chemotherapy-induced IL-6 overexpression and the subsequent activation of the ataxia-telangiectasia-mutated (ATM)-NF-κB pathway [72]. However, in most other studies, the classical IL-6/STAT3 pathway is central to the development of drug resistance (see below).

Autocrine expression of IL-6 and IL-8 by triple-negative breast cancer cells has been found to be required for growth and survival, and the simultaneous knockdown of both was required to sensitize the cells to paclitaxel- or staurosporine-induced apoptosis [73]. Trastuzumab (Herceptin) is a monoclonal antibody targeting the HER2 receptor and is commonly used to treat HER2-positive breast cancers.

Treatment of HER2+ breast cancer cells with trastuzumab induces the expression of IL-6, activating STAT3, which further upregulates IL-6 expression. This positive feedback loop has been shown to establish resistance to trastuzumab in breast [74, 75] and gastric cancer [76]. In HER2-positive cell lines, IL-6 activation of STAT3 resulted in increased S100A8/9 (calprotectin) levels, which activates proliferative and drug resistance pathways [77].

Cisplatin resistance in NSCLC has been attributed to IL-6 dependent up-regulation of a number of proteins involved in the anti-apoptotic (Bcl-2 and Mcl-1) and DNA repair (ATM, CHK1, TP73, p53, and ERCC1) pathways [78]. Knockdown of IL-6 expression in cells was achieved by lentivirus expression of IL-6 specific and control siRNAs, followed by puromycin selection. The knockdown of IL-6 increased the sensitivity of A549 cells in cell culture to cisplatin through the down-regulation of these regulatory proteins. In a xenograft mouse model using the same cell lines, the reduction in IL-6 expression in A549 cells produced tumours with a high drug sensitivity [78]. In cisplatin-resistant epithelial ovarian cancer cells, IL-6-induced activation of STAT3 is required for the repression of the microRNA, miR-204. Repression of miR-204 expression was believed to be responsible for the IL-6-induced cisplatin resistance, since active miR-204 was able to inactivate IL-6/STAT3 signalling and reduce expression of anti-apoptotic proteins. This pathway appeared relevant to chemosensitivity in patient populations as well [79]. In a separate study, cellular levels of miR-30a-5p and miR-30c-5p affected cisplatin sensitivity in A2780 ovarian cancer cells regulating DNA methylation. Cisplatin resistance was associated with downregulation of the two miRNAs due to an upregulation of the DNA methyltransferase DNMT1, the overexpression of which resulted in resistance to cisplatin [80]. In HER2-positive breast cancer patients following treatment with trastuzumab, miR-21 expression was found to be associated with residual disease and inversely correlated with PTEN expression. One target of miR-21 is the IL-6/STAT3/NF-κB signalling pathway, which is associated with drug resistance [81].

IL-6 has also been reported to either enhance chemosensitivity when suppressed, or induce drug resistance when overexpressed in numerous cancers, including colorectal cells [82] mucoepidermoid carcinoma [83], neuroblastomas [84], esophageal squamous cell carcinoma [85]and in multiple myeloma cell lines [86].

9.2.4   CXCL1 (GRO-α)

CXCL1 (growth related oncogene-α/GROα) plays a prominent role in the early stages of neutrophil recruitment during tissue inflammation [87] and activates one of the same cell surface receptors (CXCR2) as CXCL8. Production of CXCL1 in tumour cells was shown to occur in vivo after tumour-implanted mice were treated with doxorubicin, a study described later [33]. Production of this inflammatory cytokine by implanted tumours, along with CXCL8 and TNF-α, was shown to cause a number of changes to the tumour microenvironment. CXCL1 has also been suggested to induce tumour cell proliferation in an autocrine fashion, since epithelial ovarian cancer cells (SKOV3 and OVCAR-3) over-expressing CXCL1 exhibited increased proliferation rates relative to wild-type cells [88]. The shedding of EGF and activation of both EGFR and MAPK was required for the increased proliferative capacity, resulting from autocrine CXCL1 signalling through the CXCR2 G-protein-coupled receptor [88]. As reviewed by Dhawan and Richmond, CXCL1 also has strong tumourigenic potential in melanocytes [89], with the ability to promote tumour formation in mice implanted with otherwise benign immortalized melanocytes [90].

9.2.5 Transforming Growth Factor-β (TGF-β)

The effects of transforming growth factor β (TGF-β) in cancer vary, with the cytokine playing a tumour suppressive role at early stages, and promoting progression, invasion and metastasis at later stages (reviewed in [91]). More recently a role for TGF-β in drug resistance has been identified. TGF-β treatment was able to confer resistance to the anaplastic lymphoma kinase (ALK) inhibitor (crizotinib), EGFR inhibitors (gefitinib and erlotinib), a MEK inhibitor (AZD6244), a BRAF inhibitor (PLX 4032), and cisplatin in a variety of cancer cell lines. Up-regulation of TGF-β receptor-2 (TGF-βR2) expression and the subsequent activation of the MEK-ERK pathway due to the down-regulation of a component of the transcriptional regulator complex MEDIATOR (MED12) have been shown to promote drug resistance [92]. In squamous cell carcinoma stem cells, TGF-β signalling resulted in slower cell cycling and increased resistance to cisplatin, where drug resistance was independent of proliferation rate. TGF-β increased transcription of p21, leading to stabilization of NRF2 and enhanced metabolism of glutathione. This, in turn, protected cells from cisplatin-generated reactive oxygen species (ROS) [93]. In drug-resistant lung adenocarcinoma cells the up-regulation of TGF-βR2 expression by the zinc finger protein 32 (ZNF32) transcription factor promoted resistance to gefitinib and cisplatin. TGF-βR2signalling through the SMAD2 pathway was required for resistance [94]. Prostate cancer cells exposed to TGF-β exhibit increased resistance to docetaxel [95]. In docetaxel-resistant prostate cancer cells TGF-β is critical for resistance to taxanes. The transcription factors Twist1 and Y-box binding protein-1 (YB-1) both exhibit increased expression in drug resistant cell lines, and the expression and activation of both is regulated by TGF-β. Down-regulation of either transcription factor resulted in an increased drug sensitivity, further linking TGF-β to chemotherapy drug resistance [96].

Cross-talk between TGF-β and IL-6 has also been identified as a factor in drug resistance in some cancer cells. In NSCLC cells, a TGF-β mediated increase in IL-6 secretion eliminated the addiction of the cells to EGFR signalling, inducing resistance to the epidermal growth factor receptor tyrosine kinase inhibitor erlotinib [97]. In a mouse model used in the same study, induction of inflammation increased IL-6 production and produced resistance to erlotinib [97]. In biliary tract cancer, exogenously added IL-6 and TGF-β together increased the endogenous expression of both cytokines via SMAD4. Down-regulation of SMAD4 blocked invasion, EMT and gemcitabine resistance [98]. Clinically, in oral cancer samples, active TGF-β signalling has been associated with drug resistance and correlated with IL-6 pathway activation. In vitro experiments demonstrated that the knockdown of TGF-β increased sensitivity to cisplatin and radiotherapy [99]. Interestingly, in another report on bone marrow-disseminated HNSCC cells, TGF-β was responsible for the up-regulation of CXCL12/SDF-1 and its receptor, CXCR4. Resistance to cisplatin was dependent upon a positive feedback loop established by CXCL12 and CXCR4 [100]. Although the mechanisms have not been clearly delineated in all the systems studied, the development of drug resistance appears to involve, in some instances, the induction of a secondary cytokine.

9.2.6   CXCL12 (SDF-1)

CXCL12, commonly referred to as stromal cell-derived factor-1 (SDF-1), and its receptor CXCR4 are commonly overexpressed in a number of different cancer types and have been linked to proliferation, invasion, metastasis and angiogenesis. CXCL12 is also believed to play an important role in tumour/stromal environment interactions (reviewed in [101]). Moreover, as noted earlier, CXCL12 is linked to drug resistance through its regulation of anti-apoptotic pathways [101].

In pancreatic cancer explants, resistance to temsirolimus, an mTOR pathway inhibitor, is associated with increased CXCL12 expression, and inhibition of its receptor CXCR4 increased drug sensitivity [102]. In A549 cells resistant to the EGFR inhibitor gefitinib their higher expression levels of CXCL12 and CXCR4 promote resistance to the drug [103]. Silencing of CXCR4 in prostate cancer cells blocks the ability of CXCL12 to provide protection from docetaxel treatment [104, 105]. Interestingly, five different chemotherapy agents differentially regulate the expression of CXCR4 in a variety of leukemia cell lines, and the level of CXCR4 expression correlated with the degree of drug resistance. Inhibition of CXCR4 reversed the protection from drug-induced apoptosis [106]. Activation of the CXCL12-CXCR4 pathway by reactive oxygen species (ROS) promotes autophagy in mantle cell lymphomas (MCL) in the bone marrow compartment. Bortezomib-resistant MCL cells have higher levels CXCR4 than their sensitive counterparts, with stromal cells providing CXCL12. Activation of CXCR4-induced autophagy is also associated with improved survival MCL cells [107]. A CXCR4 antagonist sensitized chronic myelogenous leukemia cells to cell death induced by the receptor tyrosine kinase inhibitor imatinib. Here again, CXC12 was provided by stromal cells [108].

CXCL12, whether produced by tumour cells or, more commonly by stromal cells, regulates numerous aspects of tumour development and can also affect sensitivity to chemotherapeutic agents. CXCR4 antagonists are currently being investigated in clinical trials for their ability to sensitize leukemia, pancreatic, lung and breast cancers to specific chemotherapy regimens (reviewed in [109–112]).

9.2.7 CCL2 (MCP-1)

CCL2 (monocyte chemotactic protein 1/MCP-1) recruits monocytes and macrophages to sites of inflammation and has been described as an important factor in determining the tumour microenvironment in some cancers [113, 114]. The consistent up-regulation of IL-6, IL-8 and/or CCL2 in a series of 8 paclitaxel or doxorubicin drug-resistant cell lines, as compared to their parent cell lines, provided one of the first indications that these cytokines may have an additional role in drug resistance [60]. The cell lines studied included both ovarian and breast cell lines.

While CCL2 and CCL5 (RANTES) are barely expressed in normal breast tissue, both are up-regulated in breast tumour cells and have been clinically correlated with advanced disease and progression. Studies indicate that they mediate interactions with inflammatory cells, increasing the presence of tumour-associated macrophages (TAMs) and inhibiting anti-tumour activity by T cells. CCL2 promotes angiogenesis, while both cytokines play a role in metastasis (reviewed in [115–117]). Clinically, the expression of CCL2 has been negatively correlated with patient survival [118–120].

In a series of breast cancer cell lines, CCL2 signalling (through CCR2) induced cell migration and cell survival, both aspects of the metastatic process [121]. CCL2 was able to inhibit cell death induced by serum starvation, gentamycin or 5-fluorouracil. Cell survival was found to be dependent on activation of the MEK-ERK1/2 pathway through Smad3-dependent and Smad3-independent pathways. The Smad3-dependent pathway activated RhoA, which promoted both migration and survival. Interestingly, CCL2 had no effect on the migration or survival of "normal" MCF10A cells, suggesting a potential tumour-specific effect [121].

In ovarian cancer primary cells the expression of CCL2 was found to be associated with greater sensitivity to paclitaxel and cisplatin. CCL2 mRNA expression was similarly correlated with chemosensitivity, objective complete response and progression free survival in ovarian cancer patients [122]. Contrasting results were obtained in mouse xenografts of two paclitaxel-resistant serous ovarian cancer cell lines with an elevated CCL2 expression, where inhibition of this expression enhanced sensitivity to paclitaxel and in one case, cisplatin. In another study involving a third ovarian cancer cell line with characteristics of clear cell cancer, neither paclitaxel, CCL2 inhibition nor a combination of the two had any effect, suggesting CCL2's effect on chemotherapy sensitivity may be dependent upon the tumour subtype [123].

While less extensively investigated, there are reports of CCL2 involvement in the survival of other cancers. CCL2 has been demonstrated to up-regulate the expression of survivin, a member of the inhibitor of apoptosis (IAP) protein family, protecting a number of prostate cancer cell lines from serum starvation-induced autophagic death [124]. In addition to activation of the PI3K-Akt pathway, CCL2 also activates a separate AMP kinase/mTOR-dependent survivin expression pathway, which contributes to cell survival [125]. In acute myeloid leukemia cells, CCL2 was reported to affect transmigration and proliferation, but to have no effect on sensitivity to Ara-C-induced apoptosis [126]. In melanoma cells autocrine production of CCL2 stimulates proliferation and inhibits apoptosis. Treatment with PLX4032, a B-Raf inhibitor, induced the expression of CCL2, as well as increases in specific miRNAs associated with regulating proliferation and apoptosis. Blockade of CCL2 sensitized the cells to PLX4032. In clinical samples, treatment with vemurafenib, a B-Raf inhibitor, resulted in an increased serum CCL2, and a high serum CCL2 correlated with poorer patient response [127]. In docetaxel-resistant prostate cancer cells, docetaxel induced CCL2 expression. Inhibition of CCL2 expression sensitized the cells to low-doses of docetaxel, while overexpression of the cytokine induced cell proliferation, while protecting the cells from docetaxel-induced death. CCL2 was shown to activate ERK and PI3K pathways, while inhibiting docetaxel-induced phosphorylation of Bad and Bcl2, as well as caspase-3 activation [128]. CCL2 expression had been correlated with activation of pro-survival signalling pathways in head and neck squamous cell carcinoma (HNSCC) cells, while serving as a marker for poor prognosis in patients with HNSCC [129].

The involvement of CCL2 in breast cancer chemosensitivity and outcome illustrates the complexities of studying the role of cytokines in cancer. The cytokine is highly expressed in breast tumours, where high levels of its expression are associated with high tumour grade and poor clinical outcomes. It is highly expressed by stromal cells, where it attracts TAMs, establishing a tumourigenic microenvironment. CCL2 has also been reported to upregulate expression of the inflammatory cytokines CCL5 and TNF-β, as well as stimulating the release of angiogenic factors (reviewed in [115, 130]). Among its known tumourigenic effects, the effect of CCL2 on chemosensitivity is a more recent discovery. Identifying the relative contributions of a single cytokine in this intricate network remains a challenge.

9.2.8   CCL5 (RANTES)

CCL5, also known as RANTES (regulated on activation, normal T cell expressed and secreted), is an inflammatory cytokine that recruits leukocytes to the site of inflammation. CCL5 is expressed by numerous hematopoietic and non-hematopoietic cell types. The well-established connections between cancer and inflammation have led to studies of the role of CCL5 in tumour development and progression, particularly in breast cancer (reviewed in [115–117]).

The role of CCL5 in drug resistance is only beginning to be investigated. In a tamoxifen-resistant MCF-7 cell line, CCL5 expression establishes an autocrine loop involving STAT3 activation and the subsequent expression of anti-apoptotic genes of the Bcl-2 family. Maintenance of this autocrine loop appears essential for tamoxifen resistance, since knocking down either CCL5 or STAT3 increased tamoxifen sensitivity. The role of CCL5 was confirmed by treating the non-resistant parental MCF-7 cells with CCL5, which resulted in decreased drug sensitivity [131]. In contrast to the autocrine mechanism in MCF-7 cells, cisplatin was shown to induce the expression of CCL5 in cancer-associated fibroblasts (CAF), which, in turn, increased the resistance of ovarian cancer cells to cisplatin. CCL5 treatment of the same ovarian cancer cell line activated STAT3 and PI-3K/Akt pathways, and increased Bcl-2 expression, likely facilitating the observed cisplatin resistance [132]. The study also compared CCL5 expression in tumour biopsies from patients with platinum-sensitive and -resistant serous ovarian carcinoma and demonstrated a correlation between CCL5 expression and cisplatin resistance. These studies suggest that CCL5 can promote drug resistance through either cellular autocrine or paracrine mechanisms.

9.2.9   CCL25 (TECK)

CCL25 (TECK/Thymus-Expressed Chemokine) is the only known ligand for the receptor CCR9. In breast and ovarian cancer, CCL25/CCR9 is implicated in cell migration and invasion through the up-regulation of MMPs [133, 134]. CCL25 has also been implicated in clinical resistance to chemotherapy in patients with breast and ovarian cancer [133, 135], prostate cancer [136], non-small cell lung cancer [137] and leukemia [138]. Across a variety of cancer cell types CCL25/CCR9 engagement results in the activation of the PI3K/Akt pathway, promoting survival through down-regulation of pro-apoptotic proteins and the up-regulation of anti-apoptotic proteins [135–137, 139].

9.2.10   Interleukin-7 (IL-7)

IL-7 is a pro-inflammatory cytokine which regulates T cell development and homeostasis [140]. In a series of 12 human glioma cell lines, high expression of IL-7 was found to correlate with cisplatin resistance, as was chemoresistance in 91 clinical glioma specimens. Consistent with this view, treatment of glioma cells with IL-7 enhanced both drug resistance and cellular growth rate [141]. Since there are also reports that IL-7 expression is associated with resistance to apoptosis in T cells and NSCLC [142, 143], the role of IL-7 in chemoresistance remains to be fully explored and is likely context-dependent.

9.2.11   Interleukin-10 (IL-10/CSIF)

The cytokine IL-10 (cytokine synthesis inhibitory factor/CSIF) is generally considered to be immunosuppressive, but has complex and contrasting roles in both immunity and cancer. IL-10 seems to either stimulate or inhibit tumour development, depending upon effects on the immune system or tumour cells (reviewed in [144, 145].

Immune suppression is thought to facilitate the ability of tumours to escape the immune system, while direct promotion of drug resistance limits attempts at therapy. In lymphoma cells, autocrine/paracrine IL-10 loops have been reported to activate STAT3, leading to the expression of anti-apoptotic genes and consequent resistance to chemotherapy agents [146, 147]. Through paracrine signalling, the expression of IL-10 by TAMs has been demonstrated to elicit a paclitaxel-resistant phenotype in breast cancer cell lines, mediated by STAT3-dependent induction of Bcl-2 expression [148].

9.2.12 Interleukin-18 (IL-18/IGIF)

IL-18 was initially identified as an IFNγ-inducing factor (IGIF) and shown to play multiple roles in immune regulation. More recently the involvement of IL-18 in cancer progression has been revealed to be context dependent, producing either pro- or anti-cancer effects (reviewed in [149]). Secretion of IL-18 has been shown to contribute to doxorubicin resistance in a MCF-7 doxorubicin-resistant cell line [150]. The up-regulated expression of IL-18 was also reported to occur in drug-resistant malignant pleural mesothelioma cells and to be important in the mechanisms of resistance to the folate antimetabolite pemetrexed and the histone deacetylase inhibitor vorinostat [151]. One potential mechanism for the association with drug resistance is the down-regulated expression of multidrug resistance-associated protein-2 (MRP2/ABCC2), as demonstrated in human hepatoma HepG2 cells treated with IL-18 [152].

9.2.13 Interleukin-34 (IL-34)

IL-34 is a recently identified cytokine, shown to activate the macrophage colony-stimulating factor (M-CSF) receptor (CSF1R). To date, only one study has explored IL-34's possible role in drug resistance [153]. IL-34 is secreted by drug-resistant A549 lung cancer cells, while drug-sensitive parental cells (from which they originated) did not exhibit any expression. IL-34 has an autocrine effect in lung cancer cells, leading to the activation of the Akt pathway and chemoresistance. As a paracrine effector, IL-34 enhanced the differentiation of monocytes into M2-polarized TAMs in vitro and in vivo, increasing tumour infiltration by the M2-polarized TAMs. The M2-polarized TAMs contribute to tumour chemoresistance through the expression of immunosuppressive factors. The above studies thus suggest that IL-34 promotes drug resistance by impacting both tumour cells and the tumour microenvironment.

9.2.14   MIC-1 (GDF-15)

Macrophage inhibitory cytokine-1 (MIC-1), also known as growth and differentiation factor-15 (GDF-15), is a member of the TGF-β/bone morphogenic protein superfamily that is overexpressed in a number of cancers, including breast, ovarian, lung, colon and prostate cancer (reviewed in [154, 155]). A stress-induced cytokine, MIC-1 has been associated with disease progression, shorter patient survival and a poor response to chemotherapy [154]. In prostate cancer cell lines docetaxel treatment induced MIC-1 expression, while overexpression of MIC-1 provided protection from treatment with docetaxel and mitoxantrone [156]. In the same study, docetaxel treatment of PC3 and DU145 prostate cancer cell lines for 48 h increased expression of CXCL10, IL-1β and MIC-1 by two to eightfold, while mitoxantrone induced CXCL10 and MIC-1 expression but not IL-1β. Docetaxel treatment of mouse xenografts of LUCaP 35V cells similarly increased CXCL10, IL-1β and MIC-1 expression [156]. A PC-3 cell line selected for docetaxel resistance was found to express higher levels of MIC-1 than wild type PC-3 cells. Knockdown of MIC-1 expression in this cell line restored drug sensitivity [157]. Clinically, MIC-1 overexpression has been associated with prostate cancer progression of androgen-independent metastatic and invasive phenotypes. Down-regulation of MIC-1 has also been demonstrated to sensitize prostate cancer cells to docetaxel-induced apoptosis [158].

Cisplatin was found to increase MIC-1 expression in lung cancer cells, where expression correlated with drug resistance [159]. Cisplatin also induces MIC-1 expression in the wild type A2780 ovarian cancer cell line, but failed to do so in the cisplatin-resistant derivative cell line (A2780cis), which constitutively expresses MIC-1. Knockdown of MIC-1 expression in the A2780cis cells increased drug sensitivity in vivo, but interestingly, not in vitro. Tumour growth was suppressed by MIC-1-induced expression of p27^{Kip1}, potentially limiting cisplatin sensitivity [159]. Trastuzumab-resistant breast cancer cell lines consistently exhibited an increase in MIC-1 expression, while exogenous or overexpressed MIC-1 blocked growth inhibition by trastuzumab. Knockdown of MIC-1 sensitized resistant cells to trastuzumab. MIC-1 either produced as an autocrine factor, or by adipocytes has been demonstrated to mediate trastuzumab resistance [160, 161]. An important role for the expression of MIC-1 by cancer-associated fibroblasts has been reported to play a role in chemosensitivity for acute myeloid leukemia (AML) [162].

In contrast to the previous reports, ribosome-inactivating stress (RIS) activation reduced sensitivity to 5-fluorouracil and paclitaxel [163]. The proposed mechanism involved RIS inhibition of the p53-MIC1 positive feedback loop, resulting in a down-regulation of MIC-1 expression. In this instance, the up-regulation of MIC-1 was found to be associated with the activation of pro-apoptotic pathways, and MIC1 suppression reduced drug sensitivity [163].

9.3   Drug-Sensitizing Cytokines

While the majority of the above-described cytokines contribute to drug resistance, a subset of these cytokines clearly have effects on tumour development that can be either pro- or anti-tumourigenic. Another group of cytokines that primarily sensitize cells to drug cytotoxicity have also been identified.

9.3.1   Interleukin-24 (IL-24/Mda-7)

IL-24, also known as melanoma differentiation associated gene-7 (Mda-7), is a member of the IL-10 family. Alone, it acts as an effective anticancer agent, either when overexpressed or provided exogenously. IL-24 has also been demonstrated to increase tumour cell death synergistically when combined with chemotherapy agents (reviewed in [164]). It has been reported to increase drug sensitivity in B cell lymphoma [165], osteosarcoma [166], glioma cells [167, 168], and breast cancer [169, 170]. In glioma cells, IL-24 increases sensitivity to temozolomide by promoting the expression and activation of PKR (double-stranded RNA-activated protein kinase) and eIF-2a, while reducing expression of Bcl-2 [168]. IL-24 has also been reported to down-regulate the expression of the drug transporters P-gp (ABCB1) and BCRP1 (ABCG2) in drug-resistant cell lines [166, 170]. Paclitaxel sensitivity in MDA-MB-231 cells is increased by IL-24 treatment through the modulation of apoptotic regulatory proteins [169], while in osteosarcoma, sensitization to doxorubicin occurs both via down-regulation of P-gp and BCRP1 expression and by the reduction of autophagy [166]. IL-24 also sensitizes cells to ionizing radiation [167, 171], possibly by inhibiting survival/antiapoptotic pathways.

9.3.2   CXCL10 (IP-10)

The anthracyclines doxorubicin and mitoxantrone induce expression of type I interferons in a variety of cancer cells, including sarcomas, melanomas and leukemic cell lines. In a sarcoma cell line, exogenous type I IFNs was also found to sensitize the cells to doxorubicin and cisplatin [172]. Mechanistically, drug-induced cell death released activators of TLR3, resulting in secretion of IFNα and β. The type I IFNs, via activation of INFAR, produced a type I IFN transcriptional signature that included expression of both CXCL10 and CCL5. Through activation of the CXCR3 receptor, CXCL10 was found to be responsible for the chemosensitization [172].

9.4   Clinical Perspectives of Chemotherapy-Dependent Cytokine Production in Cancer Treatment and Patient Prognosis

The content described above reveals that, whether produced by host tissues or by the tumour cells themselves, the induced production of cytokines by chemotherapy drugs has a direct effect on patient prognosis post-treatment. In some instances, chemotherapy agents have the intended effects of reducing or halting the growth of solid or non-solid tumours. This can involve direct effects of the drugs on tumour cells, including the activation of cell death pathways or inhibition of proteins promoting cell cycle progression. Many of these mechanisms are well understood through in vitro studies and may involve the induction of cytokine production in (and secretion from) tumour cells. However, as described below, in vivo experiments or human clinical studies reveal that chemotherapy agents can have very significant effects on host tissues that affect tumour cell killing, including changes in cytokine production in host immune cells that can either augment or inhibit the ability of chemotherapy agents to kill tumours by stimulating or inhibiting anti-tumour immune responses, respectively. Chemotherapy-induced cytokine production can also have powerful effects on host tissues that dramatically affect patient treatment response and prognosis.

9.4.1   Direct and Indirect Tumour Promoting Effects of Chemotherapy-Induced Cytokines

In many instances, anti-cancer drugs can directly kill cells of the immune system, thus blocking the body's ability to detect and neutralize foreign agents or kill cancer cells. The most common form of this is chemotherapy-induced febrile neutropenia, which can be treated with colony stimulating factors [173]. In fact, a variety of chemotherapy agents for the treatment of cancer and other conditions suppress immune responses. For example, high dose cyclophosphamide can suppress both T- and B-cell function [174], while imatinib suppresses T cell proliferation and activation [175]. In some instances, this is due to the ability of chemotherapy agents to induce cytokines that block immune responses. For example, a combination of gemcitabine and 5-fluorouracil (used in a variety of cancer treatments) can activate Nlrp3 in myeloid-derived suppressor cells, leading to IL-2β production and the suppression of anti-tumour immune responses [176]. Experiments in mice have also shown that gemcitabine and 5-fluorouracil activate regulatory cells, with increased production of pro-tumourigenic cytokines [177].

9.4.2 Direct and Indirect Anti-tumour Effects of Chemotherapy-Induced Cytokines

In other instances, chemotherapy agents can promote anti-tumour immune responses. For example, neoadjuvant chemotherapy can strongly change the immune microenvironment in patients with stage IIIC/IV, high grade, serous tubo-ovarian metastatic ovarian cancer. In a recent study [178], plasma levels of several cytokines were monitored prior to and after platinum-based neoadjuvant chemotherapy for 54 patients with metastatic ovarian cancer. TNF-α, CXCL-8, and IL-6 levels decreased upon chemotherapy treatment, while IFN-γ levels increased. The increased production of IFN-γ is a known marker of T cell activation. Consistent with this view, biopsies of omental metastases from these patients showed enhanced presence after chemotherapy of both CD4+ cells (exhibiting enhanced IFN-γ production) and CD8+ T cells. T cell activation [as well as fewer FoxP3+ regulatory(T_{reg}) cells that block the action of T cells] were also found to be associated with a strong positive response to neoadjuvant chemotherapy in this study [178]. In another study, 5-fluorouracil was shown to selectively kill tumour-associated myeloid-derived suppressor cells (MDSCs). This elimination of MDSCs resulted in increased IFN-γ production by tumour-specific CD8+ T cells infiltrating the tumour. This promoted T cell-dependent anti-tumour responses in vivo [179].

Unlike the effects of high doses of cyclophosphamide on some cells, low dose cyclophosphamide can also promote immune responses by decreasing levels of T_{reg} cells [180]. The low doses of this drug promote IFN-γ production, resulting in augmented antibody responses and continued presence of memory T cells [181]. Low dose cyclophosphamide can also synergize with immunomodulators to augment tumour eradication in humans [182].

Low doses of other chemotherapy drugs (paclitaxel) can similarly augment anti-tumour immune responses by inducing T helper cell Type I cytokine production. This results in augmented cytotoxic T cell responses [183]. Studies in human myelomonocytic cells have shown that low dose paclitaxel can activate dendritic cells through its effects on toll-like receptor signalling pathways. This can then result in TNF-α production and the initiation of an innate immune response [184].

9.4.3 Direct and Indirect Effects of Chemotherapy-Induced Cytokines on Normal Host Processes

While the intent of treatment is to eliminate or reduce the growth of tumours, recent studies have elucidated the mechanisms by which chemotherapy agents exert powerful short- and long-term deleterious off-target side-effects in cancer patients. For example, treatment of patients with estrogen receptor-positive, HER2-positive breast cancer using a regimen including cyclophosphamide, doxorubicin,

5-Fluorouracil, and tamoxifen induces profound short and long-term side effects including premature death, flu-like symptoms, neutropenia, stomatitis, congestive heart failure, thromboemboli, and secondary cancers [185]. Additional side effects of chemotherapy treatment include decreased cognition and "chemobrain" [186], myelosuppression [187], and peripheral neuropathies [188]. Many of these side effects involve the induction of inflammatory cytokines and their subsequent effects on immune processes within the host.

9.4.3.1 Pro-inflammatory Cytokines and Cognitive Impairment

There is a clear association between the induction of cytokines by chemotherapy drugs and cognitive impairment. In a study of 99 patients undergoing adjuvant anthracycline-based chemotherapy for breast cancer, plasma levels of IL-6 were found to be elevated in response to treatment, and the higher concentration of IL-6 was found to be associated with more severe self-perceived cognitive disturbances [189]. Significant increases in blood levels of IL-6 and CXCL8 have been observed in response to anthracyclines in another study [190]. It is believed that these cytokines readily penetrate the blood brain barrier and bind to endothelial receptors in the brain vasculature, which further stimulate the release of other inflammatory cytokines that cause structural damage to the brain. Cytokines also destroy tight junctions between cells of the blood brain barrier through their capacity to induce the production of reactive oxygen species [191].

Supporting the role of cytokines in cognitive impairment, it has been observed that chemotherapy-induced pro-inflammatory cytokines (such as IL-1, IL-6, and TNF-α) are able to cross the blood brain barrier from the peripheral nervous system to the central nervous system, where they evoke local inflammatory responses in the brain [192]. Interestingly, release of cytokines associated with chemotherapy-induced cognitive impairment (CICI) may be regulated by Apo-lipoprotein A1, whose decreased expression is associated with neurodegenerative diseases involving cognitive impairment. ApoA1 prevents LPS-induced TNF-α release from macrophages, monocytes, and stimulated T cells [193]. Ren et al. [194] describes an interesting model for CICI, where anti-cancer drugs induce significant reactive oxygen species, which oxidize and inactivate Apo-A1, triggering LPS-induced TNF-α release from immune cells. The released TNF-α can then promote mitochondrial dysfunction and apoptotic neuronal death, as described by Tangpong et al. [195]. Anti-cancer drugs can also directly and negatively affect brain processes through their ability to reduce the density of dendritic spines [196].

9.4.3.2 Inflammatory Cytokines and Peripheral Neuropathic Pain

In addition to neuronal effects associated with cognitive impairment, chemotherapy agents can promote peripheral neuropathy. Recent investigations now provide insight in the molecular mechanisms associated with this phenomenon. In response to chemotherapy-induced injury to host and tumour tissues, macrophages are recruited to the wound site, leading to the subsequent production of various cytokines including TNF-α, IL-1β, IL-6, and CXCL-8 (reviewed recently in [197]). The induced release of TNF-α and IL-1β can directly stimulate and sensitize A- and C-type neural fibers, leading to spontaneous discharge from such fibres. This is associated with allodynia and hyperalgesia (pain) after nerve injury [198]. Moreover, TNF-α and IL-1β increase Na^+ and Ca^{++} currents at nociceptor peripheral terminals, eliciting action potentials [199, 200].

Interestingly matrix metalloproteinases (MMPs) may play critical roles in chemotherapy-induced peripheral neuropathic pain. In fact chemotherapy drugs such as taxanes can induce the expression of MMPs, which are causally linked to neurotoxicity [201]. Based on evidence from a variety of sources, Wang et al. describes a very compelling model for the role of MMPs in chemotherapy-induced peripheral neuropathy, a model that also involves release and activation of inflammatory cytokines [197]. In short, the chemotherapy-induced expression of MMPs degrades the extracellular matrix component of the basement membrane in the blood brain barrier and the myelin sheath of neurons. MMPs also promote the migration, infiltration and activation of inflammatory cells within the dorsal root ganglia and peripheral nerves. Consistent with this view, the number of activated macrophages at the sites of peripheral nerves, the dorsal root ganglia, and Schwann cells strongly increases upon administration of chemotherapy [202]. This activation promotes the release of the inflammatory cytokines described above, which directly or indirectly act on afferent neurons to induce hypersensitivity of peripheral nerves.

9.4.3.3 Chemotherapy-Induced Myelosuppression

Myelosuppression is another common side-effect of chemotherapy and involves the cessation of production of myeloid cells within the bone marrow, including platelets, red blood cells, and white blood cells (including neutrophils) [203]. Chemotherapy-induced myelosuppression has been found to be associated with enhanced production of the cytokines IL-6 and G-CSF, and the level of myelosuppression severity has been well correlated with the extent of G-CSF produced by endothelium macrophages [204]. It is possible that these cytokines play a role in the destruction of myeloid cells in a manner similar to that described above for neuronal cells. However, this is unlikely, since both IL-6 and G-CSF actually promote the synthesis of red and white blood cells, as well as platelets. Rather, it may be a compensatory mechanism by which the body attempts to compensate from the myelosuppression.

9.4.3.4 Cytokines and Chemotherapy-induced Joint Pain and Flu-Like Symptoms

Flu-like symptoms, joint pain, and fatigue are commonly observed in patients during chemotherapy with taxanes [205]. These symptoms are likely due to the release of inflammatory cytokines. In a study of 90 patients with breast cancer, plasma levels of several cytokines were quantified at baseline and at the end of one treatment cycle [67]. There were no differences in baseline cytokine levels between breast cancer patients and healthy volunteers. However, plasma levels of CXCL-8 were significantly increased (>2-fold) in response to 3-weekly paclitaxel, and weekly paclitaxel correlated with increased IL-10 levels. Interestingly, flu-like symptoms peaked 3 days after 3-weekly paclitaxel administration, while slight increases in IL-1 levels correlated with joint pain after weekly paclitaxel treatment. Increases in plasma CXCL-8 levels were also seen in patients with ovarian cancer 24 h after administration of paclitaxel/carboplatin chemotherapy [66]. No changes in TNF-α levels were observed in response to paclitaxel and no differences in cytokine levels were observed in response to chemotherapy with 5-fluorouracil, doxorubicin, and cyclophosphamide. In addition, no correlation was observed between changes in the expression of the above cytokines and fatigue after treatment. Taken together, these observations suggests that cytokine induction after chemotherapy is dependent upon the tumour cell type, the drugs administered, as well as the dose and schedule. These all have an impact on the effects of chemotherapy regimens on the patient. Likely, the ability of various chemotherapy regimens to induce side-effects like flu-like symptoms and joint pain in cancer patients are due to elevation of inflammatory cytokines from host rather than tumour tissues.

Further supporting the hypothesis that sickness behaviour (flu-like symptoms) in cancer patients undergoing chemotherapy involves the production of inflammatory cytokines are mouse studies showing that the drug etoposide (VP-16) induced strong IL-6 production in mouse macrophages and in vivo in healthy mice. Moreover, the drug induced in mice sickness-like behaviour typical of that seen when administering chemotherapy (decreased appetite, body weight, hemoglobin levels, and wheel running [206]).

9.5 Changes in Cytokine Expression Associated with Chemotherapy Resistance in Cancer Patients

While numerous studies (described above) have shown a link between the expression of specific cytokines in tumours and both chemotherapy resistance and tumour progression, the prolonged exposure of tumours to chemotherapy drugs can also result in changes in cytokine expression that promote tumour survival. For example, in a recent study of 55 patients with castration-resistant prostate cancer, blood samples were obtained prior to and 3 weeks after cycle 1 of chemotherapy.

Blood levels of several cytokines were elevated during treatment, which was associated with resistance to treatment and progressive disease [207]. These included IFN-γ, IL-4, and MIC-1. Interestingly, IL-4 is known to promote an alternative activation pathway for macrophages, creating a distinct macrophage cellular profile linked to tumour progression [207]. High levels of intra-tumoural macrophages in resected prostate cancer have been shown to correlate with increased risk of disease recurrence [208]. Supporting the view of IL-4 and promotion of tumour growth, Craig et al. showed that co-inoculation of PC3 xenograft mice with IL-4-treated macrophages resulted in augmented tumour growth [209]. As for MIC-1, its expression was found to correlate with docetaxel resistance and treatment of cells with exogenous MIC-1 increased cellular resistance to docetaxel [158]. In contrast, a siRNA against MIC-1 in docetaxel-resistant cells restored chemosensitivity [158].

9.6 Conclusions

A variety of inflammatory cytokines have been characterized for their release and subsequent autocrine and/or paracrine effects during chemotherapy treatment, mostly in an in vitro setting. Many inflammatory cytokines have been identified as playing a role in tumour drug resistance, or other cellular behaviours associated with tumour progression. Given the nature of inflammatory cytokines to induce expression of other inflammatory cytokines, tumour drug resistance is more than likely mediated by networks of cytokines in vivo. The expression of a number of cytokines by various cancer cell types has been identified, but studies typically focus on the more popular candidates, and the potential expression of other cytokines remains unexamined. The natural focus during in vitro studies has been on those cytokines with a known link to a function, such as drug resistance or tumour progression. Both the cytokines with known autocrine effects, and those that are less studied are likely to have important effects in the tumour microenvironment. While challenging, studies of these interactions are vital to understanding the origin of drug resistance.

The relevance of chemotherapy-induced cytokine pathways in tumour initiation and progression in vivo is, nevertheless, less clear. However, clinical studies have provided extensive correlational data strongly suggesting relationships between various cytokines and various aspects of tumour progression and patient prognosis. The net effect of changes in cytokine signalling pathways on tumour behaviour in vivo depends on signals from multiple cell types, involving autocrine and paracrine mechanisms that comprise complex signalling networks. These networks within the tumour microenvironment are characteristic of the cellular consortia present. They are continuously evolving as a patients' tumour progresses, as the immune system responds to this progression, and as the local and systemic effects of chemotherapy treatment run their course. The inherent complexity of signalling networks presents some difficulty for researchers. However, as discussed, some groups have begun to report paracrine cytokine signalling cascades involving tumour cells and their associated immune and endothelial cells, which drive tumour drug resistance as well as metastasis.

The immune system appears to have a duplicitous role in cancer. Whether it helps or hinders tumour progression depends upon the stimulus (tumour-derived and/or from therapy), and perhaps, most importantly, the underlying health of the patient and their immune system. Changes triggered by certain chemotherapy drugs can have significant effects on tumour behaviour either directly through their cytotoxic effects on the tumour or through their indirect effects on non-malignant cell populations within the tumour microenvironment. Taking into account each chemotherapy regimen and its effect on malignant and non-malignant cells in the tumour microenvironment appears to be critical to personalize and improve the quality of care for cancer patients undergoing chemotherapy.

Source of Funding Supported by a grant (to A.M.P.) from the Northern Cancer Foundation and a NOSM/NOSMFA Research Development Grant (to A.T.K.).

References

1. Grivennikov SI, Greten FR, Karin M (2010) Immunity, inflammation, and cancer. Cell 140(6):883–899. https://doi.org/10.1016/j.cell.2010.01.025
2. Elinav E, Nowarski R, Thaiss CA, Hu B, Jin C, Flavell RA (2013) Inflammation-induced cancer: crosstalk between tumours, immune cells and microorganisms. Nat Rev Cancer 13(11):759–771. https://doi.org/10.1038/nrc3611
3. Shalapour S, Karin M (2015) Immunity, inflammation, and cancer: an eternal fight between good and evil. J Clin Invest 125(9):3347–3355. https://doi.org/10.1172/JCI80007
4. Crusz SM, Balkwill FR (2015) Inflammation and cancer: advances and new agents. Nat Rev Clin Oncol 12(10):584–596. https://doi.org/10.1038/nrclinonc.2015.105
5. Showalter A, Limaye A, Oyer JL, Igarashi R, Kittipatarin C, Copik AJ, Khaled AR (2017) Cytokines in immunogenic cell death: applications for cancer immunotherapy. Cytokine 97:123–132. https://doi.org/10.1016/j.cyto.2017.05.024
6. Turner MD, Nedjai B, Hurst T, Pennington DJ (2014) Cytokines and chemokines: at the crossroads of cell signalling and inflammatory disease. Biochim Biophys Acta – Mol Cell Res 1843(11):2563–2582. https://doi.org/10.1016/j.bbamcr.2014.05.014
7. Akdis M, Burgler S, Crameri R, Eiwegger T, Fujita H, Gomez E, Klunker S, Meyer N, O'Mahony L, Palomares O, Rhyner C, Quaked N, Schaffartzik A, Van De Veen W, Zeller S, Zimmermann M, Akdis CA (2011) Interleukins, from 1 to 37, and interferon-γ: receptors, functions, and roles in diseases. J Allergy Clin Immunol 127(3):701–721.e770. https://doi.org/10.1016/j.jaci.2010.11.050
8. Akdis M, Aab A, Altunbulakli C, Azkur K, Costa RA, Crameri R, Duan S, Eiwegger T, Eljaszewicz A, Ferstl R, Frei R, Garbani M, Globinska A, Hess L, Huitema C, Kubo T, Komlosi Z, Konieczna P, Kovacs N, Kucuksezer UC, Meyer N, Morita H, Olzhausen J, O'Mahony L, Pezer M, Prati M, Rebane A, Rhyner C, Rinaldi A, Sokolowska M, Stanic B, Sugita K, Treis A, van de Veen W, Wanke K, Wawrzyniak M, Wawrzyniak P, Wirz OF, Zakzuk JS, Akdis CA (2016) Interleukins (from IL-1 to IL-38), interferons, transforming growth factor β, and TNF-α: receptors, functions, and roles in diseases. J Allergy Clin Immunol 138(4):984–1010. https://doi.org/10.1016/j.jaci.2016.06.033
9. Pestka S (2007) The interferons: 50 years after their discovery, there is much more to learn. J Biol Chem 282(28):20047–20051. https://doi.org/10.1074/jbc.R700004200

10. Croft M, Duan W, Choi H, Eun SY, Madireddi S, Mehta A (2012) TNF superfamily in inflammatory disease: translating basic insights. Trends Immunol 33(3):144–152. https://doi.org/10.1016/j.it.2011.10.004

11. Weiss A, Attisano L (2013) The TGFbeta superfamily signaling pathway. WIRES Dev Biol 2(1):47–63. https://doi.org/10.1002/wdev.86

12. Mukaida N, Sasaki S-i, Baba T (2014) Chemokines in cancer development and progression and their potential as targeting molecules for cancer treatment. Mediat Inflamm 2014:15. https://doi.org/10.1155/2014/170381

13. Hanahan D, Weinberg RA (2011) Hallmarks of cancer: the next generation. Cell 144:646–674

14. Goldberg JE, Schwertfeger KL (2010) Proinflammatory cytokines in breast cancer: mechanisms of action and potential targets for therapeutics. Curr Drug Targets 11(9):1133–1146

15. Korkaya H, Liu S, Wicha MS (2011) Breast cancer stem cells, cytokine networks, and the tumor microenvironment. J Clin Invest 121(10):3804–3809. https://doi.org/10.1172/JCI57099

16. Chin AR, Wang SE (2014) Cytokines driving breast cancer stemness. Mol Cell Endocrinol 382(1):598–602. https://doi.org/10.1016/j.mce.2013.03.024

17. Palacios-Arreola MI, Nava-Castro KE, Castro JI, Garcia-Zepeda E, Carrero JC, Morales-Montor J (2014) The role of chemokines in breast cancer pathology and its possible use as therapeutic targets. J Immunol Res 2014:8. https://doi.org/10.1155/2014/849720

18. Esquivel-Velazquez M, Ostoa-Saloma P, Palacios-Arreola MI, Nava-Castro KE, Castro JI, Morales-Montor J (2015) The role of cytokines in breast cancer development and progression. J Interf Cytokine Res 35(1):1–16. https://doi.org/10.1089/jir.2014.0026

19. Horwitz SB, Lothstein L, Manfredi JJ, Mellado W, Parness J, Roy SN, Schiff PB, Sorbara L, Zeheb R (1986) Taxol: mechanisms of action and resistance. Ann N Y Acad Sci 466:733–744. https://doi.org/10.1111/j.1749-6632.1986.tb38455.x

20. Edwardson D, Chewchuk S, Parissenti AM (2013) Resistance to anthracyclines and taxanes in breast cancer. In: Ahmad A (ed) Breast cancer metastasis and drug resistance. Springer New York, New York, pp 227–247. https://doi.org/10.1007/978-1-4614-5647-6_13

21. Edwardson DW, Narendrula R, Chewchuk S, Mispel-Beyer K, Mapletoft JPJ, Parissenti AM (2015) Role of drug metabolism in the cytotoxicity and clinical efficacy of anthracyclines. Curr Drug Metab 16(6):412–426

22. Bogdan C, Ding A (1992) Taxol, a microtubule-stabilizing antineoplastic agent, induces expression of tumor necrosis factor alpha and interleukin-1 in macrophages. J Leukoc Biol 52(1):119–121

23. Burkhart CA, Berman JW, Swindell CS, Horwitz SB (1994) Relationship between the structure of taxol and other taxanes on induction of tumor necrosis factor-alpha gene expression and cytotoxicity. Cancer Res 54(22):5779–5782

24. Jones VS, Huang RY, Chen LP, Chen ZS, Fu L, Huang RP (2016) Cytokines in cancer drug resistance: cues to new therapeutic strategies. Biochim Biophys Acta 1865(2):255–265. https://doi.org/10.1016/j.bbcan.2016.03.005

25. Sedgwick JD, Riminton DS, Cyster JG, Korner H (2000) Tumor necrosis factor: a master-regulator of leukocyte movement. Immunol Today 21(3):110–113. https://doi.org/10.1016/S0167-5699(99)01573-X

26. Sprowl J, Reed K, Armstrong S, Lanner C, Guo B, Kalatskaya I, Stein L, Hembruff S, Tam A, Parissenti A (2012) Alterations in tumor necrosis factor signaling pathways are associated with cytotoxicity and resistance to taxanes: a study in isogenic resistant tumor cells. Breast Cancer Res 14(1):R2

27. Edwardson DW, Boudreau J, Mapletoft J, Lanner C, Kovala AT, Parissenti AM (2017) Inflammatory cytokine production in tumor cells upon chemotherapy drug exposure or upon selection for drug resistance. PLoS One 12(9):e0183662

28. Berkova N, Page M (1995) Addition of hTNFα potentiates cytotoxicity of taxol in human ovarian cancer lines. Anticancer Res 15(3):863–866

29. Li B, Vincent A, Cates J, Brantley-Sieders DM, Polk DB, Young PP (2009) Low levels of tumor necrosis factor alpha increase tumor growth by inducing an endothelial phenotype of monocytes recruited to the tumor site. Cancer Res 69(1):338–348. https://doi.org/10.1158/0008-5472.CAN-08-1565

30. Ardestani S, Li B, Deskins DL, Wu H, Massion PP, Young PP (2013) Membrane versus soluble isoforms of TNF-a exert opposing effects on tumor growth and survival of tumor-associated myeloid cells. Cancer Res 73(13):3938–3950. https://doi.org/10.1158/0008-5472.CAN-13-0002

31. Hu G, Chong RA, Yang Q, Wei Y, Blanco MA, Li F, Reiss M, Au JLS, Haffty BG, Kang Y (2009) MTDH activation by 8q22 genomic gain promotes chemoresistance and metastasis of poor-prognosis breast cancer. Cancer Cell 15(1):9–20. https://doi.org/10.1016/j.ccr.2008.11.013

32. Morris PG, McArthur HL, Hudis CA (2009) Therapeutic options for metastatic breast cancer. Expert Opin Pharmacother 10(6):967–981. https://doi.org/10.1517/14656560902834961

33. Acharyya S, Oskarsson T, Vanharanta S, Malladi S, Kim J, Morris PG, Manova-Todorova K, Leversha M, Hogg N, Seshan VE, Norton L, Brogi E, Massague J (2012) A CXCL1 paracrine network links cancer chemoresistance and metastasis. Cell 150(1):165–178. https://doi.org/10.1016/j.cell.2012.04.042

34. Modur V, Zimmerman GA, Prescott SM, McIntyre TM (1996) Endothelial cell inflammatory responses to tumor necrosis factor alpha. Ceramide-dependent and -independent mitogen-activated protein kinase cascades. J Biol Chem 271(22):13094–13102. https://doi.org/10.1074/JBC.271.22.13094

35. Merritt WM, Lin YG, Spannuth WA, Fletcher MS, Kamat AA, Han LY, Landen CN, Jennings N, De Geest K, Langley RR, Villares G, Sanguino A, Lutgendorf SK, Lopez-Berestein G, Bar-Eli MM, Sood AK (2008) Effect of interleukin-8 gene silencing with liposome-encapsulated small interfering RNA on ovarian cancer cell growth. J Natl Cancer Inst 100(5):359–372. https://doi.org/10.1093/jnci/djn024

36. Black RA, Rauch CT, Kozlosky CJ, Peschon JJ, Slack JL, Wolfson MF, Castner BJ, Stocking KL, Reddy P, Srinivasan S, Nelson N, Boiani N, Schooley KA, Gerhart M, Davis R, Fitzner JN, Johnson RS, Paxton RJ, March CJ, Cerretti DP (1997) A metalloproteinase disintegrin that releases tumour-necrosis factor-alpha from cells. Nature 385(6618):729–733. https://doi.org/10.1038/385729a0

37. Shedden K, Taylor JMG, Enkemann SA, Tsao M-S, Yeatman TJ, Gerald WL, Eschrich S, Jurisica I, Giordano TJ, Misek DE, Chang AC, Zhu CQ, Strumpf D, Hanash S, Shepherd FA, Ding K, Seymour L, Naoki K, Pennell N, Weir B, Verhaak R, Ladd-Acosta C, Golub T, Gruidl M, Sharma A, Szoke J, Zakowski M, Rusch V, Kris M, Viale A, Motoi N, Travis W, Conley B, Seshan VE, Meyerson M, Kuick R, Dobbin KK, Lively T, Jacobson JW, Beer DG (2008) Gene expression-based survival prediction in lung adenocarcinoma: a multi-site, blinded validation study. Nat Med 14(8):822–827. https://doi.org/10.1038/nm.1790

38. Apetoh L, Ghiringhelli F, Tesniere A, Criollo A, Ortiz C, Lidereau R, Mariette C, Chaput N, Mira JP, Delaloge S, André F, Tursz T, Kroemer G, Zitvogel L (2007) The interaction between HMGB1 and TLR4 dictates the outcome of anticancer chemotherapy and radiotherapy. Immunol Rev 220:47–59. https://doi.org/10.1111/j.1600-065X.2007.00573.x

39. Apetoh L, Ghiringhelli F, Tesniere A, Obeid M, Ortiz C, Criollo A, Mignot G, Maiuri M, Ullrich E, Saulnier P, Yang H, Amigorena S, Ryffel B, Barrat F, Saftig P, Levi F, Lidereau R, Nogues C, Mira J, Chompret A, Joulin V, Clavel-Chapelon F, Bourhis J, Andre F, Delaloge S, Tursz T, Kroemer G, Zitvogel L (2007) Toll-like receptor 4-dependent contribution of the immune system to anticancer chemotherapy and radiotherapy. Nat Med 13(9):1050–1059. https://doi.org/10.1038/nm1622

40. Obeid M, Tesniere A, Ghiringhelli F, Fimia GM, Apetoh L, Perfettini J-L, Castedo M, Mignot G, Panaretakis T, Casares N, Métivier D, Larochette N, van Endert P, Ciccosanti F, Piacentini M, Zitvogel L, Kroemer G (2007) Calreticulin exposure dictates the immunogenicity of cancer cell death. Nat Med 13(1):54–61. https://doi.org/10.1038/nm1523

41. Obeid M, Panaretakis T, Tesniere A, Joza N, Tufi R, Apetoh L, Ghiringhelli F, Zitvogel L, Kroemer G (2007) Leveraging the immune system during chemotherapy: moving calreticulin to the cell surface converts apoptotic death from "Silent" to immunogenic. Cancer Res 67(17):7941–7944. https://doi.org/10.1158/0008-5472.can-07-1622

42. Ma Y, Adjemian S, Mattarollo SR, Yamazaki T, Aymeric L, Yang H, Portela Catani JP, Hannani D, Duret H, Steegh K, Martins I, Schlemmer F, Michaud M, Kepp O, Sukkurwala AQ, Menger L, Vacchelli E, Droin N, Galluzzi L, Krzysiek R, Gordon S, Taylor PR, Van Endert P, Solary E, Smyth MJ, Zitvogel L, Kroemer G (2013) Anticancer chemotherapy-induced intratumoral recruitment and differentiation of antigen-presenting cells. Immunity 38(4):729–741. https://doi.org/10.1016/j.immuni.2013.03.003

43. Kepp O, Tesniere A, Schlemmer F, Michaud M, Senovilla L, Zitvogel L, Kroemer G (2009) Immunogenic cell death modalities and their impact on cancer treatment. Apoptosis 14(4):364–375. https://doi.org/10.1007/s10495-008-0303-9

44. Xie K (2001) Interleukin-8 and human cancer biology. Cytokine Growth Factor Rev 12(4):375–391

45. Waugh DJ, Wilson C (2008) The interleukin-8 pathway in cancer. Clin Cancer Res 14(21):6735–6741. https://doi.org/10.1158/1078-0432.CCR-07-4843

46. Tanaka T, Bai Z, Srinoulprasert Y, Yang B-G, Yang B, Hayasaka H, Miyasaka M (2005) Chemokines in tumor progression and metastasis. Cancer Sci 96(6):317–322. https://doi.org/10.1111/j.1349-7006.2005.00059.x

47. Wang Y, Qu Y, Niu XL, Sun WJ, Zhang XL, Li LZ (2011) Autocrine production of interleukin-8 confers cisplatin and paclitaxel resistance in ovarian cancer cells. Cytokine 56(2):365–375. https://doi.org/10.1016/j.cyto.2011.06.005

48. Walz A, Peveri P, Aschauer H, Baggiolini M (1987) Purification and amino acid sequencing of NAF, a novel neutrophil-activating factor produced by monocytes. Biochem Biophys Res Commun 149(2):755–761. https://doi.org/10.1016/0006-291X(87)90432-3

49. Schröder JM, Christophers E (1986) Identification of C5ades arg and an anionic neutrophil-activating peptide (ANAP) in psoriatic scales. J Invest Dermatol 87(1):53–58

50. Matsushima K, Oppenheim JJ (1989) Interleukin 8 and MCAF: novel inflammatory cytokines inducible by IL 1 and TNF. Cytokine 1(1):2–13

51. Roebuck KA (1999) Regulation of Interleukin-8 gene expression. J Interf Cytokine Res 19:429–438. https://doi.org/10.1016/B978-012095440-7/50028-7

52. Xu L, Fidler IJ (2000) Interleukin 8: an autocrine growth factor for human ovarian cancer. Oncol Res 12(2):97–106

53. Murdoch C, Monk PN, Finn A (1999) Cxc chemokine receptor expression on human endothelial cells. Cytokine 11(9):704–712. https://doi.org/10.1006/cyto.1998.0465

54. Lee L-F, Haskill JS, Mukaida N, Matsushima K, Ting JPY (1997) Identification of tumor-specific paclitaxel (Taxol)-responsive regulatory elements in the Interleukin-8 promoter. Mol Cell Biol 17(9):5097–5105

55. Lee LF, Schuerer-Maly CC, Lofquist AK, Van Haaften-Day C, Ting JPY, White CM, Martin BK, Haskill JS (1996) Taxol-dependent transcriptional activation of IL-8 expression in a subset of human ovarian cancer. Cancer Res 56(6):1303–1308

56. Collins TS, Lee LF, Ting JP (2000) Paclitaxel up-regulates interleukin-8 synthesis in human lung carcinoma through an NF-kappaB- and AP-1-dependent mechanism. Cancer Immunol Immunother 49(2):78–84

57. Zhu YM, Webster SJ, Flower D, Woll PJ (2004) Interleukin-8/CXCL8 is a growth factor for human lung cancer cells. Br J Cancer 91(11):1970–1976. https://doi.org/10.1038/sj.bjc.6602227

58. Wang Y, Niu XL, Qu Y, Wu J, Zhu YQ, Sun WJ, Li LZ (2010) Autocrine production of interleukin-6 confers cisplatin and paclitaxel resistance in ovarian cancer cells. Cancer Lett 295(1):110–123. https://doi.org/10.1016/j.canlet.2010.02.019

59. Shi Z, Yang W-M, Chen L-P, Yang D-H, Zhou Q, Zhu J, Chen J-J, Huang R-C, Chen Z-S, Huang R-P (2012) Enhanced chemosensitization in multidrug-resistant human breast cancer

cells by inhibition of IL-6 and IL-8 production. Breast Cancer Res Treat 135(3):737–747. https://doi.org/10.1007/s10549-012-2196-0

60. Duan Z, Feller AJ, Penson RT, Chabner BA, Seiden MV (1999) Discovery of differentially expressed genes associated with paclitaxel resistance using cDNA array technology: analysis of interleukin (IL) 6, IL-8, and monocyte chemotactic protein 1 in the paclitaxel-resistant phenotype. Clin Cancer Res 5(11):3445–3453

61. Kassim SK, El-Salahy EM, Fayed ST, Helal SA, Helal T, EE-d A, Khalifa A (2004) Vascular endothelial growth factor and interleukin-8 are associated with poor prognosis in epithelial ovarian cancer patients. Clin Biochem 37(5):363–369. https://doi.org/10.1016/j.clinbiochem.2004.01.014

62. Herrera CA, Xu L, Bucana CD, Silva el VG, Hess KR, Gershenson DM, Fidler IJ (2002) Expression of metastasis-related genes in human epithelial ovarian tumors. Int J Oncol 20(1):5–13

63. Wilson C, Purcell C, Seaton A, Oladipo O, Maxwell PJ, O'Sullivan JM, Wilson RH, Johnston PG, Waugh DJJ (2008) Chemotherapy-induced CXC-chemokine/CXC-chemokine receptor signaling in metastatic prostate cancer cells confers resistance to oxaliplatin through potentiation of nuclear factor-kappaB transcription and evasion of apoptosis. J Pharmacol Exp Ther 327(3):746–759. https://doi.org/10.1124/jpet.108.143826

64. Lee LF, Hellendall RP, Wang Y, Haskill JS, Mukaida N, Matsushima K, Ting JP (2000) IL-8 reduced tumorigenicity of human ovarian cancer in vivo due to neutrophil infiltration. J Immunol 164(5):2769–2775. https://doi.org/10.4049/JIMMUNOL.164.5.2769

65. Huang S, Mills L, Mian B, Tellez C, McCarty M, Yang XD, Gudas JM, Bar-Eli M (2002) Fully humanized neutralizing antibodies to interleukin-8 (ABX-IL8) inhibit angiogenesis, tumor growth, and metastasis of human melanoma. Am J Pathol 161(1):125–134. https://doi.org/10.1016/S0002-9440(10)64164-8

66. Penson RT, Kronish K, Duan Z, Feller AJ, Stark P, Cook SE, Duska LR, Fuller AF, Goodman AK, Nikrui N, MacNeill KM, Matulonis UA, Preffer FI, Seiden MV (2000) Cytokines IL-1beta, IL-2, IL-6, IL-8, MCP-1, GM-CSF and TNFalpha in patients with epithelial ovarian cancer and their relationship to treatment with paclitaxel. Int J Gynecol Cancer 10(1):33–41

67. Pusztai L, Mendoza TR, Reuben JM, Martinez MM, Willey JS, Lara J, Syed A, Fritsche HA, Bruera E, Booser D, Valero V, Arun B, Ibrahim N, Rivera E, Royce M, Cleeland CS, Hortobagyi GN (2004) Changes in plasma levels of inflammatory cytokines in response to paclitaxel chemotherapy. Cytokine 25(3):94–102. https://doi.org/10.1016/j.cyto.2003.10.004

68. Hunter CA, Jones SA (2015) IL-6 as a keystone cytokine in health and disease. Nat Immunol 16(5):448–457. https://doi.org/10.1038/ni.3153

69. Ghandadi M, Sahebkar A (2016) Interleukin-6: a critical cytokine in cancer multidrug resistance. Curr Pharm Des 22(5):518–526

70. Kumari N, Dwarakanath BS, Das A, Bhatt AN (2016) Role of interleukin-6 in cancer progression and therapeutic resistance. Tumor Biol 37(9):11553–11572. https://doi.org/10.1007/s13277-016-5098-7

71. Conze D, Weiss L, Regen PS, Bhushan A, Weaver D, Johnson P, Rincón M (2001) Autocrine production of interleukin 6 causes multidrug resistance in breast cancer cells. Cancer Res 61(24):8851–8858

72. Yan HQ, Huang XB, Ke SZ, Jiang YN, Zhang YH, Wang YN, Li J, Gao FG (2014) Interleukin 6 augments lung cancer chemotherapeutic resistance via ataxia-telangiectasia mutated/NF-kappaB pathway activation. Cancer Sci 105(9):1220–1227. https://doi.org/10.1111/cas.12478

73. Hartman ZC, Poage GM, Den Hollander P, Tsimelzon A, Hill J, Panupinthu N, Zhang Y, Mazumdar A, Hilsenbeck SG, Mills GB, Brown PH (2013) Growth of triple-negative breast cancer cells relies upon coordinate autocrine expression of the proinflammatory cytokines IL-6 and IL-8. Cancer Res 73(11):3470–3480. https://doi.org/10.1158/0008-5472.CAN-12-4524-T

74. Korkaya H, Kim GI, Davis A, Malik F, Henry NL, Ithimakin S, Quraishi AA, Tawakkol N, D'Angelo R, Paulson AK, Chung S, Luther T, Paholak HJ, Liu S, Hassan KA, Zen Q, Clouthier SG, Wicha MS (2012) Activation of an IL6 inflammatory loop mediates Trastuzumab resistance in HER2+ breast cancer by expanding the cancer stem cell population. Mol Cell 47(4):570–584. https://doi.org/10.1016/j.molcel.2012.06.014
75. Li G, Zhao L, Li W, Fan K, Qian W, Hou S, Wang H, Dai J, Wei H, Guo Y (2014) Feedback activation of STAT3 mediates trastuzumab resistance via upregulation of MUC1 and MUC4 expression. Oncotarget 5(18):8317–8329. https://doi.org/10.18632/oncotarget.2135
76. Yang Z, Guo L, Liu D, Sun L, Chen H, Deng Q, Liu Y, Yu M, Ma Y, Guo N, Shi M (2015) Acquisition of resistance to trastuzumab in gastric cancer cells is associated with activation of IL-6/STAT3/Jagged-1/Notch positive feedback loop. Oncotarget 6(7):5072–5087. https://doi.org/10.18632/oncotarget.3241
77. Rodriguez-Barrueco R, Yu J, Saucedo-Cuevas LP, Olivan M, Llobet-Navas D, Putcha P, Castro V, Murga-Penas EM, Collazo-Lorduy A, Castillo-Martin M, Alvarez M, Cordon-Cardo C, Kalinsky K, Maurer M, Califano A, Silva JM (2015) Inhibition of the autocrine IL-6–JAK2–STAT3–calprotectin axis as targeted therapy for HR-/HER2+ breast cancers. Genes Dev 29(15):1631–1648. https://doi.org/10.1101/gad.262642.115
78. Duan S, Tsai Y, Keng P, Chen Y, Ok Lee S, Chen Y (2015) IL-6 signaling contributes to cisplatin resistance in non-small cell lung cancer via the up-regulation of anti-apoptotic and DNA repair associated molecules. Oncotarget 6(29):27651–27660. https://doi.org/10.18632/oncotarget.4753
79. Zhu X, Shen H, Yin X, Long L, Chen X, Feng F, Liu Y, Zhao P, Xu Y, Li M, Xu W, Li Y (2017) IL-6R/STAT3/miR-204 feedback loop contributes to cisplatin resistance of epithelial ovarian cancer cells. Oncotarget 8(24):39154–39166. https://doi.org/10.18632/oncotarget.16610
80. Han X, Zhen S, Ye Z, Lu J, Wang L, Li P, Li J, Zheng X, Li H, Chen W, Li X, Zhao L (2017) A feedback loop between miR-30a/c-5p and DNMT1 mediates cisplatin resistance in ovarian cancer cells. Cell Physiol Biochem 41(3):973–986. https://doi.org/10.1159/000460618
81. De Mattos-Arruda L, Bottai G, Nuciforo PG, Di Tommaso L, Giovannetti E, Peg V, Losurdo A, Perez-Garcia J, Masci G, Corsi F, Cortes J, Seoane J, Calin GA, Santarpia L (2015) MicroRNA-21 links epithelial-to-mesenchymal transition and inflammatory signals to confer resistance to neoadjuvant trastuzumab and chemotherapy in HER2-positive breast cancer patients. Oncotarget 6(35):37269–37280. https://doi.org/10.18632/oncotarget.5495
82. Wang Z-Y, Zhang J-A, Wu X-J, Liang Y-F, Lu Y-B, Gao Y-C, Dai Y-C, Yu S-Y, Jia Y, Fu X-X, Rao X, Xu J-F, Zhong J (2016) IL-6 inhibition reduces STAT3 activation and enhances the anti-tumor effect of carboplatin. Mediat Inflamm 2016:8. https://doi.org/10.1155/2016/8026494
83. Mochizuki D, Adams A, Warner KA, Zhang Z, Pearson AT, Misawa K, McLean SA, Wolf GT, Nor JE (2015) Anti-tumor effect of inhibition of IL-6 signaling in mucoepidermoid carcinoma. Oncotarget 6(26):22822–22835. https://doi.org/10.18632/oncotarget.4477
84. Ara T, Nakata R, Sheard MA, Shimada H, Buettner R, Groshen SG, Ji L, Yu H, Jove R, Seeger RC, DeClerck YA (2013) Critical role of STAT3 in IL-6-mediated drug resistance in human neuroblastoma. Cancer Res 73(13):3852–3864. https://doi.org/10.1158/0008-5472.CAN-12-2353
85. Suchi K, Fujiwara H, Okamura S, Okamura H, Umehara S, Todo M, Furutani A, Yoneda M, Shiozaki A, Kubota T, Ichikawa D, Okamoto K, Otsuji E (2011) Overexpression of Interleukin-6 suppresses cisplatin-induced cytotoxicity in esophageal squamous cell carcinoma cells. Anticancer Res 31(1):67–75
86. Frassanito MA, Cusmai A, Iodice G, Dammacco F (2001) Autocrine interleukin-6 production and highly malignant multiple myeloma: relation with resistance to drug-induced apoptosis. Blood 97(2):483–489. https://doi.org/10.1182/blood.V97.2.483
87. De Filippo K, Dudeck A, Hasenberg M, Nye E, van Rooijen N, Hartmann K, Gunzer M, Roers A, Hogg N (2013) Mast cell and macrophage chemokines CXCL1/CXCL2 control the early stage of neutrophil recruitment during tissue inflammation. Blood 121(24):4930–4937. https://doi.org/10.1182/blood-2013-02-486217

88. Bolitho C, Hahn MA, Baxter RC, Marsh DJ (2010) The chemokine CXCL1 induces proliferation in epithelial ovarian cancer cells by transactivation of the epidermal growth factor receptor. Endocr Relat Cancer 17(4):929–940. https://doi.org/10.1677/ERC-10-0107

89. Dhawan P, Richmond A (2002) Role of CXCL1 in tumorigenesis of melanoma. J Leukoc Biol 72(1):9–18

90. Owen JD, Strieter R, Burdick M, Haghnegahdar H, Nanney L, Shattuck-Brandt R, Richmond A (1997) Enhanced tumor-forming capacity for immortalized melanocytes expressing melanoma growth stimulatory activity/growth-regulated cytokine beta and gamma proteins. Int J Cancer 73(1):94–103

91. Lebrun J-J (2012) The dual role of TGF in human cancer: from tumor suppression to cancer metastasis. ISRN Mol Biol 2012:28. https://doi.org/10.5402/2012/381428

92. Huang S, Hölzel M, Knijnenburg T, Schlicker A, Roepman P, McDermott U, Garnett M, Grenrrum W, Sun C, Prahallad A, Groenendijk FH, Mittempergher L, Nijkamp W, Neefjes J, Salazar R, Pt D, Uramoto H, Tanaka F, Beijersbergen RL, Wessels LFA, Bernards R (2012) MED12 controls the response to multiple cancer drugs through regulation of TGF-β receptor signaling. Cell 151(5):937–950. https://doi.org/10.1016/j.cell.2012.10.035

93. Oshimori N, Oristian D, Fuchs E (2015) TGF-β promotes heterogeneity and drug resistance in squamous cell carcinoma. Cell 160(5):963–976. https://doi.org/10.1016/j.cell.2015.01.043

94. Li J, Ao J, Li K, Zhang J, Li Y, Zhang L, Wei Y, Gong D, Gao J, Tan W, Huang L, Liu L, Lin P, Wei Y (2016) ZNF32 contributes to the induction of multidrug resistance by regulating TGF-[beta] receptor 2 signaling in lung adenocarcinoma. Cell Death Dis 7:e2428. https://doi.org/10.1038/cddis.2016.328

95. Marín-Aguilera M, Codony-Servat J, Kalko SG, Fernández PL, Bermudo R, Buxo E, Ribal MJ, Gascón P, Mellado B (2012) Identification of docetaxel resistance genes in castration-resistant prostate cancer. Mol Cancer Ther 11(2):329–339. https://doi.org/10.1158/1535-7163.mct-11-0289

96. Shiota M, Kashiwagi E, Yokomizo A, Takeuchi A, Dejima T, Song Y, Tatsugami K, Inokuchi J, Uchiumi T, Naito S (2013) Interaction between docetaxel resistance and castration resistance in prostate cancer: implications of twist1, YB-1, and androgen receptor. Prostate 73(12):1336–1344. https://doi.org/10.1002/pros.22681

97. Yao Z, Fenoglio S, Gao DC, Camiolo M, Stiles B, Lindsted T, Schlederer M, Johns C, Altorki N, Mittal V, Kenner L, Sordella R (2010) TGF-β IL-6 axis mediates selective and adaptive mechanisms of resistance to molecular targeted therapy in lung cancer. Proc Natl Acad Sci U S A 107(35):15535–15540. https://doi.org/10.1073/pnas.1009472107

98. Yamada D, Kobayashi S, Wada H, Kawamoto K, Marubashi S, Eguchi H, Ishii H, Nagano H, Doki Y, Mori M (2013) Role of crosstalk between interleukin-6 and transforming growth factor-beta 1 in epithelial mesenchymal transition and chemoresistance in biliary tract cancer. Eur J Cancer 49(7):1725–1740. https://doi.org/10.1016/j.ejca.2012.12.002

99. Chen M-F, Wang W-H, Lin P-Y, Lee K-D, Chen W-C (2012) Significance of the TGF-β1/IL-6 axis in oral cancer. Clin Sci 122(10):459–472. https://doi.org/10.1042/cs20110434

100. Nakamura T, Shinriki S, Jono H, Guo J, Ueda M, Hayashi M, Yamashita S, Zijlstra A, Nakayama H, Hiraki A, Shinohara M, Ando Y (2015) Intrinsic TGF-β2-triggered SDF-1-CXCR4 signaling axis is crucial for drug resistance and a slow-cycling state in bone marrow-disseminated tumor cells. Oncotarget 6(2):1008–1019

101. Guo F, Wang Y, Liu J, Mok SC, Xue F, Zhang W (2016) CXCL12/CXCR4: a symbiotic bridge linking cancer cells and their stromal neighbors in oncogenic communication networks. Oncogene 35(7):816–826. https://doi.org/10.1038/onc.2015.139

102. Weekes CD, Song D, Arcaroli J, Wilson LA, Rubio-Viqueira B, Cusatis G, Garrett-Mayer E, Messersmith WA, Winn RA, Hidalgo M (2012) Stromal cell-derived factor 1α mediates resistance to mTOR-directed therapy in pancreatic cancer. Neoplasia 14(8):690–701

103. Jung MJ, Rho JK, Kim YM, Jung JE, Jin YB, Ko YG, Lee JS, Lee SJ, Lee JC, Park MJ (2013) Upregulation of CXCR4 is functionally crucial for maintenance of stemness in drug-resistant non-small cell lung cancer cells. Oncogene 32(2):209–221. https://doi.org/10.1038/onc.2012.37

104. Domanska UM, Timmer-Bosscha H, Nagengast WB, Oude Munnink TH, Kruizinga RC, Ananias HJ, Kliphuis NM, Huls G, De Vries EG, de Jong IJ, Walenkamp AM (2012) CXCR4 inhibition with AMD3100 sensitizes prostate cancer to docetaxel chemotherapy. Neoplasia 14(8):709–718
105. Bhardwaj A, Srivastava SK, Singh S, Arora S, Tyagi N, Andrews J, McClellan S, Carter JE, Singh AP (2014) CXCL12/CXCR4 signaling counteracts docetaxel-induced microtu-bule stabilization via p21-activated kinase 4-dependent activation of LIM domain kinase 1. Oncotarget 5(22):11490–11500. https://doi.org/10.18632/oncotarget.2571
106. Sison EAR, McIntyre E, Magoon D, Brown P (2013) Dynamic chemotherapy-induced upreg-ulation of CXCR4 expression: a mechanism of therapeutic resistance in pediatric AML. Mol Cancer Res 11(9):1004–1016. https://doi.org/10.1158/1541-7786.mcr-13-0114
107. Chen Z, Teo AE, McCarty N (2016) ROS-induced CXCR4 signaling regulates mantle cell lymphoma (MCL) cell survival and drug resistance in the bone marrow microenvironment via autophagy. Clin Cancer Res 22(1):187–199. https://doi.org/10.1158/1078-0432.ccr-15-0987
108. Beider K, Darash-Yahana M, Blaier O, Koren-Michowitz M, Abraham M, Wald H, Wald O, Galun E, Eizenberg O, Peled A, Nagler A (2014) Combination of imatinib with CXCR4 antagonist BKT140 overcomes the protective effect of stroma and targets CML in vitro and in vivo. Mol Cancer Ther 13(5):1155–1169. https://doi.org/10.1158/1535-7163. MCT-13-0410
109. Barbieri F, Bajetto A, Thellung S, Würth R, Florio T (2016) Drug design strategies focusing on the CXCR4/CXCR7/CXCL12 pathway in leukemia and lymphoma. Expert Opin Drug Discov 11(11):1093–1109. https://doi.org/10.1080/17460441.2016.1233176
110. Sleightholm RL, Neilsen BK, Li J, Steele MM, Singh RK, Hollingsworth MA, Oupicky D (2017) Emerging roles of the CXCL12/CXCR4 axis in pancreatic cancer progression and therapy. Pharmacol Ther. https://doi.org/10.1016/j.pharmthera.2017.05.012
111. Wang Z, Sun J, Feng Y, Tian X, Wang B, Zhou Y (2016) Oncogenic roles and drug target of CXCR4/CXCL12 axis in lung cancer and cancer stem cell. Tumor Biol 37(7):8515–8528. https://doi.org/10.1007/s13277-016-5016-z
112. Xu C, Zhao H, Chen H, Yao Q (2015) CXCR4 in breast cancer: oncogenic role and therapeu-tic targeting. Drug Des Dev Ther 9:4953–4964
113. Zhang J, Patel L, Pienta KJ (2010) Targeting chemokine (C-C motif) ligand 2 (CCL2) as an example of translation of cancer molecular biology to the clinic. Prog Mol Biol Transl Sci 95:31–53. https://doi.org/10.1016/B978-0-12-385071-3.00003-4
114. Lim SY, Yuzhalin AE, Gordon-Weeks AN, Muschel RJ (2016) Targeting the CCL2-CCR2 signaling axis in cancer metastasis. Oncotarget 7(19):28697–28710. https://doi.org/10.18632/ oncotarget.7376
115. Soria G, Ben-Baruch A (2008) The inflammatory chemokines CCL2 and CCL5 in breast cancer. Cancer Lett 267(2):271–285. https://doi.org/10.1016/j.canlet.2008.03.018
116. Velasco-Velazquez M, Xolalpa W, Pestell RG (2014) The potential to target CCL5/CCR5 in breast cancer. Expert Opin Ther Targets 18(11):1265–1275. https://doi.org/10.1517/1472822 2.2014.949238
117. Aldinucci D, Colombatti A (2014) The inflammatory chemokine CCL5 and cancer progres-sion. Mediat Inflamm 2014:292376. https://doi.org/10.1155/2014/292376
118. Wang J, Zhuang ZG, Xu SF, He Q, Shao YG, Ji M, Yang L, Bao W (2015) Expression of CCL2 is significantly different in five breast cancer genotypes and predicts patient outcome. Int J Clin Exp Med 8(9):15684–15691
119. Yao M, Yu E, Staggs V, Fan F, Cheng N (2016) Elevated expression of chemokine C-C ligand 2 in stroma is associated with recurrent basal-like breast cancers. Mod Pathol 29(8):810–823. https://doi.org/10.1038/modpathol.2016.78
120. Fang WB, Yao M, Brummer G, Acevedo D, Alhakamy N, Berkland C, Cheng N (2016) Targeted gene silencing of CCL2 inhibits triple negative breast cancer progression by block-ing cancer stem cell renewal and M2 macrophage recruitment. Oncotarget 7(31):49349–49367. https://doi.org/10.18632/oncotarget.9885

121. Fang WB, Jokar I, Zou A, Lambert D, Dendukuri P, Cheng N (2012) CCL2/CCR2 chemokine signaling coordinates survival and motility of breast cancer cells through Smad3 protein- and p42/44 mitogen-activated protein kinase (MAPK)-dependent mechanisms. J Biol Chem 287(43):36593–36608. https://doi.org/10.1074/jbc.M112.365999

122. Fader AN, Rasool N, Vaziri SAJ, Kozuki T, Faber PW, Elson P, Biscotti CV, Michener CM, Rose PG, Rojas-Espaillat L, Belinson JL, Ganapathi MK, Ganapathi R (2010) CCL2 expression in primary ovarian carcinoma is correlated with chemotherapy response and survival outcomes. Anticancer Res 30(12):4791–4798

123. Moisan F, Francisco EB, Brozovic A, Duran GE, Wang YC, Chaturvedi S, Seetharam S, Snyder LA, Doshi P, Sikic BI (2014) Enhancement of paclitaxel and carboplatin therapies by CCL2 blockade in ovarian cancers. Mol Oncol 8(7):1231–1239. https://doi.org/10.1016/j.molonc.2014.03.016

124. Roca H, Varsos Z, Pienta KJ (2008) CCL2 protects prostate cancer PC3 cells from autophagic death via phosphatidylinositol 3-kinase/AKT-dependent survivin up-regulation. J Biol Chem 283(36):25057–25073. https://doi.org/10.1074/jbc.M801073200

125. Roca H, Varsos ZS, Pienta KJ (2009) CCL2 is a negative regulator of AMP-activated protein kinase to sustain mTOR complex-1 activation, survivin expression, and cell survival in human prostate cancer PC3 cells. Neoplasia 11(12):1309–1317. https://doi.org/10.1593/neo.09936

126. Macanas-Pirard P, Quezada T, Navarrete L, Broekhuizen R, Leisewitz A, Nervi B, Ramírez PA (2017) The CCL2/CCR2 axis affects transmigration and proliferation but not resistance to chemotherapy of acute myeloid leukemia cells. PLoS One 12(1):e0168888. https://doi.org/10.1371/journal.pone.0168888

127. Vergani E, Guardo LD, Dugo M, Rigoletto S, Tragni G, Ruggeri R, Perrone F, Tamborini E, Gloghini A, Arienti F, Vergani B, Deho P, Cecco LD, Vallacchi V, Frati P, Shahaj E, Villa A, Santinami M, Braud FD, Rivoltini L, Rodolfo M (2016) Overcoming melanoma resistance to vemurafenib by targeting CCL2-induced miR-34a, miR-100 and miR-125b. Oncotarget 7(4):4428–4441

128. Qian DZ, Rademacher BLS, Pittsenbarger J, Huang C-Y, Myrthue A, Higano CS, Garzotto M, Nelson PS, Beer TM (2010) CCL2 is induced by chemotherapy and protects prostate cancer cells from docetaxel-induced cytotoxicity. Prostate 70(4):433–442. https://doi.org/10.1002/pros.21077

129. Ji W-T, Chen H-R, Lin C-H, Lee J-W, Lee C-C (2014) Monocyte chemotactic protein 1 (MCP-1) modulates pro-survival signaling to promote progression of head and neck squamous cell carcinoma. PLoS One 9(2):e88952. https://doi.org/10.1371/journal.pone.0088952

130. Steiner JL, Murphy EA (2012) Importance of chemokine (CC-motif) ligand 2 in breast cancer. Int J Biol Markers 27(3):179–185. https://doi.org/10.5301/JBM.2012.9345

131. Yi EH, Lee CS, Lee J-K, Lee YJ, Shin MK, Cho C-H, Kang KW, Lee JW, Han W, Noh D-Y, Kim Y-N, Cho I-H, Ye S-k (2013) STAT3-RANTES autocrine signaling is essential for tamoxifen resistance in human breast cancer cells. Mol Cancer Res 11(1):31–42. https://doi.org/10.1158/1541-7786.mcr-12-0217

132. Zhou B, Sun C, Li N, Shan W, Lu H, Guo L, Guo E, Xia M, Weng D, Meng L, Hu J, Ma D, Chen G (2016) Cisplatin-induced CCL5 secretion from CAFs promotes cisplatin-resistance in ovarian cancer via regulation of the STAT3 and PI3K/Akt signaling pathways. Int J Oncol 48(5):2087–2097. https://doi.org/10.3892/ijo.2016.3442

133. Johnson-Holiday C, Singh R, Johnson E, Singh S, Stockard CR, Grizzle WE, Lillard JW (2011) CCL25 mediates migration, invasion and matrix metalloproteinase expression by breast cancer cells in a CCR9-dependent fashion. Int J Oncol 38:1279–1285

134. Johnson EL, Singh R, Singh S, Johnson-Holiday CM, Grizzle WE, Partridge EE, Lillard JW (2010) CCL25-CCR9 interaction modulates ovarian cancer cell migration, metalloproteinase expression, and invasion. World J Surg Oncol 8(1):62. https://doi.org/10.1186/1477-7819-8-62

135. Johnson EL, Singh R, Johnson-Holiday CM, Grizzle WE, Partridge EE, Lillard JW, Singh S (2010) CCR9 interactions support ovarian cancer cell survival and resistance to cisplatin-induced apoptosis in a PI3K-dependent and FAK-independent fashion. J Ovarian Res 3:15. https://doi.org/10.1186/1757-2215-3-15

136. Sharma PK, Singh R, Novakovic KR, Eaton JW, Grizzle WE, Singh S (2010) CCR9 mediates PI3K/AKT-dependent antiapoptotic signals in prostate cancer cells and inhibition of CCR9-CCL25 interaction enhances the cytotoxic effects of etoposide. Int J Cancer 127(9):2020–2030. https://doi.org/10.1002/ijc.25219

137. Li B, Wang Z, Zhong Y, Lan J, Li X, Lin H (2015) CCR9–CCL25 interaction suppresses apoptosis of lung cancer cells by activating the PI3K/Akt pathway. Med Oncol 32(3):66. https://doi.org/10.1007/s12032-015-0531-0

138. Qiuping Z, Jei X, Youxin J, Wei J, Chun L, Jin W, Qun W, Yan L, Chunsong H, Mingzhen Y, Qingping G, Kejian Z, Zhimin S, Qun L, Junyan L, Jinquan T (2004) CC chemokine ligand 25 enhances resistance to apoptosis in CD4+ T cells from patients with T-cell lineage acute and chronic lymphocytic leukemia by means of Livin activation. Cancer Res 64(20):7579–7587. https://doi.org/10.1158/0008-5472.can-04-0641

139. Johnson-Holiday C, Singh R, Johnson EL, Grizzle WE, Lillard JW, Singh S (2011) CCR9-CCL25 interactions promote cisplatin resistance in breast cancer cell through Akt activation in a PI3K-dependent and FAK-independent fashion. World J Surg Oncol 9(1):46. https://doi.org/10.1186/1477-7819-9-46

140. Mackall CL, Fry TJ, Gress RE (2011) Harnessing the biology of IL-7 for therapeutic application. Nat Rev Immunol 11(5):330–342

141. Cui L, Fu J, Pang JC, Qiu ZK, Liu XM, Chen FR, Shi HL, Ng HK, Chen ZP (2012) Overexpression of IL-7 enhances cisplatin resistance in glioma. Cancer Biol Ther 13(7):496–503. https://doi.org/10.4161/cbt.19592

142. Sade H, Sarin A (2003) IL-7 inhibits dexamethasone-induced apoptosis via Akt/PKB in mature, peripheral T cells. Eur J Immunol 33(4):913–919. https://doi.org/10.1002/eji.200323782

143. Liu Z-H, Wang M-H, Ren H-J, Qu W, Sun L-M, Zhang Q-F, Qiu X-S, Wang E-H (2014) Interleukin 7 signaling prevents apoptosis by regulating bcl-2 and bax via the p53 pathway in human non-small cell lung cancer cells. Int J Clin Exp Pathol 7(3):870–881

144. Hamidullah, Changkija B, Konwar R (2012) Role of interleukin-10 in breast cancer. Breast Cancer Res Treat 133(1):11–21. https://doi.org/10.1007/s10549-011-1855-x

145. Mannino MH, Zhu Z, Xiao H, Bai Q, Wakefield MR, Fang Y (2015) The paradoxical role of IL-10 in immunity and cancer. Cancer Lett 367(2):103–107. https://doi.org/10.1016/j.canlet.2015.07.009

146. Alas S, Bonavida B (2001) Rituximab inactivates signal transducer and activation of transcription 3 (STAT3) activity in B-non-Hodgkin's lymphoma through inhibition of the interleukin 10 autocrine/paracrine loop and results in down-regulation of Bcl-2 and sensitization to cytotoxic drugs. Cancer Res 61(13):5137–5144

147. Danoch H, Kalechman Y, Albeck M, Longo DL, Sredni B (2015) Sensitizing B- and T- cell lymphoma cells to Paclitaxel/Abraxane–induced death by AS101 via inhibition of the VLA-4–IL10–Survivin axis. Mol Cancer Res 13(3):411–422. https://doi.org/10.1158/1541-7786.mcr-14-0459

148. Yang C, He L, He P, Liu Y, Wang W, He Y, Du Y, Gao F (2015) Increased drug resistance in breast cancer by tumor-associated macrophages through IL-10/STAT3/bcl-2 signaling pathway. Med Oncol 32(2):352. https://doi.org/10.1007/s12032-014-0352-6

149. Fabbi M, Carbotti G, Ferrini S (2015) Context-dependent role of IL-18 in cancer biology and counter-regulation by IL-18BP. J Leukoc Biol 97(4):665–675. https://doi.org/10.1189/jlb.5RU0714-360RR

150. Yao L, Zhang Y, Chen K, Hu X, Xu LX (2011) Discovery of IL-18 as a novel secreted protein contributing to doxorubicin resistance by comparative secretome analysis of MCF-7 and MCF-7/Dox. PLoS One 6(9):e24684. https://doi.org/10.1371/journal.pone.0024684

151. Yamamoto K, Seike M, Takeuchi S, Soeno C, Miyanaga A, Noro R, Minegishi Y, Kubota K, Gemma A (2014) miR-379/411 cluster regulates IL-18 and contributes to drug resistance in malignant pleural mesothelioma. Oncol Rep 32:2365–2372

152. Liu X-C, Lian W, Zhang L-J, Feng X-C, Gao Y, Li S-X, Liu C, Cheng Y, Yang L, Wang X-J, Chen L, Wang R-Q, Chai J, Chen W-S (2015) Interleukin-18 down-regulates multidrug resistance-associated protein 2 expression through Farnesoid X receptor associated

with nuclear factor kappa B and Yin Yang 1 in human hepatoma HepG2 cells. PLoS One 10(8):e0136215. https://doi.org/10.1371/journal.pone.0136215

153. Baghdadi M, Wada H, Nakanishi S, Abe H, Han N, Putra WE, Endo D, Watari H, Sakuragi N, Hida Y, Kaga K, Miyagi Y, Yokose T, Takano A, Daigo Y, Seino K-i (2016) Chemotherapy-induced IL34 enhances immunosuppression by tumor-associated macrophages and mediates survival of chemoresistant lung cancer cells. Cancer Res 76(20):6030–6042. https://doi.org/10.1158/0008-5472.can-16-1170

154. Mimeault M, Batra SK (2010) Divergent molecular mechanisms underlying the pleiotropic functions of macrophage inhibitory cytokine-1 in cancer. J Cell Physiol 224(3):626–635. https://doi.org/10.1002/jcp.22196

155. Unsicker K, Spittau B, Krieglstein K (2013) The multiple facets of the TGF-β family cytokine growth/differentiation factor-15/macrophage inhibitory cytokine-1. Cytokine Growth Factor Rev 24(4):373–384. https://doi.org/10.1016/j.cytogfr.2013.05.003

156. Huang C-Y, Beer TM, Higano CS, True LD, Vessella R, Lange PH, Garzotto M, Nelson PS (2007) Molecular alterations in prostate carcinomas that associate with in vivo exposure to chemotherapy: identification of a cytoprotective mechanism involving growth differentiation factor 15. Clin Cancer Res 13(19):5825–5833. https://doi.org/10.1158/1078-0432.ccr-07-1037

157. Zhao L, Lee BY, Brown DA, Molloy MP, Marx GM, Pavlakis N, Boyer MJ, Stockler MR, Kaplan W, Breit SN, Sutherland RL, Henshall SM, Horvath LG (2009) Identification of candidate biomarkers of therapeutic response to docetaxel by proteomic profiling. Cancer Res 69(19):7696–7703. https://doi.org/10.1158/0008-5472.can-08-4901

158. Mimeault M, Johansson SL, Batra SK (2013) Marked improvement of cytotoxic effects induced by docetaxel on highly metastatic and androgen-independent prostate cancer cells by downregulating macrophage inhibitory cytokine-1. Br J Cancer 108(5):1079–1091. https://doi.org/10.1038/bjc.2012.484

159. Meier JC, Haendler B, Seidel H, Groth P, Adams R, Ziegelbauer K, Kreft B, Beckmann G, Sommer A, Kopitz C (2015) Knockdown of platinum-induced growth differentiation factor 15 abrogates p27-mediated tumor growth delay in the chemoresistant ovarian cancer model A2780cis. Cancer Med 4(2):253–267. https://doi.org/10.1002/cam4.354

160. Joshi JP, Brown NE, Griner SE, Nahta R (2011) Growth differentiation factor 15 (GDF15)-mediated HER2 phosphorylation reduces trastuzumab sensitivity of HER2-overexpressing breast cancer cells. Biochem Pharmacol 82(9):1090–1099. https://doi.org/10.1016/j.bcp.2011.07.082

161. Griner SE, Wang KJ, Joshi JP, Nahta R (2013) Mechanisms of Adipocytokine-mediated Trastuzumab resistance in HER2-positive breast cancer cell lines. Curr Pharmacogenomics Person Med 11(1):31–41

162. Zhai Y, Zhang J, Wang H, Lu W, Liu S, Yu Y, Weng W, Ding Z, Zhu Q, Shi J (2016) Growth differentiation factor 15 contributes to cancer-associated fibroblasts-mediated chemo-protection of AML cells. J Exp Clin Cancer Res 35(1):147. https://doi.org/10.1186/s13046-016-0405-0

163. Oh C-K, Lee SJ, Park S-H, Moon Y (2016) Acquisition of chemoresistance and other malignancy-related features of colorectal cancer cells are incremented by ribosome-inactivating stress. J Biol Chem 291(19):10173–10183. https://doi.org/10.1074/jbc.M115.696609

164. Panneerselvam J, Munshi A, Ramesh R (2013) Molecular targets and signaling pathways regulated by interleukin (IL)-24 in mediating its antitumor activities. J Mol Signal 8:1750–2187. https://doi.org/10.1186/1750-2187-8-15

165. Ma M, Zhao L, Sun G, Zhang C, Liu L, Du Y, Yang X, Shan B (2016) Mda-7/IL-24 enhances sensitivity of B cell lymphoma to chemotherapy drugs. Oncol Rep 35(5):3122–3130. https://doi.org/10.3892/or.2016.4622

166. Liu Z, Xu L, Yuan H, Zhang Y, Zhang X, Zhao D (2015) Oncolytic adenovirus mediated mda7/IL24 expression suppresses osteosarcoma growth and enhances sensitivity to doxorubicin. Mol Med Rep 12(4):6358–6364. https://doi.org/10.3892/mmr.2015.4180

167. Yacoub A, Mitchell C, Hong Y, Gopalkrishnan RV, Su Z-Z, Gupta P, Sauane M, Lebedeva IV, Curiel DT, Mahasreshti PJ, Rosenfeld MR, Broaddus WC, James CD, Grant S, Fisher PB, Dent P (2004) MDA-7 regulates cell growth and radiosensitivity in vitro of primary (non-established) human glioma cells. Cancer Biol Ther 3(8):739–751. https://doi.org/10.4161/cbt.3.8.968

168. Hu CW, Yin GF, Wang XR, Ren BW, Zhang WG, Bai QL, Lv YM, Li WL, Zhao WQ (2014) IL-24 induces apoptosis via upregulation of RNA-activated protein kinase and enhances temozolomide-induced apoptosis in glioma cells. Oncol Res 22(3):159–165. https://doi.org/10.3727/096504015X14298122915628

169. Fang L, Cheng Q, Bai J, Qi YD, Liu JJ, Li LT, Zheng JN (2013) An oncolytic adenovirus expressing interleukin-24 enhances antitumor activities in combination with paclitaxel in breast cancer cells. Mol Med Rep 8(5):1416–1424. https://doi.org/10.3892/mmr.2013.1680

170. Amirzada MI, Ma X, Gong X, Chen Y, Bashir S, Jin J (2014) Recombinant human interleukin 24 reverses Adriamycin resistance in a human breast cancer cell line. Pharmacol Rep 66(5):915–919. https://doi.org/10.1016/j.pharep.2014.05.010

171. Emdad L, Sarkar D, Lebedeva IV, Su ZZ, Gupta P, Mahasreshti PJ, Dent P, Curiel DT, Fisher PB (2006) Ionizing radiation enhances adenoviral vector expressing mda-7/IL-24-mediated apoptosis in human ovarian cancer. J Cell Physiol 208(2):298–306. https://doi.org/10.1002/jcp.20663

172. Sistigu A, Yamazaki T, Vacchelli E, Chaba K, Enot DP, Adam J, Vitale I, Goubar A, Baracco EE, Remedios C, Fend L, Hannani D, Aymeric L, Ma Y, Niso-Santano M, Kepp O, Schultze JL, Tuting T, Belardelli F, Bracci L, La Sorsa V, Ziccheddu G, Sestili P, Urbani F, Delorenzi M, Lacroix-Triki M, Quidville V, Conforti R, Spano JP, Pusztai L, Poirier-Colame V, Delaloge S, Penault-Llorca F, Ladoire S, Arnould L, Cyrta J, Dessoliers MC, Eggermont A, Bianchi ME, Pittet M, Engblom C, Pfirschke C, Preville X, Uze G, Schreiber RD, Chow MT, Smyth MJ, Proietti E, Andre F, Kroemer G, Zitvogel L (2014) Cancer cell-autonomous contribution of type I interferon signaling to the efficacy of chemotherapy. Nat Med 20(11):1301–1309. https://doi.org/10.1038/nm.3708

173. Bennett CL, Djulbegovic B, Norris LB, Armitage JO (2013) Colony-stimulating factors for febrile neutropenia during cancer therapy. N Engl J Med 368(12):1131–1139. https://doi.org/10.1056/NEJMct1210890

174. Weiner HL, Cohen JA (2002) Treatment of multiple sclerosis with cyclophosphamide: critical review of clinical and immunologic effects. Multi Scler 8(2):142–154. https://doi.org/10.1191/1352458502ms790oa

175. Seggewiss R, Lore K, Greiner E, Magnusson MK, Price DA, Douek DC, Dunbar CE, Wiestner A (2005) Imatinib inhibits T-cell receptor-mediated T-cell proliferation and activation in a dose-dependent manner. Blood 105(6):2473–2479. https://doi.org/10.1182/blood-2004-07-2527

176. Bruchard M, Mignot G, Derangere V, Chalmin F, Chevriaux A, Vegran F, Boireau W, Simon B, Ryffel B, Connat JL, Kanellopoulos J, Martin F, Rebe C, Apetoh L, Ghiringhelli F (2013) Chemotherapy-triggered cathepsin B release in myeloid-derived suppressor cells activates the Nlrp3 inflammasome and promotes tumor growth. Nat Med 19(1):57–64. https://doi.org/10.1038/nm.2999

177. Shurin MR (2013) Dual role of immunomodulation by anticancer chemotherapy. Nat Med 19(1):20–22. https://doi.org/10.1038/nm.3045

178. Bohm S, Montfort A, Pearce OM, Topping J, Chakravarty P, Everitt GL, Clear A, McDermott JR, Ennis D, Dowe T, Fitzpatrick A, Brockbank EC, Lawrence AC, Jeyarajah A, Faruqi AZ, McNeish IA, Singh N, Lockley M, Balkwill FR (2016) Neoadjuvant chemotherapy modulates the immune microenvironment in metastases of tubo-ovarian high-grade serous carcinoma. Clin Cancer Res 22(12):3025–3036. https://doi.org/10.1158/1078-0432.CCR-15-2657

179. Vincent J, Mignot G, Chalmin F, Ladoire S, Bruchard M, Chevriaux A, Martin F, Apetoh L, Rebe C, Ghiringhelli F (2010) 5-fluorouracil selectively kills tumor-associated myeloid-derived suppressor cells resulting in enhanced T cell-dependent antitumor immunity. Cancer Res 70(8):3052–3061. https://doi.org/10.1158/0008-5472.CAN-09-3690

180. North RJ (1982) Cyclophosphamide-facilitated adoptive immunotherapy of an established tumor depends on elimination of tumor-induced suppressor T cells. J Exp Med 155(4):1063–1074

181. Schiavoni G, Mattei F, Di Pucchio T, Santini SM, Bracci L, Belardelli F, Proietti E (2000) Cyclophosphamide induces type I interferon and augments the number of CD44(hi) T lymphocytes in mice: implications for strategies of chemoimmunotherapy of cancer. Blood 95(6):2024–2030

182. Glaser M (1979) Regulation of specific cell-mediated cytotoxic response against SV40-induced tumor associated antigens by depletion of suppressor T cells with cyclophosphamide in mice. J Exp Med 149(3):774–779

183. Zhong H, Han B, Tourkova IL, Lokshin A, Rosenbloom A, Shurin MR, Shurin GV (2007) Low-dose paclitaxel prior to intratumoral dendritic cell vaccine modulates intratumoral cytokine network and lung cancer growth. Clin Cancer Res 13(18 Pt 1):5455–5462. https://doi.org/10.1158/1078-0432.CCR-07-0517

184. Wang J, Kobayashi M, Han M, Choi S, Takano M, Hashino S, Tanaka J, Kondoh T, Kawamura K, Hosokawa M (2002) MyD88 is involved in the signalling pathway for Taxol-induced apoptosis and TNF-alpha expression in human myelomonocytic cells. Br J Haematol 118(2):638–645

185. Albain KS, Barlow WE, Ravdin PM, Farrar WB, Burton GV, Ketchel SJ, Cobau CD, Levine EG, Ingle JN, Pritchard KI, Lichter AS, Schneider DJ, Abeloff MD, Henderson IC, Muss HB, Green SJ, Lew D, Livingston RB, Martino S, Osborne CK, Breast Cancer Intergroup of North A (2009) Adjuvant chemotherapy and timing of tamoxifen in postmenopausal patients with endocrine-responsive, node-positive breast cancer: a phase 3, open-label, randomised controlled trial. Lancet 374(9707):2055–2063. https://doi.org/10.1016/S0140-6736(09)61523-3-3

186. Argyriou AA, Assimakopoulos K, Iconomou G, Giannakopoulou F, Kalofonos HP (2011) Either called "chemobrain" or "chemofog," the long-term chemotherapy-induced cognitive decline in cancer survivors is real. J Pain Symptom Manag 41(1):126–139. https://doi.org/10.1016/j.jpainsymman.2010.04.021

187. Crawford J, Ozer H, Stoller R, Johnson D, Lyman G, Tabbara I, Kris M, Grous J, Picozzi V, Rausch G et al (1991) Reduction by granulocyte colony-stimulating factor of fever and neutropenia induced by chemotherapy in patients with small-cell lung cancer. N Engl J Med 325(3):164–170. https://doi.org/10.1056/NEJM199107183250305

188. Quasthoff S, Hartung HP (2002) Chemotherapy-induced peripheral neuropathy. J Neurol 249(1):9–17

189. Cheung YT, Ng T, Shwe M, Ho HK, Foo KM, Cham MT, Lee JA, Fan G, Tan YP, Yong WS, Madhukumar P, Loo SK, Ang SF, Wong M, Chay WY, Ooi WS, Dent RA, Yap YS, Ng R, Chan A (2015) Association of proinflammatory cytokines and chemotherapy-associated cognitive impairment in breast cancer patients: a multi-centered, prospective, cohort study. Ann Oncol 26(7):1446–1451. https://doi.org/10.1093/annonc/mdv206

190. Janelsins MC, Mustian KM, Palesh OG, Mohile SG, Peppone LJ, Sprod LK, Heckler CE, Roscoe JA, Katz AW, Williams JP, Morrow GR (2012) Differential expression of cytokines in breast cancer patients receiving different chemotherapies: implications for cognitive impairment research. Support Care Cancer 20(4):831–839. https://doi.org/10.1007/s00520-011-1158-0

191. Rochfort KD, Collins LE, Murphy RP, Cummins PM (2014) Downregulation of blood-brain barrier phenotype by proinflammatory cytokines involves NADPH oxidase-dependent ROS generation: consequences for interendothelial adherens and tight junctions. PLoS One 9(7):e101815. https://doi.org/10.1371/journal.pone.0101815

192. Watkins LR, Maier SF, Goehler LE (1995) Cytokine-to-brain communication: a review & analysis of alternative mechanisms. Life Sci 57(11):1011–1026

193. Hyka N, Dayer JM, Modoux C, Kohno T, Edwards CK 3rd, Roux-Lombard P, Burger D (2001) Apolipoprotein A-I inhibits the production of interleukin-1beta and tumor necrosis

factor-alpha by blocking contact-mediated activation of monocytes by T lymphocytes. Blood 97(8):2381–2389

194. Ren X, St Clair DK, Butterfield DA (2017) Dysregulation of cytokine mediated chemotherapy induced cognitive impairment. Pharmacol Res 117:267–273. https://doi.org/10.1016/j.phrs.2017.01.001

195. Tangpong J, Cole MP, Sultana R, Joshi G, Estus S, Vore M, St Clair W, Ratanachaiyavong S, St Clair DK, Butterfield DA (2006) Adriamycin-induced, TNF-alpha-mediated central nervous system toxicity. Neurobiol Dis 23(1):127–139. https://doi.org/10.1016/j.nbd.2006.02.013

196. Groves TR, Farris R, Anderson JE, Alexander TC, Kiffer F, Carter G, Wang J, Boerma M, Allen AR (2017) 5-fluorouracil chemotherapy upregulates cytokines and alters hippocampal dendritic complexity in aged mice. Behav Brain Res 316:215–224. https://doi.org/10.1016/j.bbr.2016.08.039

197. Wang XM, Lehky TJ, Brell JM, Dorsey SG (2012) Discovering cytokines as targets for chemotherapy-induced painful peripheral neuropathy. Cytokine 59(1):3–9. https://doi.org/10.1016/j.cyto.2012.03.027

198. Schafers M, Sorkin L (2008) Effect of cytokines on neuronal excitability. Neurosci Lett 437(3):188–193. https://doi.org/10.1016/j.neulet.2008.03.052

199. Postma TJ, Vermorken JB, Liefting AJ, Pinedo HM, Heimans JJ (1995) Paclitaxel-induced neuropathy. Ann Oncol 6(5):489–494

200. Verstappen CC, Heimans JJ, Hoekman K, Postma TJ (2003) Neurotoxic complications of chemotherapy in patients with cancer: clinical signs and optimal management. Drugs 63(15):1549–1563

201. Lisse TS, Middleton LJ, Pellegrini AD, Martin PB, Spaulding EL, Lopes O, Brochu EA, Carter EV, Waldron A, Rieger S (2016) Paclitaxel-induced epithelial damage and ectopic MMP-13 expression promotes neurotoxicity in zebrafish. Proc Natl Acad Sci U S A 113(15):E2189–E2198. https://doi.org/10.1073/pnas.1525096113

202. Peters CM, Jimenez-Andrade JM, Jonas BM, Sevcik MA, Koewler NJ, Ghilardi JR, Wong GY, Mantyh PW (2007) Intravenous paclitaxel administration in the rat induces a peripheral sensory neuropathy characterized by macrophage infiltration and injury to sensory neurons and their supporting cells. Exp Neurol 203(1):42–54. https://doi.org/10.1016/j.expneurol.2006.07.022

203. Cairo MS (2000) Dose reductions and delays: limitations of myelosuppressive chemotherapy. Oncology (Williston Park) 14(9 Suppl 8):21–31

204. Chen YM, Whang-Peng J, Liu JM, Kuo BI, Wang SY, Tsai CM, Perng RP (1996) Serum cytokine level fluctuations in chemotherapy-induced myelosuppression. Jpn J Clin Oncol 26(1):18–23

205. Weber J, Yang JC, Topalian SL, Parkinson DR, Schwartzentruber DS, Ettinghausen SE, Gunn H, Mixon A, Kim H, Cole D et al (1993) Phase I trial of subcutaneous interleukin-6 in patients with advanced malignancies. J Clin Oncol 11(3):499–506. https://doi.org/10.1200/JCO.1993.11.3.499

206. Wood LJ, Nail LM, Perrin NA, Elsea CR, Fischer A, Druker BJ (2006) The cancer chemotherapy drug etoposide (VP-16) induces proinflammatory cytokine production and sickness behavior-like symptoms in a mouse model of cancer chemotherapy-related symptoms. Biol Res Nurs 8(2):157–169. https://doi.org/10.1177/1099800406290932

207. Gordon S (2003) Alternative activation of macrophages. Nat Rev Immunol 3(1):23–35. https://doi.org/10.1038/nri978

208. Gannon PO, Poisson AO, Delvoye N, Lapointe R, Mes-Masson AM, Saad F (2009) Characterization of the intra-prostatic immune cell infiltration in androgen-deprived prostate cancer patients. J Immunol Methods 348(1–2):9–17. https://doi.org/10.1016/j.jim.2009.06.004

209. Craig M, Ying C, Loberg RD (2008) Co-inoculation of prostate cancer cells with U937 enhances tumor growth and angiogenesis in vivo. J Cell Biochem 103(1):1–8. https://doi.org/10.1002/jcb.21379

210. Levina V, Su Y, Nolen B, Liu X, Gordin Y, Lee M, Lokshin A, Gorelik E (2008) Chemotherapeutic drugs and human tumor cells cytokine network. Int J Cancer 123(9):2031–2040. https://doi.org/10.1002/ijc.23732
211. Lev DC, Onn A, Melinkova VO, Miller C, Stone V, Ruiz M, McGary EC, Ananthaswamy HN, Price JE, Bar-Eli M (2004) Exposure of melanoma cells to Dacarbazine results in enhanced tumor growth and metastasis in vivo. J Clin Oncol 22(11):2092–2100. https://doi.org/10.1200/JCO.2004.11.070
212. Lev DC, Ruiz M, Mills L, McGary EC, Price JE, Bar-Eli M (2003) Dacarbazine causes transcriptional up-regulation of interleukin 8 and vascular endothelial growth factor in melanoma cells: a possible escape mechanism from chemotherapy. Mol Cancer Ther 2. (August:753–763
213. Mahon KL, Lin HM, Castillo L, Lee BY, Lee-Ng M, Chatfield MD, Chiam K, Breit SN, Brown DA, Molloy MP, Marx GM, Pavlakis N, Boyer MJ, Stockler MR, Daly RJ, Henshall SM, Horvath LG (2015) Cytokine profiling of docetaxel-resistant castration-resistant prostate cancer. Br J Cancer 112(8):1340–1348. https://doi.org/10.1038/bjc.2015.74
214. Mahon FX, Belloc F, Lagarde V, Chollet C, Moreau-Gaudry F, Reiffers J, Goldman JM, Melo JV (2003) MDR1 gene overexpression confers resistance to imatinib mesylate in leukemia cell line models. Blood 101(6):2368–2373. https://doi.org/10.1182/blood.V101.6.2368
215. Zhang H, Wu H, Guan J, Wang L, Ren X, Shi X, Liang Z, Liu T (2015) Paracrine SDF-1α signaling mediates the effects of PSCs on GEM chemoresistance through an IL-6 autocrine loop in pancreatic cancer cells. Oncotarget 6(5):3085–3097
216. Suh Y-A, Jo S-Y, Lee H-Y, Lee C (2014) Inhibition of IL-6/STAT3 axis and targeting Axl and Tyro3 receptor tyrosine kinases by apigenin circumvent taxol resistance in ovarian cancer cells. Int J Oncol 46(3):1405–1411. https://doi.org/10.3892/ijo.2014.2808
217. Wang Y, Niu XL, Guo XQ, Yang J, Li L, Qu Y, Hu CX, Mao LQ, Wang D (2015) IL6 induces TAM resistance via kinase-specific phosphorylation of ERα in OVCA cells. J Mol Endocrinol 54(3):351–361. https://doi.org/10.1530/JME-15-0011
218. Ruffell B, Chang-Strachan D, Chan V, Rosenbusch A, Ho CM, Pryer N, Daniel D, Hwang ES, Rugo HS, Coussens LM (2014) Macrophage IL-10 blocks CD8+ T cell-dependent responses to chemotherapy by suppressing IL-12 expression in intratumoral dendritic cells. Cancer Cell 26(5):623–637. https://doi.org/10.1016/j.ccell.2014.09.006
219. Stassi G, Todaro M, Zerilli M, Ricci-Vitiani L, Di Liberto D, Patti M, Florena A, Di Gaudio F, Di Gesù G, De Maria R (2003) Thyroid cancer resistance to chemotherapeutic drugs via autocrine production of Interleukin-4 and Interleukin-10. Cancer Res 63(20):6784–6790
220. Nervi B, Ramirez P, Rettig MP, Uy GL, Holt MS, Ritchey JK, Prior JL, Piwnica-Worms D, Bridger G, Ley TJ, DiPersio JF (2009) Chemosensitization of acute myeloid leukemia (AML) following mobilization by the CXCR4 antagonist AMD3100. Blood 113(24):6206–6214. https://doi.org/10.1182/blood-2008-06-162123
221. Cho B-S, Zeng Z, Mu H, Wang Z, Konoplev S, McQueen T, Protopopova M, Cortes J, Marszalek JR, Peng S-B, Ma W, Davis RE, Thornton DE, Andreeff M, Konopleva M (2015) Antileukemia activity of the novel peptidic CXCR4 antagonist LY2510924 as monotherapy and in combination with chemotherapy. Blood 126(2):222–232. https://doi.org/10.1182/blood-2015-02-628677
222. Simstein R, Burow M, Parker A, Weldon C, Beckman B (2003) Apoptosis, chemoresistance, and breast cancer: insights from the MCF-7 cell model system. Exp Biol Med (Maywood) 228(9):995–1003
223. Van Obberghen-Schilling E, Tucker RP, Saupe F, Gasser I, Cseh B, Orend G (2011) Fibronectin and tenascin-C: accomplices in vascular morphogenesis during development and tumor growth. Int J Dev Biol 55(4–5):511–525. https://doi.org/10.1387/ijdb.103243eo

Chapter 10
Current Updates on Trastuzumab Resistance in HER2 Overexpressing Breast Cancers

Aamir Ahmad

Abstract Trastuzumab represents the predominant therapy to target breast cancer subtype marked by HER2 amplification. It has been in use for two decades and its continued importance is underlined by recent FDA approvals of its biosimilar and conjugated versions. Progression to an aggressive disease with acquisition of resistance to trastuzumab remains a major clinical concern. In addition to a number of cellular signaling pathways being investigated, focus in recent years has also shifted to epigenetic and non-coding RNA basis of acquired resistance against trastuzumab. This article provides a succinct discussion on the most recent advances in our understanding of such factors.

Keywords HER2 · Breast cancer · Trastuzumab · Epigenetic · Non-coding RNA · miRNA

10.1 HER2 Overexpressing Breast Cancers

HER2, coded by *ERBB2*, an oncogene located at the long arm of human chromosome 17(17q21-q22), was characterized initially by Coussens et al. in 1985 [1]. It derived its name from its close resemblance to EGFR (epidermal growth factor receptor), which is also known as HER1. 'Neu' in HER2/neu refers to its rodent glioblastoma cell line origin, which happens to be a kind of neural tumor [2]. HER2 is also known as "ErbB-2" because of its similarity to EGFR coding oncogene *ERBB* (avian erythroblastosis oncogene B). There are additional names for HER2 as well, such as p185 [3] and CD340.

HER2 is overexpressed or amplified in 20–30% invasive breast cancers resulting in poor prognosis [4]. Breast is not the only tissue that expresses HER2. Ovaries,

A. Ahmad (✉)
Mitchell Cancer Institute, University of South Alabama, Mobile, AL, USA
e-mail: aahmad@health.southalabama.edu

© Springer Nature Switzerland AG 2019
A. Ahmad (ed.), *Breast Cancer Metastasis and Drug Resistance*,
Advances in Experimental Medicine and Biology 1152,
https://doi.org/10.1007/978-3-030-20301-6_10

217

lungs, liver, kidneys and central nervous system also express HER2 [5]. Overexpression of HER2 results in as many as two million receptors on a single cell [4–6]. HER2 is normally associated with growth and division of breast cells and its overexpression/amplification results in abrupt and uncontrolled cell growth.

10.2 Drugs That Specifically Target HER2

Breast cancers marked by overexpression of HER2 are targeted by HER2-targeted therapies. A number of HER2-tergeting therapies have been approved by the Food and Drug Administration (FDA) for clinical use (Table 10.1). The first approved therapy was monoclonal antibody trastuzumab. Another monoclonal antibody approved for HER2 overexpressing breast cancers is pertuzumab. Lapatinib is the tyrosine kinase inhibitor that targets HER2. Other approved therapies include a conjugate of trastuzumab with emtansine and a therapy that is biosimilar to trastuzumab (Table 10.1). Readers are encouraged to have a look at the first volume of this series [2] for basic information on the two antibodies (trastuzumab and pertuzumab) and the tyrosine kinase inhibitor lapatinib.

10.3 Drug Resistance in HER2 Overexpressing Breast Cancers

As discussed previously [2], the resistance against trastuzumab, the prototype HER2-targeting drug, is both 'inherent' as well as 'developed' [6]. It is documented that not all HER2 overexpressing breast cancers respond to trastuzumab, rather, less than 35% of such breast cancer patients actually respond to trastuzumab therapy [6–8]. And, then among the patients who do respond, a big majority, close to 70% patients, develop resistance within 1 year, which invariably results in a

Table 10.1 Therapies targeted against HER2 overexpressing breast cancers

Therapy	Trade name	Type	Route	FDA approval	Mode of action
Trastuzumab	Herceptin	Monoclonal antibody	IV	Sep 1998	Directly binds to HER2 and inhibits HER2 signaling
Ogivri	Biosimilar to Trastuzumab			Dec 2017	
Lapatinib	Tykerb	Kinase inhibitor	Oral (pill)	Jan 2010	Inhibits tyrosine kinase activity of HER2
Pertuzumab	Perjeta	Monoclonal antibody	IV	June 2012	Inhibits HER2 dimerization
Ado-trastuzumab emtansine	Kadcyla/ TDM-1	Monoclonal antibody-drug conjugate	IV	Feb 2013	Combines specificity of Trastuzumab with cytotoxic activity of Emtansine

IV Intravenous

progressively aggressive and metastatic disease [9]. While resistance to lapatinib in HER2 amplified breast cancers has also been studied, trastuzumab remains the leading therapy by far for treatment of HER2 amplified breast cancers, and will remain the focus of this article.

10.4   Resistance to Trastuzumab

In the last volume [2] a discussion on mechanisms of resistance against trastuzumab was provided. The mechanisms included (a) increased expression of alternate HER family receptors which could compensate for compromised HER2 signaling [10, 11], (b) steric hindrance of HER2-trastuzumab interaction, (c) de-regulated intracellular signaling pathways [12] and (d) alterations in cell cycle regulation, particularly the inhibitory p27. Many studies in recent years have focused on these mechanisms and provided a better understanding of the trastuzumab resistance in breast cancer patients and cell lines. However, some newer areas of investigations have also opened up, such as investigations into epigenetic factors and non-coding RNAs. In the following sections, a succinct discussion on traditional as well as novel factors affecting trastuzumab resistance is being provided.

10.4.1   HER Family

As mentioned above, alternate HER family receptors have been proposed to play a role in trastuzumab resistance. There is enough evidence in literature to support this [13, 14]. For example, HER2-positive patients that are negative for HER3 have a 100% metastasis-free survival [15] i.e. absence of HER3 might actually be associated with good prognosis while HER3 positivity is a not a favorable diagnosis for patients with HER2 amplification. Further, targeting of HER3 by miRNAs (miR-125a and miR-205) increases the efficacy of trastuzumab [16]. A role of HER4 has also been suggested in trastuzumab resistance [17, 18]. Even receptors other than from HER family, such as FGFR [19] and IGF-1R [20], can play an important role in trastuzumab resistance. Thus, it seems like targeted inhibition of HER2 often results in other HER family members, or similar oncogenic receptors, stepping up to compensate for HER2 loss.

10.4.2   Other Factors/Signaling Pathways

While HER2 amplification remains the reason for initiating HER2-targeted therapy such as trastuzumab, the eventual development of resistance suggests that factors other than HER2 need to be better understood. This is exemplified by a finding [21] where it was reported that loss of PTEN expression should be an important criterion before the start of trastuzumab therapy because a little less than half of HER2 amplified breast cancer patients report a loss of PTEN. In such patients, continued administration of trastuzumab results in acquisition of EMT and stemness with loss of dependence on HER2 family receptors. The tumors essentially remind of triple negative breast cancer and continued use of trastuzumab becomes meaningless. Similar to this report, a role of stemness in trastuzumab resistance has been suggested by few investigations as well [22–27].

There is possible role of Androgen Receptor (AR) in trastuzumab resistance as infiltration of immune cells inversely correlates with AR [28]. When AR expression is high, there is low immune cells infiltration which can have profound effect on sensitivity to trastuzumab. Immune evasion in cancer cells has been demonstrated to lead to trastuzumab resistance in another study as well [29]. Other factors/signaling pathways (Table 10.2) that affect trastuzumab resistance include ATG9A [30], CD44 [27], CD147 [31], ESE-1 [32], MUC1 [33], MUC4 [34], LMO4 [35], DUSP4 [36], Src [37], STAT3 [38, 39], TGFβ-SMAD3 [40], Yes1 [41], Notch [42] and wnt/β-catenin pathway [43, 44].

In addition to identifying the molecular determinants of trastuzumab resistance, there have also been ongoing efforts to find biomarkers for predicting response to trastuzumab. Towards this end, MEL-18 has recently been proposed as a biomarker of HER2-positive breast cancers wherein its amplification has been associated with a better prognosis [45]. MEL-18 silences ADAM10/17 and depletion of MEL-18 leads to trastuzumab resistance. It has also been suggested that inducing IL21 signaling might be an effective strategy to potentiate trastuzumab effects [46]. Taken together, recent years have witnessed reports on several putative factors that potentially mediate trastuzumab resistance. Its about time to further evaluate them in clinics.

Table 10.2 Molecular factors that affect trastuzumab resistance

| Gene | Trastuzumab resistance | | Mechanism | Reference |
	Induced	Inhibited		
Androgen receptor	X		Inversely correlates with immune cell infiltration	[28]
ESE-1	X		Modulates Akt and cell cycle	[32]
HER3	X		Compensates for lost HER2 signaling	[15]
IL-21		X	Required for optimal trastuzumab activity	[46]
LMO4	X		Induces Bcl-2	[35]
MEL-18		X	Silences ADAM10/17	[45]
STAT3	X		HIF-1α upregulation and PTEN downregulation	[38]
TGFβ-SMAD3	X		Induces stemness	[40]
Wnt signaling	X		Induces EMT	[43, 44]
Yes1	X		Modulates cell cycle and apoptosis	[41]

10.4.3   Epigenetic Basis of Trastuzumab Resistance

With the knowledge that HER2 amplification confers growth advantage, and results in aggressive clinical outcome, efforts have been made to understand the epigenetic basis of this HER2 amplification in a subset of breast cancer patients [47]. It is believed that such understanding will provide rationale for designing future therapeutic regimes. Reports on epigenetic regulation of trastuzumab resistance are trickling in and are mostly indirect indications. For example, the MEL-18-mediated attenuation of trastuzumab resistance has been shown to involve epigenetic silencing of ADAM10/17 [45]. Similarly, trastuzumab resistance induced by SNHG14 long non-coding RNA has been reported to involve modulation of H3K27 acetylation [48]. Also, differential methylation of distinct genomic segments can actually be used as a tool to predict response to trastuzumab [49]. While still in its infancy, epigenetic regulation of trastuzumab is being realized. Studies focused on methylation and acetylation etc. provide direct evidence with regards to the existence of epigenetic regulation. However, regulation through non-coding RNAs is also within the broader definition of epigenetic regulation.

10.4.4   Regulation of Trastuzumab Resistance by Non-coding RNAs

Long being considered 'junk', non-coding RNAs are rapidly emerging on the forefront of contemporary cancer research [50]. A number of distinct non-coding RNAs subtypes are now known, with miRNAs being the most well-studied group. However, other non-coding RNAs are also being investigated for possible role in trastuzumab resistance.

10.4.4.1   Long Non-coding RNAs

Long non-coding (lnc) RNAs represent one distinct group of non-coding RNAs, on which several reports have emerged in recent years suggesting a possible mechanistic role in trastuzumab resistance [51]. LncRNA urothelial cancer associated 1 (UCA1) promotes trastuzumab resistance by regulating miR-18a-mediated repression of Yes-associated protein 1 (YAP1) [52] while lnc-ATB induces EMT and modulates miR-200c, resulting in trastuzumab resistance [53]. Another long noncoding RNA SNHG14 profoundly affects trastuzumab resistance. It targets Bcl-2/Bax signaling [54]. It also modulates H3K27 acetylation in the promoter of PABPC1 gene that results in increased expression of PABPC1 and eventually Nrf2 signaling, all of which leads to induced resistance to trastuzumab [48]. LncRNA GAS5, on the contrary, reverses trastuzumab resistance, by acting as a sponge for miR-21 [55]. Incidentally, miR-21 has directly been implicated in induction of EMT and resulting trastuzumab resistance [56].

10.4.4.2   Small Non-coding RNAs

Two tRNA-derived small non-coding RNAs (sncRNAs), tRF-30-JZOYJE22RR33 and tRF-27-ZDXPHO53KSN, seem to be predictive for trastuzumab resistance because patients with high expression levels of these sncRNAs were found to be less responsive to trastuzumab [57].

10.4.4.3   MicroRNAs

miRNAs have now been implicated in cancer drug resistance for many years [58]. It is, therefore, not surprising to see reports in recent years on the involvement of miRNAs in trastuzumab resistance [27, 59, 60]. miR-129-5p was predicted to play a role in trastuzumab resistance because of its down-regulation in resistant cells and its ectopic expression resulted in sensitization of resistant cells to trastuzumab [61]. Similarly, miR-542 downregulation leads to trastuzumab resistance with effects on PI3K-Akt signaling and cell cycle progression [62]. miR-7 targets multiple oncogenic pathways, including EGFR and Src, and increases sensitivity to trastuzumab [63].

miR-125a and miR-205 can potentially be effective in reversing trastuzumab resistance because they target HER3 and the silencing of HER3 by these miRNAs has been shown to improve the therapeutic efficacy of trastuzumab [16, 64]. Targeting of HER3 by miR-125b also has similar effects [65]. miR-182, miR-30b and miR-16 can similarly reverse trastuzumab resistance but their actions involve targeting of MET [66], CCNE2 [67] and FUBP1 [68] respectively.

In contrast to the miRNAs that improve sensitivity to trastuzumab, miR-21 has been shown to induce EMT and trastuzumab resistance by inhibiting PTEN and triggering IL-6/STAT3/NF-κB loop [56]. A miRNA signature, comprised of four miRNAs, miR-940 (released from tumor cells) and miR-451a, miR-16-5p and miR-17-3p (released from immune cells) has been propsed as a serum-based signature to predict response to trastuzumab [69].

Even with the limited scope of discussion here – just a few very recent years, there is clear abundance of reports discussing the role of non-coding RNAs in determination of trastuzumab resistance (Table 10.3). It is expected that in next few years, there will be a continued interest in this research area resulting in many such reports on the topic.

Table 10.3 Non-coding RNAs in Trastuzumab resistance

Non-coding RNA	Type	Role	Mechanism (if known)	Reference
ATB	lncRNA	Induces trastuzumab resistance	Induces EMT	[53]
GAS5	lncRNA	Inversely correlates with trastuzumab resistance	Sponges miR-21	[55]
miR-16-5p	miRNA	Part of miRNA signature to predict trastuzumab response		[69]
miR-17-3p	miRNA	Part of miRNA signature to predict trastuzumab response		[69]
miR-21	miRNA	Induces trastuzumab resistance	Inhibits PTEN	[56]
miR-30b	miRNA	Sensitizes cells to trastuzumab	Targets CCNE2	[67]
miR-125a	miRNA	Increases trastuzumab efficacy	Targets HER3	[16]
miR-125b	miRNA	Increases trastuzumab efficacy	Targets HER3	[65]
miR-129-5p	miRNA	Sensitizes cells to trastuzumab	Targets Rps6	[61]
miR-182	miRNA	Sensitizes cells to trastuzumab	Targets MET	[66]
miR-205	miRNA	Increases trastuzumab efficacy	Targets HER3	[16, 64]
miR-451a	miRNA	Part of miRNA signature to predict trastuzumab response		[69]
miR-940	miRNA	Part of miRNA signature to predict trastuzumab response		[69]
SNHG14	lncRNA	Induces trastuzumab resistance	Induces PABPC1	[48]
			Targets Bcl-2/ BAX signaling	[54]
tRF-30-JZOYJE22RR33	sncRNA	Predictive biomarker	Elevated in trastuzumab resistance	[57]
tRF-27-ZDXPHO53KSN	sncRNA	Predictive biomarker	Elevated in trastuzumab resistance	[57]
UCA1	lncRNA	Promotes trastuzumab resistance	Targets miR-18a-YAP1	[52]

10.5   Conclusions and Perspectives

HER2 amplified breast cancers are aggressive. They are blessed with a target for therapy, but still remain a challenge for clinicians, primarily because of the relatively quick progression to metastatic disease that results from acquisition of resistance to therapy. The mechanism(s) are under active investigation but clearly there is no final verdict yet. Among many other challenges, one is related to our rather incomplete knowledge of patient demographics. A significant proportion of breast cancer patients are aged, with almost one-third of patients being over 65 years of age. However, it has been estimated that these patients are not adequately represented in clinical trials [70]. This is clearly an area where things need to improve.

In view of the importance of trastuzumab in therapy of breast cancer patients with HER2 expression, a few other therapies have been approved by FDA which either have 'biosimilarity' to trastuzumab or have a drug conjugated to trastuzumab. It is not surprising that acquired resistance against such new therapies is already being investigated. For example, resistance against trastuzumab-emtansine therapy has been a subject of many studies [71–73] and often involves perturbed signaling such as STAT3 pathway [71] which is well known to mediate resistance against trastuzumab alone [38]. Its appears as if we are moving in circles with incremental progress at best. This calls for some radical shift in our approach. Given the role of tumor microenvironment in modulating response to therapies, including trastuzumab resistance [74], there is need to develop more robust models, such as the one recently described [75], with the goal of predicting response to therapy.

References

1. Coussens L, Yang-Feng TL, Liao YC, Chen E, Gray A, McGrath J, Seeburg PH, Libermann TA, Schlessinger J, Francke U (1985) Tyrosine kinase receptor with extensive homology to EGF receptor shares chromosomal location with neu oncogene. Science 230:1132–1139
2. Ahmad A, Sarkar FH (2012) Current understanding of drug resistance mechanisms and therapeutic targets in HER2 overexpressing breast cancers. In: Ahmad A (ed) Breast cancer metastasis and drug resistance. Springer, Place Published, New York, pp 261–274
3. Stern DF, Heffernan PA, Weinberg RA (1986) p185, a product of the neu proto-oncogene, is a receptorlike protein associated with tyrosine kinase activity. Mol Cell Biol 6:1729–1740
4. Slamon DJ, Clark GM, Wong SG, Levin WJ, Ullrich A, McGuire WL (1987) Human breast cancer: correlation of relapse and survival with amplification of the HER-2/neu oncogene. Science 235:177–182
5. Browne BC, O'Brien N, Duffy MJ, Crown J, O'Donovan N (2009) HER-2 signaling and inhibition in breast cancer. Curr Cancer Drug Targets 9:419–438
6. Vu T, Claret FX (2012) Trastuzumab: updated mechanisms of action and resistance in breast cancer. Front Oncol 2:62
7. Narayan M, Wilken JA, Harris LN, Baron AT, Kimbler KD, Maihle NJ (2009) Trastuzumab-induced HER reprogramming in "resistant" breast carcinoma cells. Cancer Res 69:2191–2194
8. Wolff AC, Hammond ME, Schwartz JN, Hagerty KL, Allred DC, Cote RJ, Dowsett M, Fitzgibbons PL, Hanna WM, Langer A, McShane LM, Paik S, Pegram MD, Perez EA, Press MF, Rhodes A, Sturgeon C, Taube SE, Tubbs R, Vance GH, De Van Vijver, Wheeler TM, Hayes DF (2007) American Society of Clinical Oncology/College of American Pathologists guideline recommendations for human epidermal growth factor receptor 2 testing in breast cancer. J Clin Oncol 25:118–145
9. Gajria D, Chandarlapaty S (2011) HER2-amplified breast cancer: mechanisms of trastuzumab resistance and novel targeted therapies. Expert Rev Anticancer Ther 11:263–275
10. Nahta R, Shabaya S, Ozbay T, Rowe DL (2009) Personalizing HER2-targeted therapy in metastatic breast cancer beyond HER2 status: what we have learned from clinical specimens. Curr Pharmacogenomics Person Med 7:263–274
11. Gallardo A, Lerma E, Escuin D, Tibau A, Munoz J, Ojeda B, Barnadas A, Adrover E, Sanchez-Tejada L, Giner D, Ortiz-Martinez F, Peiro G (2012) Increased signalling of EGFR and IGF1R, and deregulation of PTEN/PI3K/Akt pathway are related with trastuzumab resistance in HER2 breast carcinomas. Br J Cancer 106:1367–1373
12. Zhang S, Huang WC, Li P, Guo H, Poh SB, Brady SW, Xiong Y, Tseng LM, Li SH, Ding Z, Sahin AA, Esteva FJ, Hortobagyi GN, Yu D (2011) Combating trastuzumab resistance

by targeting SRC, a common node downstream of multiple resistance pathways. Nat Med 17:461–469

13. Elster N, Toomey S, Fan Y, Cremona M, Morgan C, Weiner Gorzel K, Bhreathnach U, Milewska M, Murphy M, Madden S, Naidoo J, Fay J, Kay E, Carr A, Kennedy S, Furney S, Mezynski J, Breathhnach O, Morris P, Grogan L, Hill A, Kennedy S, Crown J, Gallagher W, Hennessy B, Eustace A (2018) Frequency, impact and a preclinical study of novel ERBB gene family mutations in HER2-positive breast cancer. Therapeutic advances in medical oncology 10:1758835918778297

14. Yang L, Li Y, Shen E, Cao F, Li L, Li X, Wang X, Kariminia S, Chang B, Li H, Li Q (2017) NRG1-dependent activation of HER3 induces primary resistance to trastuzumab in HER2-overexpressing breast cancer cells. Int J Oncol 51:1553–1562

15. Adamczyk A, Kruczak A, Harazin-Lechowska A, Ambicka A, Grela-Wojewoda A, Domagala-Haduch M, Janecka-Widla A, Majchrzyk K, Cichocka A, Rys J, Niemiec J (2018) Relationship between HER2 gene status and selected potential biological features related to trastuzumab resistance and its influence on survival of breast cancer patients undergoing trastuzumab adjuvant treatment. OncoTargets Ther 11:4525–4535

16. Lyu H, Huang J, He Z, Liu B (2018) Targeting of HER3 with functional cooperative miRNAs enhances therapeutic activity in HER2-overexpressing breast cancer cells. Biological Proced Online 20:16

17. Canfield K, Li J, Wilkins OM, Morrison MM, Ung M, Wells W, Williams CR, Liby KT, Vullhorst D, Buonanno A, Hu H, Schiff R, Cook RS, Kurokawa M (2015) Receptor tyrosine kinase ERBB4 mediates acquired resistance to ERBB2 inhibitors in breast cancer cells. Cell Cycle (Georgetown, Tex) 14:648–655

18. Mohd Nafi SN, Generali D, Kramer-Marek G, Gijsen M, Strina C, Cappelletti M, Andreis D, Haider S, Li JL, Bridges E, Capala J, Ioannis R, Harris AL, Kong A (2014) Nuclear HER4 mediates acquired resistance to trastuzumab and is associated with poor outcome in HER2 positive breast cancer. Oncotarget 5:5934–5949

19. Hanker AB, Garrett JT, Estrada MV, Moore PD, Ericsson PG, Koch JP, Langley E, Singh S, Kim PS, Frampton GM, Sanford E, Owens P, Becker J, Groseclose MR, Castellino S, Joensuu H, Huober J, Brase JC, Majjaj S, Brohee S, Venet D, Brown D, Baselga J, Piccart M, Sotiriou C, Arteaga CL (2017) HER2-overexpressing breast cancers amplify FGFR signaling upon acquisition of resistance to dual therapeutic blockade of HER2. Clin Cancer Res Off J Am Assoc Cancer Res 23:4323–4334

20. Lenz G, Hamilton A, Geng S, Hong T, Kalkum M, Momand J, Kane SE, Huss JM (2018) T-Darpp activates IGF-1R signaling to regulate glucose metabolism in Trastuzumab-resistant breast cancer cells. Clin Cancer Res Off J Am Assoc Cancer Res 24:1216–1226

21. Burnett JP, Korkaya H, Ouzounova MD, Jiang H, Conley SJ, Newman BW, Sun L, Connarn JN, Chen CS, Zhang N, Wicha MS, Sun D (2015) Trastuzumab resistance induces EMT to transform HER2(+) PTEN(−) to a triple negative breast cancer that requires unique treatment options. Sci Rep 5:15821

22. Kim YJ, Sung D, Oh E, Cho Y, Cho TM, Farrand L, Seo JH, Kim JY (2018) Flubendazole overcomes trastuzumab resistance by targeting cancer stem-like properties and HER2 signaling in HER2-positive breast cancer. Cancer Lett 412:118–130

23. Chong QY, You ML, Pandey V, Banerjee A, Chen YJ, Poh HM, Zhang M, Ma L, Zhu T, Basappa S, Liu L, Lobie PE (2017) Release of HER2 repression of trefoil factor 3 (TFF3) expression mediates trastuzumab resistance in HER2+/ER+ mammary carcinoma. Oncotarget 8:74188–74208

24. Rodriguez CE, Berardi DE, Abrigo M, Todaro LB, Bal de Kier Joffe ED, Fiszman GL (2018) Breast cancer stem cells are involved in Trastuzumab resistance through the HER2 modulation in 3D culture. J Cell Biochem 119:1381–1391

25. Nami B, Wang Z (2017) HER2 in breast cancer stemness: a negative feedback loop towards Trastuzumab resistance. Cancers 9

26. De Cola A, Volpe S, Budani MC, Ferracin M, Lattanzio R, Turdo A, D'Agostino D, Capone E, Stassi G, Todaro M, Di Ilio C, Sala G, Piantelli M, Negrini M, Veronese A, De Laurenzi V

(2015) miR-205-5p-mediated downregulation of ErbB/HER receptors in breast cancer stem cells results in targeted therapy resistance. Cell Death Dis 6:e1823

27. Boulbes DR, Chauhan GB, Jin Q, Bartholomeusz C, Esteva FJ (2015) CD44 expression contributes to trastuzumab resistance in HER2-positive breast cancer cells. Breast Cancer Res Treat 151:501–513

28. van Rooijen JM, Qiu SQ, Timmer-Bosscha H, van der Vegt B, Boers JE, Schroder CP, de Vries EGE (2018) Androgen receptor expression inversely correlates with immune cell infiltration in human epidermal growth factor receptor 2-positive breast cancer. Eur J Cancer (Oxford, England: 1990) 103:52–60

29. Martinez VG, O'Neill S, Salimu J, Breslin S, Clayton A, Crown J, O'Driscoll L (2017) Resistance to HER2-targeted anti-cancer drugs is associated with immune evasion in cancer cells and their derived extracellular vesicles. Oncoimmunology 6:e1362530

30. Nunes J, Zhang H, Angelopoulos N, Chhetri J, Osipo C, Grothey A, Stebbing J, Giamas G (2016) ATG9A loss confers resistance to trastuzumab via c-Cbl mediated Her2 degradation. Oncotarget 7:27599–27612

31. Xiong L, Ding L, Ning H, Wu C, Fu K, Wang Y, Zhang Y, Liu Y, Zhou L (2016) CD147 knockdown improves the antitumor efficacy of trastuzumab in HER2-positive breast cancer cells. Oncotarget 7:57737–57751

32. Kar A, Liu B, Gutierrez-Hartmann A (2017) ESE-1 knockdown attenuates growth in Trastuzumab-resistant HER2(+) breast cancer cells. Anticancer Res 37:6583–6591

33. Farahmand L, Merikhian P, Jalili N, Darvishi B, Majidzadeh AK (2018) Significant role of MUC1 in development of resistance to currently existing anti-cancer therapeutic agents. Curr Cancer Drug Targets 18:737–748

34. Mercogliano MF, De Martino M, Venturutti L, Rivas MA, Proietti CJ, Inurrigarro G, Frahm I, Allemand DH, Deza EG, Ares S, Gercovich FG, Guzman P, Roa JC, Elizalde PV, Schillaci R (2017) TNFalpha-induced mucin 4 expression elicits Trastuzumab resistance in HER2-positive breast cancer. Clin Cancer Res Off J Am Assoc Cancer Res 23:636–648

35. Ding K, Wu Z, Li X, Sheng Y, Wang X, Tan S (2018) LMO4 mediates trastuzumab resistance in HER2 positive breast cancer cells. Am J Cancer Res 8:594–609

36. Menyhart O, Budczies J, Munkacsy G, Esteva FJ, Szabo A, Miquel TP, Gyorffy B (2017) DUSP4 is associated with increased resistance against anti-HER2 therapy in breast cancer. Oncotarget 8:77207–77218

37. Jin MH, Nam AR, Park JE, Bang JH, Bang YJ, Oh DY (2017) Resistance mechanism against Trastuzumab in HER2-positive cancer cells and its negation by Src inhibition. Mol Cancer Ther 16:1145–1154

38. Aghazadeh S, Yazdanparast R (2017) Activation of STAT3/HIF-1alpha/Hes-1 axis promotes trastuzumab resistance in HER2-overexpressing breast cancer cells via down-regulation of PTEN. Biochimic Biophys Acta Gen Subj 1861:1970–1980

39. Sonnenblick A, Brohee S, Fumagalli D, Vincent D, Venet D, Ignatiadis M, Salgado R, Van den Eynden G, Rothe F, Desmedt C, Neven P, Loibl S, Denkert C, Joensuu H, Loi S, Sirtaine N, Kellokumpu-Lehtinen PL, Piccart M, Sotiriou C (2015) Constitutive phosphorylated STAT3-associated gene signature is predictive for trastuzumab resistance in primary HER2-positive breast cancer. BMC Med 13:177

40. Chihara Y, Shimoda M, Hori A, Ohara A, Naoi Y, Ikeda JI, Kagara N, Tanei T, Shimomura A, Shimazu K, Kim SJ, Noguchi S (2017) A small-molecule inhibitor of SMAD3 attenuates resistance to anti-HER2 drugs in HER2-positive breast cancer cells. Breast Cancer Res Treat 166:55–68

41. Takeda T, Yamamoto H, Kanzaki H, Suzawa K, Yoshioka T, Tomida S, Cui X, Murali R, Namba K, Sato H, Torigoe H, Watanabe M, Shien K, Soh J, Asano H, Tsukuda K, Kitamura Y, Miyoshi S, Sendo T, Toyooka S (2017) Yes1 signaling mediates the resistance to Trastuzumab/lapatinib in breast cancer. PLoS One 12:e0171356

42. Pandya K, Wyatt D, Gallagher B, Shah D, Baker A, Bloodworth J, Zlobin A, Pannuti A, Green A, Ellis IO, Filipovic A, Sagert J, Rana A, Albain KS, Miele L, Denning MF, Osipo C (2016)

PKCalpha attenuates Jagged-1-mediated notch signaling in ErbB-2-positive breast cancer to reverse Trastuzumab resistance. Clin Cancer Res Off J Am Assoc Cancer Res 22:175–186

43. Zhao B, Zhao Y, Sun Y, Niu H, Sheng L, Huang D, Li L (2018) Alterations in mRNA profiles of trastuzumabresistant Her2positive breast cancer. Mol Med Rep 18:139–146

44. Liu W, Yuan J, Liu Z, Zhang J, Chang J (2018) Label-free quantitative proteomics combined with biological validation reveals activation of Wnt/beta-Catenin pathway contributing to Trastuzumab resistance in gastric cancer. Int J Mol Sci 19

45. Lee JY, Joo HS, Choi HJ, Jin S, Kim HY, Jeong GY, An HW, Park MK, Lee SE, Kim WS, Son T, Min KW, Oh YH, Kong G (2018) Role of MEL-18 amplification in anti-HER2 therapy of breast cancer. J Natl Cancer Inst

46. Mittal D, Caramia F, Michiels S, Joensuu H, Kellokumpu-Lehtinen PL, Sotiriou C, Loi S, Smyth MJ (2016) Improved treatment of breast cancer with anti-HER2 therapy requires Interleukin-21 signaling in CD8+ T cells. Cancer Res 76:264–274

47. Singla H, Ludhiadch A, Kaur RP, Chander H, Kumar V, Munshi A (2017) Recent advances in HER2 positive breast cancer epigenetics: susceptibility and therapeutic strategies. Eur J Med Chem 142:316–327

48. Dong H, Wang W, Mo S, Liu Q, Chen X, Chen R, Zhang Y, Zou K, Ye M, He X, Zhang F, Han J, Hu J (2018) Long non-coding RNA SNHG14 induces trastuzumab resistance of breast cancer via regulating PABPC1 expression through H3K27 acetylation. J Cell Mol Med 22:4935–4947

49. Fujii S, Yamashita S, Yamaguchi T, Takahashi M, Hozumi Y, Ushijima T, Mukai H (2017) Pathological complete response of HER2-positive breast cancer to trastuzumab and chemotherapy can be predicted by HSD17B4 methylation. Oncotarget 8:19039–19048

50. Ahmad A (2016) Non-coding RNAs: a tale of junk turning into treasure. Noncoding RNA Res 1:1–2

51. Campos-Parra AD, Lopez-Urrutia E, Orozco Moreno LT, Lopez-Camarillo C, Meza-Menchaca T, Figueroa Gonzalez G, Bustamante Montes LP, Perez-Plasencia C (2018) Long non-coding RNAs as new master regulators of resistance to systemic treatments in breast cancer. Int J Mol Sci 19

52. Zhu HY, Bai WD, Ye XM, Yang AG, Jia LT (2018) Long non-coding RNA UCA1 desensitizes breast cancer cells to trastuzumab by impeding miR-18a repression of Yes-associated protein 1. Biochem Biophys Res Commun 496:1308–1313

53. Shi SJ, Wang LJ, Yu B, Li YH, Jin Y, Bai XZ (2015) LncRNA-ATB promotes trastuzumab resistance and invasion-metastasis cascade in breast cancer. Oncotarget 6:11652–11663

54. Dong H, Wang W, Chen R, Zhang Y, Zou K, Ye M, He X, Zhang F, Han J (2018) Exosome-mediated transfer of lncRNASNHG14 promotes trastuzumab chemoresistance in breast cancer. Int J Oncol 53:1013–1026

55. Li W, Zhai L, Wang H, Liu C, Zhang J, Chen W, Wei Q (2016) Downregulation of LncRNA GAS5 causes trastuzumab resistance in breast cancer. Oncotarget 7:27778–27786

56. De Mattos-Arruda L, Bottai G, Nuciforo PG, Di Tommaso L, Giovannetti E, Peg V, Losurdo A, Perez-Garcia J, Masci G, Corsi F, Cortes J, Seoane J, Calin GA, Santarpia L (2015) MicroRNA-21 links epithelial-to-mesenchymal transition and inflammatory signals to confer resistance to neoadjuvant trastuzumab and chemotherapy in HER2-positive breast cancer patients. Oncotarget 6:37269–37280

57. Sun C, Yang F, Zhang Y, Chu J, Wang J, Wang Y, Zhang Y, Li J, Li Y, Fan R, Li W, Huang X, Wu H, Fu Z, Jiang Z, Yin Y (2018) tRNA-derived fragments as novel predictive biomarkers for Trastuzumab-resistant breast cancer. Cell Physiol Biochem 49:419–431

58. Wang Z, Li Y, Ahmad A, Azmi AS, Kong D, Banerjee S, Sarkar FH (2010) Targeting miRNAs involved in cancer stem cell and EMT regulation: An emerging concept in overcoming drug resistance. Drug Resist Updat 13:109–118

59. Decker JT, Hall MS, Blaisdell RB, Schwark K, Jeruss JS, Shea LD (2018) Dynamic microRNA activity identifies therapeutic targets in trastuzumab-resistant HER2(+) breast cancer. Biotechnol Bioeng 115:2613–2623

60. von der Heyde S, Wagner S, Czerny A, Nietert M, Ludewig F, Salinas-Riester G, Arlt D, Beissbarth T (2015) mRNA profiling reveals determinants of trastuzumab efficiency in HER2-positive breast cancer. PLoS One 10:e0117818
61. Lu X, Ma J, Chu J, Shao Q, Zhang Y, Lu G, Li J, Huang X, Li W, Li Y, Ling Y, Zhao T (2017) MiR-129-5p sensitizes the response of her-2 positive breast cancer to Trastuzumab by reducing Rps6. Cell Physiol Biochem 44:2346–2356
62. Ma T, Yang L, Zhang J (2015) MiRNA5423p downregulation promotes trastuzumab resistance in breast cancer cells via AKT activation. Oncol Rep 33:1215–1220
63. Huynh FC, Jones FE (2014) MicroRNA-7 inhibits multiple oncogenic pathways to suppress HER2Delta16 mediated breast tumorigenesis and reverse trastuzumab resistance. PLoS One 9:e114419
64. Cataldo A, Piovan C, Plantamura I, D'Ippolito E, Camelliti S, Casalini P, Giussani M, Deas O, Cairo S, Judde JG, Tagliabue E, Iorio MV (2018) MiR-205 as predictive biomarker and adjuvant therapeutic tool in combination with trastuzumab. Oncotarget 9:27920–27928
65. Li X, Xu Y, Ding Y, Li C, Zhao H, Wang J, Meng S (2018) Posttranscriptional upregulation of HER3 by HER2 mRNA induces trastuzumab resistance in breast cancer. Mol Cancer 17:113
66. Yue D, Qin X (2018) miR-182 regulates trastuzumab resistance by targeting MET in breast cancer cells. Cancer Gene Ther 26(1–2):1–10
67. Tormo E, Adam-Artigues A, Ballester S, Pineda B, Zazo S, Gonzalez-Alonso P, Albanell J, Rovira A, Rojo F, Lluch A, Eroles P (2017) The role of miR-26a and miR-30b in HER2+ breast cancer trastuzumab resistance and regulation of the CCNE2 gene. Sci Rep 7:41309
68. Venturutti L, Cordo Russo RI, Rivas MA, Mercogliano MF, Izzo F, Oakley RH, Pereyra MG, De Martino M, Proietti CJ, Yankilevich P, Roa JC, Guzman P, Cortese E, Allemand DH, Huang TH, Charreau EH, Cidlowski JA, Schillaci R, Elizalde PV (2016) MiR-16 mediates trastuzumab and lapatinib response in ErbB-2-positive breast and gastric cancer via its novel targets CCNJ and FUBP1. Oncogene 35:6189–6202
69. Li H, Liu J, Chen J, Wang H, Yang L, Chen F, Fan S, Wang J, Shao B, Yin D, Zeng M, Li M, Li J, Su F, Liu Q, Yao H, Su S, Song E (2018) A serum microRNA signature predicts trastuzumab benefit in HER2-positive metastatic breast cancer patients. Nat Commun 9:1614
70. Soto-Perez-De-Celis E, Loh KP, Baldini C, Battisti NML, Chavarri-Guerra Y, De Glas NA, Hsu T, Hurria A (2018) Targeted agents for HER2-positive breast cancer in older adults: current and future perspectives. Expert Opin Investig Drugs 27:787–801
71. Wang L, Wang Q, Gao M, Fu L, Li Y, Quan H, Lou L (2018) STAT3 activation confers trastuzumab-emtansine (T-DM1) resistance in HER2-positive breast cancer. Cancer Sci 109:3305–3315
72. Sakai H, Tsurutani J, Iwasa T, Komoike Y, Sakai K, Nishio K, Nakagawa K (2018) HER2 genomic amplification in circulating tumor DNA and estrogen receptor positivity predict primary resistance to trastuzumab emtansine (T-DM1) in patients with HER2-positive metastatic breast cancer. Breast Cancer (Tokyo, Japan) 25:605–613
73. Li G, Guo J, Shen BQ, Yadav DB, Sliwkowski MX, Crocker LM, Lacap JA, Phillips GDL (2018) Mechanisms of acquired resistance to Trastuzumab Emtansine in breast cancer cells. Mol Cancer Ther 17:1441–1453
74. Mao Y, Zhang Y, Qu Q, Zhao M, Lou Y, Liu J, huang O, Chen X, Wu J, Shen K (2015) Cancer-associated fibroblasts induce trastuzumab resistance in HER2 positive breast cancer cells. Mol BioSyst 11:1029–1040
75. Tanioka M, Fan C, Parker JS, Hoadley KA, Hu Z, Li Y, Hyslop TM, Pitcher BN, Soloway MG, Spears PA, Henry LN, Tolaney S, Dang CT, Krop IE, Harris LN, Berry DA, Mardis ER, Winer EP, Hudis CA, Carey LA, Perou CM (2018) Integrated analysis of RNA and DNA from the phase III trial CALGB 40601 identifies predictors of response to Trastuzumab-based neoadjuvant chemotherapy in HER2-positive breast cancer. Clin Cancer Res Off J Am Assoc Cancer Res 24:5292–5304

Chapter 11
Non-coding RNAs as Mediators of Tamoxifen Resistance in Breast Cancers

Mohd Farhan, Mohammad Aatif, Prasad Dandawate, and Aamir Ahmad

Abstract A large proportion of breast cancer patients are estrogen receptor positive. They generally benefit from tamoxifen, the drug that targets estrogen receptor signaling. However, de novo and acquired resistance against tamoxifen is well known. A number of signaling pathways and de-regulated factors have been evaluated to better understand the mechanism(s) of tamoxifen resistance. For past several years, non-coding RNAs have also gained attention as the putative regulators and determinants of tamoxifen resistance. A number of reports have documented evidence from in vitro and/or in vivo studies, as well as from evaluation of clinical samples, to showcase the power of non-coding RNAs as mediators of tamoxifen resistance and the predictors of disease relapse. This article puts into perspective the available information on microRNAs and the long non-coding RNAs regarding their ability to tweak resistance vs. sensitivity to tamoxifen.

Keywords Tamoxifen resistance · miRNAs · Long non-coding RNAs · Breast cancer

M. Farhan (✉)
Department of Biology, College of Basic Sciences, King Faisal University,
Al-Ahsa, Kingdom of Saudi Arabia
e-mail: mfarhan@kfu.edu.sa

M. Aatif
Department of Public Health, College of Applied Medical Sciences, King Faisal University,
Al-Ahsa, Kingdom of Saudi Arabia

P. Dandawate
ISTRA, Abeda Inamdar Senior College, Pune, India

A. Ahmad (✉)
Mitchell Cancer Institute, University of South Alabama, Mobile, AL, USA
e-mail: aahmad@health.southalabama.edu

© Springer Nature Switzerland AG 2019
A. Ahmad (ed.), *Breast Cancer Metastasis and Drug Resistance*,
Advances in Experimental Medicine and Biology 1152,
https://doi.org/10.1007/978-3-030-20301-6_11

11.1   Introduction

Estrogen receptor (ER)-positive breast cancers are the most frequently diagnosed breast cancers. Tamoxifen is the oldest drug used to target breast cancers that are ER-positive. It was approved by Food and Drug Administration in 1977 for the treatment of metastatic breast cancer [1]. It is estimated that two thirds, or more, of breast tumors are positive for ER [2–4]. This underlines the proportion of breast cancer patients that can potentially benefit from the use of tamoxifen.

11.2   Tamoxifen Resistance

By some estimates, over half of the advanced ER-positive breast cancers are intrinsically resistant to tamoxifen and about 40% of patients taking tamoxifen eventually acquire resistance to it [3]. Resistance to tamoxifen can be de novo i.e. preexisting (even before the exposure to tamoxifen) or could be acquired after exposure to tamoxifen therapy [4]. The large proportion of patients developing resistance to tamoxifen therapy makes it important to understand the mechanism(s) of action thereof. A number of mechanisms can lead to acquired resistance against tamoxifen. One of these mechanisms involves regulation by 'non-coding RNAs', the RNAs that do not code for any protein. This chapter focuses on the non-coding RNAs-mediated regulation of tamoxifen resistance as such regulation is increasingly being investigated and appreciated [5].

11.3   miRNAs as Mediators of Tamoxifen Resistance

miRNAs belong to the class of 'small' non-coding RNAs that are ~18 to 25 nucleotides in length and regulate the expression of their target genes post-transcriptionally by binding to specific sites within the 3′ UTRs (untranslated regions) of their targets [6]. There are numerous reports on the role of miRNAs in tamoxifen resistance [7–12] and therefore we first discuss the role of these small non coding RNAs in progression to resistant phenotype.

miR-221/222 were the first miRNAs connected with tamoxifen resistance [13] and, to-date, they remain some of the most studied miRNAs in resistance against tamoxifen [14]. These miRNAs, along with miR-181, were up-regulated in ER-positive breast cancer cells MCF-7 cells that were tamoxifen resistant [13]. p27(kip1), the target of miR-221/222, was observed to be significantly down-regulated. The study also validated miR-21, miR-342 and miR-489 as miRNAs that were down-regulated in resistant cells. Later, miR-101 was found to target MAGI-2 (membrane-associated guanylate kinase) leading to repression of tumor suppressor PTEN (phosphatase and tensin homolog) and the resulting tamoxifen resistance [15].

Subsequently, it was shown that the down-regulation of miR-221/222, through the use of antisense oligonucleotides, sensitized MCF-7 cells to tamoxifen by up-regulation TIMP3 (tissue inhibitor of metalloproteinase-3) [16]. It was also reported that miR-221/222 could be transported in exosomes to enhance the tamoxifen resistance [17].

Most of the studies on tamoxifen resistance have been conducted using MCF-7 cells, and have listed a number of differentially expressed miRNAs in sensitive Vs. resistant cells [18, 19]. Some studies have also evaluated patient tumors to identify a miRNA signature of tamoxifen resistance [20–22]. In a study that not only evaluated tamoxifen resistant MCF-7, but also confirmed the results in tamoxifen resistant breast tumors, miR-342 was found to be down-regulated [23]. This study established the clinical relevance of miRNAs in tamoxifen resistance. Increased mir-10a and miR-126 were later found to be predictors of prolonged relapse-free time in ER-positive breast cancer patients [21] while lower expression of miR-378a-3p associated with poor prognosis of breast cancer patients who were administered tamoxifen [24]. miR-4653-3p has also been proposed as a prognostic marker with its lower levels in metastatic/recurrent tumors and its overexpression capable of decreasing the risk of relapse [25]. While most studies have employed a single cell line in the study, the MCF-7 cells, comparing the parental MCF-7 cells with their tamoxifen resistant derivatives, our own investigation revealed an HDAC4 suppressing activity of miR-10b in two different cell lines, MCF-7 and T47D [26].

Tamoxifen itself can also de-regulate miRNAs that can, in turn, confer resistance to treatment. For example, tamoxifen was shown to down-regulate miR-451 which attenuated the repression of 14-3-3ζ with profound effects on EGFR (epidermal growth factor receptor) and MAPK2 (mitogen-activated protein kinase 2) signaling along with effects on cell proliferation, apoptosis and colony formation [27]. A follow-up study [28] additionally found down-regulated ERα as a result of tamoxifen treatment, and its expression directly correlated with miR-451.

EMT (epithelial-to-mesenchymal transition) regulating miRNAs are known to regulate drug resistance [29], particularly those belonging to miR-200 and let family [18, 30, 31]. let-7b and let-7i ectopic expression in tamoxifen resistant MCF-7 cells downregulated their target ER-α36 and sensitized the resistant cells to tamoxifen [32]. Similarly, ectopic expression of miR-200b and miR-200c sensitized LY2 cells to tamoxifen that also correlated with a phenotype that was more epithelial [33].

CSC (cancer stem cell) phenotype is also associated with drug resistance [34]. Infact, there is intricate connection between CSC, miRNAs and drug resistance [35]. This is true even in the case of tamoxifen resistance. miR-375 was reported to be a suppressor of CSC phenotype and the resistance against tamoxifen [36]. As would be expected, higher expression of the target of miR-375, HOXB3 (homeobox B3), resulted in induction of CSC phenotype, EMT and the resistance to tamoxifen.

Resistance to tamoxifen is often accompanied by an aggressive phenotype. As a proof, a study that evaluated role of miR-873 in tamoxifen resistance and reported a negative correlation between miR-873 expression and tamoxifen resistance also found reduced tumor growth in nude mice [37]. Thus, miR-873 was down-regulated in tamoxifen resistant cells and functioned as tumor suppressor in vivo. Similarly, miR-196a was reported down-regulated in tamoxifen resistant cells because of the action of myc, leading to de-repression of its target HOXB7 (Homeobox B7). and use of small molecule inhibitors of myc resulted in regression of breast cancer xenografts [38].

Acquired resistance against tamoxifen involves alterations of signaling pathways with activation of alternative signaling. Activated ERBB2 (Erb-B2 receptor tyrosine kinase 2) is one such signaling that can help reduce sensitivity to tamoxifen. However, there is indication of regulation of ERBB2 signaling by miRNAs as well. In tamoxifen resistant cells, where ERBB2 expression is high, miRs-26a/b are down-regulated and their ectopic expression can reverse tamoxifen resistance [39]. miR-26a can also exert its effects on tamoxifen sensitivity through its regulation of E2F7 (E2F transcription factor 7) [40].

Recent research has unveiled the mechanisms by which certain miRNAs might be down-regulated, in the context of tamoxifen resistance. For example, miR-27b was found to be down-regulated in tamoxifen resistant MCF-7 cells through epigenetic silencing [41]. As compared to sensitive MCF-7 cells, the promoter region for miR-27b was hypermethylated in MCF-7 cells that were resistant. Further highlighting a role of miR-27b, another study found lower levels of this miRNA in tamoxifen resistant cells, compared to parental cells and in the breast cancer tissues of tamoxifen-resistant patients, compared to patients not treated with tamoxifen [42]. As a further proof of epigenetic silencing of tamoxifen resistance regulating miRNAs, demethylation restored the expression of miR-148a and miR-152, both of which are down-regulated in resistant cells [43]. As expected the target of these miRNAs, ALCAM, was found to be over-expressed in tumors of breast cancer patients that were non-responders to tamoxifen, as opposed to responders.

Other miRNAs that correlate positively with tamoxifen resistance include miR-192-5p [44], miR-335-3p/5p [45], miR-519a [46] and miR-663b [47] and those that correlate inversely with tamoxifen resistance include miR-15a [48], miR-16 [48], miR-125a-3p [49], miR-206 [50], miR-320a [51], miR-449a [52], miR-500a-3p [44], miR-542-5p [53] and miR-574-3p [19]. Based on the reports discussed in this section, there exist a number of reports in the literature on a functional role of small non-coding RNAs, the miRNAs, in resistance against tamoxifen. A summary is provided in Table 11.1.

11.4 Long Non-coding RNAs as Mediators of Tamoxifen Resistance

LncRNAs (long non-coding RNAs) are, as their name suggests, longer RNAs that do not code for any protein product. They are ~200 nucleotides long [54]. Contrary to research and knowledge on miRNAs, lncRNAs represent a rather new class of non-coding RNAs, however, they are slowly emerging as important biomarkers as well as targets for therapy in various human cancers [55–59].

Table 11.1 List of miRNAs that regulate resistance against tamoxifen

miRNA	Status	Target	Reference
Let7s	Down-regulated	ER-α36	[32]
miR-10a	Positively correlates with relapse-free time	ND	[21]
miR-10b	Up-regulated	HDAC4	[26]
miR-15a / miR-16	Down-regulated	Cyclin E1, Bcl-2	[48]
miR-18a	Down-regulated	HIF1α	[62]
miR-21	Down-regulated	ND	[13]
	Up-regulated	PI3K-AKT-mTOR signaling	[86]
miR-26a	Down-regulated	ERBB2	[39]
		E2F7	[40]
miR-26b	Down-regulated	ERBB2	[39]
miR-27b	Down-regulated	HMGB3	[41]
		NR5A2, CREB1	[42]
miR-101	Up-regulated	MAGI-2	[15]
miR-125a-3p	Down-regulated	CDK3	[49]
miR-126	Positively correlates with relapse-free time	ND	[21]
miR-148a/ miR-152	Down-regulated	ALCAM	
miR-181	Up-regulated	ND	[13]
miR-196a	Down-regulated	HOXB7	[38]
miR-200s	Down-regulated	Zeb1	[33]
miR-205	Down-regulated	ND	[73]
miR-206	Down-regulated	WBP2	[50]
miR-221/ miR-222	Up-regulated	p27 (Kip1)	[13]
		TIMP3	[16]
		p27 and ERα	[17]
miR-320a	Down-regulated	ARPP-19, ERRγ	[51]
miR-342	Down-regulated	ND	[13]
	Down-regulated	ND	[23]
miR-375	Down-regulated	Metadherin	[29]
		HOXB3	[36]
miR-378a	Down-regulated	GOLT1A	[24]
miR-449a	Down-regulated	ADAM22	[52]
miR-451	Down-regulated	14-3-3-ζ	[27, 28]
miR-489	Down-regulated	ND	[13]
miR-519a	Up-regulated	PI3K signaling	[46]
miR-574	Down-regulated	CLTC	[19]
miR-663b	Up-regulated	TP73	[47]
miR-873	Down-regulated	CDK3	[37]
miR-4653-3p	Down-regulated	FRS2	[25]

(continued)

Table 11.1 (continued)

ND Not determined

ADAM22 Disintegrin and metalloproteinase domain-containing protein 22, *ALCAM* activated leukocyte cell adhesion molecule, *ARPP-19* cAMP-regulated phosphoprotein, *CREB1* cAMP-response element binding protein 1, *CDK3* cyclin-dependent kinase 3, *E2F7* E2F transcription factor 7, *ERBB2* erb-B2 receptor tyrosine kinase 2, *ERRγ* estrogen-related receptor gamma, *CLTC* clathrin heavy chain, FRS2: fibroblast growth factor receptor substrate 2, *GOLT1A* golgi transport 1A, *HIF1α* Hypoxia-inducible factor 1-alpha, *HMGB3* high mobility group box 3, *HOXB3* homeobox B3, *HOXB7* homeobox B7, *MAGI-2* membrane-associated guanylate kinase, *NR5A2* nuclear receptor subfamily 5 group A member 2, *TIMP3* tissue inhibitor of metalloproteinase-3, *TP73* tumor protein 73, *WBP2* WW domain binding protein 2

Mechanistic studies evaluating a role of lncRNAs in resistance against tamoxifen have emerged in past few years only. HOTAIR (HOX antisense intergenic RNA) was first found to be up-regulated in tamoxifen resistant breast cancer tissues, compared to normal counterparts [60]. Interestingly, it is induced when ER signaling is blocked, such as by administration of tamoxifen. Once up-regulated, it potentiates ER signaling, enhancing ER occupancy on chromatin and the expression of downstream ER-regulated genes.

LncRNA UCA1 (Urothelial carcinoma-associated 1) is by far the most studied lncRNA in terms of its role in resistance against therapies, including tamoxifen [61]. It positively regulates the resistance against tamoxifen in a HIF1α (Hypoxia-inducible factor 1-alpha)-dependent manner [62]. It sponges miR-18a, a negative regulator of HIF1α thus de-repressing and activating HIF1α signaling. Such inhibition of miR-18a by UCA1 has been reported in a later study as well [63]. Further, inhibition of miR-18a induced resistance to tamoxifen while its expression increased sensitivity. UCA1 also activates mTOR signaling pathway as a mechanism to suppress sensitivity to tamoxifen [64]. Exosomes from tamoxifen resistant cells are rich in UCA1 and can induce resistance in otherwise sensitive cells [65]. The tamoxifen resistance inducing ability of UCA1 has also been validated in vivo [66] and this study proposed a role of induced Wnt/β-catenin signaling in tamoxifen resistance by UCA1. A recent work has proposed regulation of EZH2/miR-21 axis and the PI3K-Akt signaling as the mechanism of tamoxifen resistance by UCA1 [67].

A lncRNA profiling study, using 947 breast cancer samples, screened for 58,648 lncRNAs and DSCAM-AS1 was revealed as the top ER-regulated lncRNA that was up-regulated [68]. A more recent study [69] further validated up-regulation of DSCAM-AS1 in tamoxifen resistance. However, this report found sponging of tumor suppressor miR-137 and the up-regulation of EPS8 (epidermal growth factor receptor pathway substrate 8) as the mechanism of resistance. Another study, that used bioinformatics to predict tamoxifen resistance-related lncRNAs by matching them with known tamoxifen resistance genes, identified LINC00894-002 as the most down-regulated lncRNA in tamoxifen resistant MCF-7 cells [70].

Uc.57 lncRNA is under-expressed in tamoxifen resistant MCF7- cells, compared to the parental MCF-7 cells [71]. Its levels are lower, and those of its downstream gene BCL11A higher, in breast cancer tissues, relative to the precancerous breast cancer tissues. Further, the over-expression of uc.57 reduced resistance against tamoxifen both in vitro as well as in vivo. The study also highlighted the ability of shikonin, a component of Chinese herbal medicine, to reverse tamoxifen resistance. Similar to Uc.57, GAS5 is another lncRNA that is down-regulated in tamoxifen resistant MCF-7 cells [72]. It sponges the oncogenic and tamoxifen resistance inducing miR-222, leading to de-repression of PTEN. Accordingly, it's expression leads to sensitization to tamoxifen.

We have discussed above the importance of EMT in inducing tamoxifen resistance, and a role of miRNAs in regulating EMT. Incidentally, a lncRNA, ROR, has also been shown to correlate with increased resistance against tamoxifen with concomitant decrease in epithelial marker e-cadherin and increased mesenchymal markers vimentin, zeb1 and zeb2 [73]. The mechanism also included down-regulation of miR-205, a known tumor suppressor that functions similar to EMT inhibiting miR-200 family of miRNAs. Inhibition of lncRNA ROR has been reported to result in autophagic cell death [74] and its regulation of tamoxifen resistance has also been shown to be mediated by MAPK/ERK signaling [75]. LINC00894-002 is another lncRNA that has been linked to EMT as its down-regulation results in repression of EMT-regulating miR-200s and induction of Zeb1 and TGFβ signaling [70].

A few other lncRNAs, such as, MALAT1 [76], CCAT2 [77] and H19 [78, 79] have also been suggested to influence sensitivity and resistance to tamoxifen. H19 was found to function through induction of Notch and c-met. Expression of this lncRNA could be reduced by inhibitors of Notch and c-met, resulting in attenuation of tamoxifen resistance [78]. H19's action was also later reported to involve modulation of wnt signaling and the EMT pathway because its knockdown inhibited wnt pathway as well as EMT [79]. These two different reports on H19 lncRNA might actually have something in common, given the known connection between Notch and wnt signaling with EMT and the breast cancer relapse [80]. Clearly, such connections need to be further explored.

lncRNA signature to predict relapse-free survival in tamoxifen treated patients, through the use of GEO and TCGA databases has also been sought [81]. Another such attempt [82], which mined data from two cohorts from GEO, listed a lncRNA signature consisting of three lncRNAs for predicting distant metastasis-free survival subsequent to tamoxifen treatment. Yet another report [83] listed a six lncRNA signature for predicting similar distant metastasis-free survival. Table 11.2 summarizes our current knowledge on lncRNAs and the mechanism by which they modulate resistance against tamoxifen.

11.5   Conclusions and Perspectives

A vast majority of our genome gets transcribed into 'non-coding RNAs' which were considered 'junk' not very long ago [84]. However, their importance has only been realized in recent years. This has led to evaluation of their ability to regulate different aspects of tumorigenesis, including relapse and the resistance against

Table 11.2 List of lncRNAs that modulate resistance against tamoxifen

lncRNA	Status	Mechanism	Reference
CCAT2	Up-regulated	*ND*	[77]
DSCAM-AS1	Up-regulated	Highly up-regulated in patient samples	[68]
		Sponges miR-137 and upregulates EPS8	[69]
GAS5	Down-regulated	Sponges miR-222	[72]
H19	Up-regulated	Regulation of Notch and c-met	[78]
		Regulation of wnt and EMT	[79]
HOTAIR	Up-regulated	Induces ER signaling	[60]
LINC00894–002	Down-regulated	EMT induction	[70]
MALAT1	Up-regulated	*ND*	[76]
ROR	Up-regulated	EMT induction	[73]
		Induced MAPK/ERK signaling	[75]
Uc.57	Down-regulated	Regulation of BCL11A and AKT/MAPK signaling	[71]
UCA1	Up-regulated	miR-18a-HIF1α feedback loop	[62]
		Activates mTOR signaling	[64]
		Exosomes-mediated transport	[65]
		Activated Wnt/β-catenin signaling	[66]
		Regulation of EZH2/miR-21 axis and PI3K/Akt signaling	[67]

ND Not Determined

EPS8 epidermal growth factor receptor pathway substrate 8, *GAS5* growth arrest-specific transcript 5, *HOTAIR* HOX antisense intergenic RNA, *MALAT1* Metastasis associated in lung adenocarcinoma transcript 1, *mTOR* mechanistic target of rapamycin, *UCA1* urothelial carcinoma-associated 1

chemotherapy. While tamoxifen has been in use in clinics for many decades and the acquired resistance against it has also been investigated for a long time, there has been no major breakthrough in our understanding of the underlying mechanisms that lead to resistance. Recent years have witnessed an interest in the role of non-coding RNAs in mediating tamoxifen resistance. However, the knowledge is far from complete. As expected from any new information, there are several observations that are confusing and need explanation. As an example, miR-21 was validated to be down-regulated in tamoxifen resistant MCF-7 cells [13] even though it is a well-known oncomir [85]. Infact, a latter study found miR-21 to be overexpressed in tamoxifen resistant MCF-7 cells [24] and silencing of miR-21 was found to induce autophagic cell death [86]. On the contrary, miR-335 is a tumor suppressing miRNA but has been reported to promote tamoxifen resistance [45]. It is apparent that more comprehensive studies need to be planned to improve our understanding. Regardless, the available data seems to suggest an immense potential of non-coding RNAs, both miRNAs and the lncRNAs, as biomarkers, prognostic markers as well as targets of possible intervention, in the context of tamoxifen resistance.

Funding   M. Farhan is thankful to the Deanship of Scientific Research, King Faisal University for research grant through the Nasher track (186137).

References

1. Cohen MH, Hirschfeld S, Flamm Honig S, Ibrahim A, Johnson JR, O'Leary JJ, White RM, Williams GA, Pazdur R (2001) Drug approval summaries: arsenic trioxide, tamoxifen citrate, anastrazole, paclitaxel, bexarotene. Oncologist 6:4–11
2. Lopez-Tarruella S, Schiff R (2007) The dynamics of estrogen receptor status in breast cancer: re-shaping the paradigm. Clin Cancer Res 13:6921–6925
3. Hultsch S, Kankainen M, Paavolainen L, Kovanen RM, Ikonen E, Kangaspeska S, Pietiainen V, Kallioniemi O (2018) Association of tamoxifen resistance and lipid reprogramming in breast cancer. BMC Cancer 18:850
4. Garcia-Becerra R, Santos N, Diaz L, Camacho J (2012) Mechanisms of resistance to endocrine therapy in breast cancer: focus on signaling pathways, mirnas and genetically based resistance. Int J Mol Sci 14:108–145
5. Hayes EL, Lewis-Wambi JS (2015) Mechanisms of endocrine resistance in breast cancer: an overview of the proposed roles of noncoding rna. Breast Cancer Res: BCR 17:40
6. Tang J, Ahmad A, Sarkar FH (2012) The role of micrornas in breast cancer migration, invasion and metastasis. Int J Mol Sci 13:13414–13437
7. Zhang W, Xu J, Shi Y, Sun Q, Zhang Q, Guan X (2015) The novel role of mirnas for tamoxifen resistance in human breast cancer. Cell Mol Life Sci CMLS 72:2575–2584
8. Muluhngwi P, Klinge CM (2015) Roles for mirnas in endocrine resistance in breast cancer. Endocr Relat Cancer 22:R279–R300
9. Egeland NG, Lunde S, Jonsdottir K, Lende TH, Cronin-Fenton D, Gilje B, Janssen EA, Soiland H (2015) The role of micrornas as predictors of response to tamoxifen treatment in breast cancer patients. Int J Mol Sci 16:24243–24275
10. Joshi T, Elias D, Stenvang J, Alves CL, Teng F, Lyng MB, Lykkesfeldt AE, Brunner N, Wang J, Gupta R et al (2016) Integrative analysis of mirna and gene expression reveals regulatory networks in tamoxifen-resistant breast cancer. Oncotarget 7:57239–57253
11. Muluhngwi P, Klinge CM (2017) Identification of mirnas as biomarkers for acquired endocrine resistance in breast cancer. Mol Cell Endocrinol 456:76–86
12. Lin YS, Lin YY, Yang YH, Lin CL, Kuan FC, Lu CN, Chang GH, Tsai MS, Hsu CM, Yeh RA et al (2018) Antrodia cinnamomea extract inhibits the proliferation of tamoxifen-resistant breast cancer cells through apoptosis and skp2/micrornas pathway. BMC Complement Altern Med 18:152
13. Miller TE, Ghoshal K, Ramaswamy B, Roy S, Datta J, Shapiro CL, Jacob S, Majumder S (2008) Microrna-221/222 confers tamoxifen resistance in breast cancer by targeting p27kip1. J Biol Chem 283:29897–29903
14. Alamolhodaei NS, Behravan J, Mosaffa F, Karimi G (2016) Mir 221/222 as new players in tamoxifen resistance. Curr Pharm Des 22:6946–6955
15. Sachdeva M, Wu H, Ru P, Hwang L, Trieu V, Mo YY (2011) Microrna-101-mediated akt activation and estrogen-independent growth. Oncogene 30:822–831
16. Gan R, Yang Y, Yang X, Zhao L, Lu J, Meng QH (2014) Downregulation of mir-221/222 enhances sensitivity of breast cancer cells to tamoxifen through upregulation of timp3. Cancer Gene Ther 21:290–296
17. Wei Y, Lai X, Yu S, Chen S, Ma Y, Zhang Y, Li H, Zhu X, Yao L, Zhang J (2014) Exosomal mir-221/222 enhances tamoxifen resistance in recipient er-positive breast cancer cells. Breast Cancer Res Treat 147:423–431

18. Manavalan TT, Teng Y, Appana SN, Datta S, Kalbfleisch TS, Li Y, Klinge CM (2011) Differential expression of microrna expression in tamoxifen-sensitive mcf-7 versus tamoxifen-resistant ly2 human breast cancer cells. Cancer Lett 313:26–43

19. Ujihira T, Ikeda K, Suzuki T, Yamaga R, Sato W, Horie-Inoue K, Shigekawa T, Osaki A, Saeki T, Okamoto K et al (2015) Microrna-574-3p, identified by microrna library-based functional screening, modulates tamoxifen response in breast cancer. Sci Rep 5:7641

20. Lyng MB, Laenkholm AV, Sokilde R, Gravgaard KH, Litman T, Ditzel HJ (2012) Global microrna expression profiling of high-risk er+ breast cancers from patients receiving adjuvant tamoxifen mono-therapy: a dbcg study. PLoS One 7:e36170

21. Hoppe R, Achinger-Kawecka J, Winter S, Fritz P, Lo WY, Schroth W, Brauch H (2013) Increased expression of mir-126 and mir-10a predict prolonged relapse-free time of primary oestrogen receptor-positive breast cancer following tamoxifen treatment. Eur J Cancer (Oxford, England: 1990) 49:3598–3608

22. Miller PC, Clarke J, Koru-Sengul T, Brinkman J, El-Ashry D (2015) A novel mapk-microrna signature is predictive of hormone-therapy resistance and poor outcome in er-positive breast cancer. Clin Cancer Res 21:373–385

23. Cittelly DM, Das PM, Spoelstra NS, Edgerton SM, Richer JK, Thor AD, Jones FE (2010) Downregulation of mir-342 is associated with tamoxifen resistant breast tumors. Mol Cancer 9:317

24. Ikeda K, Horie-Inoue K, Ueno T, Suzuki T, Sato W, Shigekawa T, Osaki A, Saeki T, Berezikov E, Mano H et al (2015) Mir-378a-3p modulates tamoxifen sensitivity in breast cancer mcf-7 cells through targeting golt1a. Sci Rep 5:13170

25. Zhong X, Xie G, Zhang Z, Wang Z, Wang Y, Wang Y, Qiu Y, Li L, Bu H, Li J et al (2016) Mir-4653-3p and its target gene frs2 are prognostic biomarkers for hormone receptor positive breast cancer patients receiving tamoxifen as adjuvant endocrine therapy. Oncotarget 7:61166–61182

26. Ahmad A, Ginnebaugh KR, Yin S, Bollig-Fischer A, Reddy KB, Sarkar FH (2015) Functional role of mir-10b in tamoxifen resistance of er-positive breast cancer cells through downregulation of hdac4. BMC Cancer 15:540

27. Bergamaschi A, Katzenellenbogen BS (2012) Tamoxifen downregulation of mir-451 increases 14-3-3zeta and promotes breast cancer cell survival and endocrine resistance. Oncogene 31:39–47

28. Liu ZR, Song Y, Wan LH, Zhang YY, Zhou LM (2016) Over-expression of mir-451a can enhance the sensitivity of breast cancer cells to tamoxifen by regulating 14-3-3zeta, estrogen receptor alpha, and autophagy. Life Sci 149:104–113

29. Ward A, Balwierz A, Zhang JD, Kublbeck M, Pawitan Y, Hielscher T, Wiemann S, Sahin O (2013) Re-expression of microrna-375 reverses both tamoxifen resistance and accompanying emt-like properties in breast cancer. Oncogene 32:1173–1182

30. Fedele M, Cerchia L, Chiappetta G (2017) The epithelial-to-mesenchymal transition in breast cancer: focus on basal-like carcinomas. Cancers (Basel) 9:134

31. Ahmad A, Sarkar SH, Bitar B, Ali S, Aboukameel A, Sethi S, Li Y, Bao B, Kong D, Banerjee S et al (2012) Garcinol regulates emt and wnt signaling pathways in vitro and in vivo, leading to anticancer activity against breast cancer cells. Mol Cancer Ther 11:2193–2201

32. Zhao Y, Deng C, Lu W, Xiao J, Ma D, Guo M, Recker RR, Gatalica Z, Wang Z, Xiao GG (2011) Let-7 micrornas induce tamoxifen sensitivity by downregulation of estrogen receptor alpha signaling in breast cancer. Mol Med (Cambridge, Mass) 17:1233–1241

33. Manavalan TT, Teng Y, Litchfield LM, Muluhngwi P, Al-Rayyan N, Klinge CM (2013) Reduced expression of mir-200 family members contributes to antiestrogen resistance in ly2 human breast cancer cells. PLoS One 8:e62334

34. Prieto-Vila M, Takahashi RU, Usuba W, Kohama I, Ochiya T (2017) Drug resistance driven by cancer stem cells and their niche. Int J Mol Sci 18:2574

35. Bao B, Li Y, Ahmad A, Azmi AS, Bao G, Ali S, Banerjee S, Kong D, Sarkar FH (2012) Targeting csc-related mirnas for cancer therapy by natural agents. Curr Drug Targets 13:1858–1868

36. Fu H, Fu L, Xie C, Zuo WS, Liu YS, Zheng MZ, Yu JM (2017) Mir-375 inhibits cancer stem cell phenotype and tamoxifen resistance by degrading hoxb3 in human er-positive breast cancer. Oncol Rep 37:1093–1099
37. Cui J, Yang Y, Li H, Leng Y, Qian K, Huang Q, Zhang C, Lu Z, Chen J, Sun T et al (2015) Mir-873 regulates eralpha transcriptional activity and tamoxifen resistance via targeting cdk3 in breast cancer cells. Oncogene 34:3895–3907
38. Jin K, Park S, Teo WW, Korangath P, Cho SS, Yoshida T, Gyorffy B, Goswami CP, Nakshatri H, Cruz LA et al (2015) Hoxb7 is an eralpha cofactor in the activation of her2 and multiple er target genes leading to endocrine resistance. Cancer Discov 5:944–959
39. Tan S, Ding K, Chong QY, Zhao J, Liu Y, Shao Y, Zhang Y, Yu Q, Xiong Z, Zhang W et al (2017) Post-transcriptional regulation of erbb2 by mir26a/b and hur confers resistance to tamoxifen in estrogen receptor-positive breast cancer cells. J Biol Chem 292:13551–13564
40. Liu J, Li X, Wang M, Xiao G, Yang G, Wang H, Li Y, Sun X, Qin S, Du N et al (2018) A mir-26a/e2f7 feedback loop contributes to tamoxifen resistance in er-positive breast cancer. Int J Oncol 53:1601–1612
41. Li X, Wu Y, Liu A, Tang X (2016) Mir-27b is epigenetically downregulated in tamoxifen resistant breast cancer cells due to promoter methylation and regulates tamoxifen sensitivity by targeting hmgb3. Biochem Biophys Res Commun 477:768–773
42. Zhu J, Zou Z, Nie P, Kou X, Wu B, Wang S, Song Z, He J (2016) Downregulation of microrna-27b-3p enhances tamoxifen resistance in breast cancer by increasing nr5a2 and creb1 expression. Cell Death Dis 7:e2454
43. Chen MJ, Cheng YM, Chen CC, Chen YC, Shen CJ (2017) Mir-148a and mir-152 reduce tamoxifen resistance in er+ breast cancer via downregulating alcam. Biochem Biophys Res Commun 483:840–846
44. Kim YS, Park SJ, Lee YS, Kong HK, Park JH (2016) Mirnas involved in ly6k and estrogen receptor alpha contribute to tamoxifen-susceptibility in breast cancer. Oncotarget 7:42261–42273
45. Martin EC, Conger AK, Yan TJ, Hoang VT, Miller DF, Buechlein A, Rusch DB, Nephew KP, Collins-Burow BM, Burow ME (2017) Microrna-335-5p and -3p synergize to inhibit estrogen receptor alpha expression and promote tamoxifen resistance. FEBS Lett 591:382–392
46. Ward A, Shukla K, Balwierz A, Soons Z, Konig R, Sahin O, Wiemann S (2014) Microrna-519a is a novel oncomir conferring tamoxifen resistance by targeting a network of tumour-suppressor genes in er+ breast cancer. J Pathol 233:368–379
47. Jiang H, Cheng L, Hu P, Liu R (2018) Microrna663b mediates tam resistance in breast cancer by modulating tp73 expression. Mol Med Rep 18:1120–1126
48. Chu J, Zhu Y, Liu Y, Sun L, Lv X, Wu Y, Hu P, Su F, Gong C, Song E et al (2015) E2f7 overexpression leads to tamoxifen resistance in breast cancer cells by competing with e2f1 at mir-15a/16 promoter. Oncotarget 6:31944–31957
49. Zheng L, Meng X, Li X, Zhang Y, Li C, Xiang C, Xing Y, Xia Y, Xi T (2018) Mir-125a-3p inhibits eralpha transactivation and overrides tamoxifen resistance by targeting cdk3 in estrogen receptor-positive breast cancer. FASEB J 32:588–600
50. Ren YQ, Wang HJ, Zhang YQ, Liu YB (2017) Wbp2 modulates g1/s transition in er+ breast cancer cells and is a direct target of mir-206. Cancer Chemother Pharmacol 79:1003–1011
51. Lu M, Ding K, Zhang G, Yin M, Yao G, Tian H, Lian J, Liu L, Liang M, Zhu T et al (2015) Microrna-320a sensitizes tamoxifen-resistant breast cancer cells to tamoxifen by targeting arpp-19 and errgamma. Sci Rep 5:8735
52. Li J, Lu M, Jin J, Lu X, Xu T, Jin S (2018) Mir-449a suppresses tamoxifen resistance in human breast cancer cells by targeting adam22. Cell Physiol Biochem 50:136–149
53. Zhu QN, Renaud H, Guo Y (2018) Bioinformatics-based identification of mir-542-5p as a predictive biomarker in breast cancer therapy. Hereditas 155:17
54. Kung JT, Colognori D, Lee JT (2013) Long noncoding rnas: past, present, and future. Genetics 193:651–669
55. Aird J, Baird AM, Lim MCJ, McDermott R, Finn SP, Gray SG (2018) Carcinogenesis in prostate cancer: the role of long non-coding rnas. Noncoding RNA Res 3:29–38

56. Helsmoortel H, Everaert C, Lumen N, Ost P, Vandesompele J (2018) Detecting long non-coding rna biomarkers in prostate cancer liquid biopsies: hype or hope? Noncoding RNA Res 3:64–74

57. Balas MM, Johnson AM (2018) Exploring the mechanisms behind long noncoding rnas and cancer. Noncoding RNA Res 3:108–117

58. D'Angelo E, Agostini M (2018) Long non-coding rna and extracellular matrix: the hidden players in cancer-stroma cross-talk. Noncoding RNA Res 3:174–177

59. Fanelli GN, Gasparini P, Coati I, Cui R, Pakula H, Chowdhury B, Valeri N, Loupakis F, Kupcinskas J, Cappellesso R et al (2018) Long-noncoding rnas in gastroesophageal cancers. Noncoding RNA Res 3:195–212

60. Xue X, Yang YA, Zhang A, Fong KW, Kim J, Song B, Li S, Zhao JC, Yu J (2016) Lncrna hotair enhances er signaling and confers tamoxifen resistance in breast cancer. Oncogene 35:2746–2755

61. Wang H, Guan Z, He K, Qian J, Cao J, Teng L (2017) Lncrna uca1 in anti-cancer drug resistance. Oncotarget 8:64638–64650

62. Li X, Wu Y, Liu A, Tang X (2016) Long non-coding rna uca1 enhances tamoxifen resistance in breast cancer cells through a mir-18a-hif1alpha feedback regulatory loop. Tumour Biol J Int Soc Oncodev Biol Med 37:14733–14743

63. Li XN, Liu AH, Tang X, Ren Y (2017) Urothelial carcinoma-associated 1 enhances tamoxifen resistance in breast cancer cells through competitively inhibiting mir-18a. Beijing da xue xue bao Yi xue ban J Peking Univ Health Sci 49:295–302

64. Wu C, Luo J (2016) Long non-coding rna (lncrna) urothelial carcinoma-associated 1 (uca1) enhances tamoxifen resistance in breast cancer cells via inhibiting mtor signaling pathway. Med Sci Monit Int Med J Exp Clin Res 22:3860–3867

65. Xu CG, Yang MF, Ren YQ, Wu CH, Wang LQ (2016) Exosomes mediated transfer of lncrna uca1 results in increased tamoxifen resistance in breast cancer cells. Eur Rev Med Pharmacol Sci 20:4362–4368

66. Liu H, Wang G, Yang L, Qu J, Yang Z, Zhou X (2016) Knockdown of long non-coding rna uca1 increases the tamoxifen sensitivity of breast cancer cells through inhibition of wnt/beta-catenin pathway. PLoS One 11:e0168406

67. Li Z, Yu D, Li H, Lv Y, Li S (2019) Long noncoding rna uca1 confers tamoxifen resistance in breast cancer endocrinotherapy through regulation of the ezh2/p21 axis and the pi3k/akt signaling pathway. Int J Oncol 54:1033–1042

68. Niknafs YS, Han S, Ma T, Speers C, Zhang C, Wilder-Romans K, Iyer MK, Pitchiaya S, Malik R, Hosono Y et al (2016) The lncrna landscape of breast cancer reveals a role for dscam-as1 in breast cancer progression. Nat Commun 7:12791

69. Ma Y, Bu D, Long J, Chai W, Dong J (2019) Lncrna dscam-as1 acts as a sponge of mir-137 to enhance tamoxifen resistance in breast cancer. J Cell Physiol 234:2880–2894

70. Zhang X, Wang M, Sun H, Zhu T, Wang X (2018) Downregulation of linc00894-002 contributes to tamoxifen resistance by enhancing the tgf-beta signaling pathway. Biochem Biokhim 83:603–611

71. Zhang CH, Wang J, Zhang LX, Lu YH, Ji TH, Xu L, Ling LJ (2017) Shikonin reduces tamoxifen resistance through long non-coding rna uc.57. Oncotarget 8:88658–88669

72. Gu J, Wang Y, Wang X, Zhou D, Shao C, Zhou M, He Z (2018) Downregulation of lncrna gas5 confers tamoxifen resistance by activating mir-222 in breast cancer. Cancer Lett 434:1–10

73. Zhang HY, Liang F, Zhang JW, Wang F, Wang L, Kang XG (2017) Effects of long noncoding rna-ror on tamoxifen resistance of breast cancer cells by regulating microrna-205. Cancer Chemother Pharmacol 79:327–337

74. Li Y, Jiang B, Zhu H, Qu X, Zhao L, Tan Y, Jiang Y, Liao M, Wu X (2017) Inhibition of long non-coding rna ror reverses resistance to tamoxifen by inducing autophagy in breast cancer. Tumour Biol J Int Soc Oncodev Biol Med 39:1010428317705790

75. Peng WX, Huang JG, Yang L, Gong AH, Mo YY (2017) Linc-ror promotes mapk/erk signaling and confers estrogen-independent growth of breast cancer. Mol Cancer 16:161

76. Huang NS, Chi YY, Xue JY, Liu MY, Huang S, Mo M, Zhou SL, Wu J (2016) Long non-coding rna metastasis associated in lung adenocarcinoma transcript 1 (malat1) interacts with estrogen receptor and predicted poor survival in breast cancer. Oncotarget 7:37957–37965
77. Cai Y, He J, Zhang D (2016) Suppression of long non-coding rna ccat2 improves tamoxifen-resistant breast cancer cells' response to tamoxifen. Mol Biol 50:821–827
78. Basak P, Chatterjee S, Bhat V, Su A, Jin H, Lee-Wing V, Liu Q, Hu P, Murphy LC, Raouf A (2018) Long non-coding rna h19 acts as an estrogen receptor modulator that is required for endocrine therapy resistance in er+ breast cancer cells. Cell Physiol Biochem 51:1518–1532
79. Gao H, Hao G, Sun Y, Li L, Wang Y (2018) Long noncoding rna h19 mediated the chemosensitivity of breast cancer cells via wnt pathway and emt process. OncoTargets Ther 11:8001–8012
80. Ahmad A (2013) Pathways to breast cancer recurrence. ISRN Oncol 2013:290568
81. Wang K, Li J, Xiong YF, Zeng Z, Zhang X, Li HY (2018) A potential prognostic long noncoding rna signature to predict recurrence among er-positive breast cancer patients treated with tamoxifen. Sci Rep 8:3179
82. Liu R, Hu R, Zhang W, Zhou HH (2018) Long noncoding rna signature in predicting metastasis following tamoxifen treatment for er-positive breast cancer. Pharmacogenomics 21:277–287
83. Wang G, Chen X, Liang Y, Wang W, Fang Y, Shen K (2018) Long noncoding rna signature and disease outcome in estrogen receptor-positive breast cancer patients treated with tamoxifen. J Breast Cancer 21:277–287
84. Ahmad A (2016) Non-coding RNAs: a tale of junk turning into treasure. Noncoding RNA Res 1:1–2
85. Feng YH, Tsao CJ (2016) Emerging role of microrna-21 in cancer. Biomed Rep 5:395–402
86. Yu X, Li R, Shi W, Jiang T, Wang Y, Li C, Qu X (2016) Silencing of microrna-21 confers the sensitivity to tamoxifen and fulvestrant by enhancing autophagic cell death through inhibition of the pi3k-akt-mtor pathway in breast cancer cells. Biomed Pharmacother 77:37–44

Chapter 12
TRAIL Mediated Signaling in Breast Cancer: Awakening Guardian Angel to Induce Apoptosis and Overcome Drug Resistance

Ning Yin, Liu Yi, Sumbul Khalid, Ulku Ozbey, Uteuliev Yerzhan Sabitaliyevich, and Ammad Ahmad Farooqi

Abstract Sequencing technologies have allowed us to characterize highly heterogeneous molecular landscape of breast cancer with unprecedented details. Tremendous breakthroughs have been made in unraveling contributory role of signaling pathways in breast cancer development and progression. It is becoming progressively more understandable that deregulation of spatio-temporally controlled pathways underlie development of resistance against different drugs. TRAIL mediated signaling has attracted considerable appreciation because of its characteristically unique ability to target cancer cells while leaving normal cells intact. Discovery of TRAIL was considered as a paradigm shift in molecular oncology because of its conspicuous ability to selectively target cancer cells. There was an exponential growth in the number of high-quality reports which highlighted cancer targeting ability of TRAIL and scientists worked on the development of TRAIL-based therapeutics and death receptor targeting agonistic antibodies to treat cancer. However, later studies challenged simplistic view related to tumor targeting ability of TRAIL. Detailed mechanistic insights revealed that overexpression of anti-apoptotic

N. Yin · L. Yi
Department of Cancer Biology, Mayo Clinic Comprehensive Cancer Center, Jacksonville, FL, USA

S. Khalid
Department of Bioinformatics and Biotechnology, International Islamic University, Islamabad, Pakistan

U. Ozbey
Department of Genetics, Health High School, Munzur University, Tunceli, Turkey

U. Y. Sabitaliyevich
Kazakhstan Medical University "KSPH", Almaty, Kazakhstan

A. A. Farooqi (✉)
Institute of Biomedical and Genetic Engineering (IBGE), Islamabad, Pakistan
e-mail: ammadfarooqi@rlmclahore.com

© Springer Nature Switzerland AG 2019
A. Ahmad (ed.), *Breast Cancer Metastasis and Drug Resistance*,
Advances in Experimental Medicine and Biology 1152,
https://doi.org/10.1007/978-3-030-20301-6_12

243

proteins, inactivation of pro-apoptotic proteins and downregulation of death receptors were instrumental in impairing apoptosis in cancer cells. Therefore researchers started to give attention to identification of methodologies and strategies to overcome the stumbling blocks associated with TRAIL-based therapeutics. Subsequent studies gave us a clear picture of signaling cascade of TRAIL and how deregulation of different proteins abrogated apoptosis. In this chapter we have attempted to provide an overview of the TRAIL induced signaling, list of proteins frequently deregulated and modern approaches to strategically restore apoptosis in TRAIL–resistant breast cancers.

Keywords TRAIL · Breast cancer · Apoptosis

12.1 Introduction

Breast cancer (BCa) is a multifaceted and therapeutically challenging cancer [1, 2]). Among the leading causes of women cancer death, breast cancer accounts up to 25% of all new cancer diagnoses in women globally. Based on clinical screening, there are three major types of breast cancer: (1) Estrogen and progesterone receptor (ER and PR) positive breast cancer. (2) Epidermal growth factor receptor (HER) 2 positive breast cancer. (3) Breast cancers which did not express any ER, PR and HER-2 at all (Triple-negative) [3, 4].

While all three types of breast tumors could be treated with systemic treatments, the outcomes of treating breast cancer patients are still dramatically influenced by expression levels of ER, PR and HER-2. ER and PR positive tumors are predominately treated with hormone therapy [4]. Tumors that are HER-2 positive are treated with HER-2 inhibitors that inhibit HER-2 activity. Triple-negative tumors have a less favorable prognosis than either those with HER-2 positive or those that are ER/PR positive and predominantly treated with chemotherapy [5]. Tumor necrosis factor-related apoptosis-inducing ligand (TRAIL) emerged as a "Magical" molecule to kill BCa cells with minimum off-target effects. In this chapter, we will focus on TRAIL induced apoptotic pathway and how different oncogenic and pro-apoptotic proteins regulated TRAIL-driven apoptosis.

12.2 TRAIL Induced Signaling Pathway

TRAIL mediated signaling has emerged as one amongst the most extensively studied pathway in molecular oncology [6]. Because of its selective ability to kill cancer cells, TRAIL and its receptors attracted considerable attention and we witnessed exponential increase in high-impact publications which uncovered mechanistic insights related to TRAIL signaling [7]. Based on the insights gleaned from decades of research, it had become clear that TRAIL transduced the signals intracellularly through DR4 and DR5. TRAIL is sequestered by the DcRs and thus kept away from binding to DR4 and DR5 to induce apoptosis. Structural association of TRAIL with DCR1, DCR2 and OPG resulted in defective apoptotic signaling [8]. Therefore, ratio of TRAIL-DRs to DcRs correlated with TRAIL sensitivity in BCa cells. Trimerization of the death receptors provided platform for attachment of an adaptor molecule, Fas-associated death domain (FADD) and subsequent binding and activation of caspase-8 and caspases-3 (shown in Fig. 12.1). Functionalization of Intrinsic pathway occurred through caspases-8 mediated processing of Bid protein. Truncated Bid (tBid) moved into the mitochondrion and promoted release of cytochrome *c* and SMAC/DIABLO into the cytoplasm. In the cytoplasm, cytochrome *c* structurally interacted with adaptor APAF-1 that resulted in the formation of signalosome known as "apoptosome" that activated caspase-9. (shown in Fig. 12.1). SMAC/DIABLO promoted apoptosis by binding to inhibitor of apoptotic (IAP) proteins and prevented these molecules from exertion of inhibitory effects on caspase activation.

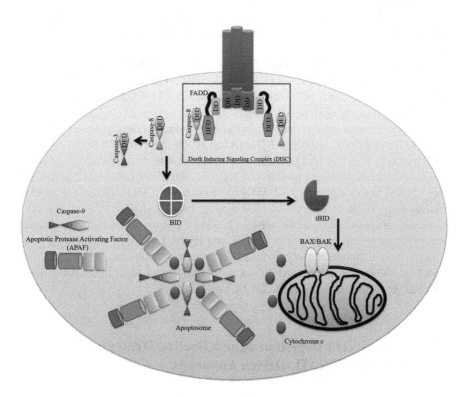

Fig. 12.1 shows TRAIL mediated signaling cascade. Interaction of TRAIL with death receptor induced receptor trimerization and formation of a Signalosome known as death inducing signaling complex (DISC). DISC promoted activation of caspase-8. Caspase8 induced activation of caspase-3. In intrinsic pathway, caspase-8 mediated processing of Bid into truncated Bid (tBid). Truncated Bid moved into the nucleus to regulate transportation of SMAC/DIABLO and cytochrome c into the cytoplasm. APAF, cytochrome-c and pro-caspase-9 formed a complex known as apoptosome

DR4 had a higher expression in better differentiated tumors and positively connected with prognostically relevant surrogate markers [9]. Expression of DR5 and decoy receptor (DcR2) correlated with higher tumor grades, higher Ki67 index and a positive nodal status. DcR2 and DR5 expression correlated negatively with overall survival (OS) of BCa patients [9]. Higher DcR1 expression in tumor epithelial cells was an independent prognostic factor for disease free survival and overall survival in BCa patients [10].

MCF7 BCa cells were found to be resistant to TRAIL mainly because of higher cell surface expression of DcR2 [11]. TRAIL resistant MCF7 cells exhibited higher DcR2 levels on surface. However, TRAIL sensitive MDA-MB-231 BCa cells displayed lower levels of DcR2. It was interesting to note that TRAIL induced apoptosis in DcR2 silenced MCF7 BCa cells [11].

DcR1 was noted to be upregulated by p53 in doxorubicin treated BCa cells. P53 used intronic p53-binding site within DcR1 to transcriptionally upregulate its expression in doxorubicin-treated BCa cells [12].

Confluence of information suggested that oncogenic proteins negatively regulated TRAIL induced apoptosis. Whereas, pro-apoptotic proteins enhanced TRAIL driven apoptosis in BCa cells.

Knock down of Crk-like protein (CRKL), Angiotensin II Receptor 2 (AGTR2), T-Box Transcription Factor 2 (TBX2) and Solute Carrier Family 26 (Sulfate Transporter), Member-2 (SLC26A2) in MDA-MB-231 BCa cells significantly reduced resistance against TRAIL [13].

Chromatin immunoprecipitation (ChIP) data provided evidence of direct binding of KDM4A to TRAIL promoter. KDM4A inhibition induced DR5 in the p53-null H1299 cells [14]. KDM4A knockdown or treatment with its inhibitor C-4 substantially enhanced mRNA and protein of CHOP in cancer cells. Anti-KDM4A ChIP also verified direct binding of KDM4A to promoter of CHOP. Notably, KDM4A inhibition significantly increased CHOP binding to the CHOP binding sites within promoter region of DR5 (shown in Fig. 12.2) [14]. C-4 treatment strongly reduced occupancy of co-repressor NCOR1/NCoR and HDAC1 at CHOP and TRAIL promoters, which simultaneously induced an increase in levels of H3K9ac and H3K27ac. Moreover, tumor growth was drastically reduced in mice xenografted with KDM4A silenced MDA-MB-231 BCa cells [14].

12.3 Amino Acid Depletion as an Effective Strategy to Induce TRAIL-Driven Apoptosis

Oncogenic transformation resulted in the alterations in metabolism of glutamine and remarkably enhanced dependency of transformed cells highly on glutamine [15]. Glutamine deprivation sensitized TNBC cells to TRAIL-induced activation of caspase-8 and consequent apoptosis. Incubation of MDA-MB4-68 BCa cells in glutamine-free conditions for 24 h induced DR5 upregulation. Moreover, cell surface appearance of DR5 was also enhanced upon deprivation of glutamine in TNBC

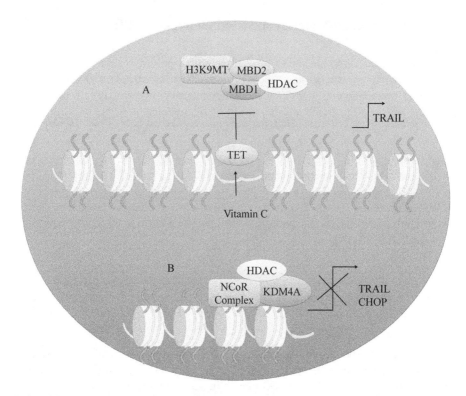

Fig. 12.2 schematically shows transcriptional regulation of TRAIL and CHOP by different transcriptional co-repressors, HDACs. (**a**) H3K9MT worked synchronously with MBD1/2 and HDAC to repress the expression of TRAIL. However, vitamin C induced activation of TET proteins inhibited accumulation of HDACs and H3K9MT at the target sites. (**b**) HDAC, NCoR complex and KDM4A worked in an orchestrated manner to inhibit the expression of CHOP and TRAIL

cells [15]. Glutamate-oxoloacetate transaminase (GOT1) transferred nitrogen to oxoloacetate to generate α-KG and aspartate. Excitingly, GOT1 inhibition significantly sensitized MDA-MB-468 BCa cells to TRAIL. Deprivation of glutamine markedly upregulated ATF4 that consequently induced CHOP mRNA and protein in MDA-MB-468 BCa cells [15].

Lexatumumab, a DR5 targeting monoclonal antibody has previously been reported to be more effective than a DR4 targeting monoclonal antibody (mapatumumab) in an orthotopic model of clinically challenging and aggressive TNBC [16]. Methionine depletion sensitized TNBC cells to lexatumumab mainly through upregulation of DR4 and DR5. MAGED2/MAGD2, a negative regulator of TRAIL-driven pathway was downregulated by methionine depletion in TNBC cells [16]. Significantly enhanced cell surface appearance of DR4 and DR5 was noticed in MAGED2 silenced MDA-MB-231 BCa cells. These findings clearly suggested that methionine depletion effectively enhanced DR4 and DR5 and simultaneously repressed MAGED2 in BCa cells [16].

12.4   Nanotechnologically Assisted Delivery of TRAIL

Hyaluronic acid (HA)-decorated polyethylenimine-poly(d,l-lactide-co-glycolide) (PEI-PLGA) nanoparticles have shown potential as remarkable delivery agents. PEI-PLGA nanoparticles were used for combinatorial delivery of TRAIL encoding plasmid and gambogic acid and found to be effective against triple-negative BCa [17]. Gambogic acid was encapsulated within core region of the PEI-PLGA nanoparticles whereas TRAIL plasmid was adsorbed to the positively charged surface of nanoparticles. Interestingly, HA coated on PEI-PLGA NPs behaved as a ligand for CD44 receptors present on surface of BCa cells [17]. TRAIL plasmid and gambogic acid co-loaded nanoparticles exhibited spherical shape and promoted release of payload into BCa cells through CD44-driven endocytic pathway. More importantly, drug-loaded nanoparticles considerably induced regression of tumor in xenografted mice [17].

12.5   Natural Products as TRAIL Sensitizers in Breast Cancer

Circumstantial evidence provided evidence of significantly enhanced killing effects of Gambogic acid in combination with TRAIL [18]. TRAIL and Gambogic acid combinatorially activated Bid (BH3 interacting-domain death agonist) and consequently functionalized intrinsic apoptotic pathway [18]. Galangin, a type of bioflavonoid isolated from the Alpinia galangal root has been reported to be effective against breast cancer [19]. TRAIL and Galangin markedly increased caspase-9, caspase-3 and Bax activity in BCa cells [19].

Three mammalian TET proteins, namely TET1, TET2 and TET3 belonged to iron and 2-oxoglutarate-dependent dioxygenase superfamily that successively oxidized 5-methylcytosine (5mC) to 5-hydroxymethylcytosine (5hmC), 5-carboxylcytosine and 5-formylcytosine [20]. Methyl CpG-binding protein-1 (MBD1) and MBD2 specifically recognized methylated DNA and recruited HDACs or H3K9MTs to 5mC (shown in Fig. 12.2). 5hmC strongly inhibited the binding of these MBD proteins to DNA and therefore triggered transcriptional upregulation of different genes. Vitamin C has recently been reported to transcriptionally stimulate TRAIL expression via TET-mediated DNA demethylation pathway in MDA-MB-231 BCa cells (shown in Fig. 12.2) [20].

12.6   Strategies to Overcome Drug Resistance

Certain hints have emerged which highlighted that BCa cell lines resistant to tamoxifen or faslodex were TRAIL- sensitive as compared to endocrine-sensitive BCa cell lines [21]. TRAIL effectively targeted CSC-like activity in tamoxifen resistant cells which resulted in prolonged remission of tumors in xenografted mice. Furthermore, TRAIL considerably reduced CSCs in endocrine-resistant BCa cells as compared to endocrine-naive tumors [21]. Additionally, systemically delivered TRAIL in endocrine-resistant patient-derived xenografts reduced CSC-like activity, tumor growth and metastases. These findings provoked additional questions related to underlying mechanism of TRAIL sensitivity in tamoxifen-resistant BCa cells [21]. Detailed mechanistic insights revealed that levels of c-FLIP were significantly reduced in tamoxifen-resistant BCa cells as compared to parental MCF-7 BCa cells [21].

TRAIL and doxorubicin were co-encapsulated in the form of ultrasound-responsive micro-bubbles which shattered into nanoshards or fragments in an ultrasound beam [22]. Micro-bubbles of different polymer shell compositions were designed and effects of both shell compositions and co-encapsulation of doxorubicin and TRAIL against MDA-MB-231 (TRAIL-sensitive) and MCF7 (TRAIL-resistant) BCa cells were tested. Data clearly suggested that shells which co-encapsulated doxorubicin and TRAIL demonstrated significantly higher killing activity against TRAIL-resistant MCF7 BCa cells [22].

12.7 Darker Side of TRAIL/DR5 Signaling in Breast Cancer

Although tremendously accumulating scientific evidence is emphasizing on apoptosis inducing role of TRAIL-driven signaling but certain hints have emerged which also provided a glimpse of darker side of TRAIL mediated signaling. Cleaved-TRAIL significantly enhanced motility of MDA-MB-231 BCa cells [23]. Deficiency in TRAIL-R2 abolished sTRAIL-driven mobility of MDA-MB-231 BCa cells [23].

Another ground-breaking discovery in solving the conundrum of TRAIL signaling associated resistance clearly suggested that DR5 and DISC constituents (FADD and caspase-8) formed the core of composite pro-apoptotic-pro-survival cell membrane-proximal platforms which promoted the apoptosis but simultaneously activated non-apoptotic pathway [24]. Immunoprecipitation technique using whole-cellular lysates and antibodies against DR4/DR5 or DcR2 revealed that these receptors formed hetero-complexes. These molecular-complexes in turn recruited FADD, caspase-8 and c-FLIP. Additionally, immunoprecipitation of caspase-8 with whole-cellular lysates verified that TRAIL induced interaction of TRAIL receptors, Receptor-interacting serine/threonine-protein kinase 1 (RIPK1), FADD and TRAF2 with initiator caspases [24]. Intriguingly, immunoprecipitation of DR5 following TRAIL treatment demonstrated that TRAF2 and RIPK1 were both recruited to TRAIL triggered multi-molecular complexes. These findings provided strong proof that both canonical DISC members (FADD, caspase-8, c-FLIP) and protein assembly earlier presumed to form a TRAIL-mediated "receptor independent-secondary complex" (TRAF2 and RIPK1) were recruited to TRAIL-specific receptors [24].

DR5 seemingly played a central role in activating the kinome of TRAIL-treated cells. Surprisingly, phosphorylation of p38, Extracellular signal regulated kinase (ERK1/2), AKT/PKB was blocked in DR5 depleted cells [24]. Moreover,

DR5-targeting TRAIL-mimetic peptides promoted p38, ERK1/2, AKT/PKB phosphorylation and comparable results were noted in DR4-DcR2 double knock-down cells after treatment with TRAIL. These findings provided sufficient evidence that DR5 had a dualistic role in pro-apoptotic and survival signaling. However, future studies must converge on investigation of this pathway in different breast cancer cell lines.

Inhibition of DR5 in osteotropic BCa cells markedly repressed their ability to form skeletal metastases after intracardiac injection [25]. Moreover, DR5 knockdown significantly decreased the migratory potential of these cells towards stromal cell-derived factor 1 (SDF1)/C-X-C motif chemokine 12 (CXCL12). However, astonishingly, intraosseus growth of BCa metastases was not found to be dependent on expression levels of DR5. Overexpression of either DR5-short or -long isoform in parental MDA-MB-231 BCa cells specifically and strongly enhanced overall expression and cell surface appearance of C-X-C chemokine receptor type 4 (CXCR4) [25].

However, this puzzling story did not end here. In a previous report it was demonstrated that TRAIL suppressed CXCR4-driven migration of MDA-MB-231 BCa cells by upregulation of microRNA-146a through NF-κB [26]. More importantly, neutralization antibody against DR4 effectively inhibited TRAIL-mediated activation of NF-κB and consequent upregulation of miR-146a [26].

Both of these conceptually related findings opened new horizons for an in-depth research related to characteristically distinct intracellular pathways triggered by DR4 and DR5 in BCa cells. It seems clear that context dependently DR4 and DR5 show different response in BCa cells. However, it still needs verification and validation using additional molecular studies.

12.8   Conclusion

Microarray-based high-throughput technologies have paradigmatically shifted our understanding characteristically unique molecular network, inactivation of tumor suppressors, overexpression of oncogenes and loss of apoptosis. TRAIL induced signaling has been deeply investigated in BCa and ground-breaking discoveries have helped us in developing a better comprehension of the proteins frequently deregulated in TRAIL induced pathway. Downregulation of death receptors, degradation of receptors, and imbalance of pro- and anti-apoptotic proteins severely compromised efficacy of TRAIL-based therapeutics in BCa.

References

1. Zardavas D, Irrthum A, Swanton C, Piccart M (2015) Clinical management of breast cancer heterogeneity. Nat Rev Clin Oncol 12(7):381–394. https://doi.org/10.1038/nrclinonc.2015.73
2. Kwa M, Makris A, Esteva FJ (2017) Clinical utility of gene-expression signatures in early stage breast cancer. Nat Rev Clin Oncol 14(10):595–610. https://doi.org/10.1038/nrclinonc.2017.74

3. Weigelt B, Reis-Filho JS (2009) Histological and molecular types of breast cancer: is there a unifying taxonomy? Nat Rev Clin Oncol 6(12):718–730. https://doi.org/10.1038/nrclinonc.2009.166
4. Lin SX, Chen J, Mazumdar M, Poirier D, Wang C, Azzi A, Zhou M (2010) Molecular therapy of breast cancer: progress and future directions. Nat Rev Endocrinol 6(9):485–493. https://doi.org/10.1038/nrendo.2010.92
5. Lee A, Djamgoz MBA (2018) Triple negative breast cancer: emerging therapeutic modalities and novel combination therapies. Cancer Treat Rev 62:110–122. https://doi.org/10.1016/j.ctrv.2017.11.003
6. Kimberley FC, Screaton GR (2004) Following a TRAIL: update on a ligand and its five receptors. Cell Res 14(5):359–372
7. von Karstedt S, Montinaro A, Walczak H (2017) Exploring the TRAILs less travelled: TRAIL in cancer biology and therapy. Nat Rev Cancer 17(6):352–366. https://doi.org/10.1038/nrc.2017.28
8. de Miguel D, Lemke J, Anel A, Walczak H, Martinez-Lostao L (2016) Onto better TRAILs for cancer treatment. Cell Death Differ 23(5):733–747. https://doi.org/10.1038/cdd.2015.174
9. Ganten TM, Sykora J, Koschny R, Batke E, Aulmann S, Mansmann U, Stremmel W, Sinn HP, Walczak H (2009) Prognostic significance of tumour necrosis factor-related apoptosis-inducing ligand (TRAIL) receptor expression in patients with breast cancer. J Mol Med (Berl) 87(10):995–1007. https://doi.org/10.1007/s00109-009-0510-z
10. Labovsky V, Martinez LM, Davies KM, de Luján Calcagno M, García-Rivello H, Wernicke A, Feldman L, Matas A, Giorello MB, Borzone FR, Choi H, Howard SC, Chasseing NA (2017) Prognostic significance of TRAIL-R3 and CCR-2 expression in tumor epithelial cells of patients with early breast cancer. BMC Cancer 17(1):280. https://doi.org/10.1186/s12885-017-3259-8
11. Sanlioglu AD, Dirice E, Aydin C, Erin N, Koksoy S, Sanlioglu S (2005) Surface TRAIL decoy receptor-4 expression is correlated with TRAIL resistance in MCF7 breast cancer cells. BMC Cancer 5:54
12. Ruiz de Almodóvar C, Ruiz-Ruiz C, Rodríguez A, Ortiz-Ferrón G, Redondo JM, López-Rivas A (2004) Tumor necrosis factor-related apoptosis-inducing ligand (TRAIL) decoy receptor TRAIL-R3 is up-regulated by p53 in breast tumor cells through a mechanism involving an intronic p53-binding site. J Biol Chem 279(6):4093–4101
13. Dimberg LY, Towers CG, Behbakht K, Hotz TJ, Kim J, Fosmire S, Porter CC, Tan AC, Thorburn A, Ford HL (2017) A genome-wide loss-of-function screen identifies SLC26A2 as a novel mediator of TRAIL resistance. Mol Cancer Res 15(4):382–394. https://doi.org/10.1158/1541-7786.MCR-16-0234. Epub 2017 Jan 20
14. Wang J, Wang H, Wang LY, Cai D, Duan Z, Zhang Y, Chen P, Zou JX, Xu J, Chen X, Kung HJ, Chen HW (2016) Silencing the epigenetic silencer KDM4A for TRAIL and DR5 simultaneous induction and antitumor therapy. Cell Death Differ 23(11):1886–1896. https://doi.org/10.1038/cdd.2016.92
15. Mauro-Lizcano M, López-Rivas A (2018) Glutamine metabolism regulates FLIP expression and sensitivity to TRAIL in triple-negative breast cancer cells. Cell Death Dis 9(2):205. https://doi.org/10.1038/s41419-018-0263-0.
16. Strekalova E, Malin D, Good DM, Cryns VL (2015) Methionine deprivation induces a targetable vulnerability in triple-negative breast cancer cells by enhancing TRAIL Receptor-2 expression. Clin Cancer Res 21(12):2780–2791. https://doi.org/10.1158/1078-0432.CCR-14-2792
17. Wang S, Shao M, Zhong Z, Wang A, Cao J, Lu Y, Wang Y, Zhang J (2017) Co-delivery of gambogic acid and TRAIL plasmid by hyaluronic acid grafted PEI-PLGA nanoparticles for the treatment of triple negative breast cancer. Drug Deliv 24(1):1791–1800. https://doi.org/10.1080/10717544.2017.1406558
18. Wang S, Xu Y, Li C, Tao H, Wang A, Sun C, Zhong Z, Wu X, Li P, Wang Y (2018. pii: S0278-6915(18)30102-9) Gambogic acid sensitizes breast cancer cells to TRAIL-induced apoptosis by promoting the crosstalk of extrinsic and intrinsic apoptotic signalings. Food Chem Toxicol. https://doi.org/10.1016/j.fct.2018.02.037

19. Song W, Yan CY, Zhou QQ, Zhen LL (2017) Galangin potentiates human breast cancer to apoptosis induced by TRAIL through activating AMPK. Biomed Pharmacother 89:845–856. https://doi.org/10.1016/j.biopha.2017.01.062
20. Sant DW, Mustafi S, Gustafson CB, Chen J, Slingerland JM, Wang G (2018) Vitamin C promotes apoptosis in breast cancer cells by increasing TRAIL expression. Sci Rep 8(1):5306. https://doi.org/10.1038/s41598-018-23714-7
21. Piggott L, da Silva AM, Robinson T, Santiago-Gómez A, Simões BM, Becker M, Fichtner I, Andera L, Piva M, Vivanco MD, Morris C, Alchami FS, Young P, Barrett-Lee PJ, Clarke RB, Gee JM, Clarkson R (2018. pii: clincanres.1381.2017) Acquired resistance of ER- positive breast cancer to endocrine treatment confers an adaptive sensitivity to TRAIL through posttranslational downregulation of c-FLIP. Clin Cancer Res. https://doi.org/10.1158/1078-0432. CCR-17-1381
22. Jablonowski LJ, Conover D, Teraphongphom NT, Wheatley MA (2018) Manipulating multifaceted microbubble shell composition to target both TRAIL-sensitive and resistant cells. J Biomed Mater Res A. https://doi.org/10.1002/jbm.a.36389
23. Dufour F, Rattier T, Constantinescu AA, Zischler L, Morlé A, Ben Mabrouk H, Humblin E, Jacquemin G, Szegezdi E, Delacote F, Marrakchi N, Guichard G, Pellat-Deceunynck C, Vacher P, Legembre P, Garrido C, Micheau O (2017) TRAIL receptor gene editing unveils TRAIL-R1 as a master player of apoptosis induced by TRAIL and ER stress. Oncotarget 8(6):9974–9985. https://doi.org/10.18632/oncotarget.14285
24. Shlyakhtina Y, Pavet V, Gronemeyer H (2017) Dual role of DR5 in death and survival signaling leads to TRAIL resistance in cancer cells. Cell Death Dis 8(8):e3025. https://doi.org/10.1038/cddis.2017.423
25. Fritsche H, Heilmann T, Tower RJ, Hauser C, von Au A, El-Sheikh D, Campbell GM, Alp G, Schewe D, Hübner S, Tiwari S, Kownatzki D, Boretius S, Adam D, Jonat W, Becker T, Glüer CC, Zöller M, Kalthoff H, Schem C, Trauzold A (2015) TRAIL-R2 promotes skeletal metastasis in a breast cancer xenograft mouse model. Oncotarget 6(11):9502–9516
26. Wang D, Liu D, Gao J, Liu M, Liu S, Jiang M, Liu Y, Zheng D (2013) TRAIL-induced miR-146a expression suppresses CXCR4-mediated human breast cancer migration. FEBS J 280(14):3340–3353. https://doi.org/10.1111/febs.12323

Chapter 13
Current State of Platinum Complexes for the Treatment of Advanced and Drug-Resistant Breast Cancers

Bernhard Biersack and Rainer Schobert

Abstract Breast cancer represents the major cause of death in female cancer patients. New efficient treatments are desperately needed, particularly especially for patients suffering from advanced stages and metastases, or those who are no longer responding to the clinically established drugs such as cisplatin or carboplatin. New promising therapy regimens and platinum complexes have emerged over the last few years that displayed efficacy in advanced platinum- and/or drug-resistant breast tumors and metastases. This chapter provides an overview of the latest developments in the field of platinum-based drugs against advanced and resistant breast cancers since 2013.

Keywords Platinum complexes · Anticancer agents · Breast cancer · Metastasis · Multidrug resistance (MDR) · Triple-negative breast cancer (TNBC)

13.1 Introduction

Rosenberg and coworkers discovered the anticancer activity of the platinum(II) complex cisplatin in 1969, and after its approval by the FDA about 10 years later cisplatin became a salient drug in the therapy of solid tumors (Fig. 13.1) [1]. DNA is the main cellular target of cisplatin which binds to it via metal coordination to the N-7 atom of purine bases such as guanine in exchange for its chlorido ligands. The resulting intra- and interstrand links lead to morphological changes of the platinated DNA eventually evoking apoptosis of the affected cells [2, 3]. Platinum therapy, however, comes at a price. Toxicity, severe side-effects and intrinsic or acquired platinum resistance confine the clinical applicability of platinum complexes [3–6]. This is true also for the second and third generation drugs carboplatin and oxaliplatin that are clinically approved in the USA and the EU (Fig. 13.1) [2–4]. Fortunately, the renaissance of interest in the medicinal chemistry of platinum opens a way out

B. Biersack (✉) · R. Schobert
Organic Chemistry Laboratory, Bayreuth, Germany
e-mail: rainer.schobert@uni-bayreuth.de

© Springer Nature Switzerland AG 2019 253
A. Ahmad (ed.), *Breast Cancer Metastasis and Drug Resistance*,
Advances in Experimental Medicine and Biology 1152,
https://doi.org/10.1007/978-3-030-20301-6_13

Fig. 13.1 Platinum
complexes in advanced
stages of investigation as
breast cancer therapeutics

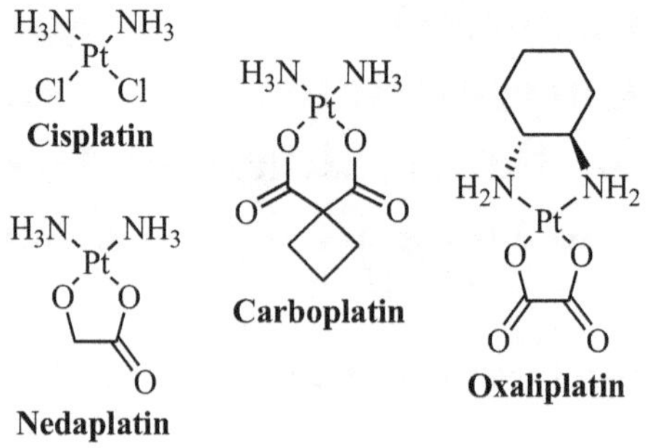

of this predicament. A plethora of new promising platinum complexes was disclosed that harness novel structural motifs, oxidation states, and conjugates with other drugs to overcome the eminent drawbacks of cisplatin, carboplatin and oxaliplatin [7–10]. Typical such examples are *trans*-Pt complexes, Pt(IV) complexes, heteronuclear complexes, and *N*-heterocyclic carbene complexes.

Breast cancer still represents the major cause of death among all female cancer patients (more than 40,000 deaths per year alone in the USA), although a reduction of the mortality rates by 36% was observed since 1989 [11, 12]. Surgery and chemotherapy as well as hormone therapy for estrogen receptor positive breast cancer represent the main treatment options for breast cancer patients. Platinum complexes such as cisplatin and its less toxic congener carboplatin appear to be promising agents against particularly aggressive triple-negative breast cancers (TNBC) [13]. The efficacy of cisplatin and carboplatin treatment against breast cancer cells seems to be regulated epigenetically and tightly correlated with certain miRNA expression profiles including tumor suppressor miRNAs and oncogenic miRNAs (oncomirs) [14, 15]. Several new platinum complexes were disclosed that proved particularly active against aggressive, metastatic and/or drug-resistant breast cancers [8, 16]. In the following, an overview is presented of platinum–based anticancer agents for the targeted treatment of drug-resistant breast cancer and breast cancer metastases, published over the last 4 years, with a focus on those breast cancers that are associated with a poor prognosis.

13.2   Platinum Complexes in Advanced Stages of Investigation for the Treatment of Aggressive and Resistant Breast Cancers

Clinically approved platinum complexes such as cisplatin and carboplatin already represent valuable options for the treatment of advanced breast cancer diseases either alone or in combination with other drugs [17]. About 15–20% of all patients are diagnosed with triple-negative breast cancer (TNBC) which lacks expression of estrogen receptor (ER) and progesterone receptor (PR) and doesn't overexpress human epidermal growth factor receptor 2 (HER2) [18]. TNBC is often associated with the development of brain and lung metastases and, thus, with a reduced overall survival rate and poor prognosis [18]. Platinum complexes have gained importance concerning the therapy of TNBC because of their DNA-damaging properties [13]. In a recent phase II trial, several patients suffering from metastatic TNBC responded well to platinum-based therapy (either cisplatin or carboplatin). In particular, patients with either germline BRCA1/2 mutations or with otherwise induced homologous recombination (HR) deficiency associated with ineffective DNA damage repair exhibited therapy response (Table 13.1) [19]. Indeed, HR deficiency on the basis of loss of heterozygosity (LOH), telomeric allelic imbalance (TAI) and large-scale state transition (LST) was discovered as a prognostic factor for BRCA1/2-mutated and sporadic TNBC response to treatment with platinum drugs [20]. In line with this finding, it was shown that the HR-repair inhibitor triapine augmented cisplatin activity in BRCA wild-type cancer cells [21]. A recent phase III trial of cisplatin in combination with gemcitabine for the treatment of metastatic TNBC revealed very promising results (median PFS/progression free survival = 7.73 months) when compared with paclitaxel plus gemcitabine (median PFS = 6.57 months), and cisplatin plus gemcitabine was suggested as the preferred first-line chemotherapy for this tumor disease in the future (Table 13.1) [22]. Another study revealed a median PFS of 4 months in patients with heavily pre-treated metastatic breast cancer who received cisplatin plus ifosfamide as salvage treatment

Table 13.1 Recent clinical studies of promising platinum complexes at advanced stages of breast cancer

Drugs	Study	Conclusion
Cisplatin or carboplatin	Phase 2, metastatic TNBC patients: RR = 25.6% (54.5% in BRCA1/2-mutant patients), CR = 3.5%, PR = 22.1%, SD = 4.7%	Germline BCRA1/1 mutation and HR-deficiency as prognostic factors for platinum response
Cisplatin plus ifosfamide	Retrospective analysis of 20 metastatic breast cancer patients: median PFS = 4 months, OS = 8.5 months	More effective than platinum monotherapy, caution: grade 3/4 toxicities
Cisplatin plus gemcitabine	Phase 3, metastatic TNBC patients: median PFS = 7.73 months	Recommended as preferred first-line therapy of TNBC
Carboplatin plus everolimus	Phase 2, metastatic TNBC patients: CBR = 36% (1 CR, 6 PRs, 7 SDs), median PFS = 3 months, OS = 16 months	Efficacious and well tolerated therapy with enduring responses
Nedaplatin plus taxanes, gemcitabine or navelbine	Analysis of 171 advanced breast cancer patients: RR = 48.2%, TTF = 13.87 months, OS = 31.53 months	Well-tolerated and suitable cisplatin surrogate with higher activity than cisplatin
Oxaliplatin plus vinorelbine	Phase 2, metastatic TNBC patients: CBR = 50.0%, RR = 31.6%, median PFS = 4.3 months, OS = 12.6 months, CR = 2.6%, PR = 28.9%, SD = 26.3%	Effective with good safety, strongly recommended for phase 3 trials

CBR clinical benefit rate, *CR* complete response, *PFS* progression free survival, *PR* partial response, *OS* overall survival, *RR* response rate, *SD* stable disease, *TTF* time to treatment failure

(Table 13.1) [23]. The combination of cisplatin with the bisphosphonate zoledronic acid (a clinically approved drug for the treatment of cancer-mediated bone diseases) exhibited synergistic effects in TNBC cells (MDA-MB-231) which was associated with suppressed Mcl-1 expression and inhibition of mTOR signalling [24].

The less toxic cisplatin congener carboplatin was investigated in combination with the mTOR inhibitor everolimus in 25 metastatic TNBC patients in a phase 2 trial (Table 13.1) [25]. Carboplatin treatment was well tolerated by the patients and one complete response, six partial responses, and seven stable diseases were observed while eight patients showed progressing disease [25]. In a study with TNBC intracranial models, the combination of carboplatin with the PARP inhibitor ABT888 showed improved survival in the BRCA-mutant intracranial TNBC models and might be a suitable therapy option for BRCA-mutant TNBC patients with brain metastases in future clinical trials [26].

The second generation platinum complex nedaplatin is a close analog of carboplatin and its activity against advanced breast cancer was evaluated and compared with cisplatin [27]. Indeed, nedaplatin-based chemotherapy (in combination with paclitaxel or docetaxel, and gemcitabine or navelbine) showed distinctly longer time-to-treatment failure (TTF) = 13.87 months and overall survival (OS) times = 31.53 months in advanced breast cancer patients when compared with cisplatin-based chemotherapy (TTF = 8.7 months, OS = 24.87 months) (Table 13.1) [27].

Oxaliplatin with the characteristic *trans*-(1*R*,2*R*)-DACH (diaminocyclohexane) ligand is approved for the therapy of colorectal cancer because it lacks cross-resistance to cisplatin and carboplatin. Thus, the effects of oxaliplatin against TNBC were evaluated in a phase 2 trial as well [28]. The biweekly administered combination of oxaliplatin and vinorelbine against pre-treated second- or third-line metastatic TNBC revealed a median PFS of 4.3 months, an OS of 12.6 months and it was characterized by a good safety profile that warrants a phase 3 study of this therapy regimen (Table 13.1) [28].

13.3   New Platinum Complexes for the Treatment of Advanced and Resistant Breast Cancers

As a suitable model for TNBC, the MDA-MB-231 breast carcinoma cell line was frequently employed in order to study the effects of new platinum complexes at the pre-clinical stage [16]. The *cis*-diphenyl pyridineamine platinum(II) complex **1** inhibited MDA-MB-231 TNBC cell growth at much lower doses (IC_{50} = 1.0 μM) than cisplatin (IC_{50} = 10 μM) (Fig. 13.2) [29]. In addition to its DNA-binding and apoptosis induction, complex **1** also suppressed the migration of MDA-MB-231 cells and, thus, has potential as an anti-metastatic agent [29]. The *trans*-2-phenylindole platinum complex **2a** and the *cis*-derivative **2b** revealed distinct growth inhibition of MDA-MB-231 cells (IC_{50} = 4.3–4.4 μM) (Fig. 13.2) [30]. While **2a** caused changes in the tertiary structure of treated plasmid DNA, **2b**

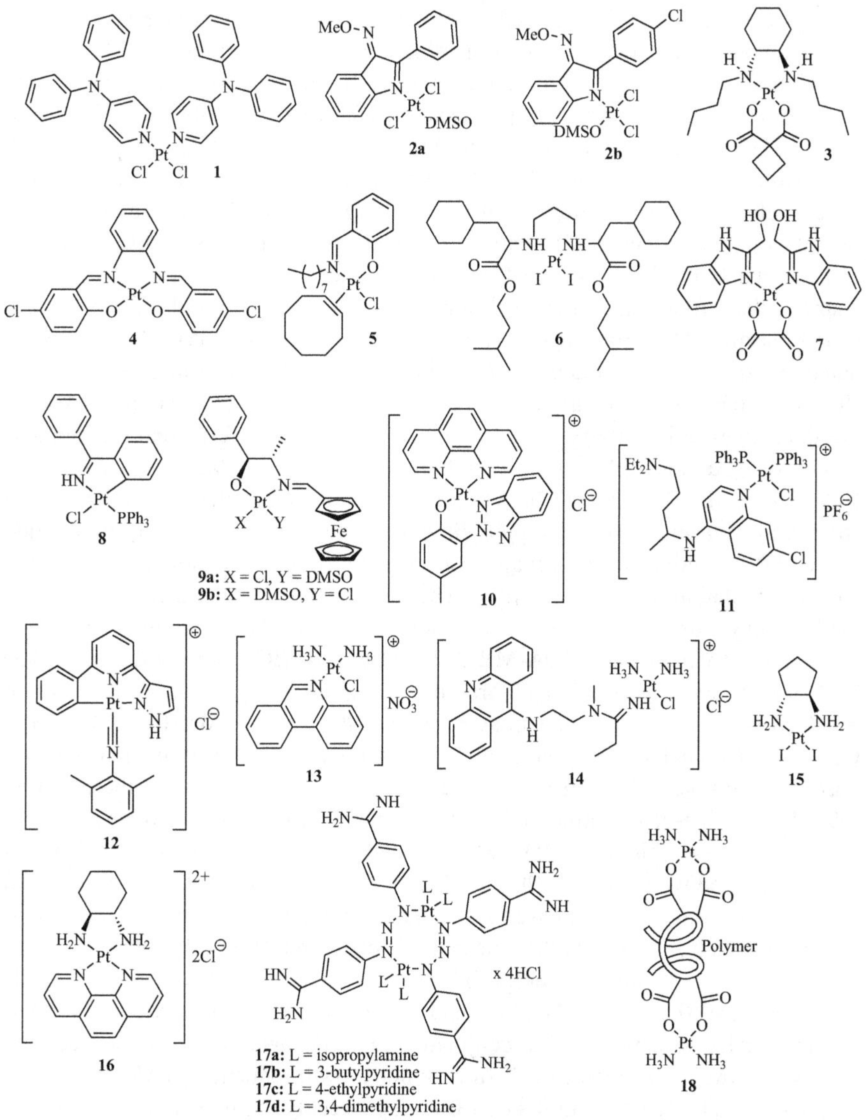

Fig. 13.2 Platinum(II) complexes with activity against the TNBC model MDA-MB-231

exerted no effects on plasmid DNA [30]. The di-*n*-butyl-DACH platinum(II) complex **3** proved more strongly growth inhibitory (IC$_{50}$ = 13.79 μM) against MDA-MB-231 cells than oxaliplatin (IC$_{50}$ = 26.82 μM) and cisplatin (IC$_{50}$ = 18.27 μM) [31]. In addition, complex **3** bound more slowly to DNA when compared with cisplatin due to sterical hindrance by the dibutyl-DACH ligand which suggests a mode of action different from cisplatin (Fig. 13.2) [31]. The Schiff base platinum(II) complex **4** was tested against MDA-MB-231 cells and showed an

IC_{50} value of 6.6 μM (Fig. 13.2) [32]. Complex **4** induced cell cycle arrest (G1-phase) and apoptosis while DNA interaction proceeded via intercalation [32]. Another Schiff base (*N*-octyl-salicylimine)(*cis*-cyclooctene)platinum(II) complex **5** was found to be a strong inducer of apoptosis in MDA-MB-231 cells (Fig. 13.2) [33]. The diiodido complex **6** inhibited MDA-MB-231 cell growth (IC_{50} = 6.6 μM) much more strongly than cisplatin (IC_{50} = 21.9 μM) due to its increased accumulation in cancer cells and to an increased DNA binding (Fig. 13.2) [34]. The 2-hydroxybenz-imidazole oxalatoplatinum(II) complex **7** showed growth inhibition in MDA-MB-231 cells similar to cisplatin and greater than carboplatin (Fig. 13.2) [35]. Complex **7** changed the tertiary structure of plasmid DNA like cisplatin and efficiently pro-tected plasmid DNA from digestion by a restriction enzyme [35]. The cycloplati-nated benzophenone imine **8** also inhibited MDA-MB-231 tumor cell growth (IC_{50} = 5.0 μM), it showed antioxidant activity, and it bound to plasmid DNA lead-ing to changes in its tertiary structure (Fig. 13.2) [36]. The ferrocene-platinum(II) complexes **9a** and **9b** strongly inhibited growth of MDA-MB-231 cells (IC_{50} = 1.4 μM) (Fig. 13.2) [37]. While **9a** initiated distinct changes in the tertiary structure of plasmid DNA, complex **9b** showed no such effects at all, which dis-proves DNA binding being a major aspect of the mode of action of these novel anticancer platinum complexes [37]. The 1,10-phenanthroline 2-(2′-hydroxy-5′-methylphenyl)-benzotriazole platinum complex **10** also showed significant growth inhibitory activity against MDA-MB-231 TNBC cells (IC_{50} = 5.2 μM) (Fig. 13.2) [38]. The triphenylphosphino chloroquine complex **11** was antiproliferative in MDA-MB-231 cells at similar concentrations (IC_{50} = 5.5 μM) (Fig. 13.2) [39]. Complex **11** bound to DNA and bovine serum albumin (BSA). When reacted with guanosine complex **11** underwent a Pt coordination to guanosine via the N7 atom [39]. The luminescent platinum(II) complex **12** featuring a pincer ligand led to a distinct growth inhibition of MDA-MB-231 cells growth inhibition (IC_{50} = 1.6 μM) when compared with cisplatin (IC_{50} = 25 μM) and it accumulated in the cancer cell lysosomes leading to an increased lysosomal membrane permeability and eventu-ally to cell death (Fig. 13.2) [40]. The cationic platinum(II) complex phenanthripla-tin (**13**) was of similar antiproliferative activity in MDA-MB-231 cells (IC_{50} = 3.1 μM) (Fig. 13.2) [41]. Its conjugation to tobacco mosaic virus (TMV) as a nano-carrier system gave a conjugate **13**-TMV with even higher activity (IC_{50} = 2.2 μM). It also led to a distinct tumor growth reduction in MDA-MB-231 tumor xenograft models at doses of 1.0 mg/kg (weekly i.v. injection) with the **13**-TMV nanoparticles accumulating in the tumor tissue [41]. The acridine-platinum(II) complex conjugate **14** inhibited MDA-MB-231 cell growth completely at doses between 5 and 10 μg/mL after 72 h (Fig. 13.2) [42]. Increased accumulation of **14** in MDA-MB-231 cells was achieved by coating of multi-walled carbon nanotubes with **14** (**14**-MWCNT) which also induced S-phase arrest and non-apoptotic cell death in MDA-MB-231 breast cancer cells [42]. The *trans*-1,2-diaminocyclopentane platinum(II) complex **15** and its conjugate with a fructose-based glyco-methacrylate-copolymer carrier (**15**-FMA) revealed potent activity against MDA-MB-231 cells (IC_{50} = 5.1 μM for **15**, IC_{50} = 4.8 μM for **15**-FMA) and the conjugate was readily taken up by breast cancer cells probably via the GLUT-5 receptor (Fig. 13.2) [43]. Reaction of *trans*-(1S,2S)-diaminocyclohexane-dichloridoplatinum(II) with 1,10-phenanthroline gave the bis-cationic complex **16** which was very active against MDA-MB-231 cells (IC_{50} = 0.64 μM) (Fig. 13.2) [44]. Intercalation of the cationic complex **16** into montmorillonite clay as a drug vehicle only slightly reduced the activity against MDA-MB-231 cells (IC_{50} = 0.9 μM) [44].

The dinuclear berenil-platinum(II) complex **17a** with isopropylamino ligands showed distinct tumor cell growth inhibition (IC_{50} = 18 μM) of MDA-MB-231 cells in contrast to cisplatin (IC_{50} = 96 μM) (Fig. 13.2) [45]. Complex **17a** increased ROS levels in MDA-MB-231 cells and decreased the cellular concentrations of antioxidants such as GSH and vitamin E [45]. The analogous berenil-complex **17b** with 3-butylpyridine ligands disclosed improved growth inhibitory activity in MDA-MB-231 cells (IC_{50} = 11 μM) when compared with complex **17a** [46]. Complex **17b** induced apoptosis in MDA-MB-231 cells in a caspase-dependent way via mitochondrial damage [46]. The new dinuclear berenil 4-ethylpyridine platinum(II) complex **17c** also exhibited stronger growth inhibition of MDA-MB-231 cells (IC_{50} = 18 μM) when compared with cisplatin (IC_{50} = 92 μM) [47]. Complex **17c** showed a more pronounced apoptosis induction in MDA-MB-231 cells (38%, 10 μM **17c**) than cisplatin (11%, 10 μM cisplatin), and the activity of **17c** was augmented by combination with anti-MUC1 antibodies (58% apoptotic cells, 10 μM **17c** and 10 μg/mL anti-MUC1) which was associated with increased levels of caspases-8, −9, and −3, and of the pro-apoptotic Bax protein [48]. More recently, another potent dinuclear berenil-platinum(II) complex **17d** with 3,4-dimethylpyridine ligands was disclosed (IC_{50} = 12 μM, MDA-MB-231 cells) which induced apoptosis both by mitochondrial damage and by the external pathway [49]. A micelles-forming carboxy-functionalized polymer was reacted with cisplatin in order to obtain the diammineplatinum(II) functionalized multinuclear polymer **18** for improved drug delivery (Fig. 13.2) [50]. Though the growth inhibitory activity of **18** (IC_{50} ca. 10 μg/mL after 48 h) was reduced in MDA-MB-231 cells when compared with cisplatin, increased platinum release was observed from the polymer micelles **18** at lower pH values (pH 5) [50].

Platinum(IV) complexes are usually more inert than platinum(II) complexes and they need to get activated by reduction to cytotoxic platinum(II) species in the hypoxic tumor environment. A prominent example is the orally applicable Pt(IV) complex satraplatin (Fig. 13.3) that had entered advanced clinical trials [51]. However, a phase 2 trial of satraplatin for the treatment of metastatic breast cancer patients dating from 2009 revealed only limited activity of satraplatin as a single agent (2 PRs, 18 SDs, from a total number of 31 metastatic breast cancer patients) [52]. A more focussed clinical study with patients suffering from advanced breast cancer characterized by HR repair deficiency would probably lead to better results for satraplatin treatment as it was the case for cisplatin and carboplatin [19, 20]. Due to the octahedral structure of Pt(IV) complexes, two more ligands can be introduced which may be applied for the fine-tuning of the biological and pharmacological properties. Inorganic chemists already took advantage of this option in designing new potent anticancer active Pt(IV) complexes [53].

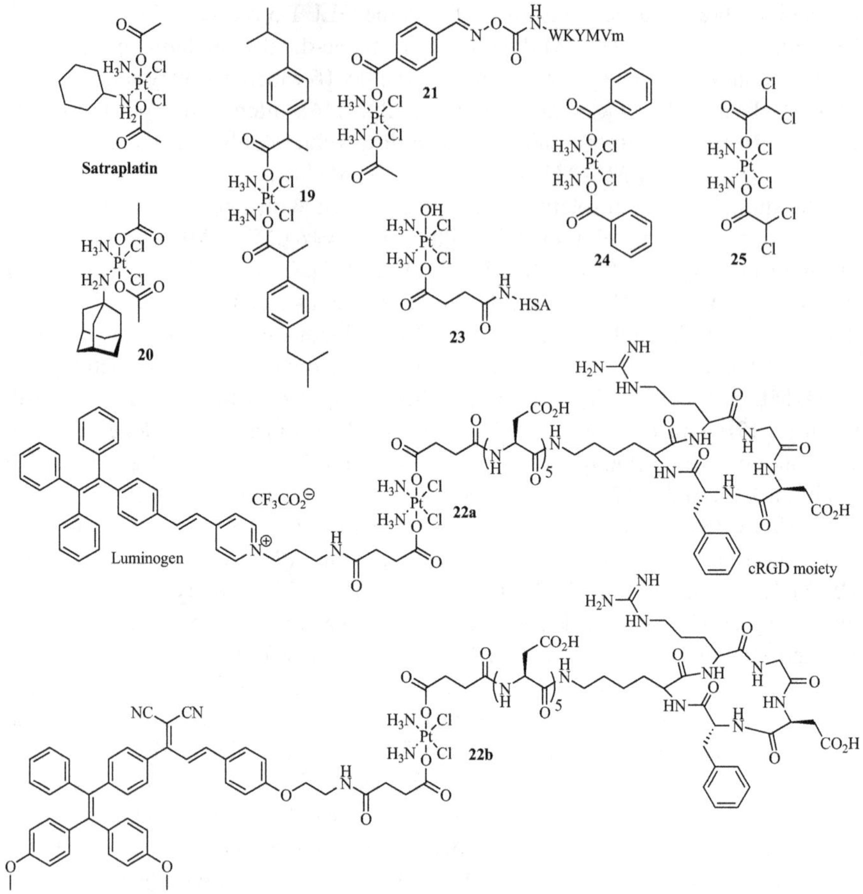

Fig. 13.3 Platinum(IV) complexes with activity against TNBC cells

The lipophilic ibuprofen platinum(IV) complex **19** revealed excellent growth inhibitory activity in MDA-MB-231 cells (IC$_{50}$ = 0.05 μM) and was much more active than the platinum(II) complex cisplatin (IC$_{50}$ = 20 μM) as a consequence of a much higher accumulation in the cancer cells (Fig. 13.3) [54]. LA-12 (**20**), a close adamantylamine analog of satraplatin, was also distinctly inhibiting the growth of MDA-MB-231 cells (IC$_{50}$ = 2.4 μM) (Fig. 13.3) [55]. Interestingly, its formulation as a tumor-targeted folate-cyclodextrin conjugate augmented its activity against MDA-MB-231 cells significantly (IC$_{50}$ = 0.7 μM) [55]. Since the FPR1/2 formyl peptide receptor is overexpressed in immune cells as well as in metastases, the Pt(IV) complex **21** was conjugated to a FPR1/2-targeting peptide (WKYMVm) in order to achieve synergy effects [56]. While **21** exhibited growth inhibitory activity against MDA-MB-231 cells in the range of cisplatin, **21** led to an enhanced secretion of TNF-α and IFN-γ in peripheral blood mononuclear cells (PBMC) when compared to cisplatin [56]. The fact that PBMCs activated by **21** efficiently inhibited

MDA-MB-231 cell growth renders this complex a promising potential immuno-modulating drug candidate [56]. Another Pt(IV) complex **22**, comprising an aggre-gation-induced emission luminogen and the integrin-targeting moiety cRGD (cyclic arginine-glycine-aspartate), was used for the study of bio-reduction of the Pt(IV) moiety [57]. The $\alpha_v\beta_3$ integrin-expressing MDA-MB-231 cells responded much bet-ter to **22a** (IC_{50} = 30.2 μM) than MCF-7 breast cancer cells with only low integrin expression (no response up to 50 μM) [57]. Following this, a similar cRGD-Pt(IV) complex **22b** linked to a photosensitizer with AIE characteristics was prepared, and irradiation with light strongly enhanced the growth inhibitory activity of **22b** in MDA-MB-231 cells (IC_{50} = 4.2 μM) when compared with its efficacy in the dark (IC_{50} = 37.1 μM) and with that of cisplatin (IC_{50} = 33.4 μM) [58]. Human serum albumin (HSA) was linked to Pt(IV) via a succinate to give complex **23** which served as starting material for the preparation of calcium phosphate(CaP)-**23** nanoparticles that release the platinum drug under acidic and hypoxic conditions [59]. Indeed, CaP-**23** exhibited better activity against MDA-MB-231 cells (IC_{50} = 1.36 μM) than cisplatin (IC_{50} = 2.66 μM) [59]. Another potent Pt(IV) com-plex is the bis-benzoyl complex **24** which was highly active against MDA-MB-231 cells (IC_{50} = 0.59 μM) [60]. Incorporation of **24** into silk fibroin nanoparticles (SNF) even augmented the activity of **24** slightly (IC_{50} = 0.39 μM) and increased its tumor selectivity [60]. MDA-MB-468 is another TNBC cell line that was applied to study the anticancer effects of mitaplatin **25** [61]. Complex **25** (1 mg/kg) inhibited the in vivo growth of MDA-MB-468 mouse xenograft tumors distinctly (tumor volume ca. 200 mm^3 for **25** vs. ca. 900 mm^3 for the control mice after 24 days) [61]. Encapsulation of **25** into polymer nanoparticles led to a similar tumor growth inhi-bition and to a prolonged drug circulation in the blood system of the treated mice while the accumulation in the kidneys was reduced [61].

ER-positive T47D breast carcinoma cells are less responsive to cisplatin than ER-positive MCF-7 breast carcinoma cells due to an enhanced glutathione-*S*-transferase (GST)-mediated drug resistance [62, 63]. However, the triazolopyrimi-dine diacetatoplatinum(II) complex **26** (Fig. 13.4) showed excellent and tumor selective activity against T47D breast cancer cells (IC_{50} = 0.26 μM) and it exceeded the activity both of cisplatin (IC_{50} = 14.4 μM) and of oxaliplatin (IC_{50} = 18.3 μM) by far [64]. A similar malonatoplatinum(II) complex **27** exhibited distinct growth inhi-bition of T47D cells (IC_{50} = 3.4 μM) while non-malignant cells were affected less (IC_{50} = 55.8 μM) [65]. A new platinum(II) conjugate **28** bearing a steroidal 7-azaindole ligand also showed increased activity against T47D cells (IC_{50} = 13 μM) when compared with cisplatin (IC_{50} = 33 μM) (Fig. 13.4) [66]. Complex **28** was also accumulated to a greater extend in the T47D cancer cells than cisplatin, and it dis-placed the intercalator ethidium bromide from plasmid DNA and inhibited cathep-sin B [66]. The analogous tri-(*p*-trifluoromethylphenyl)-phosphinoplatinum(II) complex **29** inhibited the growth of T47D cells much more strongly (IC_{50} = 1.84 μM) than cisplatin (IC_{50} = 30 μM) [67]. Complex **29** arrested the cancer cell cycle in the G0/G1 phase and it inhibited cathepsin B (IC_{50} = 8.1 μM) [67]. The *trans*-dichloridoplatinum(II) complex **30** featuring a ferrocene-based ligand was also a

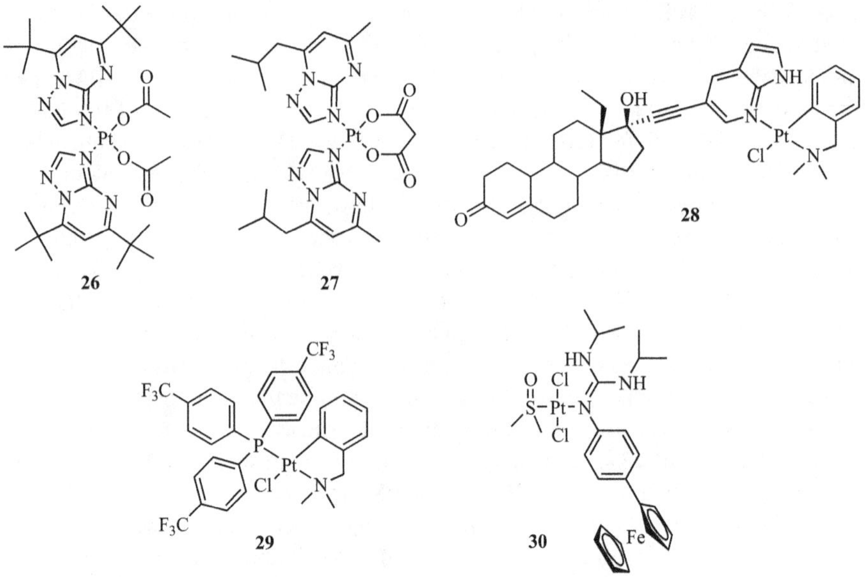

Fig. 13.4 Platinum complexes with improved activity against cisplatin-resistant T47D breast cancer cells

stronger inhibitor of the growth of T47D cells (IC_{50} = 2.4 μM) than cisplatin (IC_{50} = 15 μM) [68].

HER2 epidermal growth factor receptors are overexpressed in many aggressive tumors including breast cancer. Trastuzumab is a clinically approved monoclonal antibody that targets HER2, and a trastuzumab-platinum(IV) conjugate **31** was prepared as a tumor-targeted drug (Fig. 13.5) [69]. Complex **31** bound to HER2 and was much more active against HER2-positive SK-BR-3 breast carcinoma cells when compared with HER2-negative cell lines and it inhibited the growth of SK-BR-3 cells (IC_{50} = 21.3 μM) as effectively as cisplatin (IC_{50} = 20.7 μM) [69]. A platinum(II) conjugate **32** (Fig. 13.5) of the HER2-targeting antibody herceptin showed similar results (IC_{50} = 19.7 μM in SK-BR-3 cells) and an activity better than that of oxaliplatin (IC_{50} = 31.0 μM) [70]. In addition, a HER2-targeting affibody (= small peptidic antibody mimics) was conjugated to cisplatin-loaded liposomes, and the resulting affisome showed increased cytotoxicity and cellular accumulation in SK-BR-3 cells and it exhibited distinct tumor growth inhibition of HER2-positive TUBO breast cancer xenograft models [71].

Another study disclosed that epithelial breast cancer cells were 16-times more sensitive to complex **33** (IC_{50} = 5.3 μM) than to cisplatin (IC_{50} = 94.7 μM) (Fig. 13.5) [72]. Complex **33** reduced the expression of the anti-apoptotic Bcl-2 protein and augmented pro-apoptotic Bax expression leading to the efficient induction of apoptosis by **33** in cisplatin-resistant epithelial breast cancer cells [72].

ER-positive MCF-7 breast cancer cells under hypoxic conditions showed reduced sensitivity to cisplatin. The tetrachloridoplatinum(IV) complex **34** (Fig. 13.5)

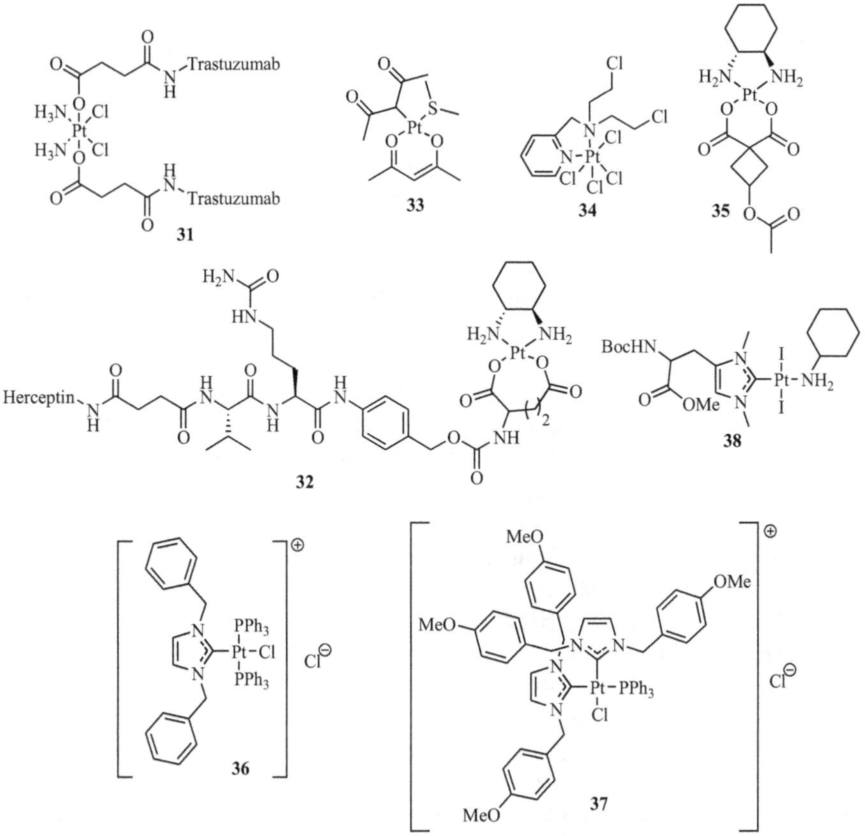

Fig. 13.5 Platinum complexes with distinct activity against various advanced or resistant breast cancers

containing the alkylating nitrogen mustard motif exhibited higher activity against MCF-7 cells both under normoxic (IC_{50} = 11.4 µM) and hypoxic conditions (IC_{50} = 8.6 µM) than cisplatin (IC_{50} = 14.1 µM under normoxic, 18.7 µM under hypoxic conditions) [73]. In addition, **34** was more efficacious in MCF-7 cells supplemented with the cisplatin-resistance factor glutathione (GSH) (IC_{50} = 12.9 µM under normoxic, 11.2 µM under hypoxic conditions) when compared with cisplatin (IC_{50} = 27.8 µM under normoxic, 29.0 µM under hypoxic conditions). **34** also showed an increased accumulation in MCF-7 cells (more than twice as high than that for cisplatin) [73]. In addition, **34** induced apoptosis and reduced the motility of MCF-7 cells [73]. The new water-soluble oxaliplatin/carboplatin analogue **35** showed growth inhibitory activity (IC_{50} = 15.0 µM) comparable with oxaliplatin (IC_{50} = 10.4 µM) and much better than carboplatin (IC_{50} = 154 µM) in multidrug-resistant MCF-7/ADR breast cancer cells (Fig. 13.5) [74]. The in vivo anticancer activity of **35** was evaluated in KM mice bearing Sarcoma 180. Complex **35** led to a greater inhibition of the tumor growth (53.2% inhibition) than oxaliplatin (32.5% inhibition) [74].

In addition, various *N*-heterocyclic carbene platinum complexes were recently investigated for their effect on multidrug-resistant MCF-7/Topo breast cancer cells which overexpress the BCRP transporter [75–77]. Complex **36** (Fig. 13.5) showed excellent and selective growth inhibition ($IC_{50} = 0.15$ μM) in MCF-7/Topo cells when compared with cisplatin ($IC_{50} = 10.6$ μM) [75]. Although **36** did not bind covalently to DNA, this complex induced DNA aggregation in addition to cell cycle arrest in the G1 phase. It also led to the disruption of blood vessels [75]. Similar DNA aggregation effects were observed for biscarbene complex **37** (Fig. 13.5), which also showed strong MCF-7/Topo cell growth inhibition ($IC_{50} = 0.52$ μM) [76]. Another *trans*-diiodidoplatinum(II) NHC complex **38** featuring a histidine-derived NHC-ligand also strongly inhibited the growth of MCF-7/Topo cells ($IC_{50} = 1.6$ μM) (Fig. 13.5) [77]. Complex **38** induced morphological changes in plasmid DNA and caused vascular disruption [77]. Its in vivo activity was evaluated in mice with cisplatin-resistant A2780cis ovarian tumors. Complex **38** (30 mg/kg, i.p.) was roughly as effective a tumor growth inhibitor as cisplatin (6 mg/kg, i.p.), yet showed a superior toxicity profile with treated mice regaining their normal weight far more quickly [77]. Hence, complex **38** is likely applicable in much higher doses than cisplatin to the effect of a significantly better tumor mass reduction.

In order to reduce the systemic toxicity of platinum complexes, a tumor-selective Pt(IV) complex conjugate **39** comprising a short self-assembling peptide sequence was prepared (Fig. 13.6) [78]. Alkaline-phosphatase (AP)-catalyzed cleavage of the phosphate group of **39** led to self-assembly and bioreduction to active platinum species in the tumor (high levels of AP are found in the environment of many tumors). Increased tumor cell accumulation as well as reduced liver and kidney toxicity were observed for 4T1-breast carcinoma xenograft models treated with **39** while the in vivo 4T1 tumor growth was inhibited by **39** similarly to cisplatin [78].

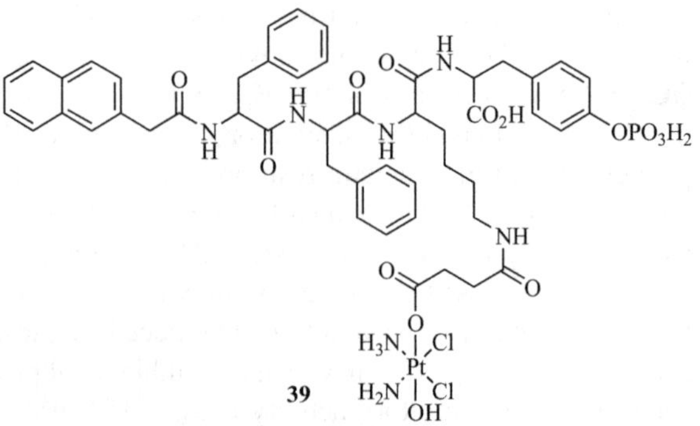

Fig. 13.6 Self-assembling Pt(IV) complex prodrug **39** for 4T1-breast cancer targeting

13.4   Conclusions

The platinum complex cisplatin has been and still is a mainstay in the therapy of solid tumors. However, meanwhile more platinum complexes have passed clinical trials and quite a few of them were found active against drug-resistant and advanced breast cancers. HR-repair deficient triple-negative breast cancers appeared to be especially sensitive to platinum drugs. Their chemical tuning in terms of structure, redox chemistry, and synergistic effects of ligands and co-conjugates has led to a plethora of new complexes with enhanced activity against and selectivity for drug-resistant and/or aggressive/metastatic breast cancers. In addition, novel delivery systems for the targeted therapy of breast cancers with platinum complexes have overcome the notorious drawbacks of the first- and second-generation platinum complexes. Taken together, there are distinct glimpses of hope that new therapies with platinum complexes will prevent or overcome drug resistance, improve prognosis and survival, reduce side-effects, and increase the quality of life of breast cancer patients in a not too distant future.

Acknowledgments   Own work referenced in this chapter was supported by grants from the Deutsche Forschungsgemeinschaft (Scho 402/8 and Scho 402/12).

References

1. Rosenberg B, VanCamp L, Trosko JE, Mansour VH (1969) Platinum compounds: a new class of potent antitumour agents. Nature 222:385–386
2. Jamieson ER, Lippard SJ (1999) Structure, recognition, and processing of cisplatin-DNA adducts. Chem Rev 99:2467–2498
3. Wang D, Lippard SJ (2005) Cellular processing of platinum anticancer drugs. Nat Rev Drug Discov 4:307–320
4. Kartalou M, Essigmann JM (2001) Mechanisms of resistance to cisplatin. Mutat Res Fundam Mol Mech Mutagen 478:23–43
5. Oh GS, Kim HJ, Shen A, Lee SB, Khadka D, Pandit A, So HS (2014) Cisplatin-induced kidney dysfunction and perspectives on improving treatment strategies. Electrolyte Blood Pressure 12:55–65
6. Dasari S, Tchounwou PB (2014) Cisplatin in cancer therapy: molecular mechanisms of action. Eur J Pharmacol 740:364–378
7. Schobert R, Biersack B, Dietrich A, Grotemeier A, Müller T, Kalinowski B, Knauer S, Voigt W, Paschke R (2007) Monoterpenes as drug shuttles: cytotoxic (6-aminomethylnicotinate) dichloridoplatinum(II) complexes with potential to overcome cisplatin resistance. J Med Chem 50:1288–1293
8. Zoldakova M, Biersack B, Kostrhunova K, Ahmad A, Padhye S, Sarkar FH, Schobert R, Brabec V (2011) (Carboxydiamine)Pt(II) complexes of a combretastatin A-4 analogous chalcone: the influence of the diamine ligand on DNA binding and anticancer effects. Med Chem Commun 2:493–499
9. Najajreh Y, Perez JM, Navarro-Ranninger C, Gibson D (2002) Novel soluble cationic *trans*-diaminedichloroplatinum(II) complexes that are active against cisplatin resistant ovarian cancer cell lines. J Med Chem 45:5189–5195

10. Liu W, Gust R (2013) Metal *N*-heterocyclic carbene complexes as potential antitumor metallodrugs. Chem Soc Rev 42:755–773

11. Ferlay J, Soerjomataram I, Dikshit R, Mathers C, Rebelo M, Parkin DM, Forman D, Bray F (2015) Cancer incidence and mortality worldwide: sources, methods and major patterns in GLOBOCAN 2012. Int J Cancer 136:E359–E386

12. DeSantis CE, Fedewa SA, Goding Sauer A, Kramer JL, Smith RA, Jemal A (2016) Breast cancer statistics, 2015: convergence of incidence rates between black and white women. CA Cancer J Clin 66:31–42

13. Petrelli F, Coinu A, Borgonovo K, Cabiddu M, Ghilardi M, Lonati V, Barni S (2014) The value of platinum agents as neoadjuvant chemotherapy in triple-negative breast cancers: a systemic review and meta-analysis. Breast Cancer Res Treat 144:223–232

14. Chen X, Lu P, Wu Y, Wang D, Zhou S, Yang S, Shen H, Zhang X, Zhao J, Tang T (2016) MiRNAs-mediated cisplatin resistance in breast cancer. Tumor Biol 37:12905–12913

15. Biersack B (2017) Interactions between anticancer active platinum complexes and non-coding RNAs/microRNAs. Non-Coding RNA Res 2:1–17

16. Biersack B, Schobert R (2013) Platinum and ruthenium complexes for the therapy of breast cancer diseases. In: Ahmad A (ed) Breast cancer metastasis and drug resistance. Springer Science+Business Media, New York

17. Cobleigh MA (2011) Other options in the treatment of advanced breast cancer. Semin Oncol Suppl 2:S11–S16

18. Lin NU, Vanderplas A, Hughes ME, Theriault RL, Edge SB, Wong YN, Blayney DW, Niland JC, Winter EP, Weeks JC (2012) Clinicopathologic features, patterns of recurrence, and survival among women with triple-negative breast cancer in the national comprehensive cancer network. Cancer 118:5463–5472

19. Isakoff SJ, Mayer EL, He L, Traina TA, Carey LA, Krag KJ, Rugo HS, Liu MC, Stearns V, Come SE, Timms KM, Hartman A-R, Borger DR, Finkelstein DM, Garber JE, Ryan PD, Winer EP, Goss PE, Ellisen LW (2015) TBCRC009: a multicenter phase II clinical trial of platinum monotherapy with biomarker assessment in metastatic triple-negative breast cancer. J Clin Oncol 33:1902–1909

20. Telli ML, Timms KM, Reid J, Hennessy B, Mills GB, Jensen KC, Szallasi Z, Barry WT, Winer EP, Tung NM, Isakoff SJ, Ryan PD, Greene-Colozzi A, Gutin A, Sangale Z, Iliev D, Neff C, Abkevich V, Jones JT, Lanchbury JS, Hartman A-R, Garber JE, Ford JM, Silver DP, Richardson AL (2016) Homologous recombination deficiency (HRD) score predicts response to platinum-containing neoadjuvant chemotherapy in patients with triple-negative breast cancer. Clin Cancer Res 22:3764–3773

21. Ratner ES, Zhu Y-L, Penketh PG, Berenblum J, Whicker ME, Huang PH, Lee Y, Ishiguro K, Zhu R, Sartorelli AC, Lin ZP (2016) Triapine potentiates platinum-based combination therapy by disruption of homologous recombination repair. Br J Cancer 114:777–786

22. Hu X-C, Zhang J, Xu B-H, Cai L, Ragaz J, Wang Z-H, Wang B-Y, Teng Y-E, Tong Z-S, Pan Y-Y, Yin Y-M, Wu C-P, Jiang Z-F, Wang X-J, Lou G-Y, Liu D-G, Feng J-F, Luo J-F, Sun K, Gu Y-J, Wu J, Shao Z-M (2015) Cisplatin plus gemcitabine versus paclitaxel plus gemcitabine as first-line therapy for metastatic triple-negative breast cancer (CBCSG006): a randomized, open-label, multicenter, phase 3 trial. Lancet Oncol 16:436–446

23. Habbel P, Kurreck A, Schulz C-O, Regierer AC, Kaul D, Scholz CW, Neumann C, Possinger K, Eucker J (2015) Cisplatin plus ifosfamide with/without etoposide as salvage therapy in heavily-pre-treated patients with metastatic breast cancer. Anticancer Res 35:5091–5096

24. Ibrahim T, Liverani C, Mercatali L, Sacanna E, Zanoni M, Fabbri F, Zoli W, Amadori D (2013) Cisplatin in combination with zoledronic acid: a synergistic effect in triple-negative breast cancer cell lines. Int J Oncol 42:1263–1270

25. Singh JC, Novik Y, Stein S, Volm M, Meyers M, Smith J, Omene C, Speyer J, Schneider R, Jhaveri K, Formenti S, Kyriakou V, Joseph B, Goldberg JD, Li X, Adams S, Tiersten A (2014) Phase 2 trial of everolimus and carboplatin combination in patients with triple negative metastatic breast cancer. Breast Cancer Res 16:R32

26. Karginova O, Siegel MB, Van Swearingen AED, Deal AM, Adamo B, Sambade MJ, Bazyar S, Nikolaishvili-Feinberg N, Bash R, O'Neal S, Sandison K, Parker JS, Santos C, Darr D, Zamboni W, Lee YZ, Miller CR, Anders CK (2015) Efficacy of carboplatin alone or in combination with ABT888 in intracranial murine models of BRCA-mutated and BRCA-wild-type triple-negative breast cancer. Mol Cancer 14:920–930

27. Pang H, Feng T, Lu H, Meng Q, Chen X, Shen Q, Dong X, Cai L (2016) Efficacy and safety of nedaplatin in advanced breast cancer therapy. Cancer Investig 34:167–172

28. Zhang J, Wang L, Wang Z, Hu X, Wang B, Cao J, Lv F, Zhen C, Zhang S, Shao Z (2015) A phase II trial of biweekly vinorelbine and oxaliplatin in second- or third-line metastatic triple-negative breast cancer. Cancer Biol Ther 16:225–232

29. Varela JG, Chatterjee AD, Guevara P, Ramirez V, Metta-Magana AJ, Villagrán D, Varela-Ramirez A, Das S, Nunez JE (2014) Synthesis, characterization, and evaluation of cis-diphenyl pyridineamine platinum(II) complexes as potential anti-breast cancer agents. J Biol Inorg Chem 19:967–979

30. Tomé M, López C, González A, Ozay B, Quirante J, Font-Bardía M, Calvet T, Calvis C, Messeguer R, Baldomá L, Badía J (2013) Trans- and cis-2-phenylindole platinum(II) complexes as cytotoxic agents against human breast adenocarcinoma cell lines. J Mol Struct 1048:88–97

31. Zhang H, Gou S, Zhao J, Chen F, Xu G, Liu X (2015) Cytotoxicity profile of novel sterically hindered platinum(II) complexes with $(1R,2R)$-N^1,N^2-dibutyl-1,2-diaminocyclohexane. Eur J Med Chem 96:187–195

32. Peng Y, Zhong H, Chen Z-F, Liu Y-C, Zhang G-H, Qin Q-P, Liang H (2014) A planar Schiff base platinum(II) complex: crystal structure, cytotoxicity and interaction with DNA. Chem Pharm Bull 62:221–228

33. Jean S, Cormier K, Patterson AE, Vogels CM, Decken A, Robichaud GA, Turcotte S, Westcott SA (2015) Synthesis, characterization, and anticancer properties of organometallic Schiff base platinum complexes. Can J Chem 93:1140–1146

34. Savic A, Filipovic L, Arandelovic S, Dojcinovic B, Radulovic S, Sabo TJ, Grguric-Sipka S (2014) Synthesis, characterization and cytotoxic activity of novel platinum(II) iodide complexes. Eur J Med Chem 82:372–384

35. Utku S, Ozcelik AB, Gümüs F, Yilmaz S, Arsoy T, Acik L, Keskin AC (2014) Synthesis, in-vitro cytotoxic activity and DNA interactions of new dicarboxylatoplatinum(II) complexes with 2-hydroxymethylbenzimidazole as carrier ligands. J Pharm Pharmacol 66:1593–1605

36. Albert J, D'Andrea L, Granell J, Pla-Vilanova P, Quirante J, Khosa MK, Calvis C, Messeguer R, Badía J, Baldomà L, Font-Bardia M, Calvet T (2014) Cyclopalladated and cycloplatinated benzophenone imines: antitumor, antibacterial and antioxidant activities, DNA interaction and cathepsin B inhibition. J Inorg Biochem 140:80–88

37. Talancón D, López C, Font-Bardía M, Calvet T, Quirante J, Calvis C, Messeguer R, Cortés R, Cascante M, Baldomà L, Badia H (2013) Diastereomerically pure platinum(II) complexes as antitumoral agents. The influence of the mode of binding {(N), (N,O)$^-$ or (C,N)}$^-$ of $(1S,2R)$-[(η^5 –C$_5$H$_5$)Fe{(η^5 –C$_5$H$_4$)-CH=N-CH(Me)-CH(OH)-C$_6$H$_5$}] and the arrangement of the auxiliary ligands. J Inorg Biochem 118:1–12

38. El-Asmy HA, Butler IS, Mouhri ZS, Jean-Claude BJ, Emmam MS, Mostafa SI (2014) Zinc(II), ruthenium(II), rhodium(III), palladium(II), silver(I), platinum(II) and MoO$_2$$^{2+}$ complexes of 2-(2'-hydroxy-5'-methylphenyl)-benzotriazole as simple or primary ligand and 2,2'-bipyridyl, 9,10-phenanthroline or triphenylphosphine as secondary ligands: structure and anticancer activity. J Mol Struct 1059:193–201

39. Villareal W, Colina-Vegas L, de Oliveira CR, Tenorio JC, Ellena J, Gozzo FC, Cominetti MR, Ferreira AG, Ferreira MAB, Navarro M, Batista AA (2015) Chiral platinum(II) complexes featuring phosphine and chloroquine ligands as cytotoxic and monofunctional DNA-binding agents. Inorg Chem 54:11709–11720

40. Tsai JL-L, Zou T, Liu J, Chen T, Chan AO-Y, Yang C, Lok C-N, Che C-M (2015) Luminescent platinum(II) complexes with self-assembly and anti-cancer properties: hydrogel, pH dependent

emission color and sustained-release properties under physiological conditions. Chem Sci 6:3823–3830

41. Czapar AE, Zheng Y-R, Riddell IA, Shukla S, Awuah SG, Lippard SJ, Steinmetz NF (2016) Tobacco mosaic virus delivery of phenanthriplatin for cancer therapy. ACS Nano 10:4119–4126

42. Fahrenholtz CD, Ding S, Bernish BW, Wright ML, Zheng Y, Yang M, Yao X, Donati GL, Gross MD, Bierbach U, Singh R (2016) Design and cellular studies of a carbon nanotube-based delivery system for a hybrid platinum-acridine anticancer agent. J Inorg Biochem 165:170–180

43. Dag A, Callari M, Lu H, Stenzel MH (2016) Modulating the cellular uptake of platinum drugs with glycopolymers. Polym Chem 7:1031–1036

44. Apps MG, Ammit AJ, Gu A, Wheate NJ (2014) Analysis of montmorillonite clay as a vehicle in platinum anticancer drug delivery. Inorg Chim Acta 421:513–518

45. Gegotek A, Cyunczyk M, Luczaj W, Bielawska A, Bielawski K, Skrzydlewska E (2014) The redox status of human breast cancer cell lines (MCF-7 and MDA-MB231) treated with novel dinuclear berenil-platinum(II) complexes. Pharmazie 69:923–928

46. Bielawski K, Czarnomysy R, Muszynska A, Bielawska A, Poplawska B (2013) Cytotoxicity and induction of apoptosis of human breast cancer cells by novel platinum(II) complexes. Environ Toxicol Pharmacol 35:254–264

47. Gornowicz A, Kaluza Z, Bielawska A, Gabryel-Porowska H, Czarnomysy R, Bielawski K (2014) Cytotoxic efficacy of a novel dinuclear platinum(II) complex used with anti-MUC1 in human breast cancer cells. Mol Cell Biochem 392:161–174

48. Gornowicz A, Bielawska A, Czarnomysy R, Gabryel-Porowska H, Muszynska A, Bielawski K (2015) The combined treatment with novel platinum(II) complex and anti-MUC1 increases apoptotic response in MDA-MB-231 breast cancer cells. Mol Cell Biochem 408:103–113

49. Czarnomysy R, Bielawski K, Muszynska A, Bielawska A, Gornowicz A (2016) Biological evaluation of dimethylpyridine-platinum complexes with potent antiproliferative activity. J Enzyme Inhib Med Chem 31:150–165

50. Shahin M, Safaei-Nikouei N, Lavasanifar A (2014) Polymeric micelles for pH-responsive delivery of cisplatin. J Drug Target 22:629–637

51. Voigt W, Dietrich A, Schmoll H-J (2006) Cisplatin und seine Analoga. Pharm Unserer Zeit 35:134–143

52. Smith JW III, McIntyre KJ, Avecedo PV, Encarnacion CA, Tedesco KL, Wang Y, Asmar L, O'Shaughnessy (2009) Results of a phase II open-label, non-randomized trial of oral satraplatin in patients with metastatic breast cancer. Breast Cancer Res Treat 118:361–367

53. Wilson JJ, Lippard SJ (2014) Synthetic methods for the preparation of platinum anticancer complexes. Chem Rev 114:4470–4495

54. Neumann W, Crews BC, Sárosi MB, Daniel CM, Ghebreselasie K, Scholz MS, Marnett LJ, Hey-Hawkins E (2015) Conjugation of cisplatin analogues and cyclooxygenase inhibitors to overcome cisplatin resistance. Chem Med Chem 10:183–192

55. Giglio V, Oliveri V, Viale M, Gangemi R, Natile G, Intini FP, Vecchio G (2015) Folate-cyclodextrin conjugates as carriers of the platinum(IV) complex LA-12. Chem Plus Chem 80:536–543

56. Wong DYQ, Yeo CHF, Ang WH (2014) Immuno-chemotherapeutic platinum(IV) prodrugs of cisplatin as multimodal anticancer agents. Angew Chem Int Ed 53:6752–6756

57. Yuan Y, Chen Y, Tang BZ, Liu B (2014) A targeted theranostic platinum(IV) prodrug containing a luminogen with aggregation-induced emission (AIE) characteristics for in situ monitoring of drug activation. Chem Commun 50:3868–3870

58. Yuan Y, Zhang C-J, Liu B (2015) A platinum prodrug conjugated with a photosensitizer with aggregation-induced emission (AIE) characteristics for drug activation monitoring and combinatorial photodynamic-chemotherapy against cisplatin resistant cancer cells. Chem Commun 51:8626–8629

59. Shi H, Cheng Q, Yuan S, Ding X, Liu Y (2015) Human serum albumin conjugated nanoparticles for pH and redox-responsive delivery of a prodrug of cisplatin. Chem Eur J 21:16547–16554

60. Lozano-Pérez AA, Gil AL, Pérez SA, Cutillas N, Meyer H, Pedreno M, Aznar-Cervantes SD, Janiak C, Cenis JL, Ruiz J (2015) Antitumor properties of platinum(IV) prodrug-loaded silk fibroin nanoparticles. Dalton Trans 44:13513–13521

61. Johnstone TC, Kulak N, Pridgen EM, Farokhzad OC, Langer R, Lippard SJ (2013) Nanoparticle encapsulation of mitaplatin and the effect thereof on in vivo properties. ACS Nano 7:5675–5683

62. Ang WH, Khalaila I, Allardyce CS, Juillerat-Jeanneret L, Dyson PJ (2005) Rational design of platinum(IV) compounds to overcome glutathione-*S*-transferase mediated drug resistance. J Am Chem Soc 127:1382–1383

63. LaPensee EW, Schwemberger SJ, LaPensee CR, Bahassi EM, Afton SE, Ben-Jonathan N (2009) Prolactin confers resistance against cisplatin in breast cancer cells by activating glutathione-*S*-transferase. Carcinogenesis 30:1298–1304

64. Hoffmann K, Lakomska I, Wisniewska J, Kaczmarek-Kedziera A, Wietrzyk J (2015) Acetate platinum(II) compound with 5,7-ditertbutyl-1,2,4-triazolo[1,5-a]pyrimidine that overcomes cisplatin resistance: structural characterization, in vitro cytotoxicity, and kinetic studies. J Coord Chem 68:3193–3208

65. Lakomska I, Hoffmann K, Wojtczak A, Sitkowski J, Maj E, Wietrzyk J (2014) Cytotoxic malonate platinum(II) complexes with 1,2,4-triazolo[1,5-a]pyrimidine derivatives: structural characterization and mechanism of the suppression of tumor cell growth. J Inorg Biochem 141:188–197

66. Zamora A, Rodríguez V, Cutillas N, Yellol GS, Espinosa A, Samper K, Capdevila M, Palacios O, Ruiz J (2013) New steroidal 7-azaindole platinum(II) antitumor complexes. J Inorg Biochem 128:48–56

67. Cutillas N, Mart'nez A, Yellol GS, Rodríguez V, Zamora A, Pedreno M, Donaire A, Janiak C, Ruiz J (2013) Anticancer C,N-cycloplatinated(II) complexes containing fluorinated phosphine ligands: synthesis, structural characterization, and biological activity. Inorg Chem 52:13529–13535

68. Nieto D, Bruna S, González-Vadillo AM, Perles J, Carillo-Hermosilla F, Antinolo A, Padrón JM, Plata GB, Cuadrado I (2015) Catalytically generated ferrocene-containing guanidines as efficient precursors for new redox-active heterometallic platinum(II) complexes with anticancer activity. Organometallics 34:5407–5417

69. Huang R, Wang Q, Zhang X, Zhu J, Sun B (2015) Trastuzumab-cisplatin conjugates for targeted delivery of cisplatin to HER2-overexpressing cancer cells. Biomed Pharmacother 72:17–23

70. Huang R, Sun Y, Zhang X, Sun B, Wang Q, Zhu J (2015) Biological evaluation of a novel Herceptin-platinum(II) conjugate for efficient and cancer cell specific delivery. Biomed Pharmacother 73:116–122

71. Alavizadeh SH, Akhtari J, Badiee A, Golmohammadzadeh S, Jaafari MR (2015) Improved therapeutic activity of HER2 affibody-targeted cisplatin liposomes in HER2-expressing breast tumor models. Exp Opin Drug Deliv 13:325–336

72. Muscella A, Vetrugno C, Fanizzi FP, Manca C, De Pascali SA, Marsigliante S (2013) A new platinum(II) compound anticancer drug candidate with selective cytotoxicity for breast cancer cells. Cell Death Dis 4:e796

73. Karmakar S, Chatterjee S, Purkait K, Mukherjee A (2016) Anticancer activity of a chelating nitrogen mustard bearing tetrachloroplatinum(IV) complex: better stability yet equipotent to the Pt(II) analogue. Dalton Trans 45:11710–11722

74. Liu W, Ye Q, Jiang J, Lou L, Xu Y, Xie C, Xie M (2013) *cis*-[Pt^{II}(1*R*,2*R*-DACH)(3-acetoxy-1,1-cyclobutanedicarboxylato)], a water-soluble, oxalate-free and stable analogue of oxaliplatin: synthesis, characterization, and biological evaluations. Chem Med Chem 8:1465–1467

75. Muenzner JK, Rehm T, Biersack B, Casini A, de Graaf IAM, Worawutputtapong P, Noor A, Kempe R, Brabec V, Kasparkova J, Schobert R (2015) Adjusting the DNA interaction and anticancer activity of Pt(II) N-heterocyclic carbene complexes by steric shielding of the *trans* leaving group. J Med Chem 58:6283–6292

76. Rehm T, Rothemund M, Muenzner JK, Noor A, Kempe R, Schobert R (2016) Novel *cis*-[(NHC)^{1}(NHC)^{2}(L)Cl]platinum(II) complexes – synthesis, structures, and anticancer activities. Dalton Trans 45:15390–15398

77. Schmitt F, Donnelly K, Muenzner JK, Rehm T, Novohradsky V, Brabec V, Kasparkova J, Albrecht M, Schobert R, Mueller T (2016) Effects of histidine-2-ylidene vs. imidazole-2-ylidene ligands on the anticancer and antivascular activity of complexes of ruthenium, iridium, platinum, and gold. J Inorg Biochem 163:221–228

78. Liu H, Li Y, Lyu Z, Wan Y, Li X, Chen H, Chen H, Li X (2014) Enzyme-triggered supramolecular self-assembly of platinum prodrug with enhanced tumor-selective accumulation and reduced systemic toxicity. J Mater Chem B 2:83038309

Chapter 14
Targeting of JAK-STAT Signaling in Breast Cancer: Therapeutic Strategies to Overcome Drug Resistance

Sobia Tabassum, Rashda Abbasi, Nafees Ahmad, and Ammad Ahmad Farooqi

Abstract Rapidly emerging ground-breaking discoveries have provided near to complete resolution of breast cancer signaling landscape and scientists have mapped the knowledge gaps associated with proteins encoded by the human genome. Based on the insights gleaned from decades of research, it seems clear that ligands transmit distinct information through specific receptors that is processed into characteristically unique biological outputs. Advances in imaging, structural biology, proteomics and genome editing have helped us to gain new insights into JAK-STAT signaling and how alterations in this pathway contributed to development of breast cancer and metastatic spread. Data obtained through high-throughput technologies has started to shed light on signal–transducer complexes formed during JAK-STAT signaling. Pharmacologists and molecular biologists are focusing on the strategies to therapeutically target this pathway to overcome drug resistance associated with breast cancer.

Keywords Janus Kinase · STAT · Cancer · Signaling · Apoptosis

14.1 Introduction

Wealth of information unequivocally illustrated instrumental role of JAK–STAT signaling cascade in breast cancer development and progression. Janus kinases (JAKs) are activated by cytosolically located domains of cytokine receptors upon cytokine binding. Granulocyte/macrophage colony-stimulatory factor (GM-CSF),

S. Tabassum
Department of Bioinformatics and Biotechnology, International Islamic University, Islamabad, Pakistan

R. Abbasi · N. Ahmad · A. A. Farooqi (✉)
Institute of Biomedical and Genetic Engineering (IBGE), Islamabad, Pakistan
e-mail: ammadfarooqi@rlmclahore.com

© Springer Nature Switzerland AG 2019
A. Ahmad (ed.), *Breast Cancer Metastasis and Drug Resistance*,
Advances in Experimental Medicine and Biology 1152,
https://doi.org/10.1007/978-3-030-20301-6_14

thrombopoietin, Erythropoietin, IL-3 and IL-5 transduce the signals through JAK2. While IFN-γ, IL-6, IL-10, IL-11, IL-19, IL-20 and IL-22 transmitted the signals through JAK1 and JAK2. JAK2-driven STAT phosphorylation resulted in homodimerization and heterodimerization of STAT proteins. STAT dimers moved into the nucleus and transcriptionally controlled expression of target genes. Suppressor of cytokine signaling (SOCS) proteins efficiently targeted entire cytokine-receptor complex for proteasomal degradation. Both SOCS1 and SOCS3 played central role in negative modulation of JAK-STAT. Structural studies provided evidence that SOCS proteins inhibited kinase activities of JAKs mainly through kinase inhibitory regions (KIR). In this chapter we have comprehensively summarized most recent evidence related to instrumental role of JAKs, STATs, SOCS and PIAS in breast cancer.

14.2   Janus Kinases

Janus kinases (JAK) belong to the family of non-receptor tyrosine kinases and centrally involved in activation of STAT proteins in breast cancer. It is therefore important to focus on different strategies which can target different JAKs to shut down JAK-STAT pathway.

0.1 Gy radiation dose reduced carcinogenesis by inhibition of the JAK1/STAT3 pathway [1]. Additionally, low-dose radiation exposure also reduced sphere formation and inhibited the self-renewal capacity of BCa cells, resulting in a significant reduction in $CD44^+/CD24^-$ population [1]. Secretion of IL-6 from non-stem cells was essential in the transformation of non-CSCs into CSCs by activating JAK1-STAT3-Oct-4 signaling axis [2].

Penta-O-galloyl-β-D-glucose   (PGG)   significantly   reduced   p-JAK1   in MDA-MB-231 BCa cells [3]. Shown in Fig. 14.1. Oral administration of 10 mg PGG/kg induced regression of tumors (49.3%) in mice xenografted with MDA-MB-231 BCa cells whereas intraperitoneally injected Taxol at the same dosage reduced tumor growth by 21.4% [3].

C-28 methyl ester of the oleane triterpenoid 2-cyano-3,12-dioxooleana-1,9-dien-28-oic acid (CDDO-Me) was very effective against JAK1-STAT3 pathway in BCa cells [4]. Shown in Fig. 14.1. Incubation of MDA-MB-468 BCa cells provided proof of binding of biotinylated- CDDO-Me to JAK1. Structural analysis suggested that kinase domain (KD) of JAK1 contained a cysteine residue at 1077th position. Expectedly, binding of biotinylated- CDDO-Me with purified recombinant JAK1-KD was noted [4].

It has previously been reported that targeting of IL-6/JAK2/STAT3/calprotectin signaling axis with FDA-approved agents, alone or combinatorially with HER2 inhibitors substantially repressed the tumorigenic properties of $HR^-/HER2^+$ BCa [5].

Methylsulfonylmethane and tamoxifen synergistically reduced phosphorylated levels of JAK2 in MCF-7 and T47D BCa cells [6]. Shown in Fig. 14.1. Both agents

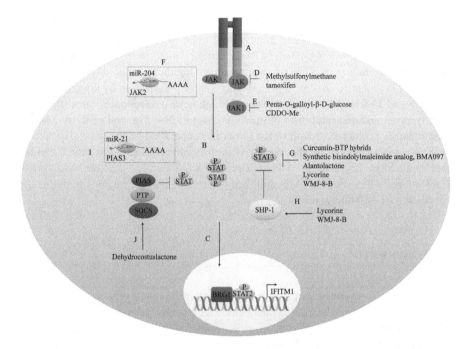

Fig. 14.1 Schematically represents JAK-STAT pathway. (**a, b**) JAK mediated phosphorylation of STAT proteins facilitated their accumulation in the nucleus to trigger expression of target genes. (**c**) BRG1 worked synchronously with STAT2 to stimulate expression of IFITM1. (**d**) Methylsulfonylmethane and tamoxifen inhibited JAK. (**e**) Penta-O-galloyl-β-D-glucose and CDDO-Me inhibited JAK1. (**f**) JAK2 was directly targeted by miR-204. (**g**) Different agents have been shown to reduce phosphorylated-STAT3 levels. (**h**) SHP-1, a negative regulator of STAT signaling was stimulated by Lycorine and WMJ-8-B. (**i**) PIAS3, another negative regulator of STAT signaling is also quantitatively controlled by miR-21. (**j**) SOCS can be stimulated by different agents

markedly reduced tumor growth in mice xenografted with MCF-7 BCa cells. Relative pulmonary metastases were also found to be significantly reduced in sections of the lungs excised from the orthotopic animal models [6].

Pre-treatment with the AG490 (JAK2 inhibitor) inhibited CXCL12-mediated STAT3 phosphorylation. Data clearly indicated that JAK2 mediated CXCR4-regulated STAT3 activation [7]. In the absence of CXCL12, JAK2 was immune-precipitated with CXCR4. After treatment with CXCL12, there was a remarkable increase in the binding of JAK2 to CXCR4, accompanied by increased level of p-STAT3, which suggested that CXCR4 directly activated JAK2 [7].

miR-204 directly targeted JAK2 in breast cancer [8]. Shown in Fig. 14.1. Apoptotic rate was dramatically enhanced in MCF-7 and MDA-MB-231 BCa cells transfected with miR-204 mimics [8]. Reconstitution of miR-204 can be an effective strategy to inhibit breast cancer progression but it still needs detailed research.

Previously published high-quality research clearly demonstrated that miRNA-23a/27a/24-2 cluster was downregulated in tumor associated macrophages (TAMs).

However, upregulation of the miRNA-23a/27a/24-2 clusters in macrophages induced regression of tumors in xenografted mice [9]. Binding of NF-κB to the promoter region of miRNA-23a/27a/24-2 cluster resulted in transcriptional repression whereas, binding of STAT6 to the promoter region stimulated the expression. MiRNA-27a and miRNA-23a inhibited macrophage polarization by targeting IRF4/ PPAR-γ and JAK1/STAT6, respectively, through negative feedback loops [9]. Data clearly explained that inhibition of miRNA-23a, miRNA-27a, and miRNA-24-2 in macrophages promoted growth of the tumor in xenografted mice.

Following section deals specifically with different STAT proteins which can be therapeutically targeted in breast cancer. STAT-family proteins are post-translationally modified by JAKs and then translocate into the nucleus to modulate expression of different genes.

14.3   STAT1

Molecular studies indicated that tyrosine kinases relied on a core set of signaling intermediates for transduction of oncogenic signals. One such scaffolding protein, Shc1 (ShcA) had been reported to structurally interact with different tyrosine kinases and played central role in tumor development, progression and metastatic spread in breast cancer models [10]. Mechanistically, it was shown that tyrosine kinases engaged Y239/240-ShcA phosphorylation sites to trigger STAT3-mediated-immunosuppressive signals and used Y313-ShcA sites to inhibit STAT1-dependent anti-tumor immunity. ShcA mutant mouse models were used for the study because all cell types in $ShcA^{2F/2F}$ and $ShcA^{313F/313F}$ animals lacked wild-type ShcA. Moreover, $ShcA^{313F/313F}$ and $ShcA^{2F/2F}$ female mice had the ability to undergo normal mammary gland development [10]. ShcA$^{+/+}$ cells model breast tumors had functionally active tyrosine kinase/ShcA axis, which simultaneously repressed STAT1 and activated STAT3 for immunosuppression. Shc$^{2F/2F}$ tumors represented those breast cancers which had low tyrosine kinase/ShcA signaling. STAT3 loss in Shc$^{313F/313F}$ mammary tumors did not affect tumor onset but delayed the growth of established tumors, specifically in a CD8$^{+/+}$ background. Thus, STAT3 contributed partially to the establishment of an immunosuppressive microenvironment in Shc$^{313F/313F}$ tumors. STAT1 deficiency in STAT3^{Low} tumors (Shc$^{2F/2F}$) significantly accelerated their growth, suggesting that STAT1 selectively conferred an immuno-surveillance response in mammary tumors which had lower STAT3 activity [10]. Development of inhibitors against Y239/240-ShcA phosphorylation site/s may prove to be an effective strategy to inhibit STAT3 activation and improve sensitivity to immunotherapeutics.

Coactivator protein SRC-1 (NCOA1), a versatile regulator was noted to be involved in modulation of molecular mechanisms related to endocrine therapy resistance in breast cancer [11]. SRC-1 worked synchronously with STAT1 for transcriptional regulation of TF/chromatin remodeler target genes. FIMO motif based sequence analyses and BioMART databases were used for better understanding and identification of loading of the SRC-1-binding molecules 10kb upstream to transcriptional start sites of target genes. H2AF2, STAT1 and H1-Histone Family, member (H1FX) binding sites were reported in the enhancer and promoter regions of different SRC-1 regulated genes, but astonishingly, only STAT1 response elements (SRE) were present upstream to various SRC-1 target genes. Immunoprecipitation assay was carried out for analysis of SRC-1-STAT1 interactions [11]. Moreover, positioning strategies of STAT1 individually and synchronously with SRC-1 to the binding regions in promoters of target genes were experimentally verified. ChIP and ChIP-re-ChIP qPCR methodologies were used for in-depth analysis of STAT1-SRC-1 in therapeutically resistant LY2 cells [11].

Certain hints have emerged which highlighted that VEGF fueled migratory and invasive potential of MDA-MB-231 cells. Accordingly, p-STAT1 and p-STAT3 levels were found to be enhanced and noted to be under control of VEGF in MDA-MB-231 cells [12]. Expectedly, reduction in the levels of p-STAT1 and p-STAT3 was noticed in VEGF silenced MDA-MB-231 cells. miR-20b was noted to directly target VEGF in MDA-MB-231 cancer cells. However, long noncoding RNA CAMTA1 protected VEGF from targeting by miR-20b by competitively binding with miR-20b [12].

Expression levels of STAT1 and alpha-smooth muscle actin (ACTA2) were noted to be upregulated in EGFR-positive BCa cells which transiently or stably overexpressed HER2 [13]. Basal ACTA2 expression was downregulated by treatment with fludarabine (STAT1 inhibitor) or AG490 (JAK2 inhibitor). Conversely, STAT1 overexpression triggered an increase in ACTA2 expression. There was a noteworthy reduction in the number of lung metastatic nodules in ACTA2 knockdown mice. Considerable reduction in metastatic sites in mice xenografted with ACTA2 silenced cancer cells [13].

14.4 Non-canonical Activation of STAT1 Is Useful

Tannic acid, a pharmacologically active polyphenol efficiently modulated non-canonical and canonical activation of STAT [14]. Phosphorylated JAK2, STAT1 and STAT3 were found to be significantly reduced in tannic acid-treated breast cancer cells. However, surprisingly, tannic acid induced an increase in phosphorylated p38 MAPK in a concentration-dependent manner. Data clearly provided a clue of tight association between p38MAPK activation and phosphorylation of STAT1 at 727th serine residue [14]. Nuclear extracts also provided evidence of reduced p-STAT3 and STAT1 tyrosine phosphorylation, whereas total STAT1 and p-STAT1 (serine 727) were noted to be enhanced. Tannic acid was unable to arrest STAT1 silenced breast cancer cells in G1 phase. Markedly enhanced levels of CDK4 and significantly reduced $p27^{Kip}$ and $p21^{Waf1/Cip1}$ were noticed in STAT1 silenced cancer cells. STAT1 binding sites were identified in promoter region of $p21^{Waf1/Cip1}$ [14]. Overall tannic acid enhanced p38MAPK/STAT1 signaling pathway to inhibit proliferation of breast cancer cells.

14.5 STAT2

Inflammatory breast cancer (IBC), a lethal and aggressive sub-type of breast cancer. Constitutive overexpression of Interferon-induced transmembrane protein 1 (IFITM1) has previously been reported in SUM149 IBC cells [15]. IFITM1 was dramatically reduced in STAT2 silenced SUM149 cells. Detailed mechanistic insights revealed that STAT2 promoted binding of brahma-related gene 1 (BRG1) to promoter region of IFITM1. Shown in Fig. 14.1. Data clearly suggested that increased expression of IFITM1 markedly promoted aggressive behavior of triple-negative SUM149 cells and STAT2/BRG1 worked in an orchestrated manner to trigger expression of IFITM1 [15].

14.6 STAT3

JAK2 and STAT3 showed an excessively high rate of protein-truncating mutations, such as nonsense base substitutions, splice site mutations and frameshift indels in breast cancer [16]. All such mutations were identified in ER+ BCa as compared to JAK2 amplifications which were identified in triple-negative BCa. JAK2 and STAT3 mutations were found to be more frequent in distant metastasis samples [16].

14.7 Natural and Synthetic Inhibitors of STAT3

Curcumin-BTP hybrids were found to be effective against STAT3 [17]. Curcumin-BTP hybrids exerted repressive effects on STAT3 phosphorylation, nuclear accumulation and inhibited STAT3-regulated target genes [17].

Synthetic bisindolylmaleimide analog, BMA097 directly interacted with SH2 (Src Homology 2) domain of STAT3 and inhibited STAT3 phosphorylation and activation, leading to downregulation of STAT3 driven genes [18]. Two new cis-clerodane-type furanoditerpenes, crispenes F and G obtained from the stems of *Tinospora crispa* inhibited STAT3 dimerization in MDA-MB-231 BCa cell line [19]. Alantolactone, a sesquiterpene lactone derived from *Inula helenium* dose-dependently reduced p-STAT3 in MDA-MB-231 BCa cells [20]. Lycorine, a pyrrolo[de]phenanthridine ring-type alkaloid obtained from Amaryllidaceae effectively inhibited phosphorylation of STAT3 and transcriptional activity via upregulation of SHP-1 [21]. Furthermore, SHP-1 was also noted to be stimulated by different other agents. Nintedanib, a multikinase inhibitor was found to efficiently reduce p-STAT3 levels mainly through SHP-1 [22]. Interestingly, Nintedanib mediated inhibitory effects on p-STAT3 were drastically impaired in SHP-1 silenced BCa cells [22]. WMJ-8-B, a novel hydroxamate derivative also promoted SHP-1 driven reduction in p-STAT3 levels in MDA-MB-231 cells [23]. WMJ-8-B induced regression of tumors in mice xenografted with MDA-MB-231 cells [23]. Galiellalactone-based STAT3-selective inhibitors inhibited phosphorylation of STAT3 at 705th tyrosine residue [24].

14.8 Crosstalk of STAT3 with GLI1/tGLI1 Facilitated Breast Carcinogenesis

SHH/GLI pathway played contributory role in breast cancer development and progression. Truncated GLI1.

(tGLI1) is a splice variant of GLI1 and contains a small in-frame deletions. tGLI1 retained all functionally active domains of GLI1, accumulated in the nucleus and transcriptionally controlled an array of genes [25]. STAT3 structurally associated with both GLI1 and tGLI1 in MDA-MB-468 BCa cells. STAT3 worked synergistically with GLI1/tGLI1 and promoted mammosphere-forming capacity of BCa cells and immortalized mammary epithelial cells [25].

14.9 STAT3 as a Regulator of Apoptosis: Reality or Fiction

RDD648 is a pharmacologically active derivative of riccardin D. RDD648 induced endoplasmic reticulum stress and lysosomal damage, as evidenced by formation of vacuoles and lysosomal membrane permeabilization [26]. RDD648 triggered activation of STAT3 and T-cell Transcription Factor-EB (TFEB). STAT3 partially inhibited TFEB driven transcriptional regulation of different genes. Partial inhibition of TFEB severely impaired its ability to facilitate lysosomal repair and biogenesis that consequently contributed to further lysosomal instability [26]. Overall these findings provided clues that STAT3 contributed to lysosomal-modulated cell death in BCa cells treated with RDD648.

14.10 Negative Regulator of JAK-STAT Signaling

It has earlier been reported that higher mRNA levels of SOCS1, 3, 4 and 7 were found to be significantly correlated with earlier stage of tumor and better clinical outcomes in BCa [27].

STAT proteins are also phosphorylated by Breast tumor kinase (Brk) in BCa cells [28]. Binding of SOCS3 to the Tyrosine Kinase Domain of Brk was noted in MDA-MB-231 BCa cells. SH2 domain of SOCS3 structurally interacted with phospho-tyrosines in the Brk tyrosine kinase domain. This binding facilitated re-orientation of SOCS3 and resulted in closer positioning of KIR domain to exert inhibitory effects on Brk [28]. Dehydrocostuslactone (DHE), a sesquiterpene lactone time-dependently enhanced SOCS-1 and SOCS-3 in MDA-MB-231 BCa cells [29].

Reduction in p-STAT3 levels promoted an increase in the expression of chemo-attractants Regulated on activation, normal T cell expressed and secreted (RANTES) and IP-10 in MCF-7 BCa cells and an increased migration of lymphocytes [30]. miR-21 was noted to directly target PIAS3. Shown in Fig. 14.1. Repression of PIAS3 triggered an increase in p-STAT3 levels. Therefore, targeted inhibition of miR-21 chaperoned PIAS3 from repression and promoted secretion of RANTES and IP-10 from MCF-7 BCa cells [30].

14.11   STAT4

Hepatitis B X-interacting protein (HBXIP) worked synchronously with STAT4 and stimulated expression of S100A4 in BCa cells [31]. Tumor growth was considerably enhanced in mice xenografted with HBXIP overexpressing MCF-7 BCa cells, whereas knockdown of S100A4 induced regression of tumors in xenografted mice [31].

14.12   STAT5

PR-domain containing protein-14 (PRDM14) is reportedly involved in repression of differentiation. STAT5 was noted to stimulate PRDM14 [32]. More importantly, CDC42 through phosphorylation of p-21 activated kinase (PAK1) promoted STAT5 activation and consequently STAT5 mediated upregulation of PRDM14. Certain hints have pointed towards central role of STAT5 in CDC42–PRDM14 signaling axis. Targeted inhibition of miRNA-424 induced an increase in transcript levels of PRDM14 by eightfolds, while STAT5 inhibition resulted in repression of PRDM14 by threefolds. Localization of STAT5 was noticed in nucleus in anti-miR-424-MDA231 BCa cells [32]. Phosphorylated-PAK1 co-localized with STAT5 and facilitated its nuclear accumulation. Data clearly suggested that CDC42 activated STAT5, through phosphorylation of PAK1 that resulted in PRDM14 activation [32]. Mechanistically it was revealed that miR-424–CDC42–PRDM14 axis contributed to BCa metastases under hyperglycemic situation through enhanced invasion and hyper-activation of breast cancer stem cells pool.

Overexpression of CUB and zona pellucida-like domain-containing protein-1 (CUZD1) in non-transformed mammary epithelial cells significantly enhanced tumorigenic potential of these cells [33]. Orthotopic inoculation of these cells in mouse mammary glands triggered formation of adenocarcinomas, increased quantities of p-STAT5 and EGF cascade activation. Chemical blockade of STAT5 by pimozide considerably repressed the production of growth factors of EGF family and inhibited PRL-mediated proliferation of cancer cells. Pimozide induced regression of CUZD1-driven mammary tumorigenesis in xenografted mice. Both p-STAT5 and CUZD1 were reduced in the nucleus in PRLR silenced cells [33]. Chromatin immunoprecipitation for p-STAT5 and CUZD1 demonstrated that the loss of Prolactin receptor (PRLR) markedly reduced loading of STAT5/CUZD1 at promoter region of epiregulin. It seems encouraging that knockdown of CUZD1 and STAT5 can prove to be helpful in the treatment of breast cancer.

14.13 Conclusion

Recent functional studies of JAK-STAT pathway with the use of structural biology approaches and functional genomics have helped us in developing a better understanding of contributory role played by this cascade in breast cancer development and progression. We have witnessed tremendous breakthroughs in molecular oncology and it is now more understandable that deregulation of spatio-temporally controlled JAK-STAT pathway is therapeutically challenging. Substantial fraction of information has been added related to different JAKs, STATs, SOCS in breast cancer. Moreover, pharmacologists and natural product researchers are focusing on identification of bioactive molecules which can effectively target JAK-STAT pathway with minimum off-target effects.

References

1. Kaushik N, Kim MJ, Kim RK, Kumar Kaushik N, Seong KM, Nam SY, Lee SJ (2017) Low-dose radiation decreases tumor progression via the inhibition of the JAK1/STAT3 signaling axis in breast cancer cell lines. Sci Rep 7:43361. https://doi.org/10.1038/srep43361
2. Kim SY, Kang JW, Song X, Kim BK, Yoo YD, Kwon YT, Lee YJ (2013) Role of the IL-6-JAK1-STAT3-Oct-4 pathway in the conversion of non-stem cancer cells into cancer stem-like cells. Cell Signal 25(4):961–969. https://doi.org/10.1016/j.cellsig.2013.01.007
3. Lee HJ, Seo NJ, Jeong SJ, Park Y, Jung DB, Koh W, Lee HJ, Lee EO, Ahn KS, Ahn KS, Lü J, Kim SH (2011) Oral administration of penta-O-galloyl-β-D-glucose suppresses triple-negative breast cancer xenograft growth and metastasis in strong association with JAK1-STAT3 inhibition. Carcinogenesis 32(6):804–811. https://doi.org/10.1093/carcin/bgr015
4. Ahmad R, Raina D, Meyer C, Kufe D (2008) Triterpenoid CDDO-methyl ester inhibits the Janus-activated kinase-1 (JAK1)-->signal transducer and activator of transcription-3 (STAT3) pathway by direct inhibition of JAK1 and STAT3. Cancer Res 68(8):2920–2926. https://doi.org/10.1158/0008-5472.CAN-07-3036
5. Rodriguez-Barrueco R, Yu J, Saucedo-Cuevas LP, Olivan M, Llobet-Navas D, Putcha P, Castro V, Murga-Penas EM, Collazo-Lorduy A, Castillo-Martin M, Alvarez M, Cordon-Cardo C, Kalinsky K, Maurer M, Califano A, Silva JM (2015) Inhibition of the autocrine IL-6-JAK2-STAT3-calprotectin axis as targeted therapy for HR-/HER2+ breast cancers. Genes Dev 29(15):1631–1648. https://doi.org/10.1101/gad.262642.115
6. Nipin SP, Darvin P, Yoo YB, Joung YH, Kang DY, Kim DN, Hwang TS, Kim SY, Kim WS, Lee HK, Cho BW, Kim HS, Park KD, Park JH, Chang SH, Yang YM (2015) The combination of methylsulfonylmethane and tamoxifen inhibits the Jak2/STAT5b pathway and synergistically

inhibits tumor growth and metastasis in ER-positive breast cancer xenografts. BMC Cancer 15:474. https://doi.org/10.1186/s12885-015-1445-0

7. Liu X, Xiao Q, Bai X, Yu Z, Sun M, Zhao H, Mi X, Wang E, Yao W, Jin F, Zhao L, Ren J, Wei M (2014) Activation of STAT3 is involved in malignancy mediated by CXCL12-CXCR4 signaling in human breast cancer. Oncol Rep 32(6):2760–2768. https://doi.org/10.3892/or.2014.3536. Epub 2014 Oct 10

8. Wang X, Qiu W, Zhang G, Xu S, Gao Q, Yang Z (2015) MicroRNA-204 targets JAK2 in breast cancer and induces cell apoptosis through the STAT3/BCl-2/survivin pathway. Int J Clin Exp Pathol 8(5):5017–5025. eCollection 2015

9. Ma S, Liu M, Xu Z, Li Y, Guo H, Ge Y, Liu Y, Zheng D, Shi J (2016) A double feedback loop mediated by microRNA-23a/27a/24-2 regulates M1 versus M2 macrophage polarization and thus regulates cancer progression. Oncotarget 7(12):13502–13519. https://doi.org/10.18632/oncotarget.6284

10. Ahn R, Sabourin V, Bolt AM, Hébert S, Totten S, De Jay N, Festa MC, Young YK, Im YK, Pawson T, Koromilas AE, Muller WJ, Mann KK, Kleinman CL, Ursini-Siegel J (2017) The Shc1 adaptor simultaneously balances Stat1 and Stat3 activity to promote breast cancer immune suppression. Nat Commun 8:14638. https://doi.org/10.1038/ncomms14638

11. Browne AL, Charmsaz S, Varešlija D, Fagan A, Cosgrove N, Cocchiglia S, Purcell S, Ward E, Bane F, Hudson L, Hill AD, Carroll JS, Redmond AM, Young LS (2018) Network analysis of SRC-1 reveals a novel transcription factor hub which regulates endocrine resistant breast cancer. Oncogene. https://doi.org/10.1038/s41388-017-0042-x

12. Lu P, Gu Y, Li L, Wang F, Yang X, Yang Y (2017) Long noncoding RNA CAMTA1 promotes proliferation and mobility of human breast cancer cell line MDA- MB-231 via targeting miR-20b. Oncol Res. https://doi.org/10.3727/096504017X14953948675395

13. Jeon M, You D, Bae SY, Kim SW, Nam SJ, Kim HH, Kim S, Lee JE (2016) Dimerization of EGFR and HER2 induces breast cancer cell motility through STAT1-dependent ACTA2 induction. Oncotarget 8(31):50570–50581. https://doi.org/10.18632/oncotarget.10843

14. Darvin P, Joung YH, Kang DY, Sp N, Byun HJ, Hwang TS, Sasidharakurup H, Lee CH, Cho KH, Park KD, Lee HK, Yang YM (2017) Tannic acid inhibits EGFR/STAT1/3 and enhances p38/STAT1 signalling axis in breast cancer cells. J Cell Mol Med 21(4):720–734. https://doi.org/10.1111/jcmm.13015

15. Ogony J, Choi HJ, Lui A, Cristofanilli M, Lewis-Wambi J (2016) Interferon-induced trans-membrane protein 1 (IFITM1) overexpression enhances the aggressive phenotype of SUM149 inflammatory breast cancer cells in a signal transducer and activator of transcription 2 (STAT2)-dependent manner. Breast Cancer Res 18(1):25. https://doi.org/10.1186/s13058-016-0683-7

16. Yates LR, Knappskog S, Wedge D, Farmery JHR, Gonzalez S, Martincorena I, Alexandrov LB, Van Loo P, Haugland HK, Lilleng PK, Gundem G, Gerstung M, Pappaemmanuil E, Gazinska P, Bhosle SG, Jones D, Raine K, Mudie L, Latimer C, Sawyer E, Desmedt C, Sotiriou C, Stratton MR, Sieuwerts AM, Lynch AG, Martens JW, Richardson AL, Tutt A, Lønning PE, Campbell PJ (2017) Genomic evolution of breast cancer metastasis and relapse. Cancer Cell 32(2):169–184.e7. https://doi.org/10.1016/j.ccell.2017.07.005

17. Zhang W, Guo J, Li S, Ma T, Xu D, Han C, Liu F, Yu W, Kong L (2017) Discovery of monocarbonyl curcumin-BTP hybrids as STAT3 inhibitors for drug-sensitive and drug-resistant breast cancer therapy. Sci Rep 7:46352. https://doi.org/10.1038/srep46352

18. Li X, Ma H, Li L, Chen Y, Sun X, Dong Z, Liu JY, Zhu W, Zhang JT (2018b) Novel synthetic bisindolylmaleimide alkaloids inhibit STAT3 activation by binding to the SH2 domain and suppress breast xenograft tumor growth. Oncogene. https://doi.org/10.1038/s41388-017-0076-0

19. Noman MAA, Hossain T, Ahsan M, Jamshidi S, Hasan CM, Rahman KM (2018) Crispenes F and G, cis-clerodane furanoditerpenoids from tinospora crispa, inhibit STAT3 dimerization. J Nat Prod 81(2):236–242. https://doi.org/10.1021/acs.jnatprod.7b00377

20. Cui L, Bu W, Song J, Feng L, Xu T, Liu D, Ding W, Wang J, Li C, Ma B, Luo Y, Jiang Z, Wang C, Chen J, Hou J, Yan H, Yang L, Jia X (2017) Apoptosis induction by alantolactone in breast cancer MDA-MB-231 cells through reactive oxygen species-mediated mitochondrion-dependent pathway. Arch Pharm Res. https://doi.org/10.1007/s12272-017-0990-2

21. Wang J, Xu J, Xing G (2017) Lycorine inhibits the growth and metastasis of breast cancer through the blockage of STAT3 signaling pathway. Acta Biochim Biophys Sin Shanghai 49(9):771–779. https://doi.org/10.1093/abbs/gmx076
22. Liu CY, Huang TT, Chu PY, Huang CT, Lee CH, Wang WL, Lau KY, Tsai WC, Chao TI, Su JC, Chen MH, Shiau CW, Tseng LM, Chen KF (2017) The tyrosine kinase inhibitor nintedanib activates SHP-1 and induces apoptosis in triple-negative breast cancer cells. Exp Mol Med 49(8):e366. https://doi.org/10.1038/emm.2017.114
23. Chuang YF, Huang SW, Hsu YF, Yu MC, Ou G, Huang WJ, Hsu MJ (2017) WMJ-8-B, a novel hydroxamate derivative, induces MDA-MB-231 breast cancer cell death via the SHP-1-STAT3-survivin cascade. Br J Pharmacol 174(17):2941–2961. https://doi.org/10.1111/bph.13929
24. Kim HS, Kim T, Ko H, Lee J, Kim YS, Suh YG (2017) Identification of galiellalactone-based novel STAT3-selective inhibitors with cytotoxic activities against triple-negative breast cancer cell lines. Bioorg Med Chem 25(19):5032–5040. https://doi.org/10.1016/j.bmc.2017.06.036
25. Sirkisoon SR, Carpenter RL, Rimkus T, Anderson A, Harrison A, Lange AM, Jin G, Watabe K, Lo HW (2018) Interaction between STAT3 and GLI1/tGLI1 oncogenic transcription factors promotes the aggressiveness of triple-negative breast cancers and HER2-enriched breast cancer. Oncogene. https://doi.org/10.1038/s41388-018-0132-4
26. Li L, Sun B, Gao Y, Niu H, Yuan H, Lou H (2018a) STAT3 contributes to lysosomal-mediated cell death in a novel derivative of riccardin D-treated breast cancer cells in association with TFEB. Biochem Pharmacol 150:267–279. https://doi.org/10.1016/j.bcp.2018.02.026. [Epub ahead of print]
27. Sasi W, Jiang WG, Sharma A, Mokbel K (2010) Higher expression levels of SOCS 1,3,4,7 are associated with earlier tumour stage and better clinical outcome in human breast cancer. BMC Cancer 10:178. https://doi.org/10.1186/1471-2407-10-178
28. Gao Y, Cimica V, Reich NC (2012) Suppressor of cytokine signaling 3 inhibits breast tumor kinase activation of STAT3. J Biol Chem 287(25):20904–20912. https://doi.org/10.1074/jbc.M111.334144
29. Kuo PL, Ni WC, Tsai EM, Hsu YL (2009) Dehydrocostuslactone disrupts signal transducers and activators of transcription 3 through up-regulation of suppressor of cytokine signaling in breast cancer cells. Mol Cancer Ther 8(5):1328–1339. https://doi.org/10.1158/1535-7163.MCT-08-0914
30. Wang Z, Han J, Cui Y, Zhou X, Fan K (2013) miRNA-21 inhibition enhances RANTES and IP-10 release in MCF-7 via PIAS3 and STAT3 signalling and causes increased lymphocyte migration. Biochem Biophys Res Commun 439(3):384–389. https://doi.org/10.1016/j.bbrc.2013.08.072
31. Liu S, Li L, Zhang Y, Zhang Y, Zhao Y, You X, Lin Z, Zhang X, Ye L (2012) The oncoprotein HBXIP uses two pathways to up-regulate S100A4 in promotion of growth and migration of breast cancer cells. J Biol Chem 287(36):30228–30239. https://doi.org/10.1074/jbc.M112.343947
32. Nandy SB, Orozco A, Lopez-Valdez R, Roberts R, Subramani R, Arumugam A, Dwivedi AK, Stewart V, Prabhakar G, Jones S, Lakshmanaswamy R (2017) Glucose insult elicits hyperactivation of cancer stem cells through miR-424-cdc42-prdm14 signalling axis. Br J Cancer 117(11):1665–1675. https://doi.org/10.1038/bjc.2017.335
33. Mapes J, Anandan L, Li Q, Neff A, Clevenger CV, Bagchi IC, Bagchi MK (2018) Aberrantly high expression of the CUB and zona pellucida-like domain-containing protein 1 (CUZD1) in mammary epithelium leads to breast tumorigenesis. J Biol Chem 293(8):2850–2864. https://doi.org/10.1074/jbc.RA117.000162

Chapter 15
Role of mTORC1 and mTORC2 in Breast Cancer: Therapeutic Targeting of mTOR and Its Partners to Overcome Metastasis and Drug Resistance

Ghazala Butt, Durray Shahwar, Muhammad Zahid Qureshi, Rukset Attar, Misbah Akram, Yelda Birinci, Gokce Seker Karatoprak, Maria Luisa Gasparri, and Ammad Ahmad Farooqi

G. Butt (✉)
Department of Botany, GCU, Lahore, Pakistan
e-mail: dr.ghazalayasmeen@gcu.edu.pk

D. Shahwar
Lahore College for Women University, Lahore, Pakistan

M. Z. Qureshi
Department of Chemistry, GCU, Lahore, Pakistan

R. Attar (✉)
Department of Obstetrics and Gynecology, Faculty of Medicine, Yeditepe University, Istanbul, Turkey

M. Akram
Department of Bioinformatics and Biotechnology, International Islamic University, Islamabad, Pakistan

Y. Birinci
Faculty of Engineering and Natural Sciences, Sabanci University, Istanbul, Turkey

G. S. Karatoprak
Department of Pharmacognosy, Faculty of Pharmacy, Erciyes University, Kayseri, Turkey

M. L. Gasparri
Department of Gynecology and Obstetrics, University Hospital of Bern and University of Bern, Bern, Switzerland

Department of Gynecology and Obstetrics, "Sapienza" University of Rome, Rome, Italy

Surgical and Medical Department of Translational Medicine, "Sapienza" University of Rome, Rome, Italy

A. A. Farooqi
Laboratory for Translational Oncology and Personalized Medicine, RLMC, Lahore, Pakistan

© Springer Nature Switzerland AG 2019
A. Ahmad (ed.), *Breast Cancer Metastasis and Drug Resistance*,
Advances in Experimental Medicine and Biology 1152,
https://doi.org/10.1007/978-3-030-20301-6_15

Abstract Based on the insights gleaned from decades of research, it seems clear that mechanistic target of rapamycin (mTOR) is an essential signaling node that integrates environmental clues for regulation of cell survival, metabolism and proliferation of the cells. However, overwhelmingly increasing scientific evidence has added a new layer of intricacy to already complicated and versatile signaling pathway of mTOR. Deregulation of spatio-temporally controlled mTOR-driven pathway played contributory role in breast cancer development and progression. Pharmacologists and molecular biologists have specifically emphasized on the identification and development of mTOR-pathway inhibitors. In this chapter we have attempted to provide an overview of the most recent findings related to therapeutic targeting of mTOR-associated mTORC1 and mTORC2 in breast cancer. We have also comprehensively summarized regulation of mTOR and its partners by microRNAs in breast cancer.

Keywords mTOR · Signaling · Therapy · Apoptosis

15.1 Introduction

Mechanistic target of rapamycin (mTOR) has emerged as a master regulator and proteomic studies have helped in identification of binding partners of mTOR. Detailed mechanistic insights revealed that mTOR worked synchronously with different proteins which assembled to form a signalosome. mTOR strategically formed functionally distinct and characteristically unique mTOR complexes: mTORC1 and mTORC2. mTORC1 multi-component machinery contained RAPTOR (regulatory-associated protein of mTOR). Phosphatidylinositol-3-kinase (PI3K) and PKB/AKT inhibited RHEB (Ras-homolog enriched in brain), which resulted in the activation of mTORC1 (Shown in Fig. 15.1). Eukaryotic translation initiation factor 4E (eIF4E)-binding protein 1 (4E-BP1) belongs to the family of translational repressors and a direct target of mTOR. Booth 4E-BP1 and ribosomal protein S6 kinase-1 (S6K1) were found to be phosphorylated by mTOR. mTORC2 complex contained RICTOR (rapamycin-insensitive companion of mTOR) and phosphorylated at 473rd serine residue and increased degree of activation of AKT (Shown in Fig. 15.1). AKT had a linchpin role in mTOR-induced pathway because it acted as a downstream effector of mTORC2 and an upstream activator of mTORC1. FKBP8 and PRAS40 were found to negatively modulate mTOR –mediated signaling. FKBP8 prevented RHEB from activation of mTORC1 and PRAS40 competed with RAPTOR for binding to 4E-BP1 and S6K1 (Shown in Fig. 15.1). Rapidly emerging experimentally verified data has demystified additional proteins complexes which played critical role in regulation of mTOR pathway. GATOR (GTPase-activating protein (GAP) activity toward RAGs) complex critically regulated the pathway which signaled amino acid sufficiency to mTORC1. GATOR is composed of two sub-complexes, GATOR1 and GATOR2. More importantly, when amino acids were low, mTOR-driven signaling was inhibited by GATOR1. Inhibition of the molecules

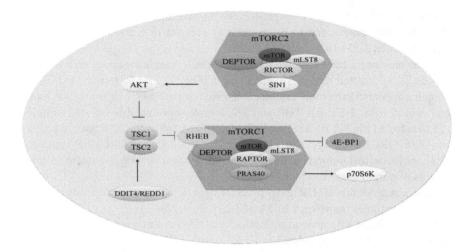

Fig. 15.1 schematically represents mTOR–driven signaling. mTOR transduced the signals through mTORC1 and mTORC2. PKB/AKT inhibited TSC and facilitated activation of mTORC1, a multi-protein signalosome. RAPTOR was a major component of mTORC1, whereas, PRAS40 negatively regulated mTORC1. mTORC1 activated p70S6K and inhibited 4E-BP1. mTORC2 activated AKT. RICTOR was an important member of mTORC2. Tuberous sclerosis complex (TSC), Mechanistic target of rapamycin (mTOR), Regulatory-associated protein of mTOR (RAPTOR), Rapamycin-insensitive companion of mammalian target of rapamycin (RICTOR), Proline-rich Akt substrate of 40 kDa (PRAS40), DNA-damage-inducible transcript 4 (DDIT4)

of GATOR1 multi-protein assembly, nitrogen permease regulator proteins (NPRL2, NPRL3) and DEP domain-containing protein-5 (DEPDC5) made mTORC1-driven pathway resistant to amino acid deprivation.

The main aim of this chapter is, firstly, to review our recently evolving knowledge about signaling downstream of mTOR to the translational machinery and, secondly, to schematically represent how mTORC1 and mTORC2 played contributory role in breast cancer development and progression and how these signalosomes can be therapeutically targeted. In the upcoming section we will discuss how microRNAs played versatile role in regulation of mTOR-triggered pathway.

15.2 miRNA Regulation of mTOR Pathway in Breast Cancer

MicroRNAs are non-coding RNAs which have emerged as key players in the field of molecular oncology. miRNAs are broadly characterized into oncogenic and tumor suppressor miRNAs. Discovery of miRNAs has doubtlessly re-shaped our concepts related to central dogma of molecular biology. miRNA regulation has revolutionized our existing concepts related to mTOR signaling and molecular biologists have started to unveil how different miRNAs post-transcriptionally controlled various proteins of mTORC1 and mTORC2 in different cancers. These regulations are also studied in breast cancer but the available data is insufficient.

miR-184 was noted to be epigenetically inactive in breast cancer. AKT2 and PRAS40 levels were found to be remarkably reduced in miR-184 mimics transfected MDA-MB-231 BCa cells [20].

It has previously been reported that TSC1/TSC2 complex induced activation of mTORC2 and exerted repressive effects on mTORC1 [13]. Seemingly, mTORC2 signaling appeared to be more prominent in ERα^+ and mTORC1 signaling was more prevalent in ERα^- BCa. RICTOR and TSC1 levels were notably reduced in miR-155 transfected MCF-7 BCa cells which highlighted that miR-155 triggered activation of mTORC1. Findings clearly suggested that miR-155/mTORC1/ER signaling axis contributed to development of hormone independent phenotype evident through the loss of progesterone receptor (PgR) [13].

Levels of p-AKT, p-mTOR and p-p70S6K were found to be dramatically reduced in miR-10a mimics transfected MDA-MB-231 BCa cells [7].

Deregulation of long noncoding RNAs (lncRNAs) is a major stumbling block in standardization of therapy related to HER2-positive BCa [8, 9]. GAS5, a lncRNA was found to be downregulated BCa cells. Lapatinib upregulated GAS5 in trastuzumab-resistant BCa cells via inhibition of mTOR pathway. GAS5 competitively binds to miR-21 and sequesters it away from PTEN. PTEN is a negative regulator of PI3K/AKT pathway. İnhibition of mTOR by rapamycin induced an increase in GAS5 expression [8, 9].

Recently accumulating evidence has highlighted newer roles of integrins and integrin-dependent signaling cascade in BCa. Furthermore, recent reports have also uncovered new functions of core adhesion molecules in BCa-related cascades distal to cell–extracellular matrix (ECM) contacts and this was exemplified by the core adhesome kinase, FAK. Focal adhesion kinase (FAK), a focal adhesion-localized protein was found to be functionally active in response to ECM-integrin interaction and prolonged integrin–ECM-initiated signals following internalization of receptors to promote anchorage-independent growth of BCa cells and to fuel metastases.

V-ets erythroblastosis virus E26 oncogene homolog-1 (ETS-1) played significant role in breast cancer progression [8, 9]. ETS-binding sites have previously been identified in promoter of β1 integrin and inhibition of ETS-1 markedly reduced expression of β1-integrin. Mechanistically, miRNA-199a-5p directly targeted ETS-1 in BCa cells. ETS-1 expression was observed to be downregulated in miR-199a-5p overexpressing MDA-MB-231 BCa cells. More importantly, FAK/Src/AKT/mTOR axis was noted to be inactive in miR-199a-5p overexpressing BCa cells [8, 9]. miR-147 also exerted inhibitory effects on of AKT/mTOR pathway in BCa cells [25].

On the basis of the high-quality research and the above discussion, we propose two areas which need detailed research. (1) Since its discovery, field of microRNAs has undergone substantial broadening, however, we still have to see how different miRNAs regulated positive and negative regulators of mTORC1 and mTORC2 in breast cancer. (2) Can mTOR inhibitors be used in combination with miRNA mimics in breast cancer?

15.3 Therapeutic Targeting of mTOR Pathways

MAPK-interacting kinases (MNKs) phosphorylated 209th serine residue of eIF4E and promoted expression of oncogenic proteins, whereas mTORC1 phosphorylated and inhibited 4E-BP1 to re-activate translational of different oncogenes [10]. Pyrimidine derivative, PP242 (torkinib) effectively reduced phosphorylated levels of 4E-BP1 and mTORC1-downstream targets, including p70S6K and ribosomal protein S6. Inhibition of PI3K/AKT/mTOR and MNK-eIF4E pathways significantly impaired migratory potential of MDA-MB-231 BCa cells [10].

In a model of breast cancer, RICTOR inhibition resulted in repression of phosphorylation at 473rd serine residue in AKT which delayed tumor latency and burden. PP242 and lapatinib reduced p-AKT levels in SKBR3, BT474 and MDA-MB-361 BCa cells [17].

mTORC1/2 inhibitor vistusertib (AZD2014) and palbociclib (CDK4/6 inhibitor) synergistically reduced tumor growth and decreased transcriptional upregulation of E2F-target genes [16]. RAPTOR and RHEB were found to be reduced in EVI1 depleted cells [14]. Chromatin immunoprecipitation (ChIP) analysis provided evidence of accumulation of EVI1 at promoter region of SOX9 in untreated HCC1937 and everolimus-adapted cell models [14]. TSC1 formed a complex with TSC2 and inhibited mTOR-induced downstream signaling. In untreated cancer, lower levels of TSC1/2 were found to be correlated with enhanced activity of mTORC1 and with a primary metastatic phenotype. EVI1 and SOX9 were noted to be functionally active in cancer cells treated with mTOR inhibitors and strategically sustained mTOR signaling through upregulation of RAPTOR and RHEB [14].

Estrogen stimulated nuclear accumulation of RAPTOR in BT474 BCa cells [1]. Nuclear interaction between ERα and RAPTOR occurred rapidly within 10 min after estrogen treatment. mTOR physically interacted and phosphorylated ERα. Mechanistically it was shown that ERα physically associated with RAPTOR and recruited mTORC1 to the nucleus where mTOR phosphorylated ERα, which resulted in transcriptional upregulation of target genes [1].

AKT phosphorylated 40 kDa Proline-rich AKT1 substrate (PRAS40/AKT1S1) at 246th threonine residue and sequestered it away from mTOR and blocked PRAS40-modulated repressive effects on mTORC1 [15]. Interestingly, mTORC1 phosphorylated on 183rd serine residue in PRAS40. Phosphorylated levels of 4E-BP1, p70S6K and S6 were notably enhanced in PRAS40-knockdown MCF7 BCa cells. AKT inhibitor (MK2206) and rapamycin synergistically reduced phosphorylated levels of PRAS40 and 4E-BP1 [15].

RICTOR overexpression significantly enhanced metastases in spontaneous and intravenously seeded models of HER2-overexpressing BCa [18]. RICTOR inhibition markedly suppressed migration and invasion of HER2-amplified BCa cells. It was intriguing to note that active Rac1 played central role in RICTOR-dependent invasion and motility, and it also rescued invasive potential of RICTOR depleted cells. RICTOR/mTORC2 mediated inhibition of RhoGDI2 (Rac1 inhibitor), promoted Rac1 activity and invasion of tumor cells [18]. T-lymphoma invasion and metastasis-inducing protein-1 (TIAM1) activated Rac1 by promoting the exchange of Rac1 bound GDP for GTP. mTORC2 substrate PKB/AKT did not affect RhoGDI2 inhibition, but partially increased Rac1 activity through TIAM1, thus partially rescuing cellular invasion. mTORC2 effector, PKCα rescued RICTOR-mediated RhoGDI2 inhibition, partially rescued Rac-GTP and migration of BCa cells [18]. In the upcoming section we will conceptually summarize how natural products have played their role in effective targeting of mTOR –driven pathway.

15.4   Natural Products Mediated Targeting of mTOR and Its Complexes

Nordihydroguaiaretic acid (NDGA), isolated from the creosote bush Larrea divaricate efficiently exerted inhibitory effects on basal levels of mTORC1 but mTORC2 activity remained unchanged in BCa cells [24]. Though NDGA stimulated AMPK/TSC2 pathway, which negatively regulated mTORC1, but astonishingly, NDGA mediated inhibitory effects on mTORC1 were not impaired in AMPK and TSC2 depleted BCa cells. Mechanistically, NDGA directly targeted mTORC1 complex because NDGA suppressed amino acids- and insulin-triggered mTORC1 and behaved like rapamycin to interfere with mTOR-RAPTOR interactions [24]. Anthricin (deoxypodophyllotoxin), derived from *Anthriscus sylvestris* (L.) markedly inhibited phosphorylated AKT and mTORC1 in BCa cells [6]. 20 μM of piperlongumine significantly reduced phosphorylated levels of TSC2, 4E-BP1 and p70S6K in MCF-7 BCa cells [12]. Rottlerin exerted inhibitory effects on phospho-P70S6K (70 kDa) and phospho-S6 (32 kDa) in MDA-MB-231 and T-47D BCa cells [11]. DNA damage-inducible transcript-4 (DDIT4) was noted to inhibit mTORC1 activity in BCa cells [22]. Baicalein, a natural flavone markedly upregulated DDIT4 in MDA468 and SKBR3 BCa cells (Shown in Fig. 15.2). Baicalein was intraperitoneally injected into tumor bearing mice. Data clearly suggested that Baicalein induced regression of tumors in SCID mice xenografted with MDA468 BCa cells. Baicalein suppressed phosphorylation of both S6K1 and S6 in MDA468 BCa cells. mTORC1 activity was not inhibited in DDIT4 knockdown BCa cells [22].

Secalonic acid-D (SAD), a mycotoxin significantly inhibited mTOR-driven downstream proteins such as p70S6K and 4E-BP1 in MCF-7 BCa cells [5]. Extract of *Astragalus membranaceus* efficiently repressed p-PI3K, p-AKT and p-mTOR in MCF-7, MDA-MB-231 and SK-BR-3 BCa cells [27]. Delphinidin notably inhibited phospho-AKT and phospho-mTOR in BT474 and MDA-MB-453 BCa cells [4]. Eriocalyxin B time-dependently reduced the phosphorylation of AKT/PKB, mTOR and p70S6K leading to the inactivation of AKT/mTOR/p70S6K signal transduction cascade in BCa cells (Shown in Fig. 15.2) [26].

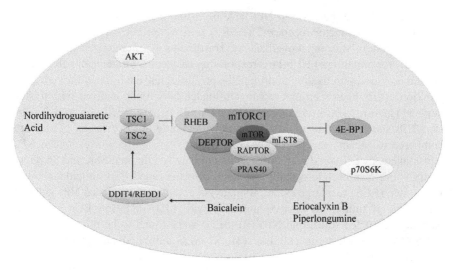

Fig. 15.2 shows natural products mediated targeting of mTOR pathway. Different natural products targeted different proteins of mTOR pathway

Natural products mediated targeting of mTORC1 has been extensively studied. However, targeting of mTORC2 by different phytochemicals needs detailed research. It will also be essential to demystify negative regulators of mTORC1 and mTORC2 in different cancers and how these proteins can be effectively targeted by different natural products.

15.5   Nano-formulated Drugs for Targeting of mTOR Pathway in Breast Cancer

It is well known that mTOR Complexes activation stimulates tumor progression and malignancy of breast cancer cells. mTOR inhibitors have been noted to show less efficiency because of their limited pharmacokinetic properties such as poor solubility, low bioavailability, and uncontrolled release. For example, rapamycin and its analogs are frequently being used as inhibitors for mTOR signaling. When it is systemically administered to the patient it can easily diffuse and accumulate in vital tissues. Thus, it may cause serious side effects since rapamycin is a strong immunosuppressant by itself. Recently, rapamycin has been formulated as a nano-formulation to overcome its limited administration and to reduce its systemic side effects. Another important contribution of nanoformulated drug usage in cancer treatment is providing a unique opportunity to improve efficacy and biodistribution of the drugs. In accordance with this concept, rapamycin loaded glyceryl monooleate (GMO) based-lipid-NPs have been found to be useful against human epidermal growth factor receptor-2 (HER2) positive SKBR3 BCa cells by [19]. The nanosystem was functionalized by Trastuzumab, a humanized monoclonal antibody, for targeting of HER2 overexpressing BCa cells. Strategically, this nanosystem provided stabilization of drug in the physiological environment for a longer duration. It has been seen that rapamycin-loaded NPs functionalized with trastuzumab (Tmab-rapa-NPs) are more effective for killing cancer cells. Overall, Tmab-rapa-NPs showed significant activity in downregulation of expression of markers compared to rapamycin effect only [19]. Rapamycin and paclitaxel loaded NPs advantageously delivered both drugs and significantly inhibited S6K and S6 phosphorylation. Nanotechnologically delivered drugs escaped from reticuloendothelial system (RES) to a large extent. Rapamycin and paclitaxel loaded NPs induced regression of tumors in mice xenografted with MDA-MB-468 BCa cells [3]. Rapamycin-loaded solid lipid NPs (RP-SLN) were found to be effective against SH-SY5Y neuroblastoma cell line (3). RP-SLN inhibited phosphorylation of p70S6K in SH-SY5Y [21].

Curcumin-loaded and calcium-doped dendritic mesoporous silica NPs modified with folic acid were also found to be effective against MCF-7 BCa cells [23]. Bioavailability, plasma concentrations and tumor distributions of curcumin were significantly higher in mice intraperitoneally injected with curcumin loaded NPs [23]. Gold nanoparticles-conjugated quercetin inhibited mTOR pathway in MCF-7 and MDA-MB-231 BCa cells [2].

As a future perspective in breast cancer treatment, these nanosystems and the like which have shown strong inhibitory activities against mTOR complexes can be developed in optimum nanoformulations for efficient targeting of breast cancer cells.

15.6   Conclusion

It seems clear that substantial fraction of information has been added into the existing pool of knowledge related to mTOR-driven pathway and how mTOR formed assemblies with different proteins to modulate different mechanisms. However, various facets of mTOR driven pathway are superficially studied in breast cancer. How different members of mTORC1 and mTORC2 can be targeted by different natural products needs detailed research. We have also incomplete understanding about microRNA regulation of positive and negative regulators of mTOR complexes. Future studies must converge on mechanistic insights related to role of mTORC1 and mTORC2 in regulation of epithelial-to-mesenchymal transition.

Better and sharper conceptualization of these aspects will prove to be helpful in getting a step closer to individualized medicine.

References

1. Alayev A, Salamon RS, Berger SM, Schwartz NS, Cuesta R, Snyder RB, Holz MK (2016) mTORC1 directly phosphorylates and activates ERα upon estrogen stimulation. Oncogene 35(27):3535–3543. https://doi.org/10.1038/onc.2015.414
2. Balakrishnan S, Mukherjee S, Das S, Bhat FA, Raja Singh P, Patra CR, Arunakaran J (2017) Gold nanoparticles-conjugated quercetin induces apoptosis via inhibition of EGFR/PI3K/ Akt-mediated pathway in breast cancer cell lines (MCF-7 and MDA-MB-231). Cell Biochem Funct 35(4):217–231. https://doi.org/10.1002/cbf.3266
3. Blanco E, Sangai T, Wu S, Hsiao A, Ruiz-Esparza GU, Gonzalez-Delgado CA et al (2014) Colocalized delivery of rapamycin and paclitaxel to tumors enhances synergistic targeting of the PI3K/Akt/mTOR pathway. Mol Ther 22(7):1310–1319
4. Chen J, Zhu Y, Zhang W, Peng X, Zhou J, Li F, Han B, Liu X, Ou Y, Yu X (2018) Delphinidin induced protective autophagy via mTOR pathway suppression and AMPK pathway activation in HER-2 positive breast cancer cells. BMC Cancer 18(1):342. https://doi.org/10.1186/ s12885-018-4231-y
5. Guru SK, Pathania AS, Kumar S, Ramesh D, Kumar M, Rana S, Kumar A, Malik F, Sharma PR, Chandan BK, Jaglan S, Sharma JP, Shah BA, Tasduq SA, Lattoo SK, Faruk A, Saxena AK, Vishwakarma RA, Bhushan S (2015) Secalonic acid-D represses HIF1α/VEGF-mediated angiogenesis by regulating the Akt/mTOR/p70S6K signaling cascade. Cancer Res 75(14):2886–2896. https://doi.org/10.1158/0008-5472.CAN-14-2312
6. Jung CH, Kim H, Ahn J, Jung SK, Um MY, Son KH, Kim TW, Ha TY (2013) Anthricin isolated from *Anthriscus sylvestris* (L.) Hoffm. Inhibits the growth of breast cancer cells by inhibiting Akt/mTOR signaling, and its apoptotic effects are enhanced by autophagy inhibition. Evid Based Complement Alternat Med 2013:385219. https://doi.org/10.1155/2013/385219
7. Ke K, Lou T (2017) MicroRNA-10a suppresses breast cancer progression via PI3K/Akt/ mTOR pathway. Oncol Lett 14(5):5994–6000. https://doi.org/10.3892/ol.2017.6930.
8. Li W, Wang H, Zhang J, Zhai L, Chen W, Zhao C (2016a) miR-199a-5p regulates β1 integrin through Ets-1 to suppress invasion in breast cancer. Cancer Sci 107(7):916–923. https://doi. org/10.1111/cas.12952
9. Li W, Zhai L, Wang H, Liu C, Zhang J, Chen W, Wei Q (2016b) Downregulation of LncRNA GAS5 causes trastuzumab resistance in breast cancer. Oncotarget 7(19):27778–27786. https:// doi.org/10.18632/oncotarget.8413
10. Lineham E, Tizzard GJ, Coles SJ, Spencer J, Morley SJ (2018) Synergistic effects of inhibiting the MNK-eIF4E and PI3K/AKT/ mTOR pathways on cell migration in MDA-MB-231 cells. Oncotarget 9(18):14148–14159. https://doi.org/10.18632/oncotarget.24354
11. Lu W, Lin C, Li Y (2014) Rottlerin induces Wnt co-receptor LRP6 degradation and suppresses both Wnt/β-catenin and mTORC1 signaling in prostate and breast cancer cells. Cell Signal 26(6):1303–1309. https://doi.org/10.1016/j.cellsig.2014.02.018
12. Makhov P, Golovine K, Teper E, Kutikov A, Mehrazin R, Corcoran A, Tulin A, Uzzo RG, Kolenko VM (2014) Piperlongumine promotes autophagy via inhibition of Akt/mTOR signalling and mediates cancer cell death. Br J Cancer 110(4):899–907. https://doi.org/10.1038/ bjc.2013.810
13. Martin EC, Rhodes LV, Elliott S, Krebs AE, Nephew KP, Flemington EK, Collins-Burow BM, Burow ME (2014) microRNA regulation of mammalian target of rapamycin expression and activity controls estrogen receptor function and RAD001 sensitivity. Mol Cancer 13:229. https://doi.org/10.1186/1476-4598-13-229
14. Mateo F, Arenas EJ, Aguilar H, Serra-Musach J, de Garibay GR, Boni J, Maicas M, Du S, Iorio F, Herranz-Ors C, Islam A, Prado X, Llorente A, Petit A, Vidal A, Català I, Soler T, Venturas G, Rojo-Sebastian A, Serra H, Cuadras D, Blanco I, Lozano J, Canals F, Sieuwerts AM, de Weerd V, Look MP, Puertas S, García N, Perkins AS, Bonifaci N, Skowron M, Gómez-Baldó L et al (2017) Stem cell-like transcriptional reprogramming mediates metastatic resistance to mTOR inhibition. Oncogene 36(19):2737–2749. https://doi.org/10.1038/onc.2016.427

15. Mi W, Ye Q, Liu S, She QB (2015) AKT inhibition overcomes rapamycin resistance by enhancing the repressive function of PRAS40 on mTORC1/4E-BP1 axis. Oncotarget 6(16):13962–13977

16. Michaloglou C, Crafter C, Siersbæk R, Delpuech O, Curwen JO, Carnevalli LS, Staniszewska AD, Polanska UM, Cheraghchi-Bashi A, Lawson M, Chernukhin I, McEwen R, Carroll JS, Cosulich SC (2018. pii: molcanther.0537.2017) Combined inhibition of mTOR and CDK4/6 is required for optimal blockade of E2F function and long term growth inhibition in estrogen receptor positive breast cancer. Mol Cancer Ther. https://doi.org/10.1158/1535-7163.MCT-17-0537

17. Morrison Joly M, Hicks DJ, Jones B, Sanchez V, Estrada MV, Young C, Williams M, Rexer BN, Sarbassov dos D, Muller WJ, Brantley-Sieders D, Cook RS (2016) Rictor/mTORC2 drives progression and therapeutic resistance of HER2-amplified breast cancers. Cancer Res 76(16):4752–4764. https://doi.org/10.1158/0008-5472.CAN-15-3393

18. Morrison Joly M, Williams MM, Hicks DJ, Jones B, Sanchez V, Young CD, Sarbassov DD, Muller WJ, Brantley-Sieders D, Cook RS (2017) Two distinct mTORC2-dependent pathways converge on Rac1 to drive breast cancer metastasis. Breast Cancer Res 19(1):74. https://doi.org/10.1186/s13058-017-0868-8.

19. Parhi P, Sahoo SK (2015) Trastuzumab guided nanotheranostics: a lipid based multifunctional nanoformulation for targeted drug delivery and imaging in breast cancer therapy. J Colloid Interface Sci 451:198–211

20. Phua YW, Nguyen A, Roden DL, Elsworth B, Deng N, Nikolic I, Yang J, Mcfarland A, Russell R, Kaplan W, Cowley MJ, Nair R, Zotenko E, O'Toole S, Tan SX, James DE, Clark SJ, Kouros-Mehr H, Swarbrick A (2015) MicroRNA profiling of the pubertal mouse mammary gland identifies miR-184 as a candidate breast tumour suppressor gene. Breast Cancer Res 17:83. https://doi.org/10.1186/s13058-015-0593-0

21. Polchi A, Magini A, Mazuryk J, Tancini B, Gapinski J, Patkowski A et al (2016) Rapamycin loaded solid lipid nanoparticles as a new tool to deliver mTOR inhibitors: formulation and in vitro characterization. Nanomaterials (Basel) 6(5):87

22. Wang Y, Han E, Xing Q, Yan J, Arrington A, Wang C, Tully D, Kowolik CM, Lu DM, Frankel PH, Zhai J, Wen W, Horne D, Yip MLR, Yim JH (2015) Baicalein upregulates DDIT4 expression which mediates mTOR inhibition and growth inhibition in cancer cells. Cancer Lett 358(2):170–179. https://doi.org/10.1016/j.canlet.2014.12.033

23. Wang J, Wang Y, Liu Q, Yang L, Zhu R, Yu C, Wang S (2016) Rational design of multifunctional dendritic mesoporous silica nanoparticles to load curcumin and enhance efficacy for breast cancer therapy. ACS Appl Mater Interfaces 8(40):26511–26523

24. Zhang Y, Xu S, Lin J, Yao G, Han Z, Liang B, Zou Z, Chen Z, Song Q, Dai Y, Gao T, Liu A, Bai X (2012) mTORC1 is a target of nordihydroguaiaretic acid to prevent breast tumor growth in vitro and in vivo. Breast Cancer Res Treat 136(2):379–388. https://doi.org/10.1007/s10549-012-2270-7

25. Zhang Y, Zhang HE, Liu Z (2016) MicroRNA-147 suppresses proliferation, invasion and migration through the AKT/mTOR signaling pathway in breast cancer. Oncol Lett 11(1):405–410

26. Zhou X, Yue GG, Chan AM, Tsui SK, Fung KP, Sun H, Pu J, Lau CB (2017a) Eriocalyxin B, a novel autophagy inducer, exerts anti-tumor activity through the suppression of Akt/mTOR/p70S6K signaling pathway in breast cancer. Biochem Pharmacol 142:58–70. https://doi.org/10.1016/j.bcp.2017.06.133

27. Zhou R, Chen H, Chen J, Chen X, Wen Y, Xu L (2018) Extract from Astragalus membranaceus inhibit breast cancer cells proliferation via PI3K/AKT/mTOR signaling pathway. BMC Complement Altern Med 18(1):83. https://doi.org/10.1186/s12906-018-2148-2

Chapter 16
Epigenetics of Breast Cancer: Clinical Status of Epi-drugs and Phytochemicals

Samriddhi Shukla, Dhanamjai Penta, Priya Mondal, and Syed Musthapa Meeran

Abstract Epigenetics refers to alterations in gene expression due to differential histone modifications and DNA methylation at promoter sites of genes. Epigenetic alterations are reversible and are heritable during somatic cell division, but do not involve changes in nucleotide sequence. Epigenetic regulation plays a critical role in normal growth and embryonic development by controlling transcriptional activities of several genes. In last two decades, these modifications have been well recognized to be involved in tumor initiation and progression, which has motivated many investigators to incorporate this novel field in cancer drug development. Recently, growing number of epigenetic changes have been reported that are involved in the regulations of genes involved in breast tumor growth and metastasis. Drugs possessing epigenetic modulatory activities known as epi-drugs, mainly the inhibitors of histone deacetylases (HDACs) and DNA methyltransferases (DNMTs). Some of these drugs are undergoing different clinical trials for breast cancer treatment. Several phytochemicals such as green tea polyphenols, curcumin, genistein, resveratrol and sulforaphane have also been shown to alter epigenetic modifications in multiple cancer types including breast cancer. In this chapter, we summarize the role of epigenetic changes in breast cancer progression and metastasis. We have also discussed about various epigenetic modulators possessing chemopreventive and therapeutic efficacy against breast cancer with future perspectives.

Keywords Epigenetics · Breast cancer · Phytochemicals · DNA methylation · Histone modifications · Epi-drugs

S. Shukla
Department of Paediatrics, Cincinnati Children's Hospital Medical Center, Cincinnati, OH, USA

D. Penta · P. Mondal · S. M. Meeran (✉)
Laboratory of Cancer Epigenetics, Department of Biochemistry, CSIR-Central Food Technological Research Institute, Mysore, India
e-mail: s.musthapa@cftri.res.in

© Springer Nature Switzerland AG 2019
A. Ahmad (ed.), *Breast Cancer Metastasis and Drug Resistance*,
Advances in Experimental Medicine and Biology 1152,
https://doi.org/10.1007/978-3-030-20301-6_16

293

16.1   Introduction

Breast carcinogenesis was previously considered as a complex multistep process driven by a series of genetic abnormalities such as 'loss of function' mutations in tumor suppressor genes (TSGs) and 'gain of function' mutations in cellular proto-oncogenes. However, discovery of different epigenetic mechanisms and proof of their contribution in aberrant gene expression established role of epigenetic changes as important contributors of breast carcinogenesis. In addition to driving breast cancer initiating changes such as acquired mutations in key TSGs such as *BRCA1* or proto-oncogenes such as *c-MYC*; epigenetic aberrations (epimutations) also contribute equally in breast carcinogenesis. The aberrant transcriptional regulation results in distorted patterns of expressions of genes involved in the process of cell division, differentiation and survival. Epigenetic changes function at chromosomal levels in breast cancer cells, as a regulatory layer, coordinating all the crucial biological processes to maintain cellular homeostasis. Loss of this dynamic equilibrium results in development of disease states. Well-studied epigenetic changes in cancer include altered patterns of DNA methylation and histone modifications, which regulate nucleosomal assembly and chromatin remodelling, thereby determining binding or removal of different DNA binding proteins. In addition, microRNAs (miRNAs) are a class of RNA epigenetic regulators with capabilities to alter gene expression at both post-transcriptional and translational levels. These molecules bind to their target mRNA sites and lead to degradation of mRNA by double-stranded RNA degrading enzyme [91]. DNA methylation is defined as covalent addition of a methyl group to the 5th carbon of the cytosine (C) nucleotide in the CpG dinucleotide sequences, mediated mainly by two types of DNA methyltransferases (DNMTs). The maintenance of methylations pattern is carried by maintenance methyltransferase such as DNMT1, and the de novo methylations by the de novo methyltransferases such as DNMT3a and DNMT3b as depicted in Fig.16.1.

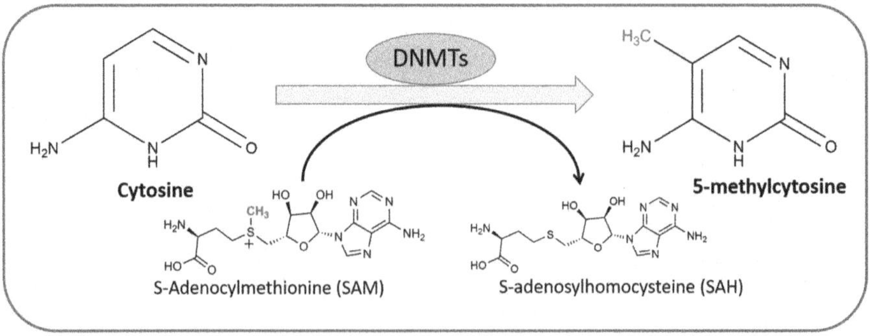

Fig. 16.1 DNA methylation. DNA methylation is one of the major epigenetic modification occurs on the 5th carbon of cytosine nucleotide present in the CpG Island at the core promoter of the gene. A group of enzymes known as DNA methyltransferases (DNMTs) mediates the DNA methylation where S-adenosyl methionine (SAM) donates methyl group for this reaction. DNA methylation plays a critical role in the transcriptional regulations of genes involved in cancer

S-adenosyl methionine (SAM) functions as a universal methyl group donor. DNA methylation is important in many imperative biological events such as X-chromosome inactivation, genomic imprinting as well as many developmental processes. Lower promoter methylation status is a characteristic of constitutively expressed genes, for example housekeeping genes. Genes with regulative expression have been reported to display higher promoter methylation. Breast cancer cells, similar to other cancers display global hypomethylation and focal (gene-specific) hypermethylation [6, 29, 42, 79, 95]. Global hypomethylation tends to increase with age and facilitates genomic instability as well as activation of oncogenes [24, 82]. On the other hand, focal hypermethylation mostly functions in epigenetic silencing of different TSGs [22, 29, 85]. Post-translational histone modifications are vital epigenetic modifications, which modulate the structure of the chromatin, thereby altering accessibility of DNA [28]. The histone code of any organism is set and modified by a set of enzymes known as histone modifying enzymes such as histone acetyltransferases (HATs), histone deacetylases (HDACs) and histone methyl transferases (HMTs). DNA methylation is also associated with specific histone modifications, which together affect the chromatin structure leading to transcriptional gene silencing [4, 28]. MicroRNAs interact with a variety of genes involved in multiple cellular pathways such as proliferation, migration and survival. Depending on their gene targets, miRNAs have an ability to function as tumor suppressors or oncogenic miRNAs [91]. In the following sections, we have discussed the roles of these epigenetic modifications in course of breast carcinogenesis. We have also discussed breast cancer epigenetic targets and their targeting epigenetic modulatory compounds in breast cancer chemoprevention and therapeutics.

16.2 The Breast Cancer Methylome

DNA methylation is one of the three known epigenetic regulatory layers of spatial and temporal patterns of gene expression. Hypermethylation plays a fundamental role in the process of genomic imprinting, which refers to methylation-induced silencing of one of the two parental alleles of a gene to ascertain mono-allelic gene expression, X-chromosome inactivation in female foetus occurs through a parallel imprinting mechanism [31, 80]. By definition, DNA methylation is a heritable epigenetic mechanism, which regulates gene expression, and is restricted to covalent addition of a methyl group to the 5th carbon of cytosine in a CpG dinucleotide. During evolution, the frequency of CpG dinucleotide sequences have been severely decreased to approximately 20% of the predicted frequency in the vertebrate genome, and among the remaining CpG dinucleotides, more than 70% are methylated [104]. Analysis of the human methylome has revealed that distribution of CpG dinucleotides is far from random, and some of them cluster together to form CpG-rich DNA regions, known as CpG islands. Most often, CpG islands are located in the upstream promoter and first exonic region of over half of human genes [98]. Under normal circumstances, CpG islands in the actively expressed genes are unmethylated. However, during the process of neoplastic transformation, DNA methylation in cancer cells is different as compared to normal cells with focal hypermethylation of CpG islands in many genes [4, 28]. Thus, an altered DNA methylation profile is a hallmark of almost all types of human cancers, including breast cancer. A whole genome high-throughput methylation sequencing study validated a global promoter hypomethylation and a cell type-specific regulation of promoter methylation in a panel of breast cancer cell lines [85].

The process of DNA methylation is catalyzed by DNMTs that catalyze transfer of methyl group from SAM to cytosine in the CpG dinucleotide. To date, five different DNMTs have been identified DNMT1, DNMT2, DNMT3a, DNMT3b and DNMT3L. Maintenance of established methylation patterns in hemi-methylated genes are mediated by DNMT1, which copies pre-existing methylation patterns from parental DNA strand to daughter DNA strand [97]. DNMT1 has been reported to be overexpressed in pre-invasive breast tumors [105]. De novo DNA methylation is mediated by three DNMTs; DNMT3a, DNMT3b and DNMT3L [16, 74]. However, DNMT3L lacks the ability to bind directly to SAM, and is responsible for increasing the binding of DNMT3a to SAM, thereby indirectly assisting de novo methylation [1, 16]. DNMT2, the small 391-amino-acid enzyme, has been reported to possess a feeble DNMT activity, but its biological function is not well known [21]. Studies have reported that Dicer-mediated miRNA biogenesis is indirectly involved in modulation of DNA methylation by regulating the expression of *DNMT3* genes [5, 94]. Dicer belongs to RNase III family of enzymes and is known to be involved in biosynthesis of small RNA species such as small interfering RNAs (siRNAs) and miRNAs [53]. In Dicer-deficient cells, miRNAs of miR-290 cluster are less expressed and expression of their target retinoblastoma-like protein (Rbl2) is increased. Rbl2-mediated transcriptional repression leads to downregulation of DNMT3 expression resulting in global hypomethylation [5, 94]. In breast tumors, *DNMT3b* mRNA overexpression has been reported, which correlates well with focal hypermethylated phenotype and poor prognosis [38, 83].

16.2.1 Focal Hypermethylation Profiles of Breast Tumors

Gene promoters containing CpG-islands are generally unmethylated in normal cells to maintain transcriptionally active euchromatic conformation, allowing gene expression. However, in breast cancer cells, many of these genes get hypermethylated at their CpG-islands leading to inactivation of their expression by changing open euchromatic conformation to compact heterochromatic conformation [28]. Most often, genes that are selectively hypermethylated during tumorigenesis are functionally involved in restriction of cellular proliferation. Some gene promoters, which are hypermethylated in different human cancers, belong to classical TSGs with one inherited mutated allele. Knudson's two-hit hypothesis states that complete inactivation of a TSG requires 'loss of function' of both alleles [55]. Therefore, hypermethylation-assisted silencing of the remaining active allele of TSG can function as the second hit. Accordingly, some well-known breast cancer TSGs, such as $p16^{INK4a}$, *APC* and *BRCA1*, mutated in the germline sporadically, display functional inactivation of remaining functional allele in transformed breast cells through focal DNA methylation [10, 50, 93]. Till now, multiple methylated tumor suppressors have been identified in breast cancer, which perform a plethora of biological functions, encompassing cell cycle regulation ($p14^{ARF}$, $p16^{INK4a,}$ $p57^{KIP2}$ *cyclin D2, 14–3–3σ*), growth-inhibitory signaling (*RARβ, SYK, RASSF1A, TGFβR-II, HIN1, SOCS1, NES1, SFRP1, WIF1*), apoptosis (*DAPK1, APC, HOXA5, HIC1, TWIST, TMS1*), DNA repair (*GSTP1, BRCA1, MGMT*), hormonal receptors (*ERα, ERβ, PR*), cell adhesion and invasion (*CDH1, CDH13, APC, prostasin, BCSG1, TIMP-3*), angiogenesis (*maspin, THBS1*), and so on [13, 104]. In addition, studies have reported DNA methylation-mediated silencing of miRNAs with tumor suppressor function [59]. Levels of miRNA methylation increase with increase in aggressiveness of the breast tumors. Promoter hypermethylation of genes encoding tumor suppressor miRNAs such as let-7 family, miR-206, miR-17-5p, miR-125a, miR-125b, miR-200, miR-34, and miR-31, is a common occurrence in breast tumors [73, 101]. Genome methylation patterns have been developed as markers for early detection and classification of subtype of breast tumors, as predictors for risk assessment and monitoring prognosis, and indicators of susceptibility or response to therapy [104]. These advances in knowledge of breast cancer methylome robustly indicate crucial role of DNA hypermethylation, which synergistically interacts with other genetic alterations to promote breast cancer development. For example, human mammary epithelial cells (HMECs) with decreased $p16^{INK4A}$ expression, resulting from hypermethylation of $p16^{INK4A}$ promoter, achieved growth competence by effectively bypassing senescence [100, 104]. Since $p16^{INK4A}$ has been known to regulate the polycomb-mediated methylation patterns in normal human mammary epithelium; aberration of the cell cycle control by inhibiting the cell cycle regulatory TSG $p16^{INK4A}$ could create a context for uncontrolled cell division in cells at risk for cancer [54, 81]. In addition to cell-cycle regulatory genes, promoter hypermethylation-mediated silencing of genes involved in DNA repair, such as *BRCA1* and *MGMT*, could also result in inactivation of other TSGs or activation of oncogenes driving the process of breast tumorigenesis [27]. Inhibitors of the oncogenic Wnt signaling, such as *WIF1* and *SFRP1*, have been reported to be recurrently epigenetically silenced in primary breast tumors, silencing being attributable to promoter hypermethylation [2, 63]. Promoter hypermethylation of some key breast cancer regulatory genes can be utilized as an early biomarker of breast carcinogenesis. Focal hypermethylation may also function in differentiating pre-invasive and invasive breast tumors [13, 22]. Breast CpG island methylator phenotype (bCIMP) indicating a genome-wide higher proportion of hypermethylated genes can be utilized as a predictor of disease progression, where higher methylation indicates lower risk of breast cancer metastasis [30]. Conclusively, focal hypermethylation-mediated silencing contributes to the process of breast carcinogenesis not only through silencing of TSGs, but also by silencing inhibitors of different oncogenic pathways.

16.2.2   Global Hypomethylation Profiles of Breast Tumors

Repetitive DNA sequence elements are generally silenced by promoter methylation to avoid disruptive chromosomal rearrangements such as gene translocations and insertion of reactivated transposable elements resulting in gene disruptions [24, 52]. However, in cancer cells, global genomic hypomethylation leads to activation of these repetitive elements, chromosomal aberrations, disruption of genomic imprinting and increase in chromosomal instability [62]. In addition, promoter hypomethylation of numerous proto-oncogenes implicated in cellular processes of proliferation and metastasis (for example *synuclein C* and *urokinase*) and development of drug resistance (*N-cadherin, β-catenin, annexin A4, ID4* and *WNT11*) also facilitates process of breast carcinogenesis [62]. In addition, *BRCA1* mutations are also associated with aberrant regulation of DNMTs resulting in global hypomethylation profiles and hypomethylation-induced expression of various proto-oncogenes in breast carcinogenesis [90]. Global genomic hypomethylation and hypomethylation of CpG sequences in satellite DNA has been established as an early event during breast carcinogenesis [48]. Methylation analysis of repetitive DNA elements long interspersed repetitive DNA elements (LINE1), satellite DNA elements (SAT2) and short interspersed repetitive DNA elements (ALU) indicated that these elements are significantly hypomethylated in breast tumors compared to adjacent normal breast tissue [19].

16.3   Breast Cancer Histone Code

Aberrations in normal patterns of covalent histone modifications function as another important epigenetic hallmark of cancer. Among multiple histone modifications, histone acetylation and methylation are relatively stable histone modifications. These modifications have been considered as prospective histone modification marks that are carried over through multiple cell cycles. Histone modifications determine chromatin conformation by regulating chromatin-remodelling events as depicted in Fig. 16.2. Open chromatin state renders DNA sequences approachable to transcriptional complexes resulting in a transcriptionally active chromatin known as the euchromatin. Closed chromatin state is transcriptionally inactive and is known as heterochromatin. Generally, histone acetylation at lysine (K) H3K5, H3K8, H3K9, H3K12, H3K18 and H4K16; lysine methylation at H3K4 and arginine dimethylation at H4R3 are considered as euchromatic histone modification marks [8, 28, 87, 88]. Heterochromatic histone modification marks include mono-, di, or tri-methylations at lysines H3K9, H3K20 and H4K27 [28, 49, 57, 62]. One classical example of aberrant histone modifications is global reduction in trimethylation of H4K20 (H4K20me3) and acetylation of H4K16 (H4K16Ac), along with DNA hypomethylation at repetitive sequence elements in many primary tumors including breast tumors [34]. Furthermore, alterations in expression of histone

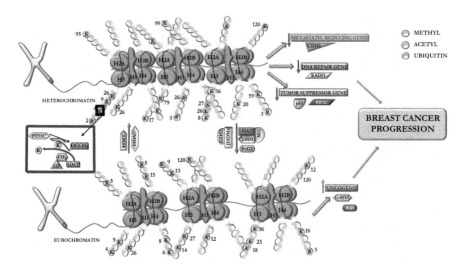

Fig. 16.2 Role of histone modifications in the transcriptional regulation of genes involved in the breast cancer progression. Schematic diagram demonstrating that the histone acetyltransferases (HATs) transfer the acetyl groups into the specific positions of lysine (K), arginine (R) residues present in the tail of the histone protein. Acetylation of histone unwind the DNA into the transcriptionally active state called as euchromatin. In contrast, histone deacetylases (HDACs) remove the acetyl groups from the tail of the histones and bring them into the transcriptionally repressive state called as heterochromatin. HDACs also helps to histone methyltransferases (HMTs) to transfer methyl groups into the specific K and R residues in the histone tail. Methylation of histone also inactivates the chromatin. The heterochromatin state of chromatin, in general, represses the transcription of tumor suppressor genes (*p53, BRCA*), DNA repair genes (*RAD51*) etc. Activation of oncogenes and inactivation of tumor-suppressor genes, in general, contribute to the breast cancer progression. *LSD1* Lysine-specific histone demethylase 1, *HP* Histone protein

modifying enzymes modify patterns of histone modifications in breast cancer cells. Chromosomal translocations involving HATs such as cAMP response element–binding binding protein (CREBBP), E1A-binding protein p300 (EP300), nuclear receptor coactivator-2 (NCOA2), MYST3 and MYST4 have been identified in different cancers including breast cancer [47]. In different types of cancers, binding of adenoviral oncoproteins E1A and SV40T to HATs lead to oncogenic transformation through global deacetylation of H3K18, with concomitant activation of genes inducing cell growth and proliferation [32, 78]. Truncating mutations in EP300 and monoallelic loss of lysine acetyltransferase-5 (KAT5) increases potential of cancer cells for malignant transformation [37, 39]. Overexpression of different HDACs, such as HDAC1, HDAC2, HDAC3 and HDAC6 have also been reported in tumors [11, 67, 75]. Class I HDACs (except HDAC8) have been observed to be upregulated in breast cancer. Alterations in class II HDACs modify patterns of cell cycle proliferation, apoptosis, gene expression and ER signaling in breast cancer cells [23]. Overexpression of HDACs-1, 6 and 8 induces breast cancer invasion and expression of matrix metallopeptidase-9 (MMP-9) [75]. Functional role of HDAC2 in tumor promotion is controversial, as truncating mutations in this gene have been reported to confer resistance against HDAC inhibitors [84]. Sirtuins are also known to be overexpressed in a wide variety of tumors [86]. Overexpression of SIRT1, SIRT2, SIRT3 and SIRT7 is a frequent event during breast carcinogenesis [3]. Therefore, targeting these enzymes might be a successful approach against cancers with sirtuins overexpression. Mysteriously, inhibition of SIRT1 expression led to partial reactivation of TSGs, without any change in the heavily methylated promoters [77].

Altered expression or activity of lysine methyl transferases (KMTs) and lysine demethylases (KDMs), resulting from chromosomal translocation, gene amplification, deletion, overexpression or methylation-mediated silencing is also evident in human cancers. The H3K27-specific KMT, EZH2 is overexpressed in solid tumors including breast cancer [12, 58]. However, a few studies have shown inactivating mutations in EZH2 observed in cancers. A KMT involved in methylation of H3K36 and H4K20, known as nuclear receptor–binding SET domain protein-1 (NSD1) has been reported to be silenced by promoter hypermethylation. Heterozygous mutation or loss of heterozygosity in this gene leads to a childhood overgrowth syndrome with a high risk of tumorigenesis known as Sotos syndrome [7, 103]. Role of KDMs in cancer has recently been investigated. Enigmatically, overexpression as well as 'loss of function' mutations in various genes of Jumonji/ARID domain containing protein 1 (JARID1) family of H3K4me2/3 KDMs has been shown to add in the process of tumorigenesis in breast cancer [43]. Low-level detection of histone modifications was found to be associated with adverse prognosis in breast cancer. Histone acetylations at H4K16 and methylations at H3K4 as well as H4K20 were considerably higher in normal breast cells than corresponding breast tumors. Overall increased levels of histone acetylation at H3K9 and H3K18 and methylation at H4R3 led to prolonged disease-free survival. Moderate to low levels of histone acetylation at H3K9, H3K18 and H4K12, histone methylation at H3K4 and H4K20, and arginine methylation at H4R3 were correlated with poorer disease prognosis [26]. Thus, histone modifying enzymes constitute interesting epigenetic targets in breast carcinogenesis and histone modification marks might as well function as diagnostic and prognostic markers of breast cancer.

16.4   Breast Cancer miRNA Epigenome

Alterations in pattern of miRNA expression have been established very well in human breast cancer [15, 46]. These miRNAs function in inhibition of genes involved in different cellular pathways, for example genes involved in cellular proliferation and regulation of cell cycle. Regulation of miRNA expression may take place either through promoter hypermethylation in miRNA-encoding genes, or through copy number variations. In the miRNAs known to be altered in breast cancer, a substantial proportion has been aligned to genomic fragile sites or regions associated with cancers [46]. Significant alterations in expression of miRNA-processing enzymes Dicer and AGO1 have been observed during the processes of

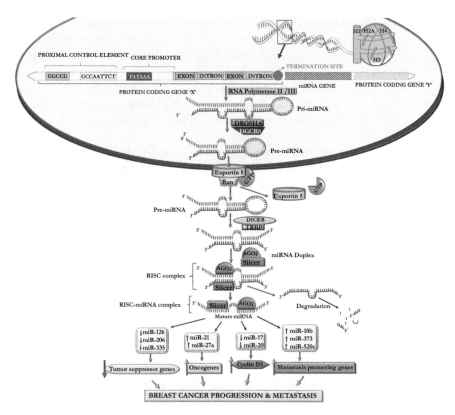

Fig. 16.3 MicroRNA (miRNA) regulations in breast cancer progression and metastasis. Post-transcriptional modifications control the expression of different genes. miRNA is synthesized in the form of primary microRNA (Pri-miRNA). A complex of the nuclear enzyme, drosha, and microprocessor complex subunit, DGCR8 that produce a short size precursor miRNA (pre-miRNA) from pri-miRNA. Exportin 5, a nuclear membrane protein, transfers pre-miRNA from the nucleus into cytoplasm. Cytoplasmic enzyme dicer with TRBP cleave hair-pin loop structure of the pre-miRNA and generate double-stranded RNA without hair-pin called as 'miRNA duplex'. Argonaut, an RNase H type endonuclease, along with slicer binds to miRNA duplex and create the RISC-complex, which eventually cleaved into the mature miRNA. Mature miRNA binds to target sequence of mRNA of the specific gene and inhibits its transcriptional expressions. miRNA regulates the expression of tumor suppressor genes, oncogenes, metastatic genes and cell cycle-regulating genes, and thereby contributes to the breast cancer progression and metastasis. *RISC* RNA-induced silencing complex, *AGO2* Argonaut 2, *DGCR 8 DiGeorge syndrome chromosomal region 8, TRBP* HIV-1 TAR RNA binding protein

breast carcinogenesis as shown in Fig. 16.3. The alterations in miRNA processing machinery can also cause miRNA deregulation [107].

The most studied family of breast tumor suppressor miRNAs, Let-7 family has been involved in targeting of RAS, caspase-3 and HMGA2 genes and disruption of Let-7 expression causes oncogenic transformation [51, 65]. Let-7 family of miR-NAs represses many important cell cycle regulatory TSGs; for example Cyclin A, CDC25A, Cyclin D1, Cyclin D3, CDK4, CDK6, CDK8 and CCNA2 [51, 89]. Loss of heterozygosity at human genomic location of miR-17/20 cluster at chromosome 13q31 is frequent in a number of different cancer types including breast cancer [25, 61]. In human breast tumors, decreased miR-17/20 expression induced higher Cyclin D1 expression compared with matching normal breast tissues [102]. Other major tumor suppressor miRNAs downregulated in course of breast cancer include miR-145, miR-205, miR-206 etc. Tumor suppressor miRNAs (miR-126, miR-206 and miR-335) have been observed to be breast cancer metastasis-suppressor miR-NAs [99].

Frequent overexpression of oncogenic miRNA miR-21 has been observed in breast tumors. MiR-21 is an oncogenic miRNA, which targets multiple TSGs involved in *p53* suppression pathway and promotes invasion and metastasis in breast cancer [35]. miR-27a is a breast oncogenic miRNA, which functions in down-regulation of multiple cell cycle inhibitors leading to deregulated cell proliferation [66]. Up-regulation of miR-10b, miR-373 and miR-520c induces processes of breast cancer invasion and metastasis [45, 64]. The regulation of miRNA expression by annotated genes indicates significance of miRNA promoters and new possibilities for therapeutic intervention by using compounds to regulate miRNA expression. Because, miRNAs are involved in breast cancer initiation as well as metastatic progression, these molecules can be used as ideal targets for development of new therapies against breast cancer.

16.5 Epigenetic Drugs (Epi-drugs) Against Breast Cancer

In contrast to genetic mutations, the epimutations are reversible. This reversibility has attracted researchers to go on a quest for epigenetic drugs, which can restore normal epigenetic landscapes in cancer cells by inhibiting epigenetic modulatory enzymes. The US-Food and Drug Administration (USFDA) have approved four epigenetic inhibitors for the treatment of specific hematologic malignancies. Two DNMT inhibitors, 5-azacytidine and 5-aza-2′-deoxycytidine (trade names, vidaza and decitabine, respectively) have been approved for treatment of higher-risk myelodysplastic syndrome. Two HDAC inhibitors, suberoylanilide hydroxamic acid and FK-228 (trade names, vorinostat and romidepsin, respectively) have been approved for rare cutaneous T cell lymphoma (CTCL) and other hematological cancers [14, 36, 71, 76]. In 2014, another HDAC inhibitor PXD101 Belinostat (trade name, Beleodaq) has been approved by the USFDA for treatment of aggressive form of non-Hodgkin's lymphoma [33, 72]. Recently, quest of epigenetic therapies has widened and in addition to these DNMT and HDAC inhibitors, inhibition of HATs, class I, II and IV-specific HDACs, class III HDACs (sirtuins), KMTs, KDMs and multiple kinases is being considered. Due to ever-changing expression patters of cancer cells, these epigenetic drugs will potentially become a vital part of therapeutic regime in the near future against all cancer types.

Another cytidine analog stable in aqueous solution, 5-fluoro-2′-deoxycytidine, is undergoing clinical trials in combination with other therapeutic agents for treatment of various tumors [41, 69]. Similarly, another orally active DNMT inhibitor zebularine has shown therapeutic promise against multiple cancer types in pre-clinical studies [68, 106]. Some novel non-nucleoside analog DNMT inhibitors have also shown potent DNA demethylation activity against cancer [17, 40]. The HDAC inhibitors include compounds that can be divided into four distinct chemical classes: short-chain fatty acids, hydroxamic acids, cyclic peptides and benzamide derivatives. HDAC inhibitors are characterized by the unique presence of a Zn-binding domain that can block substrate-Zn chelation at the HDAC active sites. Since sirtuins require NAD+ at their active sites, these HDACs are unaffected by these inhibitors. HDAC inhibitors suppress carcinogenesis by inducing G1 or G2-M phase cell cycle arrest, differentiation and/or apoptosis, by inhibiting angiogenesis and metastasis. HDAC inhibitors also enhance tumor sensitivity to chemotherapy.

16.6   Selective Epigenetic Modifying Phytochemicals Against Breast Cancer

Interest has been growing in recent years for the use of epigenetic modulatory phytochemicals against many human diseases including cancer. Many of the bioactive phytochemicals have shown to inhibit multiple epigenetic targets and thereby alter the expressions of key genes involved in tumor, as shown in Fig. 16.4. The

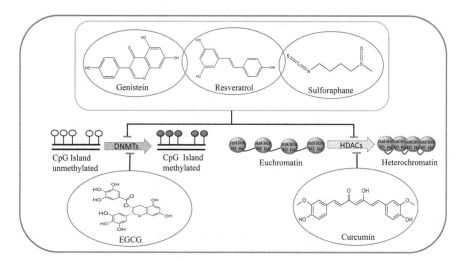

Fig. 16.4 Natural dietary bioactive phytochemicals and their epigenetic modulatory effects. Natural bioactive phytochemicals act as anticancer agents by regulating some of the major epigenetic modifications like DNA methylation and histone modification. DNA methyltransferases (DNMTs), enzyme mediate the methylation at the CpG island located at the promoter, whereas histone deacetylases (HDACs) deacetylate the histone tail in the core histone. Inhibition of DNA methylation and induction of histone acetylation play a major role in cancer prevention and therapy

preferential use of phytochemicals may be due to various reasons including natural origin, wider availability, lesser adverse effects and most importantly, easy to adopt in the regular diet. The dietary phytochemicals are the bioactive plant secondary metabolites belongs to the classes include polyphenols, alkaloids, nitrogen compounds and carotenoids mostly found in fruits, vegetables and other plant products. Experimental evidence and traditional knowledge reveal that many bioactive dietary phytochemicals act as antiproliferative, antiangiogenic, antimetastatic and pro-apoptotic molecules implies through genetic and epigenetic mechanisms.

Green tea (*Camellia sinensis*) is a universal beverage consumed worldwide and more commonly in Asia and North America. Apart from basic nutrients like protein, carbohydrates and minerals, green tea contains a higher amount of bioactive polyphenols such as epigallocatechin-3-gallate (EGCG), epicatechin-3-gallate (ECG), epicatechin (EC) and epigallocatechin (ECG). Among, EGCG is the most abundant and well-studied for its anti-cancerous activity. EGCG has been shown to attributes its anti-cancer activity through various mechanisms including inhibition of epigenetic modulatory enzymes such as DNMTs and HATs [92]. In addition to its preclinical evidences, clinical trials have also supported the anti-cancer effect of green tea in humans. A double–blind placebo controlled trail evidenced a significant reduction in tumor incidence in patients who were taken 600 mg./day green tea catechins orally for 1 year compared to control-patients [9]. Many other case-control studies have also supported that the consumption of green tea reduced the risk of cancer incidence in human [44]. Resveratrol, a phytoalexin found in many fruits but most abundant in the grape skin and berries. One of the herbaceous perennial, *Polygonum cuspidatam,* is the richest natural source of resveratrol and has been traditionally used for the treatment of inflammation and dermatitis. Previous studies have shown that resveratrol act as an anticancer molecule in different tumors in multiple stages including cancer initiation and progression through several mechanisms. Supplementation of resveratrol and its therapeutic effect against breast cancer patients is well documented. A recent phase I randomized double-blind pilot study showed that women with higher consumption of resveratrol decrease the risk of breast cancer through the inhibition of hypermethylation of key genes associated for cancer progression [108]. Furthermore, a case-control study showed that consumption of resveratrol reduces the risk of breast cancer compared with people who have consumed less than the former one [60].

Curcumin is a bright yellow-pigmented plant polyphenol; it is a principal curcuminoid derived from the rhizome of the perennial turmeric (*Curcuma onga*) plant. Several preclinical studies have shown that curcumin inhibits the cell proliferation, metastasis, angiogenesis and induces apoptosis in cancer cells through different mechanisms including inhibition of key epigenetic modulatory enzymes such as DNMTs and HDACs [92]. Recent studies imply that curcumin can interact with many tumor-suppressive and tumor-promotive miRNA's involved in the various stages of breast tumors [70]. Many preclinical studies have suggested that the consumption of curcumin is beneficial to fight against human neoplasia [44]. It has been demonstrated that the intake of curcumin suppresses the progressions of bladder cancer, intestinal neoplasia and pancreatic cancer in humans [18, 20]. Randomized clinical trials have documented that the oral intake of 500 mg–8 g per day curcumin shown a beneficial effect in cancer patients [44]. A phase I clinical study showed that the liposomal-encapsulated curcumin with single doses of 10–400 mg/m^2 had a dose-dependent increase of plasma curcumin level with no clinical side effects. However, some morphological changes in the red blood cells were observed after 120 mg/m^2, which is likely indicating the dose-limiting sign of toxicity [96]. Lycopene is a one of the plant accessory pigment belongs to the carotenoid family found in many fruits and vegetables. Several experimental studies revealed that lycopene is a potent antioxidant, it protects the biomolecules by reducing the intracellular ROS generation. Nearly 21 observational studies revealed that consumption of moderate and higher lycopene-rich diets decreases the risk of prostate cancer by 6% and 11%, respectively [56]. However, no clinical studies with the epigenetic modulatory effect of lycopene have been reported yet. In accordance, many other bioactive phytochemicals are also yet to be clinically validated through they have been reported to have epigenetic modulatory potential in preclinical models.

16.7 Conclusion

DNA methylation, histone modifications and miRNA mediated gene-silencing play a major role in the neoplastic transformation of cells. In general, DNA methylation and hypo-acetylation at histones silence the transcriptional expressions of key genes involved in tumor progressions. Synthetic DNMTs and HDACs inhibitors have opened a new avenue in the field of drug discovery against cancer. However, many epigenetic modulatory compounds are under various stages of clinical trials, but so far, very few drugs have been approved for the treatment of cancer, especially for the treatment of haematological cancer. Many of these available synthetic compounds show various limitations such as higher cost, limited bioavailability, lack of target specificity and adverse side effects. In addition, these synthetic compounds can produce mutagenic bi-products inside the body. Taken together, the higher cost and the adverse side effects associated with the synthetic epigenetic modulatory compounds necessitate the use of natural bioactive phytochemicals as epigenetic modulator against cancer. Preclinical as well as clinical studies have provided strong evidences that bioactive natural compounds possess potent anti-cancer properties and some of these effects are coordinated via modulation of the epigenetic machinery of the transformed cells. However, very limited informations are only available on the clinical usage of epigenetic-modulatory phytochemicals against human breast cancer. Further clinical trials are required to validate the preclinical knowledge and transform these epigenetic modulators from the bench to bedside.

References

1. Aapola U, Kawasaki K, Scott HS et al (2000) Isolation and initial characterization of a novel zinc finger gene, DNMT3L, on 21q22.3, related to the cytosine-5-methyltransferase 3 gene family. Genomics 65:293–298
2. Ai L, Tao Q, Zhong S, Fields CR, Kim WJ, Lee MW, Cui Y, Brown KD, Robertson KD (2006) Inactivation of Wnt inhibitory factor-1 (WIF1) expression by epigenetic silencing is a common event in breast cancer. Carcinogenesis 27:1341–1348
3. Ashraf N et al (2006) Altered sirtuin expression is associated with node-positive breast cancer. Br J Cancer 95(8):1056–1061
4. Baylin SB, Ohm JE (2006) Epigenetic gene silencing in cancer – a mechanism for early oncogenic pathway addiction? Nat Rev Cancer 6(2):107–116
5. Benetti R, Gonzalo S, Jaco I et al (2008) A mammalian microRNA cluster controls DNA methylation and telomere recombination via Rbl2-dependent regulation of DNA methyltransferases. Nat Struct Mol Biol 15:268–279
6. Benevolenskaya EV, Islam AB, Ahsan H et al (2016) DNA methylation and hormone receptor status in breast cancer. Clin Epigenetics 8:17
7. Berdasco M, Ropero S, Setien F, Fraga MF, Lapunzina P, Losson R, Alaminos M, Cheung NK, Rahman N, Esteller M (2009) Epigenetic inactivation of the Sotos overgrowth syndrome gene histone methyltransferase NSD1 in human neuroblastoma and glioma. Proc Natl Acad Sci U S A 106:21830–21835
8. Bernstein BE, Kamal M, Lindblad-Toh K et al (2005) Genomic maps and comparative analysis of histone modifications in human and mouse. Cell 120:169–181
9. Bettuzzi S et al (2006) Chemoprevention of human prostate cancer by oral administration of green tea catechins in volunteers with high-grade prostate intraepithelial neoplasia: a preliminary report from a one-year proof-of-principle study. Cancer Res 66(2):1234–1240
10. Birgisdottir V, Stefansson OA, Bodvarsdottir SK, Hilmarsdottir H, Jonasson JG, Eyfjord JE (2006) Epigenetic silencing and deletion of the BRCA1 gene in sporadic breast cancer. Breast Cancer Res 8:R38
11. Bolden JE, Peart MJ, Johnstone RW (2006) Anticancer activities of histone deacetylase inhibitors. Nat Rev Drug Discov 5:769–784
12. Bracken AP, Helin K (2009) Polycomb group proteins: navigators of lineage pathways led astray in cancer. Nat Rev Cancer 9(11):773–784
13. Brooks J, Cairns P, Zeleniuch-Jacquotte A (2009) Promoter methylation and the detection of breast cancer. Cancer Causes Control 20:1539–1550
14. Byrd JC, Marcucci G, Parthun MR et al (2005) A phase 1 and pharmacodynamic study of depsipeptide (FK228) in chronic lymphocytic leukemia and acute myeloid leukemia. Blood 105:959–967
15. Calin GA (2009) MicroRNAs and cancer: what we know and what we still have to learn. Genome Med 1:78
16. Chedin F, Lieber MR, Hsieh CL (2002) The DNA methyltransferase-like protein DNMT3L stimulates de novo methylation by Dnmt3a. Proc Natl Acad Sci U S A 99:16916–16921
17. Chen S, Wang Y, Zhou W et al (2014) Identifying novel selective non-nucleoside DNA methyltransferase 1 inhibitors through docking-based virtual screening. J Med Chem 57:9028–9041
18. Cheng AL et al (2001) Phase I clinical trial of curcumin, a chemopreventive agent, in patients with high-risk or pre-malignant lesions. Anticancer Res 21(4B):2895–2900
19. Cho YH, Yazici H, Wu HC, Terry MB, Gonzalez K, Qu M, Dalay N, Santella RM (2010) Aberrant promoter hypermethylation and genomic hypomethylation in tumor, adjacent normal tissues and blood from breast cancer patients. Anticancer Res 30:2489–2496
20. Dhillon N et al (2008) Phase II trial of curcumin in patients with advanced pancreatic cancer. Clin Cancer Res 14(14):4491–4499

21. Dong A, Yoder JA, Zhang X, Zhou L, Bestor TH, Cheng X (2001) Structure of human DNMT2, an enigmatic DNA methyltransferase homolog that displays denaturant-resistant binding to DNA. Nucleic Acids Res 29:439–448

22. Dulaimi E, Hillinck J, Ibanez de Caceres I, Al-Saleem T, Cairns P (2004) Tumor suppressor gene promoter hypermethylation in serum of breast cancer patients. Clin Cancer Res 10:6189–6193

23. Duong V, Bret C, Altucci L et al (2008) Specific activity of class II histone deacetylases in human breast cancer cells. Mol Cancer Res 6:1908–1919

24. Eden A, Gaudet F, Waghmare A, Jaenisch R (2003) Chromosomal instability and tumors promoted by DNA hypomethylation. Science 300:455

25. Eiriksdottir G, Johannesdottir G, Ingvarsson S et al (1998) Mapping loss of heterozygosity at chromosome 13q: loss at 13q12-q13 is associated with breast tumour progression and poor prognosis. Eur J Cancer 34:2076–2081

26. Elsheikh SE, Green AR, Rakha EA et al (2009) Global histone modifications in breast cancer correlate with tumor phenotypes, prognostic factors, and patient outcome. Cancer Res 69:3802–3809

27. Esteller M (2000) Epigenetic lesions causing genetic lesions in human cancer: promoter hypermethylation of DNA repair genes. Eur J Cancer 36(18):2294–2300

28. Esteller M (2007) Cancer epigenomics: DNA methylomes and histone-modification maps. Nat Rev Genet 8(4):286–298

29. Esteller M et al (2001) DNA methylation patterns in hereditary human cancers mimic sporadic tumorigenesis. Hum Mol Genet 10(26):3001–3007

30. Fang F, Turcan S, Rimner A et al (2011) Breast cancer methylomes establish an epigenomic foundation for metastasis. Sci Transl Med 3:75ra25

31. Ferguson-Smith AC, Surani MA (2001) Imprinting and the epigenetic asymmetry between parental genomes. Science 293:1086–1089

32. Ferrari R, Pellegrini M, Horwitz GA, Xie W, Berk AJ, Kurdistani SK (2008) Epigenetic reprogramming by adenovirus e1a. Science 321:1086–1088

33. Foss F, Advani R, Duvic M et al (2015) A Phase II trial of Belinostat (PXD101) in patients with relapsed or refractory peripheral or cutaneous T-cell lymphoma. Br J Haematol 168:811–819

34. Fraga MF et al (2005) Loss of acetylation at Lys16 and trimethylation at Lys20 of histone H4 is a common hallmark of human cancer. Nat Genet 37(4):391–400

35. Frankel LB, Christoffersen NR, Jacobsen A, Lindow M, Krogh A, Lund AH (2008) Programmed cell death 4 (PDCD4) is an important functional target of the microRNA miR-21 in breast cancer cells. J Biol Chem 283:1026–1033

36. Garcia JS, Jain N, Godley LA (2010) An update on the safety and efficacy of decitabine in the treatment of myelodysplastic syndromes. Oncol Targets Ther 3:1–13

37. Gayther SA, Batley SJ, Linger L et al (2000) Mutations truncating the EP300 acetylase in human cancers. Nat Genet 24:300–303

38. Girault I, Tozlu S, Lidereau R, Bièche I (2003) Expression analysis of DNA methyltransferases 1, 3A, and 3B in sporadic breast carcinomas. Clin Cancer Res 9:4415–4422

39. Gorrini C et al (2007) Tip60 is a haplo-insufficient tumour suppressor required for an oncogene-induced DNA damage response. Nature 448(7157):1063–1067

40. Gros C, Fleury L, Nahoum V et al (2015) New insights on the mechanism of quinoline-based DNA methyltransferase inhibitors. J Biol Chem 290:6293–6302

41. Guo D, Myrdal PB, Karlage KL, O'Connell SP, Wissinger TJ, Tabibi SE, Yalkowsky SH (2010) Stability of 5-fluoro-2′-deoxycytidine and tetrahydrouridine in combination. AAPS PharmSciTech 11:247–252

42. Hon GC, Hawkins RD, Caballero OL et al (2012) Global DNA hypomethylation coupled to repressive chromatin domain formation and gene silencing in breast cancer. Genome Res 22:246–258

43. Horton JR, Engstrom A, Zoeller EL, Liu X, Shanks JR, Zhang X, Johns MA, Vertino PM, Fu H, Cheng X (2016) Characterization of a linked Jumonji domain of the KDM5/JARID1 family of histone H3 lysine 4 demethylases. J Biol Chem 291:2631–2646

44. Hosseini A, Ghorbani A (2015) Cancer therapy with phytochemicals: evidence from clinical studies. Avicenna J Phytomed 5(2):84–97
45. Huang Q, Gumireddy K, Schrier M et al (2008) The microRNAs miR-373 and miR-520c promote tumour invasion and metastasis. Nat Cell Biol 10:202–210
46. Iorio MV, Casalini P, Piovan C, Braccioli L, Tagliabue E (2011) Breast cancer and microRNAs: therapeutic impact. Breast 20(Suppl 3):S63–S70
47. Iyer NG, Ozdag H, Caldas C (2004) p300/CBP and cancer. Oncogene 23:4225–4231
48. Jackson K, Yu MC, Arakawa K, Fiala E, Youn B, Fiegl H, Müller-Holzner E, Widschwendter M, Ehrlich M (2004) DNA hypomethylation is prevalent even in low-grade breast cancers. Cancer Biol Ther 3:1225–1231
49. Jenuwein T, Allis CD (2001) Translating the histone code. Science 293(5532):1074–1080
50. Jin Z, Tamura G, Tsuchiya T, Sakata K, Kashiwaba M, Osakabe M, Motoyama T (2001) Adenomatous polyposis coli (APC) gene promoter hypermethylation in primary breast cancers. Br J Cancer 85:69–73
51. Johnson SM, Grosshans H, Shingara J, Byrom M, Jarvis R, Cheng A, Labourier E, Reinert KL, Brown D, Slack FJ (2005) RAS is regulated by the let-7 microRNA family. Cell 120:635–647
52. Jones PA (2002) DNA methylation and cancer. Oncogene 21:5358–5360
53. Kim VN (2005) MicroRNA biogenesis: coordinated cropping and dicing. Nat Rev Mol Cell Biol 6:376–385
54. Kiyono T, Foster SA, Koop JI, McDougall JK, Galloway DA, Klingelhutz AJ (1998) Both Rb/p16INK4a inactivation and telomerase activity are required to immortalize human epithelial cells. Nature 396:84–88
55. Knudson AG (2000) Chasing the cancer demon. Annu Rev Genet 34:1–19
56. Kotecha R, Takami A, Espinoza JL (2016) Dietary phytochemicals and cancer chemoprevention: a review of the clinical evidence. Oncotarget 7(32):52517–52529
57. Kouzarides T (2007) Chromatin modifications and their function. Cell 128:693–705
58. Kunju LP, Cookingham C, Toy KA, Chen W, Sabel MS, Kleer CG (2011) EZH2 and ALDH-1 mark breast epithelium at risk for breast cancer development. Mod Pathol 24:786–793
59. Lehmann U, Hasemeier B, Christgen M, Müller M, Römermann D, Länger F, Kreipe H (2008) Epigenetic inactivation of microRNA gene hsa-mir-9-1 in human breast cancer. J Pathol 214:17–24
60. Levi F et al (2005) Resveratrol and breast cancer risk. Eur J Cancer Prev 14(2):139–142
61. Lin YW, Sheu JC, Liu LY, Chen CH, Lee HS, Huang GT, Wang JT, Lee PH, Lu FJ (1999) Loss of heterozygosity at chromosome 13q in hepatocellular carcinoma: identification of three independent regions. Eur J Cancer 35:1730–1734
62. Lo PK, Sukumar S (2008) Epigenomics and breast cancer. Pharmacogenomics 9:1879–1902
63. Lo PK, Mehrotra J, D'Costa A, Fackler MJ, Garrett-Mayer E, Argani P, Sukumar S (2006) Epigenetic suppression of secreted frizzled related protein 1 (SFRP1) expression in human breast cancer. Cancer Biol Ther 5:281–286
64. Ma L, Teruya-Feldstein J, Weinberg RA (2007) Tumour invasion and metastasis initiated by microRNA-10b in breast cancer. Nature 449:682–688
65. Mayr C, Hemann MT, Bartel DP (2007) Disrupting the pairing between let-7 and Hmga2 enhances oncogenic transformation. Science 315:1576–1579
66. Mertens-Talcott SU et al (2007) The oncogenic microRNA-27a targets genes that regulate specificity protein transcription factors and the G2-M checkpoint in MDA-MB-231 breast cancer cells. Cancer Res 67(22):11001–11011
67. Müller BM, Jana L, Kasajima A, Lehmann A, Prinzler J, Budczies J, Winzer KJ, Dietel M, Weichert W, Denkert C (2013) Differential expression of histone deacetylases HDAC1, 2 and 3 in human breast cancer--overexpression of HDAC2 and HDAC3 is associated with clinico-pathological indicators of disease progression. BMC Cancer 13:215
68. Nakamura K, Nakabayashi K, Htet Aung K, Aizawa K, Hori N, Yamauchi J, Hata K, Tanoue A (2015) DNA methyltransferase inhibitor zebularine induces human cholangiocarcinoma cell death through alteration of DNA methylation status. PLoS One 10:e0120545

69. Newman EM, Morgan RJ, Kummar S et al (2015) A phase I, pharmacokinetic, and pharmacodynamic evaluation of the DNA methyltransferase inhibitor 5-fluoro-2′-deoxycytidine, administered with tetrahydrouridine. Cancer Chemother Pharmacol 75:537–546
70. Norouzi S et al (2018) Curcumin as an adjunct therapy and microRNA modulator in breast cancer. Curr Pharm Des 24(2):171–177
71. O'Connor OA (2006) Pralatrexate: an emerging new agent with activity in T-cell lymphomas. Curr Opin Oncol 18(6):591–597
72. O'Connor OA, Horwitz S, Masszi T et al (2015) Belinostat in patients with relapsed or refractory peripheral T-cell lymphoma: results of the pivotal phase II BELIEF (CLN-19) study. J Clin Oncol 33:2492–2499
73. O'Day E, Lal A (2010) MicroRNAs and their target gene networks in breast cancer. Breast Cancer Res 12(2):201
74. Okano M, Bell DW, Haber DA, Li E (1999) DNA methyltransferases Dnmt3a and Dnmt3b are essential for de novo methylation and mammalian development. Cell 99:247–257
75. Park SY, Jun JA, Jeong KJ, Heo HJ, Sohn JS, Lee HY, Park CG, Kang J (2011) Histone deacetylases 1, 6 and 8 are critical for invasion in breast cancer. Oncol Rep 25:1677–1681
76. Piekarz RL, Frye R, Turner M et al (2009) Phase II multi-institutional trial of the histone deacetylase inhibitor romidepsin as monotherapy for patients with cutaneous T-cell lymphoma. J Clin Oncol 27:5410–5417
77. Pruitt K, Zinn RL, Ohm JE, McGarvey KM, Kang SH, Watkins DN, Herman JG, Baylin SB (2006) Inhibition of SIRT1 reactivates silenced cancer genes without loss of promoter DNA hypermethylation. PLoS Genet 2:e40
78. Rasti M et al (2005) Recruitment of CBP/p300, TATA-binding protein, and S8 to distinct regions at the N terminus of adenovirus E1A. J Virol 79(9):5594–5605
79. Rauscher GH, Kresovich JK, Poulin M et al (2015) Exploring DNA methylation changes in promoter, intragenic, and intergenic regions as early and late events in breast cancer formation. BMC Cancer 15:816
80. Reik W, Lewis A (2005) Co-evolution of X-chromosome inactivation and imprinting in mammals. Nat Rev Genet 6(5):403–410
81. Reynolds PA, Sigaroudinia M, Zardo G, Wilson MB, Benton GM, Miller CJ, Hong C, Fridlyand J, Costello JF, Tlsty TD (2006) Tumor suppressor p16INK4A regulates polycomb-mediated DNA hypermethylation in human mammary epithelial cells. J Biol Chem 281:24790–24802
82. Richardson BC (2002) Role of DNA methylation in the regulation of cell function: autoimmunity, aging and cancer. J Nutr 132:2401S–2405S
83. Roll JD, Rivenbark AG, Jones WD, Coleman WB (2008) DNMT3b overexpression contributes to a hypermethylator phenotype in human breast cancer cell lines. Mol Cancer 7:15
84. Ropero S, Fraga MF, Ballestar E et al (2006) A truncating mutation of HDAC2 in human cancers confers resistance to histone deacetylase inhibition. Nat Genet 38:566–569
85. Ruike Y, Imanaka Y, Sato F, Shimizu K, Tsujimoto G (2010) Genome-wide analysis of aberrant methylation in human breast cancer cells using methyl-DNA immunoprecipitation combined with high-throughput sequencing. BMC Genomics 11:137
86. Saunders LR, Verdin E (2007) Sirtuins: critical regulators at the crossroads between cancer and aging. Oncogene 26(37):5489–5504
87. Schneider R, Bannister AJ, Myers FA, Thorne AW, Crane-Robinson C, Kouzarides T (2004) Histone H3 lysine 4 methylation patterns in higher eukaryotic genes. Nat Cell Biol 6:73–77
88. Schübeler D, MacAlpine DM, Scalzo D et al (2004) The histone modification pattern of active genes revealed through genome-wide chromatin analysis of a higher eukaryote. Genes Dev 18:1263–1271
89. Schultz J et al (2008) MicroRNA let-7b targets important cell cycle molecules in malignant melanoma cells and interferes with anchorage-independent growth. Cell Res 18(5):549–557
90. Shukla V, Coumoul X, Lahusen T et al (2010) BRCA1 affects global DNA methylation through regulation of DNMT1. Cell Res 20:1201–1215

310 S. Shukla et al.

91. Shukla S, Khan S, Tollefsbol TO et al (2013) Genetics and epigenetics of lung cancer: mechanisms and future perspectives. Curr Cancer Ther Rev 9:97–110
92. Shukla S, Meeran SM, Katiyar SK (2014) Epigenetic regulation by selected dietary phytochemicals in cancer chemoprevention. Cancer Lett 355(1):9–17
93. Silva J, Silva JM, Domínguez G, García JM, Cantos B, Rodríguez R, Larrondo FJ, Provencio M, España P, Bonilla F (2003) Concomitant expression of p16INK4a and p14ARF in primary breast cancer and analysis of inactivation mechanisms. J Pathol 199:289–297
94. Sinkkonen L, Hugenschmidt T, Berninger P, Gaidatzis D, Mohn F, Artus-Revel CG, Zavolan M, Svoboda P, Filipowicz W (2008) MicroRNAs control de novo DNA methylation through regulation of transcriptional repressors in mouse embryonic stem cells. Nat Struct Mol Biol 15:259–267
95. Song FF, Xia LL, Ji P et al (2015) Human dCTP pyrophosphatase 1 promotes breast cancer cell growth and stemness through the modulation on 5-methyl-dCTP metabolism and global hypomethylation. Oncogene 4:e159
96. Storka A et al (2015) Safety, tolerability and pharmacokinetics of liposomal curcumin in healthy humans. Int J Clin Pharmacol Ther 53(1):54–65
97. Tajima S, Suetake I (1998) Regulation and function of DNA methylation in vertebrates. J Biochem 123(6):993–999
98. Takai D, Jones PA (2002) Comprehensive analysis of CpG islands in human chromosomes 21 and 22. Proc Natl Acad Sci U S A 99(6):3740–3745
99. Tavazoie SF, Alarcón C, Oskarsson T, Padua D, Wang Q, Bos PD, Gerald WL, Massagué J (2008) Endogenous human microRNAs that suppress breast cancer metastasis. Nature 451:147–152
100. Tlsty TD et al (2004) Genetic and epigenetic changes in mammary epithelial cells may mimic early events in carcinogenesis. J Mammary Gland Biol Neoplasia 9(3):263–274
101. Veeck J, Esteller M (2010) Breast cancer epigenetics: from DNA methylation to microRNAs. J Mammary Gland Biol Neoplasia 15(1):5–17
102. Ventura A, Young AG, Winslow MM et al (2008) Targeted deletion reveals essential and overlapping functions of the miR-17 through 92 family of miRNA clusters. Cell 132:875–886
103. Wang GG, Allis CD, Chi P (2007) Chromatin remodeling and cancer, Part I: Covalent histone modifications. Trends Mol Med 13:363–372
104. Widschwendter M, Jones PA (2002) DNA methylation and breast carcinogenesis. Oncogene 21(35):5462–5482
105. Xu X, Gammon MD, Hernandez-Vargas H, Herceg Z, Wetmur JG, Teitelbaum SL, Bradshaw PT, Neugut AI, Santella RM, Chen J (2012) DNA methylation in peripheral blood measured by LUMA is associated with breast cancer in a population-based study. FASEB J 26:2657–2666
106. Yang PM, Lin YT, Shun CT, Lin SH, Wei TT, Chuang SH, Wu MS, Chen CC (2013) Zebularine inhibits tumorigenesis and stemness of colorectal cancer via p53-dependent endoplasmic reticulum stress. Sci Rep 3:3219
107. Zhang L, Coukos G (2006) MicroRNAs: a new insight into cancer genome. Cell Cycle 5:2216–2219
108. Zhu W et al (2012) Trans-resveratrol alters mammary promoter hypermethylation in women at increased risk for breast cancer. Nutr Cancer 64(3):393–400

Chapter 17
Targeting CSC in a Most Aggressive Subtype of Breast Cancer TNBC

Bin Bao and Ananda S. Prasad

Abstract Triple negative breast cancer (TNBC) is a more aggressive subtype of breast cancer and is characteristic of the absence of the expressions of estrogen receptor, progesterone receptor, and human epithelial growth factor receptor 2 in breast tumor tissues. This subtype of breast cancer has the poorest prognosis, compared to other subtypes of breast cancer. TNBC is heterogeneous by showing several different histo-pathological and molecular subtypes with different prognosis and is more commonly found in younger age of women, especially African-American and Hispanic women. Recent epidemiological data indicate that TNBC is highly associated with overweight/obesity. Due to the absence of the common tumor biomarkers of breast cancer, the current molecular target therapy is not effective. TNBC patients have a shorter survival rate and an increased tumor recurrence. The concept of cancer stem cells (CSC), also called tumor initiating cells (TIC) has been more and more accepted and considered to contribute to aggressive phenotypes of many tumors including breast cancer. Moreover, CSC/TIC has been identified in the tumor tissues of breast cancer including TNBC. These rare subpopulations of CSC/TIC cells might be one of the key contributors to the aggressive phenotypes of TNBC such as drug treatment resistance, metastasis, and tumor recurrence. Therefore, targeting these CSC/TIC cells will provide a new therapeutic strategy for the treatment of TNBC.

Keywords Obesity/Overweight · Triple Negative Breast Cancer · Cancer Stem Cells

B. Bao (✉) · A. S. Prasad
Department of Oncology, School of Medicine, Wayne State University, Detroit, MI, USA
e-mail: baob@karmanos.org

© Springer Nature Switzerland AG 2019
A. Ahmad (ed.), *Breast Cancer Metastasis and Drug Resistance*,
Advances in Experimental Medicine and Biology 1152,
https://doi.org/10.1007/978-3-030-20301-6_17

17.1   Introduction

Breast cancer is one of the most common malignant diseases in women across the world including the USA, with approximately 1.7 million of new cases of breast cancer diagnosed each year, which accounts for about 12% of all new cancer cases and 25% of all cancers in women. According to WHO, there are approximately 500,000 deaths due to breast cancer in the world every year. Breast cancer has been the second leading cause of cancer-related death in women with the highest amount of newly diagnosed cases over the decades in the USA [1]. It has been reported that on average, one of eight women develop breast cancer in their life-time [1]. Aging has been believed as a major risk factor for the development of breast cancer. However, women between the ages of 20 and 59 are at highest risk for the cancer-related death in the UAS [2]. It has been estimated that breast cancer affects about 121 per 100,000 women and its incidence rate is reported more frequently in African American women than in European American or other ethnic women in the USA [1]. It is reported that the survival rates of breast cancer have increased between 1987 and 2007 from 84% to 90% [2], due to early detection and effective treatment options. Many factors such dietary pattern, life-styles, tumor screen behaviors, and socio-economic status might impact overall survival of breast cancer (Dal 2008). For example, dietary patterns of breast cancer patients containing fruits, whole grains and fish, and vegetables but lacking animal fats and red meats has been highly associated with the overall survival of breast cancer [3]. After diagnosis of breast cancer, patient survival rates are also dependent on appropriateness of treatment and tumor characteristics [3]. Overall, breast cancer has been considered as an aging-related disease and is much more commonly seen in post-menopausal than in pre-menopausal women except certain subtypes of breast cancer. However, other factors such as genetics, hormones or its receptors, environmental factors, and socio-economic status also greatly contribute to the development of breast cancer.

Breast cancer is characterized by its heterogeneity and complexity, due to the structure of the mammary glands and status of hormones, growth factors, or receptors in the body and is mainly classified into four subtypes based on the status of hormone receptors such estrogen receptor (ER) and progesterone receptor (PR), and one oncogenic biomarker human epithelial growth factor receptor 2 (HER2). Triple negative breast cancer (TNBC, defined as ER-/PR-HER2-) is one common subtype of breast cancer, due to the lack of these three common tumor biomarkers, which accounts for 10–25% of breast cancer. This subtype of breast cancer is the most aggressive subtype of breast cancer with the poorest prognosis, due to the lack of molecular targeted treatment. The incidence of TNBC is prevalent worldwide. However, TNBC is more frequently seen in young ages of women, especially more in African ancestry than other racial or ethnic groups. It is also reported that TNBC is more seen in Ashkenazi Jewish ancestry [4]. This subtype of breast cancer is also highly associated with obesity or overweight, a similar phenomenon observed in other subtypes of breast cancer.

Although a great effort has been made on the investigation of breast cancer biology over several decades, the molecular mechanism of tumorigenesis of breast cancer including TNBC is still not fully understood. The concept of cancer stem cells (CSC) or tumor initiating cells (TIC) has been more and more accepted in the field of cancer biology since the first identification of CSC cells in the bone marrow of acute myeloid leukemia (AML) patients in 1993 [5]. The rare subpopulations of CSC cells have been identified and characterized with tumor aggressive phenotypes in many different cancers, including breast cancer, and have been shown to have very important clinical implications. In this article, we will discuss the role of CSC and its different markers in breast cancer including TNBC. We will also discuss the role of several molecular signaling pathways such as Wnt/β-catenin, Notch, hedgehog, and STAT3 in the regulation of CSC characteristics in breast cancer including TNBC. Finally, we will discuss the significance of targeting CSC as a new therapeutic treatment strategy for breast cancer including TNBC.

17.2   Breast Cancer

Breast cancer is one of the most challengeable public health issues in the world. According to a recent report of cancer statistics by the American Cancer Society, there are approximately 252,710 newly diagnosed breast cancers in the USA in 2017. From 2005 to 2014, overall breast cancer incidence rates increased among African, Hispanic, and Asian American women but are stable in European American women in the USA [1, 6]. The incidence rates of hormone receptor-positive breast cancer increased among all racial/ethnic groups, whereas rates of hormone receptor-negative breast cancers decreased. Currently, it is estimated that on average, 25% women will develop breast cancer over their life-time. If they have inherited gene mutations such as BRCA1, BRCA2, and p53, their risk will be greatly increased. Breast cancer affects 121 per 100,000 people, with a greater incidence among African Americans than other ethnic groups. It is estimated that there are 40,610 deaths due to breast cancer in the USA, the second leading cause of cancer-related death among women in the USA [1].

Thanks to the early detection and more effective treatment options, the mortality of breast cancer greatly decreased and the disease survival rate of breast cancer increased, compared to the past several decades [1]. It has been reported that from 1989 to 2015, breast cancer death rates decreased by 39% in the USA [1]. However, more than 20% of breast cancer patients still develop treatment resistance, tumor recurrence, and metastasis, especially for those breast cancer patients diagnosed at advanced stages of the disease [7, 8].

Due to the complexity and heterogeneity of breast cancer, it can be classified into several different subtypes based on the histo-morphology and the status of major tumor markers of breast cancer such as ER, PR, and/or HER2 protein. Different subtypes of breast cancer have different prognosis in clinic. For example,

HR+/HER2- subtype breast cancer has the best prognosis and is the most common for all races, with the highest rates among non-Hispanic European American women in the USA. This subtype of breast cancer is strongly correlated with the use of mammography. Another subtype of breast cancer, triple-negative (ER-/PR-/HER2-) breast cancer has the highest incidence rate with the worst prognosis among non-Hispanic African American women, compared to other ethnic women in the USA [9].

Traditionally, breast cancer is classified into two subtypes, hormone receptor (HR, estrogen receptor/progesterone, namely ER/PR) positive group and HR negative group, which account for 60–70% and 30–40% of breast cancer, representatively. The status of ER expression in breast cancers is strongly associated with the status of PR expression [10]. HR-positive breast cancer patients typically respond to HR-targeted therapy such as tamoxifen, a selective ER inhibitor, and other HR inhibitors with the best prognosis. HR-negative breast cancer is more aggressive, and is not responsive to HR-targeted therapy [10].

In order to better understand the pathogenesis of breast cancer and explore more effective treatment options for breast cancer, breast cancers have been currently separated into four subtypes according to hormone receptor expressions (negative or positive, namely HR+/−) and/or epithelial cell of origin (luminal or basal) by the analysis of gene expression profiling. There are two groups of HR+ breast cancers, namely luminal A and luminal B, and other two groups of HR- breast cancer, namely human growth factor receptor 2 (HER2)-enriched and HER2 negative basal-like breast cancer. Thus, the breast cancer subtypes can be classified into [1]: luminal A (HR+/HER2-); [2]: luminal B (HR+/HER2+); [3]: HER2-enrich (HR-/HER2+), and [4]: triple negative basal-like (HR-/HER2-) [9]. TNBC tissues usually express basal marker proteins. Thus, triple negative subtype of breast cancer is frequently taken as a surrogate marker of basal-like breast cancer or sometimes called as triple negative basal-like breast cancer. However, it has been noted that triple-negative breast cancer and basal-like breast cancer are separated into different subtypes of breast cancer by some investigators [11]. The gene expression profiling analysis is not currently standard clinical practice. However, within the past 10 years, the examinations of HR/HER2 status in breast cancer have been become routine practice, which might provide an effective treatment strategy for breast cancer [9].

Even though a great progress has been achieved leading to a decrease in the mortality of breast cancer over the past decades, the detailed mechanisms of the development and progress of breast cancer including TNBC is not full understood. It has been reported that the risk factor for the development of breast cancer is associated with aging, oral contraceptive use, less physical activity, obesity, high-energy food intakes, life habits, family history of breast cancer, reproductive experiences such as parity, and breastfeeding. For example, women with family history of breast cancer, especially with inherited gene mutations such as BRCA1, BRCA2, and p53 have a greater risk for the development of breast cancer [7, 10, 12].

17.3   Race Disparity and Breast Cancer

Breast cancer still remains as one of the leading cause of cancer-related death in women in the world even though a significant decrease in the mortality rate of breast cancer. However, race disparity in breast cancer-related death has been observed in Western countries. In the USA, African American women have 40% higher death rate of breast cancer, compared to European white American women [1, 6, 13]. Similar findings have been found in European countries. For example, a prospective study with 3000 breast cancer patients including European white women, African black women, and Asian ethnic women in the United Kingdom (UK) shows that overall breast cancer is more seen in African women [14]. More specifically, ER-/PR-/HER2-negative breast cancer is more frequently seen in African black women (26.1%) than European white women (18.6%, $P = 0.043$). Despite equal access to health care, young African black patients in the UK have a significantly poorer outcome than European white patients. African ethnicity is an independent risk factor for decreased distant relapse-free survival (DRFS) particularly in ER-positive patients [14]. These race disparities in breast cancer have been considered to link several different factors such as the availability of early clinical detection, access to clinical diagnosis and treatment, lifestyle cultures, socioeconomic differences, and biological/genetic feature differences [15].

17.4   TNBC, a most Aggressive Subtype of Breast Cancer

As described earlier, TNBC is the most aggressive subtype of breast cancer and is characteristic of the absence of the expressions of ER, PR, and human HER2 in breast tumor tissues. From histo-pathological views, the majority of TNBC show to have higher grade features such as a high nuclear grade, increased mitotic activity, higher nuclear-to-cytoplasmic ratio, and increased tumor proliferation rate, although a small percentage of TNBC show a lower grade feature [10, 11].

Clinically, TNBC has a poorer prognosis, especially for basal-like subtype, with more aggressive phenotypes such as higher rates of tumor metastasis and recurrence. The most common locations of metastases are in the brain and lung. For example, one cohort study reports that five 5 year-follow-up studies from 231 breast cancers including 17.3% TNBC in China report that the tumor size, recurrence rate, and metastasis rate were significantly increased in TNBC patients, compared to non-TNBC patients [16]. The TNBC patients also had a lower rate of 5 year survival, compared to non-TNBC patients, suggesting that TNBC has the worse clinical outcomes, compared to non-TNBC [16].

17.5 Classifications of TNBC and Its Implication in Clinic

Currently, TNBC is routinely diagnosed based on the accurate assessment of ER/PR protein expression levels by IHC (immuno-histo-chemistry) and the protein level of HER2 by IHC and/or fluorescent in situ hybridization (FISH), but not based on the gene expression profiling analysis, even though gene expression profiling has been used to confirm it by some researchers [11]. The accurate assessment of these three biomarkers is very critical to avoid a risk of the false diagnosis of TNBC so that physicians/oncologists might provide an effective treatment strategy for TNBC patients. The definition of ER negative and PR negative breast cancer has been recommended to those breast cancers that express less than 1% immunoreactive cells to ER and HR staining. However, it has been noted that some clinical trials and epidemiological studies use a threshold of more than 10% immuno-reactive cells to define ER- and PR-positive [11].

Overall, breast cancer is characteristic of heterogeneity and complexity clinically. Beyond the requirement for an accurate diagnosis of TNBC, this subtype breast cancer still has heterogeneous clinical features and behaviors. Further classifications for better understanding the molecular basis of TNBC heterogeneity would provide a new opportunity to discover an actionable molecular targeted treatment strategy for TNBC. Currently, there are two classification mechanisms of TNBC categories by different analysis approaches, namely histological classification and molecular classifications. By histological classification, the majority of TNBC (95%) are classified as invasive ductal carcinoma. Another subtype of TNBC is classified as invasive lobular carcinoma (1–2%). These invasive subtypes of TNBC are mostly associated with poor prognosis. The remaining subtypes, which are rare, are classified as metaplastic carcinoma with squamous differentiation (<1%), spindle-cell metaplastic carcinoma (<1%), adenoid cystic carcinoma (<1%), secretory carcinoma (<1%), typical medullary carcinoma (<1%), atypical medullary carcinoma (<1%), and apocrine carcinoma (<1%), respectively [11]. The rare subtypes of medullary carcinomas in TNBC are characteristic of highly lymphoplasmacytic infiltration and a good prognosis compared to other subtypes of TNBC [17]. It is also noted that other rare TNBC subtypes such as adenosquamous carcinoma, adenoid cystic carcinoma, and fibromatosis-like spindle-cell metaplastic carcinoma are less aggressive and only capable of local recurrence [18].

The molecular classification TNBC is based on the results from transcriptomic and genomic analysis studies, which would provide a good opportunity to find an effective therapeutic strategy aiming at a more specific target for the treatment of TNBC. At present, six different subtypes of TNBC by the molecular classification have been proposed by the use of a meta-analysis study (including 21 breast cancer data sets with 587 cases of TNBC) of the gene expression profiling data, namely, (1): basal-like 1, (2): basal-like 2, (3): mesenchymal, (4): mesenchymal stem-like, (5): immunomodullary, and (6): luminal androgen receptor [19]. It has been noted that some subtypes of TNBC by molecular classification are closely linked to some subtypes of TNBC by the histological classification [19]. These subtypes of TNBC based on the molecular classification have been used for the assessment of differential chemotherapeutic sensitivity in 130 patients with TNBC [20].

17.6 Epidemiology and Etiology of TNBC

TNBC is characteristic of higher cell proliferation, poor cellular differentiation, increased recurrence copy number gene imbalances, and gene mutations in p53 tumor suppressor protein. As currently known, TNBC is one common subtype of breast cancer worldwide, including North America, Asia, Africa, and Europe, which accounts for 10–25% of breast cancer. However, there are still race disparities for TNBC. A large number of epidemiological studies reveal that the incidence rate for TNBC is higher women of African ancestry, especially for women of younger ages. Although the incidence rates of TNBC are different across regional populations of women of African ancestry, it is consistently higher than that reported in comparison to other racial or ethnic original groups such as Asian ancestry, American ancestry, and European ancestry [10]. It is also reported that TNBC is more frequently seen in Ashkenazi Jewish ancestries [4].

Currently, the pathogenesis of TNBC is not fully understood. Increased numbers of epidemiological studies have provided the evidence showing that the risk factors of the development of TNBC might be associated with higher parity, or having more than one child, and shorter duration of breastfeeding [21–23]. It has been noted that oral contraceptive use is also associated with the development of TNBC [10, 23].

It has been widely accepted that overweight/obesity is one of the key risk factors of the development of breast cancer including TNBC. Although one early study among African women showed a conflicting conclusion of the relationship between obesity and TNBC, this may have been due to its small sample size [24]. In 2013, a meta-analysis study of case-case and case-control studies including women of African ancestry demonstrated that obesity is associated with the development of TNBC for all women [25]. Further studies have also provided clear evidence to support the concept that obesity is a high risk factor for the development of TNBC.

Socioeconomic status might play an important role in the development of TNBC. It has been found that low socioeconomic status is positively associated with development of TNBC. Socioeconomic status is strongly associated with race, lifestyles, obesity, reproductive experiences such as high parity, and tumor screening behaviors [10]. Of course, genetic susceptibility such as the gene mutations in BRCA1, BRCA2, and p53 is one of the major risk factors in developing TNBC [4, 10, 11, 26, 27]. However, more studies including epidemiological and basic science studies are required to provide more evidence and better understanding of TNBC pathogenesis in future.

17.7 Treatment of TNBC

Currently, cytotoxic chemotherapy such as anthracyline and taxaned-based chemotherapeutic drugs has been the first choice for treatment of TNBC over the past decades. Despite lack of known molecular targets and the more aggressive courses of TNBC, this subtype of breast cancer is highly responsible for cytotoxic chemotherapeutic drugs, compared to other subtypes of breast cancer. The response rates of TNBC patients who achieve a pathological complete response after the treatment with neoadjuvant chemotherapy ranges from 30% to 45% [20, 28, 29]. The combination of standard chemotherapy with other chemotherapeutic drugs such as platinum salts has been reported to increase a complete pathological response in TNBC [10]. Thus, platinum salts are widely used as an optional treatment for TNBC in clinical settings. Despite its worse clinical outcomes, TNBC patients who achieve a complete pathological response have a better long-term clinical outcome, with overall survival rate of more than 94% [30]. However, TNBC still has higher rates of recurrence after chemotherapy.

Although there is a lack of expression of three known biomarkers in TNBC for the targeted therapy, a great effort has been continuously taken to explore new targeted therapies for the treatment of TNBC. Currently, applications of several selective targeted therapeutic drugs aiming molecular signaling pathways such as PARP, PI3K/mTOR, cell-cycle, JAK/STAT, Notch, RAS/RAF/MEK, HIF-1α, and androgen receptor have been reported for the treatment of TNBC in preclinical and clinical trials [10].

17.8 Obesity and TNBC

Obesity is widely prevalent across the world. It has been reported by the World Health Organization (WHO) that more than 700 million people are obese in the world each year [31, 32]. It is estimated that 65% of the population in the USA are considered obese or overweight [33–35]. Therefore, obesity and overweight adults have become a major public health concern. According to the Food and Agriculture Organization (FAO)/WHO, obesity and overweight conditions are diagnosed by body mass index (BMI), which is calculated by dividing kilograms of body weight into meters squared of height. The current categories of BMI are referred as severely obese ($\geq$35.0), obese (30.0–34.9), overweight (25.0–29.9), normal weight (18.5–24.9), and underweight (<18.5) [34, 36, 37].

It is clearly accepted that being obese or overweight highly increases the risk of several chronic degenerative diseases such as hypertension, diabetes mellitus, and cardiovascular disease. Similarly, high BMI or obesity is positively associated with an increased risk of several common cancers including breast cancer [38–47]. High BMI/obesity has been under study as a risk factor for the development of breast cancer including TNBC for several decades [39, 41, 48, 49]. A majority of epidemiological and clinical studies have revealed that high BMI/obesity is associated with an increased risk or mortality of breast cancer [49–54].

In 2004, a large population-based prospective study with 495,477 women demonstrated that obese women, with BMI ≥35.0, had double the mortality rate from breast cancer when compared to women in the lowest BMI category [55]. More several studies have revealed that high BMI is positively associated with breast cancer in post-menopausal women, but not breast cancer in pre-menopausal women [56, 57]. However, once breast cancer has developed, high BMI has adverse clinical consequences regardless of their pre-menopausal or post-menopausal state [3, 50, 56]. These findings clearly suggest that obesity is associated with the development and progression of breast cancer.

Increasing numbers of epidemiological and clinical studies have provided evidence that obesity is also associated with the development and progression of TNBC. One recent clinical observation study with 1106 TNBC patients, including 656 normal body weight subjects and 450 overweight subjects (BMI greater than 24), revealed that high BMI is highly associated with overall survival (hazard ratio (HR): 1.46; CI: 1.04–2.06) in all the TNBC patients, but not breast cancer-specific survival. In the pre-menopausal group, overweight/obesity is found to be associated with both breast cancer-specific survival and overall survival [58]. However, overweight/obesity is not associated with breast cancer-specific survival and overall survival in the post-menopausal patients with TNBC [58]. More recently, one prospective study with 206 of TNBC patients shows that the breast cancer patients with obesity (BMI = or >25) had larger tumor size, poor overall survival rate, and poor disease-free survival rate [59]. These findings strongly suggest that obesity is an independent prognostic factor for TNBC.

Besides obesity being a poor clinical prognostic factor for breast cancer including TNBC, more evidence indicates that obesity is also a higher risk factor for the development of breast cancer including TNBC [14, 25]. In 2013, one meta-analysis report including 11 original articles (11 case-case studies and 5 case-control studies) with a total of 24,479 breast cancer patients including 3845 the subjects diagnosed with TNBC reveals that there is a significant association between TNBC and obesity [25]. The pooled odds ratios (OR) were 1.2 and 1.24 from case-case and case-control studies, respectively. Moreover, in the pre-menopausal group, there is a significant association between BMI and TNBC. The OR and 95% confidence interval were 1.43 and 1.23–1.65, respectively. These findings clearly suggest that women with overweight/obesity, especially pre-menopausal women have increased risk of developing TNBC, compared to non-obese women [25]. These findings strongly suggest that overweight/obesity plays an important role in the development and progression of TNBC. However, the molecular insight of the role of obesity in the development of TNBC is still not fully elucidated. More studies are required for further investigation of the molecular role of obesity in TNBC in the future.

17.9   Clinical Implications of CSC in Breast Cancer Including TNBC

Although the concept of CSCs or tumor initiating cells (TICs) as special small sub-populations of tumor cells contributing to the initiation and development of cancer was proposed more than several decades ago, it is still in its infancy. Significant progress in the concept and molecular biology of CSC has not been elucidated until the small sub-population of CSCs was first isolated and characterized from the bone marrow of acute myeloid leukemia (AML) patients in 1997 [5]. The implantation of 5000 of these isolated CSC cells with CD34+/CD38- phenotype induced human-like AML in mice whereas the implantation of more than 100,000 unsorted primitive hematopoietic cells from the same patients of AML was required for this induction of human-like AML in the animals [5]. In 2003, the isolation and identification of CSC cells (CD44+/CD24−/low or CD44+/CD24−/low/ESA+) with characteristics of greater tumorigenic potenial and tumor aggressive phenotype from tumor tissues of breast cancer patients provided the first direct evidence of the existenace of CSC cells or CSC-like cells in solid tumors [60]. Since then, these small sub-populations of CSCs have been identified and substantially characterized from a variety of different malignant diseases such as gastric, prostate, pancreatic, lung, colon, and brain tumors as well as leukemia and melanoma. Similar to normal stem cells, for instance, fetal and adult stem cells, CSCs share common features such as dormancy, long life-span, self-renewal capacity, over-expression of stem cell genes, and the potential of its differentiation into multiple cell lineages, all of which contribute to the development and progression of tumors including breast cancer. It has been believed that normal adult stem cells such as mesenchymal stem cells including mammary stem cells are capable of being reprogrammed into CSC cells due to the aberrations of certain micro-environments such as hypoxia, chronic inflammation, and defective DNA repair systems in the body, eventually leading to tumorigenesis [61].

Currently CSCs have been identified to account for a very small percentage (0.05–1%) of tumor bulk cells in a tumor tissue, or in a tumor micro-environment, and have the greatest ability of CSC self-renewal and the higher potential of unlimited differentiation capacity into heterogeneous tumor cell populations, consistent with the higher potential of tumor formation in vivo, all of which contribute to tumor aggressive phenotypes [62–66]. Increasing evidence indicates that the concept of CSCs has great clinical implications because the small sub-populations of CSCs have been identified in many different tumor tissues and are highly associated with poorer clinical outcome such as short disease-free survival time, increased tumor recurrent rate, and remarkable resistance to chemo-radiation therapy [62–64, 67]. For example, one clinical study has shown that the small sub-populations of CSC cells identified by either CD44+/CD24- or aldehyde dehydrogenase 1 positive (ALDH1+) stem cell markers are significantly increased in breast cancer patients after chemotherapy. The patients with increased sub-populations of CD44+/

CD24- CSCs after chemotherapy have the high values of ki67 proliferation index in post-chemotherapy tumor tissues. The patients with increased sub-populations of ALDH1-positive CSCs after chemotherapy are also associated with estrogen receptor negativity and p53 over-expression in the post-chemotherapy tumor samples [68]. Furthermore, the patients with such an increased CSC sub-population after chemotherapy has shown to have a significantly poor clinical outcome such as shorter disease-free survival period [68]. Another clinical study reveals that CD44+/CD24- CSC ratio in breast tumor tissues collected from 1350 of breast cancer patients, accompanied by histological grades, molecular types, and clinical stages is independent factors of clinical outcomes in breast cancer patients, and it is significantly associated with tumor aggressive phenotypes including ER, PR, and Ki67, a known proliferation index [69]. Moreover, the sub-populations of CD44+/CD24- CSC cells are highly associated with a five-year disease-free survival rate of breast cancer. The breast cancer patients who had high values of CD44+/CD24- CSC ratio have poor clinical outcomes such as higher distant tumor recurrence rate compared to those patients with lower values of CD44+/CD24- CSC ratio [69]. Moreover, human breast cancer cells containing ALDH positive CSC cells have an increased capacity of metastasis with distinct CSC molecular phenotypes, e.g., ALDH, Notch-2, and CXCR1 [70]. Furthermore, it is noted that the CSC-like (Aldefluor +) cells of breast cancer including TNBC had increased potential of metastasis in vivo [70–72]. These findings suggest that CSCs might be involved in the promotion of treatment resistance and metastasis in breast cancer including TNBC. The concept of CSC also provides a good explanation for clinical observations of why tumor shrinkage alone by treatments may not be linked to the disease-free survival rate of cancer patients [67], which is partially due to the presence of these small sub-populations of CSCs with the tumor aggressive phenotypes after conventional treatments. It has been noted from experimental studies that inhibition of CSC characteristics results in the suppression of tumor development and progression in vivo [73]. Therefore, inhibition or elimination of CSCs would likely become a new and targeted therapeutic strategy for the treatment of aggressive breast cancer including TNBC.

17.10 Identification of CSC in Breast Cancer Including TNBC by Stem Cell Markers

The identification and characterization of CSCs in breast cancer including TNBC provides insight into ways in which to selectively inhibit or eradicate CSCs as a treatment for tumor aggressive phenotypes. Several common stem cell markers, including CSC-specific markers such as CD34, CD44, CD123, CD133, Oct4, Sox2, Nanog, c-kit, ABCG2, and ALDH have been identified in the CSC subpopulations isolated from a wide variety of solid tumor tissues.

Breast CSCs are a small subpopulation (0.1–1%) of breast cancer cells in primary tumors. A rare subset of breast CSC has a high capacity for self-renewal and is able to initiate tumorigenesis when transplanted into NOD/SCID mice [60, 74]. Several common stem cell markers, including CSC-specific markers such as CD24, CD44, CD133, ALDH, epithelial specific antigen (ESA, also called as EpCAM), c-kit, ABCG2, and ALDH have been identified in primary tumor specimens of breast cancer [75]. A critical role for CD44$^+$ in the development of breast cancer has been indicated by the finding that injection of less than 100 breast CSCs with the phenotype of CD44$^+$/CD24$^-$ or CD44+/CD24-/ESA+ can result in 85% tumor formation in xenograft models, while injection of more than 10,000 non-CSC breast adenocarcinoma cells or tumor cells with other phenotypes fails to form tumors in vivo [60, 76]. Moreover, the cancer cells with the phenotype of CD133$^+$ have CSC characteristics in vitro and in vivo similar to CD44$^+$/CD24$^-$ or CD44+/CD24-/ESA+ CSCs while CD133$^-$ breast adenocarcinoma cells do not generate tumors in mouse tumor xenograft models [74]. As there is no overlap in cell surface marker proteins between CD133$^+$ and CD44$^+$/CD24$^-$ or CD44+/CD24-/ESA+ CSCs [60, 76], there is no universal CSC marker for each type of breast cancer. However, there is some overlap of CSCs among tumor patients between ALDH$^+$ and CD44$^+$/CD24$^-$ cell subpopulations [77]. One experimental study indicates that breast cancer CSCs with a CD44$^+$/CD24$^-$/ALDH$^+$ phenotype have greater tumorigenic potential than CSCs with the CD44$^+$CD24$^-$ or ALDH$^+$ phenotype [78]. Recently, we isolated the triple marker-positive (CD44+/CD133+/EpCAM+) CSC cells of breast cancer from MDA-MB-468 TNBC cells by FACS technique. These rare subpopulations of CSC cells, accounting for less than 0.1% of cancer cells, display CSC characteristics with increased capacity of self-renewal, cell viability, and erlotinib treatment resistance, suggesting the important role of stem markers CD44, CD133, and ESA in maintaining CSC characteristics in TNBC [79]. As ALDH is not expressed with CD44 and CD133 in ovarian tumors, it appears that CSCs with the phenotypes of CD44$^+$, CD24$^-$, CD133$^+$, and ALDH$^+$ have the most pronounced tumorigenic potential in breast cancer, conferring these CSC subpopulations as attractive targets for the treatment of breast cancer including TNBC.

17.11   The Role of Molecular Signaling Pathways in the Regulation of CSC in TNBC

It has been noted that many different molecular signaling pathways might be associated with the maintenance of CSC phenotypes and functions in many different cancers including breast cancer. Here, we will discuss several molecular signaling pathways such as Notch, Wnt/β-catenin, STAT3, and Hedgehog, which are closely associated with CSC characteristics in breast cancer including TNBC, as described below.

17.11.1 Notch

It has been known that Notch signaling pathway plays a pivotal role in the regulation of a wide variety of fundamental biological and cellular processes such as proliferation, stem cell maintenance, differentiation during embryonic and adult development and homeostasis of adult self-renewing organs [80–82]. To date, there are four family members of the Notch receptor proteins (namely Notch-1, 2, 3, 4) encoded by its individual Notch receptor genes, which can be activated by interacting with a family of its Delta/Serrate/LAG-2 (DSL) ligands. The extra-cellular domain of Notch receptors consists of multiple tandemly arranged epithelial growth factor (EGF)-like repeats, which participate in receptor-ligand binding. Notch receptor signaling pathway is initially activated through the receptor-ligand interaction between two neighboring cells (signaling sending cell and signaling receiving cell). Upon activation, the Notch receptor is cleaved through a cascade of proteolytic cleavages by the metalloprotease such as TNF-α-converting enzyme (TACE) and a γ-secretase complex, followed by the release of the intracellular domain of Notch (NICD). The released NICD is then translocated into the nucleus for trans-activation of Notch target genes such as Hes1, Hey1, and cyclin D1 [83]. The endogenous γ-secretase inhibitors (GSI) can down-regulate the Notch receptor signaling pathway by its binding to γ-secretase complex, which leads to the inactivation of γ-secretase enzyme activity [83]. The evidence from a large number of experimental studies suggests that Notch receptor signaling pathway plays a pivotal role in tumor aggressive phenotypes by regulating cell proliferation, apoptosis, invasion, as well as the induction of EMT and CSC functions [82, 84–86]. EMT is a biological process originally involved in the embryonic development and tissue remodeling and is widely considered to have a pivotal role in tumor aggressiveness mediated via induction of cancer cell invasion and migration, and the characteristics of CSCs, which lead to tumor treatment resistance, metastasis, and tumor recurrence [87]. There are some limited reports showing that Notch proteins could exert tumor suppressive effects in few cancers such as lung and skin cancers. However, a large number of studies have revealed that Notch receptor proteins have oncogenic effects in a wide variety of cancers including breast cancer. Oncogenic or tumor suppressive activities of Notch proteins are cellular context-dependent [85].

It has been clear that the Notch signaling pathway provides a great role in the development of mammary glands by the regulation of stem cell maintenance and differentiation of mammary luminal progenitor cells [88]. Moreover, evidence reveals that the Notch signaling pathway is positively associated with the tumor development and progression of breast cancer including TNBC. It is noted that increased expression of Notch 3 receptor is linked to TNBC [89]. Furthermore, several experimental studies indicate that the Notch signaling pathway might regulate characteristics of CSC/TIC cells in breast cancer [90]. One report reveals that Notch 1 and Notch 4 signaling activities are significantly higher in the CSC/TIC-like

(ESA+/CD44+/CD24−/low) cells of breast cancer cells including TNBC cells [91]. The treatment with several different Notch signaling inhibitors (namely γ secretase inhibitors) decreased breast CSC/TIC number and activity as well as tumor formation in vitro and in vivo. The functional loss of Notch 1 or Notch 4 by its shRNA also significantly impacts breast CSC/TIC activity [91]. It has been recently found that TNBC is intrinsically linked to an adult mammary stem cell population signature [88]. This signaling signature predisposes CSC subpopulation of breast cancer cells including TNBC [92]. More evidence shows that increased expressions of Notch receptors 1–4 are found in TNBC basal like cells along with the expression of ALDH1, a known stem cell marker, but not in other subtypes of breast cancer cell lines, mediating the regulation of CSC characteristics [93]. These findings suggest a potential role of Notch receptor signaling pathway in the regulation of CSC characteristics in breast cancer including TNBC.

17.11.2 Wnt/β-catenin

Wnt/β-catenin signalling pathway modulates cell growth by the up-regulation of β-catenin protein expression, nuclear localization of β-catenin protein, and its binding to the lymphoid-enhancing factor (LEF)/TCF family of transcription factors, which leads to the expression of its target genes in controlling cell growth and proliferation [94–98]. A number of experimental studies have provided supportive evidence for a direct role of Wnt/β-catenin signaling pathway in the development of embryonic and adult stem cells through the regulation of phenotype and self-renewal capacity of stem cells in some organs including mammary gland [98]. Moreover, deregulation of Wnt/β-catenin signaling pathway has been observed in many different cancers including breast cancer [99, 100]. The activation of the Wnt/β-catenin signaling pathway in epidermal stem cells of transgenic mice can result in epithelial cancers [101], and induce EMT phenotype [87, 101–104]. Therefore, Wnt/β-catenin signaling pathway plays an important role in the regulation of CSCs and EMT characteristics in many different cancers including breast cancer [87, 103, 105–111].

One early in vivo experimental study shows that primary breast tumor xenografted from TNBC cells such as SUM-149 cells have over-expression of several genes of Wnt/β-catenin signaling pathway such as LRP5, FZD9, WISP2, and CCND3, compared to their corresponding metastatic tumor to lung. The over-expression of DKK, an endogenous inhibitor protein of Wnt/β-catenin signaling pathway or the functional loss of LRP6 by its shRNA results in the reduction of CSC self-renewal capacity in TNBC cells [112]. These inhibitions of Wnt/β-catenin signaling pathway also result in the increased gene expression of epithelial marker of epithelial-to-mesenchymal transition (EMT) and the reduced gene expression of EMT transcription factors, which results in the inhibition of EMT. EMT characteristics have shown to be highly associated with CSC characteristics, contributing to tumor aggressive phenotypes [112]. It is reported that the Wnt/β-catenin signaling pathway is activated in TNBC, and is associated with poor clinical outcomes in breast cancer. For example, The Wnt receptors such as low-density lipoprotein receptor-related protein 6 (LRP6) and frizzed-7 (FZD7) are found to be up-regulated in TNBC [113]. The functional loss of LRP6 or FZD7 in TNBC cells results in the suppression of tumor growth in vivo. A selective breast cancer stem cell inhibitor, salinomycin (also previously considered as Wnt/β-catenin signaling inhibitor), results in the inhibition of CSC functions by the induction of LRP6 degradation in TNBC cells [113]. These findings support that Notch receptor signaling pathway might play a key role in the regulation of CSC characteristics in breast cancer including TNBC.

17.11.3   STAT3

Signal transducer and activation of transcription 3 (STAT3) is a key mediator of pro-inflammatory cytokine signal pathway, which involves the regulation of cell growth, proliferation, and differentiation [114]. After the activation of STAT3 protein responsive to various extra-cellular stimuli such as cytokines and growth factors, STAT3 protein becomes a phosphorylated form, an active form, undergoes nuclear transduction, binds to STAT3 DNA binding sites, and eventually activates the expression of target genes that regulate cell growth and differentiation [114]. Aberrations of the STAT3 signaling pathway are associated with the development and progression of many different tumors including breast cancer [114]. Evidence shows that STAT3 is constitutively activated in all breast cancer subtypes. Additionally, this aberrant activation is most often associated with TNBC as the poorer prognosis [114].

Increasing evidence shows that STAT3 signaling pathway might play an important role in maintaining CSC phenotypes and functions in breast cancer including TNBC. It has been noted that the over-expression of STAT3 increases the gene expression of stem cell markers such as Oct4, Nanog, and Sox2 in breast cancer MCF-7 cells [115]. The inhibition of STAT3 activity by activation of tumor suppressor LKB1 abrogates CSC phenotypes in breast cancer cells [115]. The functional loss of STAT3 in stem cells results in the decrease in expression of neural stem cell marker nestin in neural precursor cells [116]. A further study shows that STAT3 directly binds to the promoter region of Sox2 gene, leading to the high level of Sox2 expression and subsequent high level of nestin expression [116]. Recently, the data from experimental studies demonstrated that the CSC-like (CD44+/CD24-) cells of breast cancer cells in primary human tumors had significantly higher levels of IL-6/JAK2/STAT3 signaling pathway, compared to non-CSC-like tumor cells of breast cancer [117]. These findings suggest a potential role of STAT3 signaling pathway in the regulation of CSC characteristics in breast cancer including TNBC.

17.11.4 Hedgehog

Another important molecular signaling pathway highly associated with the regulation of CSC characteristics is the Hedgehog signaling pathway. The hedgehog signaling pathway is a major regulator of cell differentiation, tissue polarity and cell proliferation [118, 119]. To date, there are three secreted proteins of hedgehog family members, namely, sonic hedgehog (Shh), desert hedgehog (Dhh), and indian hedgehog (Ihh). The hedgehog proteins are activated by several steps of processes such as cleavage and lipid modification. The binding of lipid-modified hedgehog proteins to its receptors such as either patched1 or patched2 (PTCH1 or PTCH2), an inhibitor of smoothened (Smo) leads to the loss of PTCH activity, and consequent activation of Smo, which in turn transduces the hedgehog signal to the cytoplasm. Subsequently, the activated Smo causes the activation of Gli (glioma-associated oncogene family protein) family of transcriptional effectors through complex interactions with costal2 (Cos2), fused (Fu) and suppressor of fu (Sufu), leading to the up-regulation of gene expression of downstream targets such as PTCH, Wnt, N-Myc, cyclin D/E, FoxM1, and bone morphogenetic protein (BMP). Therefore, the hedgehog ligands such as Shh, Dhh and Ihh stimulate Gli transcription factors, which constitute the final effectors of the hedgehog signaling pathway in controlling cell proliferation and differentiation.

It has been known that hedgehog signaling pathway plays a pivotal role in the development of mammary gland through the regulation of embryonic and adult mammary stem cells. Increasing evidence clearly suggests the activation of hedgehog signaling pathway in many different human cancers including breast cancer [120–122]. Furthermore, because hedgehog signaling pathway plays a central role in the control of cell proliferation and differentiation of both embryonic stem cells and adult stem cells, the aberrant activation of hedgehog signaling pathway could lead to the generation of CSCs from normal stem cells and the development of tumor [111]. Recent studies have shown that activation of hedgehog signaling pathway is critically related to the characteristics of CSCs and EMT in many different of cancers [118, 119, 123], which suggests that hedgehog signaling pathway may play a pivotal role in regulating CSC characteristics within the tumor microenvironment of breast cancer including TNBC.

One experimental study shows that the gene expression of hedgehog signaling components such as PTCH1, Gli1, and Gli2 are highly expressed in normal human mammary stem cells-like cells cultured as mammosphere cells, compared to those cells of differentiated mammary cells by using mammosphere-derived cells grown in suspension culture condition (FBS-free) vs a collagen substratum (5% FBS media) [124]. The activation of hedgehog signaling pathway by its agonists increased the number and size of mammosphere cells. However, the inactivation of hedgehog signaling pathway by its antagonist decreased its number and size. Furthermore, the activation of the hedgehog signaling pathway is found in human breast CSC/TIC cells (CD44+/CD24−/low cells derived from primary human breast tumor tissues, compared to non-CSC/TIC tumor cells (CD44-/CD24+) of primary human breast tumor. A few number of these CSC/TIC cells increased tumorigenesis with the activation of hedgehog signaling pathway in vivo [124]. These findings clearly suggest that hedgehog signaling pathway might play a very important role in the maintenance of CSC phenotypes and functions in breast cancer including TNBC.

17.12 Targeting Treatment Strategy of TNBC by Targeting CSC

Due to the lack of molecular targeted treatment therapy for TNBC and rapid development of drug resistance, TNBC has the worst clinical outcomes, as described earlier. The concept of CSC has been more and more widely accepted within a decade. The rare sub-population of CSC cells has been identified in many different tumor tissues including breast cancer. More evidence shows that the sub-population of CSC cells has been associated with the tumorigenesis and progression of TNBC with the worse clinical outcomes. Therefore, targeting this small sub-population of CSC would provide a new therapeutic strategy for the treatment of TNBC. In our recent experimental report, we conducted flow cytometry analysis based on three different cancer stem cell markers, namely CD44, CD133, and EpCAM in TNBC cells such as MDA-MB-468 cells. We found that the triple-marker positive (CD44+/CD133+/EpCAM+) cells (defined as CSC-like cells) accounts for less than 0.1% in MDA-MB-468 cells. We isolated a few of these triple-marker positive CSC cells by FACS technique, and maintained these CSC cells in FBS-free CSC media to sustain its undifferentiated status. We also found that CSC-like cells grow faster than the triple-marker negative (CD44-/CD133-/EpCAM-) cells of MDA-MB-468 cells and have a high resistant capacity to chemotherapeutical drug erlotinib treatment. However, a newly designed catalase-based agent (CAT-SKL) specifically inhibits cell viability and CSC self-renewal capacity in these CSC-like cells of MDA-MB-468 cells [79]. Metformin has been used as classical anti-diabetic drug for the treatment of DM, especially for DM type II for over several decades. A large number of clinical studies indicate that metformin might be acted as a potent anti-tumor drug for the treatment or prevention of some cancers such as pancreatic cancer and breast cancer [125] even though the detailed mechanism of its anti-tumor effect is not fully elucidated. One recent experimental study shows that metformin inhibits CSC phenotypes and functions by the suppression of PKA/GSK3β/KLF5 axis in TNBC cells [126]. The expression levels of PKA/GSK3β are positively correlated with the expression of KLF5, a known stem cell transcription factor in human TNBC tumor tissues [126]. These findings suggest targeting CSC characteristics might provide a new selective therapeutic strategy for the treatment of TNBC (Fig. 17.1).

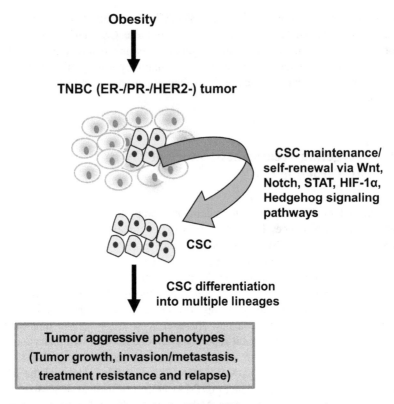

Fig. 17.1 A putative relationship of obesity, TNBC, CSC, and tumor aggressiveness

17.13   Conclusion

TNBC is a common subtype of breast cancer, accounting for about 10–25% cases of invasive breast cancer, with complexity and heterogeneity. Due to the absence of three most common cancer biomarkers, ER, PR, and HER2 in breast cancer, the current targeted therapy for TNBC is not effective, which leads to its poorest clinical outcomes such as a shorter survival rate, tumor recurrence, and metastasis, compared to other non-TNBC subtypes of breast cancer. Its etiology is not clear. However epidemiological data indicate that TNBC is more frequently seen found in Hispanic and African-American women, especially in women of younger ages. Increasing evidence indicates that TNBC is highly associated with overweight/obesity. However, the detailed mechanisms of TNBC pathogenesis are not fully understood. Recently, the concept of CSC/TIC is more and more accepted and considered to contribute to tumor aggressive phenotypes such as drug treatment resistance, tumor recurrence, and metastasis. Moreover, rare subpopulations of CSC/TIC cells have been identified with the greatest capacity of tumorigenesis in vivo from the tumor tissues of breast cancer, including TNBC. Therefore, targeting these small subpopulations of CSC/TIC in TNBC will provide a new therapeutic strategy for the treatment of breast cancer, including TNBC.

References

1. Siegel RL, Miller KD, Jemal A (2017) Cancer statistics, 2017. CA Cancer J Clin 67:7–30
2. Siegel R, Naishadham D, Jemal A (2012) Cancer statistics, 2012. CA Cancer J Clin 62:10–29
3. Dal ML, Zucchetto A, Talamini R, Serraino D, Stocco CF, Vercelli M et al (2008) Effect of obesity and other lifestyle factors on mortality in women with breast cancer. Int J Cancer 123:2188–2194
4. Afghahi A, Telli ML, Kurian AW (2016) Genetics of triple-negative breast cancer: implications for patient care. Curr Probl Cancer 40:130–140
5. Bonnet D, Dick JE (1997) Human acute myeloid leukemia is organized as a hierarchy that originates from a primitive hematopoietic cell. Nat Med 3:730–737
6. DeSantis CE, Ma J, Goding SA, Newman LA, Jemal A (2017) Breast cancer statistics, 2017, racial disparity in mortality by state. CA Cancer J Clin 67:439–448
7. Cadoo KA, Fornier MN, Morris PG (2013) Biological subtypes of breast cancer: current concepts and implications for recurrence patterns. Q J Nucl Med Mol Imaging 57:312–321
8. Cadoo KA, Traina TA, King TA (2013) Advances in molecular and clinical subtyping of breast cancer and their implications for therapy. Surg Oncol Clin N Am 22:823–840
9. Kohler BA, Sherman RL, Howlader N, Jemal A, Ryerson AB, Henry KA et al (2015) Annual report to the nation on the status of cancer, 1975–2011, featuring incidence of breast cancer subtypes by race/ethnicity, poverty, and state. J Natl Cancer Inst 107:djv048
10. Brewster AM, Chavez-MacGregor M, Brown P (2014) Epidemiology, biology, and treatment of triple-negative breast cancer in women of African ancestry. Lancet Oncol 15:e625–e634
11. Bianchini G, Balko JM, Mayer IA, Sanders ME, Gianni L (2016) Triple-negative breast cancer: challenges and opportunities of a heterogeneous disease. Nat Rev Clin Oncol 13:674–690
12. Cabodi S, Taverna D (2010) Interfering with inflammation: a new strategy to block breast cancer self-renewal and progression? Breast Cancer Res 12:305
13. DeSantis CE, Fedewa SA, Goding SA, Kramer JL, Smith RA, Jemal A (2016) Breast cancer statistics, 2015: convergence of incidence rates between black and white women. CA Cancer J Clin 66:31–42
14. Copson E, Maishman T, Gerty S, Eccles B, Stanton L, Cutress RI et al (2014) Ethnicity and outcome of young breast cancer patients in the United Kingdom: the POSH study. Br J Cancer 110:230–241
15. Newman LA, Griffith KA, Jatoi I, Simon MS, Crowe JP, Colditz GA (2006.;%20) Meta-analysis of survival in African American and white American patients with breast cancer: ethnicity compared with socioeconomic status. J Clin Oncol 24:1342–1349
16. Ma JG, Wang NJ, Yu WJ (2011) Comparison of biological behavior between triple-negative breast cancer and non-triple- negative breast cancer. Nan Fang Yi Ke Da Xue Xue Bao 31:1729–1732
17. Huober J, Gelber S, Goldhirsch A, Coates AS, Viale G, Ohlschlegel C et al (2012) Prognosis of medullary breast cancer: analysis of 13 International Breast Cancer Study Group (IBCSG) trials. Ann Oncol 23:2843–2851
18. Wetterskog D, Lopez-Garcia MA, Lambros MB, A'Hern R, Geyer FC, Milanezi F et al (2012) Adenoid cystic carcinomas constitute a genomically distinct subgroup of triple-negative and basal-like breast cancers. J Pathol 226:84–96
19. Lehmann BD, Bauer JA, Chen X, Sanders ME, Chakravarthy AB, Shyr Y et al (2011) Identification of human triple-negative breast cancer subtypes and preclinical models for selection of targeted therapies. J Clin Invest 121:2750–2767
20. Masuda H, Baggerly KA, Wang Y, Zhang Y, Gonzalez-Angulo AM, Meric-Bernstam F et al (2013) Differential response to neoadjuvant chemotherapy among 7 triple-negative breast cancer molecular subtypes. Clin Cancer Res 19:5533–5540
21. Shinde SS, Forman MR, Kuerer HM, Yan K, Peintinger F, Hunt KK et al (2010) Higher parity and shorter breastfeeding duration: association with triple-negative phenotype of breast cancer. Cancer 116:4933–4943

22. Phipps AI, Chlebowski RT, Prentice R, McTiernan A, Wactawski-Wende J, Kuller LH et al (2011) Reproductive history and oral contraceptive use in relation to risk of triple-negative breast cancer. J Natl Cancer Inst 103:470–477

23. Ma H, Wang Y, Sullivan-Halley J, Weiss L, Marchbanks PA, Spirtas R et al (2010) Use of four biomarkers to evaluate the risk of breast cancer subtypes in the women's contraceptive and reproductive experiences study. Cancer Res 70:575–587

24. Stead LA, Lash TL, Sobieraj JE, Chi DD, Westrup JL, Charlot M et al (2009) Triple-negative breast cancers are increased in black women regardless of age or body mass index. Breast Cancer Res 11:R18

25. Pierobon M, Frankenfeld CL (2013) Obesity as a risk factor for triple-negative breast cancers: a systematic review and meta-analysis. Breast Cancer Res Treat 137:307–314

26. Kumar P, Aggarwal R (2016) An overview of triple-negative breast cancer. Arch Gynecol Obstet 293:247–269

27. Stevens KN, Vachon CM, Couch FJ (2013) Genetic susceptibility to triple-negative breast cancer. Cancer Res 73:2025–2030

28. von MG, Untch M, Blohmer JU, Costa SD, Eidtmann H, Fasching PA et al (2012.;%20) Definition and impact of pathologic complete response on prognosis after neoadjuvant chemotherapy in various intrinsic breast cancer subtypes. J Clin Oncol 30:1796–1804

29. Cortazar P, Zhang L, Untch M, Mehta K, Costantino JP, Wolmark N et al (2014) Pathological complete response and long-term clinical benefit in breast cancer: the CTNeoBC pooled analysis. Lancet 384:164–172

30. Liedtke C, Mazouni C, Hess KR, Andre F, Tordai A, Mejia JA et al (2008) Response to neoadjuvant therapy and long-term survival in patients with triple-negative breast cancer. J Clin Oncol 26:1275–1281

31. Schuster DP (2010) Obesity and the development of type 2 diabetes: the effects of fatty tissue inflamation, vol 3. Dovepress, New Zealand, pp 253–262

32. WHO (2006) World Health Organization fact sheet for world wide prevalence of obesity. https://www.who.int/topics/obesity/en/

33. Chang S, Masse LC, Moser RP, Dodd KW, Arganaraz F, Fuemmler BF et al (2008) State ranks of incident cancer burden due to overweight and obesity in the United States, 2003. Obesity (Silver Spring) 16:1636–1650

34. Flegal KM, Carroll MD, Kuczmarski RJ, Johnson CL (1998) Overweight and obesity in the United States: prevalence and trends, 1960–1994. Int J Obes Relat Metab Disord 22:39–47

35. Perks CM, Holly JM (2011) Hormonal mechanisms underlying the relationship between obesity and breast cancer. Endocrinol Metab Clin N Am 40:485–507, vii

36. FAO/WHO/UN (1985) Energy and protein requirements: report of a joint expert consultation. WHO TR 724. WHO, Geneva

37. Flegal KM, Carroll MD, Ogden CL, Curtin LR (2010) Prevalence and trends in obesity among US adults, 1999–2008. JAMA 303:235–241

38. Anderson AS, Caswell S (2009) Obesity management – an opportunity for cancer prevention. Surgeon 7:282–285

39. Bianchini F, Kaaks R, Vainio H (2002) Overweight, obesity, and cancer risk. Lancet Oncol 3:565–574

40. Bu-Abid S, Szold A, Klausner J (2002) Obesity and cancer. J Med 33:73–86

41. Calle EE, Thun MJ (2004) Obesity and cancer. Oncogene 23:6365–6378

42. Gumbs AA (2008) Obesity, pancreatitis, and pancreatic cancer. Obes Surg 18:1183–1187

43. Hsing AW, Sakoda LC, Chua S Jr (2007) Obesity, metabolic syndrome, and prostate cancer. Am J Clin Nutr 86:s843–s857

44. Kuriyama S, Tsubono Y, Hozawa A, Shimazu T, Suzuki Y, Koizumi Y et al (2005) Obesity and risk of cancer in Japan. Int J Cancer 113:148–157

45. Percik R, Stumvoll M (2009) Obesity and cancer. Exp Clin Endocrinol Diabetes 117:563–566

46. Pischon T, Nothlings U, Boeing H (2008) Obesity and cancer. Proc Nutr Soc 67:128–145

47. Teucher B, Rohrmann S, Kaaks R (2010) Obesity: focus on all-cause mortality and cancer. Maturitas 65:112–116

48. Brown KA, Simpson ER (2010) Obesity and breast cancer: progress to understanding the relationship. Cancer Res 70:4–7
49. Carroll KK (1998) Obesity as a risk factor for certain types of cancer. Lipids 33:1055–1059
50. Barnett GC, Shah M, Redman K, Easton DF, Ponder BA, Pharoah PD (2008) Risk factors for the incidence of breast cancer: do they affect survival from the disease? J Clin Oncol 26:3310–3316
51. Boyle P, Ferlay J (2005) Cancer incidence and mortality in Europe, 2004. Ann Oncol 16:481–488
52. Carmichael AR (2006) Obesity and prognosis of breast cancer. Obes Rev 7:333–340
53. Carter JC, Church FC (2009) Obesity and breast cancer: the roles of peroxisome proliferator-activated receptor-gamma and plasminogen activator inhibitor-1. PPAR Res 2009:345320
54. Rapp K, Schroeder J, Klenk J, Stoehr S, Ulmer H, Concin H et al (2005) Obesity and incidence of cancer: a large cohort study of over 145,000 adults in Austria. Br J Cancer 93:1062–1067
55. Calle EE, Rodriguez C, Walker-Thurmond K, Thun MJ (2003) Overweight, obesity, and mortality from cancer in a prospectively studied cohort of U.S. adults. N Engl J Med 348:1625–1638
56. Reeves GK, Pirie K, Beral V, Green J, Spencer E, Bull D (2007) Cancer incidence and mortality in relation to body mass index in the Million Women Study: cohort study. BMJ 335:1134
57. van den Brandt PA, Spiegelman D, Yaun SS, Adami HO, Beeson L, Folsom AR et al (2000) Pooled analysis of prospective cohort studies on height, weight, and breast cancer risk. Am J Epidemiol 152:514–527
58. Hao S, Liu Y, Yu KD, Chen S, Yang WT, Shao ZM (2015) Overweight as a prognostic factor for triple-negative breast cancers in Chinese women. PLoS One 10:e0129741
59. Chen HL, Ding A, Wang ML (2016) Impact of central obesity on prognostic outcome of triple negative breast cancer in Chinese women. Springerplus 5:594. https://doi.org/10.1186/s40064-016-2200-y. eCollection;%2016.:594-2200
60. Al-Hajj M, Wicha MS, Benito-Hernandez A, Morrison SJ, Clarke MF (2003) Prospective identification of tumorigenic breast cancer cells. Proc Natl Acad Sci U S A 100:3983–3988
61. Bao B, Ahmad A, Li Y, Azmi AS, Ali S, Banerjee S et al (2012) Targeting CSCs within the tumor microenvironment for cancer therapy: a potential role of mesenchymal stem cells. Expert Opin Ther Targets 16:1041–1054
62. Hermann PC, Bhaskar S, Cioffi M, Heeschen C (2010) Cancer stem cells in solid tumors. Semin Cancer Biol 20:77–84
63. Ischenko I, Seeliger H, Kleespies A, Angele MK, Eichhorn ME, Jauch KW et al (2010) Pancreatic cancer stem cells: new understanding of tumorigenesis, clinical implications. Langenbeck's Arch Surg 395:1–10
64. Lee CJ, Dosch J, Simeone DM (2008) Pancreatic cancer stem cells. J Clin Oncol 26:2806–2812
65. Xu Q, Wang L, Li H, Han Q, Li J, Qu X et al (2012) Mesenchymal stem cells play a potential role in regulating the establishment and maintenance of epithelial-mesenchymal transition in MCF7 human breast cancer cells by paracrine and induced autocrine TGF-beta. Int J Oncol 41:959–968
66. Xu Y, Hu YD (2009) Lung cancer stem cells research. Clues from ontogeny. Saudi Med J 30:1381–1389
67. Creighton CJ, Chang JC, Rosen JM (2010) Epithelial-mesenchymal transition (EMT) in tumor-initiating cells and its clinical implications in breast cancer. J Mammary Gland Biol Neoplasia 15:253–260
68. Lee HE, Kim JH, Kim YJ, Choi SY, Kim SW, Kang E et al (2011) An increase in cancer stem cell population after primary systemic therapy is a poor prognostic factor in breast cancer. Br J Cancer 104:1730–1738
69. Liu C, Luo Y, Liu X, Lu P, Zhao Z (2012) Clinical implications of CD44+/. Cancer Biother Radiopharm 27:324–328
70. Charafe-Jauffret E, Ginestier C, Iovino F, Wicinski J, Cervera N, Finetti P et al (2009) Breast cancer cell lines contain functional cancer stem cells with metastatic capacity and a distinct molecular signature. Cancer Res 69:1302–1313

71. Charafe-Jauffret E, Ginestier C, Birnbaum D (2009) Breast cancer stem cells: tools and models to rely on. BMC Cancer 9:202

72. Charafe-Jauffret E, Ginestier C, Iovino F, Tarpin C, Diebel M, Esterni B et al (2010) Aldehyde dehydrogenase 1-positive cancer stem cells mediate metastasis and poor clinical outcome in inflammatory breast cancer. Clin Cancer Res 16:45–55

73. Bao B, Azmi A, Aboukameel A, Ahmad A, Bolling-Fischer A, Sethi S et al (2014) Pancreatic cancer stem-like cells display aggressive behavior mediated via activation of FoxQ1. J Biol Chem 289:14520–14533

74. Klonisch T, Wiechec E, Hombach-Klonisch S, Ande SR, Wesselborg S, Schulze-Osthoff K et al (2008) Cancer stem cell markers in common cancers – therapeutic implications. Trends Mol Med 14:450–460

75. Prud'homme GJ (2012) Cancer stem cells and novel targets for antitumor strategies. Curr Pharm Des 18:2838–2849

76. Patrawala L, Calhoun T, Schneider-Broussard R, Zhou J, Claypool K, Tang DG (2005) Side population is enriched in tumorigenic, stem-like cancer cells, whereas ABCG2+ and A. Cancer Res 65:6207–6219

77. Yu C, Yao Z, Jiang Y, Keller ET (2012) Prostate cancer stem cell biology. Minerva Urol Nefrol 64:19–33

78. Ginestier C, Hur MH, Charafe-Jauffret E, Monville F, Dutcher J, Brown M et al (2007) ALDH1 is a marker of normal and malignant human mammary stem cells and a predictor of poor clinical outcome. Cell Stem Cell 1:555–567

79. Bao B, Mitrea C, Wijesinghe P, Marchetti L, Girsch E, Farr RL et al (2017) Treating triple negative breast cancer cells with erlotinib plus a select antioxidant overcomes drug resistance by targeting cancer cell heterogeneity. Sci Rep 7:44125. https://doi.org/10.1038/srep44125.:44125

80. Artavanis-Tsakonas S, Rand MD, Lake RJ (1999) Notch signaling: cell fate control and signal integration in development. Science 284:770–776

81. Bray SJ (2006) Notch signalling: a simple pathway becomes complex. Nat Rev Mol Cell Biol 7:678–689

82. Lino MM, Merlo A, Boulay JL (2010) Notch signaling in glioblastoma: a developmental drug target? BMC Med 8:72

83. Miele L (2006) Notch signaling. Clin Cancer Res 12:1074–1079

84. Ellisen LW, Bird J, West DC, Soreng AL, Reynolds TC, Smith SD et al (1991) TAN-1, the human homolog of the Drosophila notch gene, is broken by chromosomal translocations in T lymphoblastic neoplasms. Cell 66:649–661

85. Radtke F, Raj K (2003) The role of Notch in tumorigenesis: oncogene or tumour suppressor? Nat Rev Cancer 3:756–767

86. Weng AP, Ferrando AA, Lee W, Morris JP, Silverman LB, Sanchez-Irizarry C et al (2004) Activating mutations of NOTCH1 in human T cell acute lymphoblastic leukemia. Science 306:269–271

87. Jing Y, Han Z, Zhang S, Liu Y, Wei L (2011) Epithelial-mesenchymal transition in tumor microenvironment. Cell Biosci 1:29

88. Rangel MC, Bertolette D, Castro NP, Klauzinska M, Cuttitta F, Salomon DS (2016) Developmental signaling pathways regulating mammary stem cells and contributing to the etiology of triple-negative breast cancer. Breast Cancer Res Treat 156:211–226

89. Turner N, Lambros MB, Horlings HM, Pearson A, Sharpe R, Natrajan R et al (2010) Integrative molecular profiling of triple negative breast cancers identifies amplicon drivers and potential therapeutic targets. Oncogene 29:2013–2023

90. Farnie G, Clarke RB (2007) Mammary stem cells and breast cancer – role of Notch signalling. Stem Cell Rev 3:169–175

91. Harrison H, Farnie G, Howell SJ, Rock RE, Stylianou S, Brennan KR et al (2010) Regulation of breast cancer stem cell activity by signaling through the Notch4 receptor. Cancer Res 70:709–718

92. Soady KJ, Kendrick H, Gao Q, Tutt A, Zvelebil M, Ordonez LD et al (2015) Mouse mammary stem cells express prognostic markers for triple-negative breast cancer. Breast Cancer Res 17:31. https://doi.org/10.1186/s13058-015-0539-6.:31-0539

93. D'Angelo RC, Ouzounova M, Davis A, Choi D, Tchuenkam SM, Kim G et al (2015) Notch reporter activity in breast cancer cell lines identifies a subset of cells with stem cell activity. Mol Cancer Ther 14:779–787

94. DeSano JT, Xu L (2009) MicroRNA regulation of cancer stem cells and therapeutic implications. AAPS J 11:682–692

95. Perera RJ, Ray A (2007) MicroRNAs in the search for understanding human diseases. BioDrugs 21:97–104

96. Bienz M, Clevers H (2003) Armadillo/beta-catenin signals in the nucleus – proof beyond a reasonable doubt? Nat Cell Biol 5:179–182

97. Peifer M, Polakis P (2000) Wnt signaling in oncogenesis and embryogenesis – a look outside the nucleus. Science 287:1606–1609

98. Yu QC, Verheyen EM, Zeng YA (2016) Mammary development and breast cancer: a Wnt perspective. Cancers (Basel) 8:cancers8070065

99. Doucas H, Garcea G, Neal CP, Manson MM, Berry DP (2005) Changes in the Wnt signalling pathway in gastrointestinal cancers and their prognostic significance. Eur J Cancer 41:365–379

100. Kang CM, Kim HK, Kim H, Choi GH, Kim KS, Choi JS et al (2009) Expression of Wnt target genes in solid pseudopapillary tumor of the pancreas: a pilot study. Pancreas 38:e53–e59

101. Honeycutt KA, Roop DR (2004) C-Myc and epidermal stem cell fate determination. J Dermatol 31:368–375

102. Honeycutt KA, Koster MI, Roop DR (2004) Genes involved in stem cell fate decisions and commitment to differentiation play a role in skin disease. J Investig Dermatol Symp Proc 9:261–268

103. Takebe N, Harris PJ, Warren RQ, Ivy SP (2011) Targeting cancer stem cells by inhibiting Wnt, Notch, and Hedgehog pathways. Nat Rev Clin Oncol 8:97–106

104. Katoh M, Katoh M (2007) WNT signaling pathway and stem cell signaling network. Clin Cancer Res 13:4042–4045

105. Jiang YG, Luo Y, He DL, Li X, Zhang LL, Peng T et al (2007) Role of Wnt/beta-catenin signaling pathway in epithelial-mesenchymal transition of human prostate cancer induced by hypoxia-inducible factor-1alpha. Int J Urol 14:1034–1039

106. Hugo H, Ackland ML, Blick T, Lawrence MG, Clements JA, Williams ED et al (2007) Epithelial – mesenchymal and mesenchymal – epithelial transitions in carcinoma progression. J Cell Physiol 213:374–383

107. Luo Y, He DL, Ning L, Shen SL, Li L, Li X et al (2006) Over-expression of hypoxia-inducible factor-1alpha increases the invasive potency of LNCaP cells in vitro. BJU Int 98:1315–1319

108. Liu S, Dontu G, Wicha MS (2005) Mammary stem cells, self-renewal pathways, and carcinogenesis. Breast Cancer Res 7:86–95

109. de Sousa EM, Vermeulen L, Richel D, Medema JP (2011) Targeting Wnt signaling in colon cancer stem cells. Clin Cancer Res 17:647–653

110. Katoh M (2011) Network of WNT and other regulatory signaling cascades in pluripotent stem cells and cancer stem cells. Curr Pharm Biotechnol 12:160–170

111. Oishi N, Wang XW (2011) Novel therapeutic strategies for targeting liver cancer stem cells. Int J Biol Sci 7:517–535

112. DiMeo TA, Anderson K, Phadke P, Fan C, Perou CM, Naber S et al (2009) A novel lung metastasis signature links Wnt signaling with cancer cell self-renewal and epithelial-mesenchymal transition in basal-like breast cancer. Cancer Res 69:5364–5373

113. King TD, Suto MJ, Li Y (2012) The Wnt/beta-catenin signaling pathway: a potential therapeutic target in the treatment of triple negative breast cancer. J Cell Biochem 113:13–18

114. Banerjee K, Resat H (2016) Constitutive activation of STAT3 in breast cancer cells: a review. Int J Cancer 138:2570–2578

115. Sengupta S, Nagalingam A, Muniraj N, Bonner MY, Mistriotis P, Afthinos A et al (2017) Activation of tumor suppressor LKB1 by honokiol abrogates cancer stem-like phenotype in breast cancer via inhibition of oncogenic Stat3. Oncogene 36:5709–5721

116. Foshay KM, Gallicano GI (2008) Regulation of Sox2 by STAT3 initiates commitment to the neural precursor cell fate. Stem Cells Dev 17:269–278

117. Marotta LL, Almendro V, Marusyk A, Shipitsin M, Schemme J, Walker SR et al (2011) The JAK2/STAT3 signaling pathway is required for growth of CD44(+)CD24(−) stem cell-like breast cancer cells in human tumors. J Clin Invest 121:2723–2735

118. Gritli-Linde A, Bei M, Maas R, Zhang XM, Linde A, McMahon AP (2002) Shh signaling within the dental epithelium is necessary for cell proliferation, growth and polarization. Development 129:5323–5337

119. Yang L, Xie G, Fan Q, Xie J (2010) Activation of the hedgehog-signaling pathway in human cancer and the clinical implications. Oncogene 29:469–481

120. Chaudary N, Pintilie M, Hedley D, Fyles AW, Milosevic M, Clarke B et al (2011) Hedgehog pathway signaling in cervical carcinoma and outcome after chemoradiation. Cancer 118:3105–3115

121. Dormoy V, Danilin S, Lindner V, Thomas L, Rothhut S, Coquard C et al (2009) The sonic hedgehog signaling pathway is reactivated in human renal cell carcinoma and plays orchestral role in tumor growth. Mol Cancer 8:123

122. Katoh Y, Katoh M (2009) Hedgehog target genes: mechanisms of carcinogenesis induced by aberrant hedgehog signaling activation. Curr Mol Med 9:873–886

123. Choi SS, Omenetti A, Witek RP, Moylan CA, Syn WK, Jung Y et al (2009) Hedgehog pathway activation and epithelial-to-mesenchymal transitions during myofibroblastic transformation of rat hepatic cells in culture and cirrhosis. Am J Physiol Gastrointest Liver Physiol 297:G1093–G1106

124. Liu S, Dontu G, Mantle ID, Patel S, Ahn NS, Jackson KW et al (2006) Hedgehog signaling and Bmi-1 regulate self-renewal of normal and malignant human mammary stem cells. Cancer Res 66:6063–6071

125. Bao B, Wang Z, Li Y, Kong D, Ali S, Banerjee S et al (2011) The complexities of obesity and diabetes with the development and progression of pancreatic cancer. Biochim Biophys Acta 1815:135–146

126. Shi P, Liu W, Tala WH, Li F, Zhang H et al (2017) Metformin suppresses triple-negative breast cancer stem cells by targeting KLF5 for degradation. Cell Discov 3:17010. https://doi.org/10.1038/celldisc.2017.10. eCollection;%2017.:17010

Chapter 18
Cross-Roads to Drug Resistance and Metastasis in Breast Cancer: miRNAs Regulatory Function and Biomarker Capability

Nataly Naser Al Deen, Farah Nassar, Rihab Nasr, and Rabih Talhouk

Abstract Breast cancer and specifically metastatic breast cancer (mBC) constitutes a major health burden worldwide with the highest number of cancer-related mortality among women across the globe. Despite having similar subtypes, breast cancer patients present with a spectrum of aggressiveness and responsiveness to therapy due to cancer heterogeneity. Drug resistance and metastasis contribute to therapy failure and cancer recurrence. Research in the past two decades has focused on microRNAs (miRNAs), small endogenous non-coding RNAs, as active players in tumorigenesis, therapy resistance and metastasis and as novel non-invasive cancer biomarkers. This is due to their unique dysregulated signatures throughout tumor progression and their tumor suppressive/oncogenic roles. Identifying miRNAs signatures capable of predicting therapy response and metastatic onset in breast cancer patients might improve prognosis and offer prolonged median and relapse-free survival rate. Despite the growing reports on miRNAs as novel non-invasive biomarkers in breast cancer and as regulators of breast cancer drug resistance or metastasis, the quest on whether some miRNAs are capable of regulating both simultaneously is inevitable, yet understudied. This chapter will review the role of miRNAs as biomarkers and as active players in inducing/reversing anti-cancer drug resistance, driving/blocking metastasis or regulating both simultaneously in breast cancer.

N. Naser Al Deen · R. Talhouk (✉)
Department of Biology, Faculty of Arts and Sciences, American University of Beirut, Beirut, Lebanon
e-mail: rtalhouk@aub.edu.lb

F. Nassar
Department of Internal Medicine, Faculty of Medicine, American University of Beirut, Beirut, Lebanon

R. Nasr (✉)
Department of Anatomy, Cell Biology and Physiological Sciences, Faculty of Medicine, American University of Beirut, Beirut, Lebanon
e-mail: rn03@aub.edu.lb

© Springer Nature Switzerland AG 2019
A. Ahmad (ed.), *Breast Cancer Metastasis and Drug Resistance*,
Advances in Experimental Medicine and Biology 1152,
https://doi.org/10.1007/978-3-030-20301-6_18

335

Keywords Breast cancer · Metastatic breast cancer · miRNA · Drug resistance · Metastasis · Biomarker · Prognostic · Therapy-predictive · Multi-drug resistance

Abbreviations

BC	Breast cancer
CTCs	Circulating tumor cells
DCIS	Ductal carcinoma in situ
DFS	Disease-free survival
ER	Estrogen receptor
mBC	Metastatic breast cancer
MDR	Multidrug resistance
microRNAs	miRNAs or miRs
OS	Overall survival
PFS	Progression-free survival
TNBC	Triple negative breast cancer

18.1   Introduction

18.1.1   Overview on Breast Cancer and Its Metastasis

Breast cancer is a global public health burden, constituting the highest cancer incidence in females and the second most common cancer diagnosed worldwide, with around 1.7 million new cases each year. In the U.S., almost one in eight females fall victims of invasive breast cancer throughout their lifetime [1]. Recent statistics by the American Cancer Society reported breast cancer to be amongst the three most commonly diagnosed female cancers, along with lung and bronchus cancer and colorectal cancer, all of which comprise 50% of all female cancer cases and contribute to most cancer deaths in women [1]. Breast cancer is a heterogeneous disease with various subtypes, conventionally classified according to histology (most common types are ductal carcinoma in situ, invasive ductal carcinoma and invasive lobular carcinoma), immunopathology (estrogen receptor, progesterone receptor and human epidermal growth factor receptor 2 (HER2) status) and molecular signature (luminal A, luminal B, triple-negative/basal-like, HER2-enriched or normal-like) [2–4]. Despite having similar subtypes, breast cancer patients present with a spectrum of aggressiveness and responsiveness to therapy [5]. This questioned the efficacy of the mentioned conventional classification methods and the available prognostic and diagnostic tests for breast cancer. Hence, recent studies are focusing on complementing the conventional breast cancer classification tools using patients' distinct signature of microRNAs (miRNAs), small non-coding single-stranded nucleotides [6]. For instance, Bhattacharyya et al. [7] used fivefold cross-validation techniques in an attempt to sub-classify breast cancer using miRNA signatures compared to pre-existing clinical records. Their results not only validated that miRNA can corroborate the conventional molecular subtype classification, but also proposed the existence of further subtypes through using hierarchical clustering.

Metastatic breast cancer (mBC) is the most aggressive form of breast cancer, which affects 10–15% of patients within 3 years from diagnosis and is characterized by increased tumor burden and its spread to distal regions [8]. The metastatic cascade begins with tumor dissemination, denoted by local invasion of neighboring tissues, intravasation into the blood or lymph, persistence of the escaped cells in the circulation and subsequent extravasation. It is then followed by colonization, where the escaped cells adjust to the new microenvironment [9]. Epithelial to mesenchymal transition (EMT), an inherent developmental process, necessary for the proper morphogenesis of tissues, is one key step in driving invasion and metastasis. Epithelial cancer cells devise EMT to provoke motility, migration and invasion, switch to a mesenchymal phenotype to lose epithelial polarity and cellular interactions [10]. Developing better diagnostic and therapeutic interventions for mBC is fundamental. miRNAs play key regulatory roles along all stages of the metastatic cascade whereby McGuire et al. [11] summarized the different miRNAs in mBC implicated in invasion (miR-199a, miR-214, miR-200a/b/c, miR-141 and miR-429), dissemination (miR-31), extravasation (miR-10b, miR-373, miR-20a, miR-214 and miR-31) and proliferation (miR-10b, miR-34a, miR-155, miR-200a/b/c, miR-141 and miR-429).

Drug resistance and metastasis continue to pose a challenge in breast cancer and mBC treatment due, in part, to the limitations that entail the available prognostic and diagnostic tests, which range from having low sensitivity, to being highly invasive, to yielding high false positive rates and over-diagnosis [12]. For instance, first, the use of serum carbohydrate antigens such as carcinoembryonic antigen (CEA) and cancer antigen 153 (CA153) as biomarkers is limited by its low sensitivity [13]. Second, there exists few available multi-gene expression DNA microarrays based testing, like Oncotype DX, MammaPrint, Veridex 76-gene and MapQuant Dx. Oncotype DX test, which estimates the recurrence likelihood through assessing 16 cancer-related genes, 5 reference genes and whether patients are eligible for chemotherapy [14], MammaPrint, a prognostic test that analyzes 70 genes and identifies patients with stage 1 or 2, node negative, invasive breast cancer <5 cm in size. Veridex 76-gene signature, a diagnostic test that predicts distant metastasis in ER-positive (ER+) patients within 5 years of diagnosis through a signature of 60 genes for ER+ patients and 16 for ER-negative (ER-) patients [15]. MapQuant Dx, which further classifies grade II tumors into grade I-like (low chance of distant relapses) and grade III-like (clinically similar to grade III) and predicts chemotherapeutic benefit, but can only be used as prognostic tool for ER+ tumors [15]. However, all these tests necessitate patient tissue samples, and thus are highly invasive. Third, mammograms not only exhibit high false positive rates and are incapable of detecting mBC and cause over-diagnosis, but patients below the age of 40 are not recommended to undergo mammography screening because of their dense breast tissue architecture [16, 17]. Additionally, the conventional diagnostic tool for mBC, sentinel lymph node biopsy (SLNB), only detects local but not distal metastasis [11]. Thus, the limitations of the conventional classification tools along with the unavailability of non-invasive, highly sensitive and highly specific mBC diagnostic, prognostic and therapy predictive tests called for the investigation of miRNAs; to better understand their regulatory role in drug resistance and distant metastasis and their biomarker potential.

18.1.2   miRNAs Biogenesis

miRNAs are small (16–29 nucleotides) endogenous, non-coding, single-stranded RNAs that negatively regulate gene expression at the post-transcriptional level [6]. Around half of miRNAs exist in clusters with other miRNAs and are transcribed as polycistronic precursor miRNAs, while others reside within exons and the 3′-untranslated region (UTR) of mRNAs [18]. Various miRNAs promoters transcribe their own miRNAs in intergenic sites, whereas, the majority of miRNAs are transcribed by their host gene promoters when they reside in the introns of protein coding or non-coding host genes. miRNAs biogenesis undertakes a sequence of processes, where RNA polymerase II/III first transcribes miRNAs into primary transcripts (pri-miRNAs) which are several kilobases long. pri-miRNAs in the nucleus are then cleaved by RNase III endonuclease Drosha and DGCR8 protein into intermediate (60–70 nucleotide-long stem loop) precursor miRNAs (pre-miRNAs). The latter are exported to the cytoplasm via exportin-5 (XPO5) complexed with Ran-GTP, and undergo cleavage into mature length by Dicer, another RNase III endonuclease together with the double-stranded RNA-binding protein TRBP [19]. At this stage, the mature miRNA strand unwinds from its complementary strand (passenger strand), and is normally targeted for degradation. The mature strand gets presented onto the RNA-induced silencing complex (RISC), a ribonucleoprotein complex comprised of the mature miRNAs and Argonaute (AGO2) proteins [19, 20]. However, recent studies have shown that the passenger strand can also be loaded onto RISC and therefore can have regulatory function [21]. The RISC complex preferentially binds the seed-matching sequence of the 3′-UTR of target protein-coding mRNA genes, whereby perfect complementarity leads to mRNA degradation by AGO2 via the induction of RNA-mediated interference (RNAi) pathway. Imperfect complementarity leads to translational repression of the target mRNA or mRNA degradation as a result of deadenylation by the CAF1-CCR4-NOT1 de-adenylase complex and subsequent de-capping of the target mRNA [22, 23] (Fig. 18.1). Although miRNAs are known to silence their target mRNA, studies shed light on few miRNAs that promote the expression of their target mRNA, a mechanism termed "RNA activation" (RNAa), majorly attributed to epigenetic regulation of AGO2 [24]. A single miRNA can regulate many genes, which normally exhibit cellular regulatory roles including proliferation, metabolism,

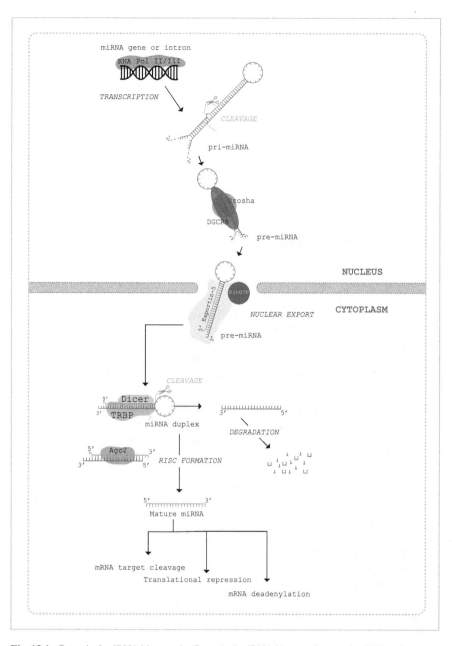

Fig. 18.1 Canonical miRNA biogenesis. Canonical miRNA biogenesis starts by RNA polymerase II/III transcribing miRNAs into primary transcripts (pri-miRNAs) in the nucleus, which are then cleaved by Drosha and DGCR8 protein into intermediate precursor miRNAs (pre-miRNAs). Pre-miRNAs are exported to the cytoplasm via exportin-5 (XPO5) complexed with Ran-GTP, and undergo cleavage into mature length by Dicer complexed with TRBP. The mature miRNA strand is unwound from its complementary strand (passenger strand), which gets degraded, while the mature strand is presented onto the RNA-induced silencing complex (RISC), comprised of the mature miRNAs and AGO2 proteins. The RISC complex preferentially binds the seed-matching sequence of the 3′-UTR of target protein-coding mRNA genes and perfect complementarity leads to mRNA degradation while imperfect complementarity leads to translational repression or deadenylation, which results in degradation of the target mRNA. (Modified from: Winter et al. [19])

differentiation, cell death or aging [25]. Various miRNAs exhibit oncogenic or tumor suppressive roles during cancer pathogenesis, and hence, play part in cancer progression, drug resistance or metastasis. However, deciphering miRNAs that concurrently control drug resistance and metastasis is fundamental, yet understudied [26]. Due to their dysregulation along the different stages of tumorigenesis and their presence and stability in bodily fluids, miRNAs have gained much attention in the past decade. Several studies reported miRNAs diagnostic, prognostic and therapy predictive biomarker potential in breast cancer and others discuss their role as active players in drug resistance and metastasis, all of which will be discussed thereof.

18.1.3   Circulating miRNAs Origin and Function

miRNAs were first detected in bodily fluids by Chim et al. [27] who discovered circulating placental miRNA in pregnant women plasma. Soon after, Lawrie et al. [28] identified the first miRNA signature in patients with diffuse large B-cell lymphoma with elevated serum miR-155, miR-210 and miR-21. Circulating miRNAs were then found in blood and plasma, colostrum and breast milk, tears, bronchial lavage and in amniotic, peritoneal, seminal, pleural and cerebrospinal fluids [29]. Previous studies by Lima et al. [30] related the stability of miRNAs in the circulation to their encapsulation in microvesicles or in exosomes. Turchinovich et al. [31] showed that some circulating miRNAs are generated from dead cells, while Merkerova et al. [32] attributed a portion of circulating miRNAs to have originated from blood or immune cells. Recent studies mainly attribute the origin of circulating miRNAs to their passive out-flow from dead cells or active secretion in exosome by tumor and other cell types. Wu et al. [33] characterized exosome-derived miR-19a as a key player in breast cancer metastasis to the bones through facilitating breast cancer and osteoclast cellular communication. Zhong et al. [34] argued that drug resistance can be transmitted from resistant to sensitive breast cancer cells through exosomal miRNA discharge. Similarly, Le et al. [35] showed that transferring cells expressing miR-200 and extracellular vesicles from tumors into murine and human cancer xenografts resulted in acquisition of metastatic potential in weakly metastatic cells, both locally and distally.

Circulating miRNAs harbor a plethora of non-invasive biomarkers and warrant more extensive investigation due to their ease of accessibility in bodily fluids, stability, resistance to RNase digestion and extreme conditions and withstanding long storage [33, 36]. Many studies bid the urge of using miRNAs as novel non-invasive biomarkers for prognosis, diagnosis and therapy prediction in breast cancer and mBC [12, 33] while others discuss the role miRNAs play in controlling metastasis [37–41] inducing and/or reversing breast cancer drug resistance [26, 42, 43], setting new patient selection criteria for clinical trials [44], characterizing new breast cancer subtypes [7] and identifying miRNAs that have both therapy-sensitizing and metastasis blocking roles in breast cancer [26]; most of which will be discussed hereafter. This chapter will highlight the biomarker roles of miRNAs in breast cancer and mBC and will review the regulatory role of miRNAs in causing or reversing drug resistance, metastasis, or both simultaneously.

18.2   miRNAs as Diagnostic, Prognostic and Therapy Predictive Biomarkers in Breast Cancer

McGuire et al. [11] reviewed the essential role circulating miRNAs play as mBC diagnostic or prognostic biomarkers in discriminating non-metastatic from metastatic tumors to guide mBC early diagnosis and monitor disease progression. For instance, circulating miR-10b, miR-34a and miR-155 were elevated in mBC patients [45] and circulating miR-10b and miR-373 [46] as well as miR-20a and miR-214 [47] were upregulated in patients with lymph node positive breast cancer as opposed to patients with no lymph node involvement. Moreover, miR-10b has been reported as a potential mBC biomarker to the brain and bones [48, 49] while miR-141, miR-200a, miR-200b, miR-200c, miR-203, miR-210, miR-375 and miR-801 were significantly upregulated in plasma of mBC patients with circulating tumor cells, CTC [50]. Upregulation in miR-105 predicted metastasis in early onset breast cancer [51], while elevation in miR-17 and miR-155 discriminated metastatic from non-metastatic breast cancers [52]. Moreover, metastasis as a result of primary breast tumors correlated with over-expression of miR-34a and miR-155 in the serum, while upregulated miR-34a predicted increased aggressiveness [53].

Nassar et al. [12] shed light in their review on prognostic miRNAs in breast cancer in terms of predicting the overall survival (OS), disease outcome and recurrence in patients. Out of the prognostic biomarkers, miR-106b, found in serum and tissues, predicted risk of high recurrence and shorter OS [54], while miR-122, which was over-expressed in serum of relapsed patients, served as metastasis predictive miRNA. Sahlberg et al. [55] reported that miR-18b, miR-103, miR-107 and miR-652 predicted recurrence and decreased OS in triple negative breast cancer (TNBC) patients. Recent study by Halvorsen et al. [56] was the first to characterize miRNAs profiled from tumor interstitial fluid (TIF) as prognostic and diagnostic biomarkers and as potential bridges between tumor cells and their micro-environment. The authors profiled TIF, normal interstitial fluid, tumor tissues and serum samples from breast cancer patients and a corresponding validation cohort. The results identified upregulation of 266 miRNAs in TIF, of which 61 were present in more than three quarters of the serum samples. Seven miRNAs of the latter predicted poor survival rate and 23 miRNAs were linked to immune cells and adipocyte existence in the serum. Furthermore, Lánczky et al. [57] devised an integrated platform that can search for all documented miRNAs through GEO, EGA, TCGA and PubMed database to arrive at survival analysis capable of predicting the efficiency of miRNAs acting as prognostic biomarkers. Importantly, via this platform, miR-210, miR-328, miR-484 and miR-874 were shown to be capable of predicting prognosis or risk of recurrence [11].

Dysregulation of miRNAs could also predict the therapy outcome and patient's sensitivity or resistance to a specific treatment, which is the leading cause of recurrence and poor prognosis in breast cancer patients [58]. Chen et al. [59] showed in breast cancer formalin-fixed paraffin-embedded (FFPE) tissues that miR-222, miR-29a, miR-34a, miR-423, miR-140, miR-3178, miR-574, miR-6780b and miR-744 were significantly associated with drug resistance and that miR-222, miR-29a, miR-140, miR-574, miR-6780b, miR-7107 and miR-744 were correlated with poor prognosis. Moreover, some miRNAs were associated with radioresistance, like the over-expression of miR-21, miR-144 and miR-27a and the down-regulation of miR-205, miR-200c and miR-302 [12]. Gasparri et al. [53] reviewed urinary miRNAs in breast tumors, wherein miR-125b predicted resistance to chemotherapy while miR-21, miR-34a, miR-125b, miR-155, miR-195, miR-200b, miR-200c, miR-375 and miR-451 were specific to breast cancer patients and were capable of predicting therapy outcome [60]. Other miRNAs offer potential therapeutic roles in addition to their therapy predictive roles, like the case with miR-200 family, which inhibits angiogenesis through targeting EMT [61]. However, drug resistance remains the leading cause of therapy failure, cancer recurrence and metastasis in breast cancer patients, and thus, understanding its underlying mechanisms along with miRNAs regulatory function holds major promises.

18.3   miRNAs and Drug Resistance in Breast Cancer

18.3.1   Mechanisms of Drug Resistance in Breast Cancer

The conventional treatment regimens for breast cancer, and mBC, include a combination of surgery with chemotherapeutic agents [mostly anthracyclines (doxorubicin and epirubicin), taxanes (paclitaxel and docetaxel), fluorouracil (5-FU) and cyclophosphamide], hormonal therapies [estrogen antagonists: tamoxifen, toremifene and fulvestrant that compete with estrogen to bind and block its receptor or aromatase inhibitors (AIs): letrozole, anastrozole, exemestane, which stop estrogen production], targeted therapy (trastuzumab against HER2+) or a combination thereof. Despite the available treatment regimens, breast cancer drug resistance is amongst the leading causes of therapy futility, cancer recurrence and distant metastasis worldwide [11, 26, 42, 62]. One in two breast cancer patients are expected to present with therapy failure or acquire chemotherapy resistance with aggressive malignancy [63, 64]. Anti-cancer therapy resistance can be classified into intrinsic and acquired, wherein pre-existing resistance mechanisms render the patient unresponsive or resistant to cancer therapy (intrinsic resistance), while acquired selection pressure along the course of treatment might tilt the balance from initially-responsive to resistant variants (acquired resistance) [65]. Various mechanisms contribute to cancer drug resistance including reduction in the intracellular drug concentrations brought by aberrant drug transport and metabolism (less drug reaching the cells or higher drug efflux), deregulation in cell cycle, apoptosis and/or DNA repair machineries, overexpression of oncogenic signaling pathways responsible for tumor transformation, dysregulation in DNA methylation and histone modifications and changes in drug target expression and/or availability [20, 65]. All of which have been implicated in breast cancer and have been shown to be regulated in part by miRNAs. In this regard, miRNAs have been studied as potential biomarkers, to predict treatment response and as master regulators in chemotherapy, hormonal, targeted and radiotherapy resistance.

18.3.2   Role of miRNA in Chemotherapy and in Multidrug Resistance

Breast cancer drug resistance poses a threat through therapy failure, cancer recurrence and distant metastasis. One major hurdle in chemotherapeutic response is cancer cells acquisition of multidrug resistance (MDR), a phenomenon cancer cells develop upon exposure to one chemotherapeutic agent that renders them unresponsive and resistant to various drugs, subjecting breast cancer patients to treatment futility, poor prognosis and cancer-related deaths [66]. MDR is classified into non-classical and transport-based classical MDR phenotypes. Changes in enzymatic activity of glutathione S-transferase and topoisomerase or alteration in apoptotic proteins are responsible for the non-classical phenotype, while reduced uptake of the drug by cancer cells or increased drug efflux out of the cell represent classical MDR.

The major players in classical MDR are comprised of one or more ATP binding cassette (ABC) transporters, which are ABCB1 (MDR-1/P-pg), multidrug resistance-associated protein ABCC1 (MRP-1) and breast cancer-resistant protein ABCG2 (BCRP), all of which possess hydrophobic elements that compete with drug transport across the cellular membrane [66]. For instance, an upregulation of miR-130 and consequent downregulation of PTEN was detected in tumor tissues as compared to normal adjacent tissues as well as in MCF-7 breast cancer cells resistant to adriamycin (MCF-7/ADR) as compared to sensitive MCF-7 and MCF-10A cells, a non-malignant breast epithelial cell line [43]. Increased drug resistance and proliferation and decreased apoptotic levels were observed upon over-expression of miR-130b in MCF-7/ADR cells, while downregulation of miR-130b showed opposite patterns. The authors also noted along with the downregulation of PTEN an induction of MDR through activation of the PI3K/Akt pathway and linked it to the upregulation of miR-130b, which in turn induced proliferation and apoptosis. Another example of MDR was reported in doxorubicin-resistant (MCF-7/DOX) breast cancer cells that exhibited low levels of miR-451 compared to DOX-sensitive cells and resulted in increased MDR1 levels, hence increased DOX resistance [67]. By rescuing the levels of miR-451, DOX sensitivity increased through bypassing MDR. Furthermore, MRP-1-mediated MDR can be regulated by miR-326, particularly, in VP-16 (Etoposide)-resistant MDR cell line (MCF-7/VP), where MRP-1 was the only over-expressed ABC transporter protein [66]. A downregulation of miR-326 and up-regulation of MRP-1 were reported in MCF-7/VP cells as well as in different tissues of advanced breast cancer, while a decrease in MRP-1 expression and an increase in VP-16 and DOX sensitivity were identified upon transfection with miR-326 mimics [67].

In non-classical MDR, Glutathione S-transferase P1 (GSTP1) was studied in tissue samples and exosomes from sera of patients with advanced breast cancer pre-and-post anthracycline/taxane-based neoadjuvant chemotherapy to reduce the tumor burden and block metastasis [68]. GSTP1, a member of the phase II metabolic enzymes, can drive chemoresistance through conjugating various anti-cancer drugs with glutathione, resulting in their detoxification. After therapy, levels of GSTP1 were elevated in advanced patients compared to responsive patients with partial re-localization of cellular GSTP1 to the cytoplasm, both in tissue and exosomal samples. The same pattern was seen in the exosomal marker, tumor susceptibility gene 101 protein (TSG101). This proposed the use of GSTP1-containing exosomes in predicting/transferring chemo-resistance. Therefore, future studies could develop exosomal miRNA biomarkers for MDR prediction, to prevent chemoresistance beforehand, and anti-cancer treatments could govern a merge between the already available therapies and ones that take into consideration preventing/reversing MDR, including exosomal miRNAs [69].

As for the role of miRNAs in chemoresistance, miRNAs are shown either to exhibit a confirmed involvement in chemoresistance, thus increasing the value of IC_{50} *in vitro* or drug resistance *in vivo* or to serve as a biomarker of chemoresistance [65]. For instance *in vitro* analysis showed that miR-451 was downregulated in MCF-7/DOX-resistant breast cancer cells and was involved in DOX-resistance through targeting P-glycoprotein (MDR1 gene) [67], while the up-regulation of miR-221-222 served as biomarkers for Tamoxifen resistance via targeting p27(Kip1) in MCF-7 and T47D cells [70]. The same pattern was seen with miR-449a/b upregulation in Tamoxifen resistance in frozen breast cancer tissues. In addition, an increase in miR-449a/b levels was shown in tamoxifen-sensitive ZR75 cells while decreased levels of miR-449a/b conferred chemo-resistance in tamoxifen-resistant AK47 cells and other resistant cell lines, which is possibly a consequence of repression of miR-449a/b through DNA methylation [71].

Moreover, aggressive TNBC cells exhibited higher survival and metastatic potential as a result of miR-181a upregulation upon Dox treatment, which is in line with the poor disease free survival and overall survival noticed in TNBC patients that have high levels of miR-181a upon DOX treatment [42]. Hong et al. [72] discussed one of the most studied miRNAs in breast cancer, oncomiR miR-21. miR-21 upregulation infers chemoresistance, possibly through either enhancing proliferation and suppressing tumor suppressor programmed cell death 4 (PDCD4), thus inhibiting apoptosis, or through repressing PTEN, therefore boosting growth and invasion [73, 74]. A combination therapy of miR-21 inhibitors with paclitaxel was shown to be more efficacious than paclitaxel alone [75]. Zhou et al. [76] characterized a crucial role upregulation of miR-125b plays in paclitaxel-resistant breast cancer cells, by directly downregulating pro-apoptotic Bcl-2 antagonist killer 1 (Bak1), which in turn is partially responsible for paclitaxel cellular uptake. Rescuing the sensitivity of breast cancer cells to paclitaxel was attained through re-expressing Bak1, or inhibiting miR-125b.

18.3.3   Role of miRNAs in Hormonal Therapy Response/ Resistance

miRNAs also play important regulatory roles in hormonal and targeted therapy resistance that might also be breast cancer sub-type specific. As for ER+ breast tumors, treatment regimens typically rely on decreasing (both endogenous or circulating) estrogen levels or on blocking ER using tamoxifen. Although tamoxifen is widely used, ER- breast cancer patients, which comprise 20–30% of breast cancer cases, cannot benefit from this endocrine therapy, neither do a large number of ER+ patients that display intrinsic resistance to endocrine therapy. Unfortunately, most of the patients who primarily respond to endocrine therapy acquire resistance along the way due to the evasion of cancer cells to endocrine regulatory effect by means of estrogen-independent ER constitutive activation, estrogen/ER-independent growth pathway activation, EMT or miRNAs aberrant expression. While remission is documented in post-menopausal women who receive aromatase inhibitors or other post-tamoxifen therapies, the majority fall victims to relapse and metastasis. This reflects one of the limitations in the conventional staging tools that are incapable of stratifying patients with more stringent differential prognosis and predicting their likelihood to respond to endocrine therapy. Thus, the latter is now accompanied by further cancer subtype classification methods such as the Oncotype DX and MapQuant Dx, which should also be coupled by characterizing the patient's miRNAs signature for enhanced therapy response prediction [77].

miRNAs regulatory role was studied in three tamoxifen-resistant breast cancer cell lines (TamRs) and their tamoxifen-sensitive counterparts in a pursuit to interpret the molecular machineries behind tamoxifen resistance [78]. Out of the 131 dysregulated miRNAs in TamRs, 22 miRNAs showed comparative expression levels among all TamRs, and were shown to affect common underlying pathways, despite regulating different target genes. Of the regulated gene targets *ESR1*, *PGR1*, *FOXM1* and *14-3-3* family genes were noted. Integrational and functional analysis revealed two significantly upregulated target genes, *SNAI2* (a member of the Snail superfamily which can repress E-cadherin, plays a role in EMT and has an anti-apoptotic activity) and *FYN* (a proto-oncogene tyrosine-protein kinase and a member of the Src family of kinases) in all TamRs, with the downregulation of their regulatory miRNAs and a growth regulatory effect on TamRs. To corroborate the results, combination of miR-190b and miR-516a-5p expression (out of the 131 dysregulated miRNAs in TamRs) exhibited a therapy predictive role in ER+ breast cancer patient cohort who underwent adjuvant tamoxifen treatment. Moreover, transfection of miR-101 in tamoxifen sensitive MCF-7 cells rendered them resistant to tamoxifen and enhanced their growth, independent of estrogen, via AKT activation and Magi-2 suppression [79].

18.3.4 Role of miRNAs in Targeted- and Immune-Therapy Response/Resistance

Trastuzumab (HER2 monoclonal antibody) resistance is correlated with poor prognosis in HER2+ breast cancer patients [80]. Downregulation of tumor suppressor PTEN, a key regulator of apoptosis and cell invasion, is related to the up-regulation of miR-21. Treatment of breast cancer cells that are resistant to Trastuzumab therapy with antisense oligonucleotides against miR-21 re-sensitized cells through prompting cell death and arresting cell cycle [81]. Moreover, overexpression of miR-125a and miR-125b in SKBR3 cell lines, which overexpress HER2 (ErbB2), efficiently decreased mRNA and protein levels of ErbB2 and ErbB3. It also suppressed anchorage-dependent growth, migration and invasion, subsequently, suppressing MAPK and PI3K/Akt pathways [82]. This is of importance since many studies have been working on the inhibition of PI3K/Akt/mTOR pathway in an effort to target ErbB2 overexpression for the treatment of HER2+ tumors [83]. Studies have also characterized the miRNAs profile specific to HER2 status in breast tumors represented by miR-520d, miR-181c, miR-302c, miR-376b, miR-30e as well as let-7f, let-7g, miR-107, mir-10b, miR-126, miR-154 and miR-195 [84, 85].

Interestingly, not only do miRNAs take part in drug resistance of different breast cancer types, but they can also help cancer cells escape immunosurveillance and acquire therapy resistance in aggressive breast tumors via regulating apoptosis and immune detection. Elevated levels of miR-519a-3p in breast cancer is correlated to poor survival and breast cancer resistance through regulating TRAIL-R2, FasL and granzyme B/perforin and enhancing apoptosis. By directly repressing TRAIL-R2 and caspase-8 and indirectly repressing caspase-7, miR-519a-3p increases breast cancer cell resistance to therapy and hinders their responsiveness to apoptotic stimuli. As for its role in evading immunosurveillance, miR-519a-3p impairs the recognition of tumor cells by natural killer (NK) cells by means of decreasing the expression of NKG2D ligands ULBP2 and MICA present on tumor cell surface, necessary for cancer cell recognition [86].

18.3.5 Role of miRNAs in Radioresistance

miRNAs also play part in breast cancer radioresistance. For instance, miR-21 overexpression plays a major role in radioresistance in breast cancer cells through inducing DNA damage-G2 checkpoint upon irradiation, subsequently, aiding tumor cell survival [87]. A transient upregulation of miR-21 in radioresistant T47D breast cancer cells was reported upon 5 Gy irradiation compared to a downregulation in radiosensitive MDA-MB-361 cells. Inhibiting miR-21 pre-irradiation resulted in DNA damage-G2 checkpoint decrease and increase in apoptosis both in T47D cells (7–27%) and in MDA-MB-361 cells (18–30%). In a validation cohort of 86 invasive breast cancer patient samples and their normal adjacent tissues, miR-21 was overexpressed in the cancerous tissues and associated with decreased metastases-free survival. This proposed the potential of combining anti-miR-21 with radiotherapy to avoid radioresistance. Moreover, downregulation of miR-302 correlated with radioresistance, because rescuing of its expression in breast cancer cells increased their radiosensitivity. miR-302 acts as a key player in sensitizing radioresistant breast cancer cells to radiotherapy through downregulating key regulators in radioresistance, AKT1 and RAD52, both *in vitro* and *in vivo* [88].

Thus, studying the miRNome of breast cancer patients will help discover predictive biomarkers to circumvent unnecessary toxic treatments, and using miRNAs in combination with conventional therapy may reverse subsequent drug resistance. Deciphering the roles miRNAs play in drug (chemo/hormonal/targeted/radio therapy) resistance across different breast cancer types is of great importance.

18.4   miRNAs and Metastasis in Breast Cancer

18.4.1   Circulating miRNAs as Biomarkers for Metastasis in Breast Cancer

Breast cancer morbidity and mortality is generally consequent to distant metastasis rather than the primary tumor per se, constituting 90% of mortality in solid tumors [89, 90]. mBC usually manifests in the lungs, liver, brain or bones. Almost half of mBC patients suffer from distal metastasis to the bones, the most common site, followed by lungs, liver and brain, respectively. Moreover, breast cancer relapse as a result of therapy failure results in metastasis, whereby around 22% of relapsed patients present with various metastatic sites. Different breast cancer molecular subtypes metastasize into distinct sites. For instance, luminal A, B and HER2+ breast cancers metastasize mostly to the bones while basal breast cancers metastasize mainly to the lungs. While luminal tumors rarely metastasis to the brain, HER2+ cancers do [11].

Despite the significant drop in deaths from breast cancer in the last two decades, the majority of female cancer mortality is attributed to breast cancer, specifically mBC. The continuous follow-up on patient's prognosis, through predicting progression-free survival (PFS) and OS tailored to a patients' unique profile is key for personalized medicine, which can increase patient's overall quality of life. CTC are FDA-approved mBC prognostic markers. To date, clinicopathological characteristics including patient's age at diagnosis, size of the tumor, number and types of metastatic sites, receptor status, distant disease-free survival (DDFS), among others are used for metastasis and patient survival prediction. Circulating miRNAs are promising biomarkers for mBC. For instance, elevated levels of miR-141, miR-200a, miR-200b, miR-200c, miR-203, miR-375, miR-210 and miR-801 not only predicted mBC onset, but also correlated with CTC status and predicted PFS, OS and metastasis 2 years prior to onset [39]. Markou et al. [40] studied the expression level of a panel of miRNAs (miR-21, miR-146a, miR-200c and miR-210) in primary breast tumors from formalin-fixed, paraffin-embedded tissues (89 FFPE samples) compared to normal breast tissues (30 samples) and in CTCs as well as in the plasma of mBC patients (55 donors) compared to healthy subjects (20 donors). CTCs, plasma and primary tumor tissues were studied concurrently from more than half [30] of the metastatic patients under study. Results revealed a differential expression in all metastatic miRNAs between the normal and mBC tissues and an upregulation of all metastatic miRNAs in CTC and matching plasma samples (especially miR-21 in CTCs). More so, overexpression of miR-21 and miR-146a and down-regulation in miR-200c and miR-210 were noted in tumor tissues, while miR-21, miR-146a, and miR-210 were exclusively dysregulated in plasma of breast cancer patients, but not healthy subjects. Another study characterized the miRNome of 40 mBC patients, confirmed it in another patient cohort and found a panel of 16 prognostic miRNAs that correlated with overall survival, of which 11 related to progression-free survival [39]. Importantly, 6 miRNAs (miR-200a, miR-200b, miR-200c, miR-210, miR-215 and miR-486-5p) were identified as early detection markers for metastasis, up to 2 years before its clinical manifestation. Thus, identifying miRNAs signature capable of predicting metastatic onset might offer prolonged median and relapse-free survival rates and might enhance prognosis in breast cancer and mBC patients.

18.4.2   miRNAs as Active Players/Regulators of Breast Cancer Along the Metastatic Cascade

miRNAs, through regulating genes involved in breast tumorigenesis, have been reported to play crucial roles in the genetic and epigenetic alterations along the metastatic cascade. miRNAs can play a dichotomous role as metastasis promoters, like the scenario with miR-373, miR-151, miR-520, miR-143 or miR-10b or as metastasis suppressors, as with miR-9, miR-139, miR-335, miR-125 or miR-206 [89]. Ma et al. [91] correlated the increase in migration and invasion in mBC cells to the upregulation of miR-10b, which is transcriptionally controlled by TWIST, basic helix–loop–helix protein. Recent studies showed that restoration of tumor-suppressor miR-340 in metastatic MDA-MB-231 cells drastically suppressed migration, invasion and metastasis through targeting the Wnt signaling pathway [38].

miRNAs contribute to metastasis first by priming cells to adopt an EMT phenotype, thus rendering them more motile and invasive. EMT regulatory miRNAs are miR-7, miR-124, miR-145, miR-200 family, miR-205, miR-375 and miR-448 [92]. EMT is characterized by the loss of cells to their epithelial features like apical-basal polarity and tight cell-cell adhesion and the subsequent acquisition of mesenchymal ones via development of extensions, loosened cell-cell adhesion and actin cytoskeletal reorientation. Key players in EMT are Snail (SNAI1), Slug, ZEB (ZEB1 and ZEB2/SIP1) and TWIST1 and E47, all of which act towards the suppression of E-cadherin. miRNAs not only control the initial step of metastasis, EMT, but they also contribute to intravasation of cancer cells into the circulation and the successive extravasation and survival in the metastatic sites. For instance, in SUM149 breast cancer cells, miR-9 was shown to regulate E-cadherin coding gene, CDH1, thus increased EMT, cell motility and invasiveness [93]. In ER- breast cancer cells, miR-520/373 family repressed invasion and intravasation *in vitro* and *in vivo*, respectively. Moreover, in patients with ER- breast tumors, miR-520c suppression was indicative of lymph node metastasis. After cancer cells undergo EMT, intravasation, extravasation and manage to survive and disseminate to the appropriate distal organ, the final step towards metastasis is the cells' proper colonization at the metastatic site. This is defined as the well-known seed-and-soil hypothesis, implying that cancer cells or "seed" grow in fertile or appropriate tumor microenvironment, the "soil" [9]. For instance, miR-200 through directly regulating the metastasis suppressor Sec23a contributes to breast tumor cells colonization [94].

McGuire et al. [11] summarized different miRNAs implicated in invasion (miR-199a, miR-214, miR-200a/b/c, miR-141, miR-429), dissemination (miR-31), extravasation (miR-10b, miR-373, miR-20a, miR-214, miR-31) and proliferation (miR-10b, miR-34a, miR-155, miR-200a/b/c, miR-141, miR-429). Moreover, antagonistic effects of miRNAs were studied for miR-214 and miR-148b that act as pro-metastatic and anti-metastatic miRNAs in mBC dissemination through dictating the interactions between tumor and endothelial cells. Metastatic dissemination was blocked through dual alteration; downregulating miR-214 and upregulating miR-148b, resulted in downregulation of cell adhesion genes ITGA5 and ALCAM, subsequently blocked tumor escape through blood endothelial vessels *in vitro*, *in vivo* and in primary breast cancer patient samples [95].

miR-22/SIRT1 (Sirtuin1) axis was linked to breast cancer growth and metastatic suppression and proposed it as a potential therapeutic target against mBC [96]. Notably, miR-22 directly suppresses SIRT1 in MCF-7 breast cancer cells. The suppression of miR-22 and significant upregulation of SIRT1 was revealed in breast cancer tissues as compared to normal tissues and in stage III-IV breast tumors as compared to stage I-II breast tumors. Thus, miR-22 downregulation was indicative of poor differentiation, metastasis and progressive breast cancer stages. On the contrary, overexpression of miR-22 attenuated proliferation, migration and invasion in MCF-7 cells, while overexpressing SIRT1 reversed the tumor-suppressive and metastasis-suppressive role of up-regulated miR-22 in the cells. Moreover, Li et al. [97] related breast cancer metastatic initiation to the downregulation of miR-452 and the resulting upregulation in RAB11A, both in breast cancer tissues and cell lines. miR-452 acts a tumor suppressor through downregulating RAB11A and is responsible for suppressing migration and invasion in breast cancer. In addition, by upregulating the pro-metastatic gene RhoA, miR-155 promoted EMT, cell migration and invasion [98], while miR-31 blocked metastasis by inhibiting RhoA and disabling cancer cells from exiting the primary tumor site, disseminating and/or surviving in distal sites [99, 100]. miR-31 targets also include Frizzled3 (Fzd3), integrin α-5 (ITGA5), myosin phosphatase-Rho interacting protein (M-RIP), matrix metallopeptidase 16 (MMP16), radixin (RDX), as well as PKCε, which deregulates NF-κB signaling pathway, increase apoptosis and enhances MCF-10A and

MDA-MB-231 cells radiosensitivity [101, 102]. In MCF-7 cells, upregulation of miR-17-5P increased invasiveness and migration via targeting HBP1/β-catenin pathway [103]. In addition, miR-145, through regulating c-Myc and mucin and downregulating c-Myc downstream targets like cyclin D1 and elF4E plays a role in cancer cell motility and cell cycle progression [79].

Moreover, miRNAs not only control metastasis, but they also regulate angiogenesis. Lu et al. [104] investigated the role of the tumor suppressive miR-140-5p in breast cancer in regulating invasion and angiogenesis. Their results showed that miR-140-5p regulates the vascular endothelial growth factor VEGF-A *in vitro* and *in vivo*. Similarly, miR-378 and miR-27a have been shown to enhance angiogenesis and tumor cell survival in breast cancer [105, 106]. Moreover, downregulation of miR-140-5p was observed in breast cancer and mBC tissues as compared to their normal counterparts, and thus, might serve as a novel anti-metastatic and anti-angiogenic agent in breast cancer.

18.4.3   Examples of miRNAs Implicated in Common Sites of Breast Metastases

miRNAs can play a role in breast cancer metastasis to distal regions such as brain, bone and lung. Li et al. [37] discussed the importance of deciphering the role miR-NAs play in diagnosing and, possibly, treating breast cancers with brain metastasis. This is since (10–30%) of patients with advanced breast cancer suffer from brain metastasis with poor prognosis. The universal gene expression signatures of patients with primary in situ breast carcinoma and patients with brain metastasis were investigated in a pursuit to identify the differential expression patterns in miRNAs, their corresponding mRNA targets and the underlying signaling pathways that might serve as early detection markers for brain metastasis. Results showed a strong correlation between miR-17-5p and miR-16-5p and BCL2, SMAD3 and SOCS1 and subsequent oncogenic pathways like ones concerned with EMT, cell cycle control, adherence junctions and extracellular matrix-receptor communication. A comparison of patient samples to matched breast cancer patients from The Cancer Genome Atlas (TCGA) revealed similar expression levels in 11 miRNAs, wherein miR-17-5p was upregulated in TNBC tissues extracted from the database, with opposing patterns between miR-17-5p levels and overall survival and PTEN and BCL2 levels. Thus, devising a systems-gene expression patterns can better guide clinicians into predicting optimal treatment options specific for patients with breast cancer brain metastasis.

Soria-Valles et al. [107] linked downregulation of miR-21 to matrix metalloproteinase, collagenase-2 (MMP-8), which exhibited a tumor suppressive role and lung metastasis blockage in MDA-MB-231 breast cancer cells. The authors validated the results *in vitro* and *in vivo* and related the protective role of MMP-8 to decorin cleavage and inhibition in TGF-β signaling, which in turn downregulates miR-21.

This eventually induces tumor suppressors such as programmed cell death 4. An example of miRNAs effect on bone metastasis was discussed in a study on the stimulatory role of TWIST1 on breast cancer intravasation and dissemination to the bones using human osteotropic MDA-MB-231/B02 breast cancer cells and immunodeficient mice [108]. TWIST1 stable transfection *in vitro* showed enhancement in tumor cell invasion, but not tumor growth, and resulted in upregulation in the pro-invasive miR-10b level. *In vivo*, TWIST1 transfection caused higher osteolytic lesions, reduced bone volume and caused doubling of the tumor burden. Upon treatment with DOX, TWIST1 was suppressed, and hence, bone metastasis was blocked *in vivo*. Blocking miR-10b in the mice caused drastic reduction in TWIST1-expressing breast cancer cells found in the bone marrow. Therefore, miR-10b takes part in regulating TWIST1-induced breast cancer bone metastasis.

Bishopric et al. [109] inoculated MDA-MB-231 and MDA-MB-436 breast cancer xenografts into immunedeficient mice mammary fat pads to produce primary tumors and corresponding lymph node, liver, lung and diaphragm metastases. By comparing the miRNAs profiles of the primary and the metastatic tumors, the authors found miR-203 levels, which acts as a tumor suppressor, to be significantly associated with the size of the primary tumor at all metastatic sites. miR-203 acted by directly targeting TWF1 and APBB2. Although miR-203 was shown to be necessary for metastasis growth, its over-expression inhibited metastasis, thus implicating opposing function and a dynamic, context-dependent function of miR-203 along the metastatic cascade.

18.5 miRNAs Role in the Interplay Between Drug Resistance and Metastasis in Breast Cancer

Despite the booming reports on miRNAs that act on drug resistance or metastasis, the quest on whether some miRNAs are capable of regulating both simultaneously is fundamental, yet understudied. The rationale behind this is that the likelihood of recurrence and subsequent distant metastasis in tumor cells increases due to drug resistance. For instance, miR-644a acts pleiotropically through increasing cell death and inhibiting EMT, thus sensitizing various breast cancer subtypes to both hormonal-and-targeted therapeutic agents (like tamoxifen and gefitinib) and blocking metastasis [26]. EMT inhibition was thus proposed as the common underlying mechanism towards drug sensitization and metastasis blockade. Moreover, miR-644a was shown to directly downregulate transcriptional co-repressor C-Terminal Binding Protein 1 (CTBP1), which in turn upregulates wild type-or mutant-p53. The downregulation of CTBP1 retarded growth, metastasis and drug resistance and was validated in miR-644a CRISPR-Cas9 knockouts. Of note, only patients with mutant-p53 and upregulation in CTBP1 exhibited shorter survival, priming CTBP1 to serve as a prognostic marker for p53-mutant patients. This suggested a therapy-sensitizing and metastasis blocking potential through reactivation of miR-644a/

CTBP1/p53 axis in breast cancer along with its potential as progression and therapy predictive biomarker. Another study suggested NSC95397, a small molecule capable of obstructing transcriptional repression brought by CTBP1, as an easier drug target than miR-644a [110].

Other examples of the role miRNAs play in regulating EMT in breast cancer, leading to endocrine (hormone) therapy resistance is how breast cancer cells acquired a mesenchymal phenotype due to the upregulation of miR-9 that resulted in E-cadherin repression and vimentin overexpression [77, 93]. Moreover, miRNAs can initiate drug resistance and metastasis concomitant with cancer stem cell (CSC) characteristics. Although CSCs only constitute part of the tumor burden, they are known to initiate growth, metastasis and drug resistance in tumors [89]. While some miRNAs have been reported to control the interplay between cancer stemness and drug resistance, others reported how miRNAs control stem cell and metastatic characteristics of cancer cells via EMT regulation. For instance, compared to non-CSCs extracted from advanced mBC cells, CD24−/CD44+/ESA+ CSC population was capable of driving metastasis. When these CSC metastasize to the bones and brain, downregulation in miR-7 was noted; however, blockade of brain metastasis was possible through re-expressing miR-7 in breast CSCs, which in turn repressed stemness regulatory gene, KLF4 [111]. In addition, miRNAs can play a role in breast cancer drug resistance and metastasis through epigenetics [112]. Thus, studies are investigating the effect of differentially methylated regions (DMRs) of miRNAs loci in invasive breast cancers. For instance, analysis of DMRs and methylation patterns in miR-31, miR-135b and miR-138-1 were correlated with patterns seen in early and late postpartum breast cancer patients [113]. Moreover, a correlation was shown between aggressiveness and advanced breast cancer disease and the methylation of tumor suppressive and DNMT3b targets which are miR-124a-1, miR-124a-2 and miR-124a-3 [114]. However, while aberrant DNA methylation, in part, controls the expression of miRNAs and subsequent downstream pathways, miRNAs can also control some DNA methylators.

In addition, miRNAs can play a role in chemoresistance in aggressive TNBC, which does not respond to any targeted therapies. Niu et al. [115] showed that TNBC cells exhibited higher survival and metastatic potential as a result of miR-181a upregulation upon genotoxic DOX treatment. These results were also noticed in TNBC patients with high levels of miR-181a post-DOX treatment who had poor disease free survival and overall survival. Moreover, chemoresistance was attributed to apoptosis evasion and enhanced invasion in DOX-treated TNBC cells to the direct suppression of BAX by miR-181a. Thus, blocking miR-181a could potentially rescue DOX sensitivity in TNBC cells and alleviate metastasis. A similar pattern was observed in HER2+ breast cancer patients, with noted upregulation in miR-181a, whereby blocking miR-181a re-sensitized breast cancer cells to Trastuzumab and inhibited metastasis. Thus, inhibiting miR-181a could reverse both chemo-and-targeted therapy resistance and block metastasis in TNBC and HER2+ breast tumors, respectively. Moreover, Bai et al. [116] showed increase in EMT and TGF-β signaling with a downregulation of miR-200c in highly invasive, tumorigenic, Trastuzumab-resistant HER2+ breast cancer cells. Re-expression of miR-200c targeted both a TGF-β transcriptional activator ZNF217 and a key player in the TGF-β signaling pathway, ZEB1, thus rescuing Trastuzumab sensitivity and blocking invasion concomitantly. Alternatively, silencing of ZEB1 or ZNF217 or inhibiting TGF-β signaling exhibited same response as restoration of miR-200c in resistant cells, suggesting a miR-200c/ZEB1 and miR-200c/ZNF217/TGF-β/ ZEB1 regulatory circuits in Trastuzumab resistance and distal metastasis.

Therefore, it is vital to focus on miRNAs that act both as therapy sensitizers and metastasis blockers, for an optimal understanding of their regulatory role, and for widening their potential use as biomarkers and therapeutic tools against breast cancer. One successful promising example is oncomiR, miR-21, which is almost upregulated in most breast cancers and has been reported to drive both drug resistance and metastasis. Mei et al. [75] potentiated the simultaneous delivery of miR-21 inhibitor and paclitaxel through G5-PAMAM dendrimer, in order to impede both tumor growth and invasiveness in breast cancer. Thus, complimenting conventional therapies with miRNAs inhibitors/mimics holds hope in combating drug-resistance and circumventing metastasis in breast cancer [20].

18.6   Conclusions and Future Directions

We have highlighted thus far the novelty of utilizing miRNAs to serve not only as biomarkers for breast cancer progression, invasiveness, drug resistance and metastasis, but also as potential key players in re-sensitizing breast cancer cells to chemo/ targeted/hormonal therapies and/or potentially blocking metastasis. All the mentioned miRNAs from the literature, pooled according to their regulatory role, their biomarker capability, dysregulation pattern, target protein/pathway, sample source, breast cancer type and mode of action are presented in Tables 18.1, 18.2, 18.3, and 18.4. Moreover, QIAGEN's Ingenuity® Pathway Analysis (IPA®, QIAGEN Redwood City, www.qiagen.com/ingenuity), IPA, has a comprehensive, manually curated content of the Ingenuity Knowledge Base as well as has powerful algorithms that identify regulators, relationships, mechanisms, functions, and pathways relevant to changes observed in an analyzed dataset. A powerful feature of IPA is the MicroRNA Target Filter that finds validated and predicted miRNA-mRNA target pairings based on Ingenuity Expert Finding, Ingenuity ExpertAssist Findings, TargetScan, TarBase and miRecords and allows filtration according to diseases, cell/tissue type, location, molecule type, species, or biological pathways. Thus, through MicroRNA Target Filter, we linked the miRNAs discussed here to validated mRNAs that are part of IPA networks or canonical pathways of interest (i.e., drug resistance, breast cancer, metastasis, EMT). The validated mRNA targets were filtered according to validated databases: Human, Tarbase, miRecords, Ingenuity Expert Findings and Ingenuity ExpertAssist Findings as well as according to mammary cell/tissue type. The predicted and validated targets are tabulated (if any) in Tables 18.2, 18.3, and 18.4.

Table 18.1 Summary of miRNAs that exhibit biomarker role in BC and their dysregulation pattern versus their target protein/pathway, sample source, breast cancer type and function

Role	miRNA	sample source (cell line vs patient samples)	breast cancer type	Function	Ref.
Biomarker miRNAs	miR-10b, miR-34a, miR-155, miR-17, miR-122	patient samples	mBC	distinguishehs mBC from non-mBC patients	[45, 52]
	miR-10b, miR-373, miR-20a, miR-214	patient samples	lymph node+ BC	upregulated in patients with lymph node positive breast cancer	[46–47]
	miR-10b	patient samples	mBC	mBC biomarker to the brain and bones	[48, 49]
	miR-141, miR-200a, miR-200b, miR-200c, miR-203, miR-210, miR-375, miR-801	patient samples	BC	significantly elevated in patients with circulating tumor cells	[50]
	miR-105	patient samples	early onset BC	predicted metastasis in early onset BC	[51]
	miR-34a, miR-155	patient samples (serum)	mBC	metastasis as a result of primary BC	[48]
	miR-17-5p	TNBC tissues	TNBC	opposing patterns between miR-17-5p levels and overall survival (OS)	[37]
	266 miRs in TIF	TIF and serum from BC patients	BC	prognostic and diagnostic biomarkers	[56]
	miR-222, miR-29a, miR-140,	FFPE tissues	BC	correlated with poor prognosis	[59]
	miR-210, miR-328, miR-484, miR-874	patient samples	BC	predicting prognosis or risk of recurrence	[11]
	miR-106b	serum and tissues	BC	predicted high recurrence & shorter OS	[54]
	miR-18b, miR-103, miR-107, miR-652	patient samples	TNBC	predicted recurrence and decreased OS in TNBC	[55]

Within each cluster, upregulated miRNAs are highlighted in yellow, downregulated miRNAs in dark blue and dysregulated miRNAs (meaning miRNAs with conflicting dysregulation patterns between studies or dysregulation pattens not indicated in the study) in purple
ND Not Determined, *BC* Breast Cancer, *mBC* Metastatic Breast Cancer, *OS* overall survival, *DFS* disease-free survival, *PFS* progression-free survival, *TNBC* triple negative breast cancer, *DCIS* ductal carcinoma in situ, *CTCs* circulating tumor cells

However, a few caveats are common in most of the mentioned studies, and must be addressed. Markou et al. [40] pointed out the pitfalls underlying the lack of reproducibility across studies performed by different groups on similar patients and cancer profiles. For instance, when comparing the databases of 15 studies characterizing circulating miRNAs profiles of breast cancer patients, very little overlap was detected. The authors attributed the lack of reproducibility to variations in sample origins (plasma, serum, whole blood), variability in cohort population and inconsistencies in sample collection protocols/timings and sample processing. As for the discrepancies in miRNAs profiles reported from the same tumor, it might be partly attributed to the lack of an established endogenous miRNA for normalization [117]. Pichler and Calin [118] addressed few solutions, like the importance of designing larger prospective clinical trials that encompass the published work on candidate diagnostic or prognostic miRNAs and comparing them to the gold standard techniques in a blinded fashion. Most of the current findings were done retrospectively, were prone to error-and-selection bias and lacked long-term follow-up. Cortez et al. [44] stressed on the importance of characterizing specific panels of differentially expressed miRNAs rather than single miRNAs as exclusive biomarker panels to a certain type of cancer, stage (early vs advanced), therapy response, patient outcome, recurrence or metastatic output, which will also account for intra-tumoral and intercellular heterogeneity.

Table 18.2 Summary of miRNAs implicated in drug resistance in BC and their dysregulation pattern, their target protein/pathway, validated targets from IPA, sample source, breast cancer type and function

Role	miRNA	target protein/pathway	validated targets from IPA	sample source (cell line vs patient samples)	breast cancer type	Function	Ref.
miRNAs implicated in drug resistance	miR-21	ND	ND	ND	BC	associated with radio resistance	[12]
	miR-144		ND				
	miR-27a		FADD, FOXO1, GRB2, IGF1, MMP13, NOTCH1, PDPK1, PXN, SMAD3, SMAD4				
	miR-130	PTEN, MDR, PI3K/Akt pathway	NOTCH, SMAD3, SMAD4, SMAD5	tumor tissues and MCF-7/ADR	BC	Increased drug resistance and proliferation and decreased apoptotic levels	[43]
	miR-21	PTEN	ND	HER2+ BC patient samples	HER2+ BC	predicted Trastuzumab resistance and poor prognosis	[73, 74]
	miR-101	AKT, Magi-2	ND	MCF-7 cells	benign BC	resistance to tamoxifen and increased ER-independent growth	[79]
	miR-125b	Bak1	TP53	paclitaxel-resistant BC cells	BC	increased paclitaxel resistance	[76]
	miR-519a-3p	TRAIL, FasL, granzyme B/perforin	ND	BC cells	aggressive BC	poor survival and resistance to apoptosis and therapy	[86]
	miR-519a-3p	NKO2D, ULBP2, MICA	ND	BC cells	aggressive BC	escaping immunosurveillance and recognition by NK cells	[73]
	miR-21	PDCD4, PTEN	ND	Trastuzumab-resistant (BC cells and in vivo xenografts models)	Trastuzumab-resistant BC	chemoresistance	[73, 74]
	miR-21	G2 checkpoint	ND	radioresistant T47D cells, radiosensitive MDA-MB-361 cells, BC patients	radioresistant and invasive breast cancer	increase in DNA damage-G2 checkpoint and increased cell survival	[87]
	miR-221	p27(Kip1)	FOXO3, PIK3R1, PTEN	in vitro	BC	biomarkers for Tamoxifen resistance	[70]
	miR-222		FOXO3, PIK3R1, PTEN				
	miR-449a/b		ND				
	miR-449a	ND	ND	frozen BC tissues	BC	inverse correlation with BC grade and tamoxifin resistance	[71]
	miR-449b		ND				
	miR-451	ND	ABCB1	doxorubicin-resistant (MCF-7/DOX) BC cells	BC	increased MDR1 levels and doxorubicin resistance	[67]
	miR-326	MRP-1	SMO	VP-16-resistant MDR (MCF-7/VP) & advanced BC tissues	advanced BC	preventative and MDR-reversing role of miR-326 in MRP-1 mediated MDR BC	[67]
	miR-302	AKT1 and RAD52	ND	In vitro and in vivo	radioresistant breast cancer cells	downregulation causes radioresistance, and re-expression radiosensitivity	[88]
	miR-205	ND	PTEN	ND	BC	associated with radio resistance	[12]
	miR-200a, miR-302		ND				
	miR-222	ND	FOXO3, PIK3R1, PTEN	FFPE tissues	BC	associated with drug resistances	[59]
	miR-29a		PIK3R1, PTEN				
	miR-34a		MAP2K1, TP53				
	miR-130		HDAC4, SMAD3, VEGFA				
	miR-3178, miR-574, miR-6780b, miR-744, miR-423		ND				
	miR-21, miR-155	ND	ND	urinary miRNAs	breast and ovarian cancer	distinguishing patients with BC and miR-125b predicted resistance to chemotherapy	[60]
	miR-125b		TP53				
	miR-451		ABCB1				
	miR-190b, miR-516a-5p	ND	ND	patient cohort	ER+ BC patients with adjuvant tamoxifen treatment	therapy predictive role	[79]

Within each cluster, upregulated miRNAs are highlighted in yellow, downregulated miRNAs in dark blue and dysregulated miRNAs (meaning miRNAs with conflicting dysregulation patterns between studies or dysregulation pattens not indicated in the study) in purple. The validated pathways selected in IPA only included cancer and drug resistance pathways
ND Not Determined, *BC* Breast Cancer, *mBC* Metastatic Breast Cancer, *OS* overall survival, *DFS* disease-free survival, *PFS* progression-free survival, *TNBC* triple negative breast cancer, *DCIS* ductal carcinoma in situ, *CTCs* circulating tumor cells

One major area that requires development in miRNA-based therapies is the establishment of stable and effective delivery systems with minimal off-target and adverse effects. As exosomes house miRNAs, they have proven to be efficient in miRNAs delivery to breast cancer cells expressing EGFR. Ohno et al. [119] described how engineering protocols were capable of expressing transmembrane domain of platelet-derived growth factor receptor (PDGF) merged to GE11 peptide, a less mitogenic EGFR binding partner, on donor cells. These exosomes where then able to successfully deliver let-7a miRNA, intravenously, in RAG2$^{-/-}$ mice breast cancer xenografts that exhibited EGFR. Some successful nucleic acid therapies made it to human clinical trials, the first of which was miraversen (www.clinicaltrials.gov, study no. NCT01200420), which was designed to capture miR-122 to inhibit the

Table 18.3 Summary of miRNAs implicated in metastasis in BC and their dysregulation pattern, their target protein/pathway, validated targets from IPA, sample source, breast cancer type and function

Role	miRNA	target protein/pathway from the literature	validated targets from IPA	sample source (cell line vs patient samples)	breast cancer type	Function	Ref.
miRNAs implicated in metastasis	miR-141	ND	CTNNB1, MAP2K4, PTPRD, STAT5B, TGFB2, ZEB1, ZEB2	Circulating miRNA	Breast Cancer	predicted MBC onset, correlated with CTC status and predicted PFS and OS	[39]
	miR-200a/b/c		PLCG1, PTEN, PTPN12, PTPN13, PTPRD, ZEB1, ZEB2				
	miR-203		ABL1, SOCS3				
	miR-375, miR-210, miR-801						
	miR-10b	TWIST	ND	mBC cells	mBC	increase in migration and invasion	[38, 89]
	miR-17-5P	HBP1/β-catenin	BCL2, BMPR2, CCND1, CDKN1A, CREB1, JAK1, MAP3K12, MMP3, PTEN, STAT3, TGFBR2, TNF, VEGFA, VIM	MCF-7 cells	BC	increased invasiveness and migration	[37]
	miR-203	TWF1, APBB2	ABL1, SOCS3	MDA-MB-231 and MDA-MB-436 breast cancer xenografts	lymph node, liver, lung and diaphragm metastases	opposing function and a dynamic, context-dependent function of miR-203 in metastasis (enhancer and suppressor)	
	miR-181a	STAT3, NF-κB, IL-6	BCL2, CDKN1B, KRAS, MMP14, NOTCH4, TIMP3	TNBC patients with Dox treatment	TNBC	higher metastatic potential, and poor DFS & OS	[115]
	miR-340	Wnt pathway	ND	metastatic MDA-MB-231 cells	invasive BC	migration, invasion & metastasis suppression	[38]
	miR-17-3p	BCL2, SMAD3, SOCS1, EMT	BCL2, BMPR2, CCND1, CDKN1A, CREB1, JAK1, MAP3K12, MMP3, PTEN, STAT3, TGFBR2, TNF, VEGFA, VIM	patient samples and TCGA database	patients with DCIS or brain metastasis	devising a systems-gene expression patterns to predict cancer metastasis	[37]
	miR-16-3p		ANLN, BCL2, CCND1, CDC14B, CDC25A, CFL2, EGFR, EIF4E, FGF2, FGF7, FGFR1, GRB2, H3F3A/H3F3B, HSP90B1, IGF1, IGF1R, IGF2R, ITGA2, JUN, MAP2K1, MAP2K4, MAPK3, MCL1, PHKB, PPP2R5C, PTGS2, RAF1, RECK, RHOT1, VEGFA, WIPF1, WNT3A, ZYX				
	miR-452	RAB11A	ND	BC tissues and cell lines	BC	MBC initiation (when upregulated, acts as tumor suppressor)	[97]
	miR-520c	ND	ARHGEF3, CCND1, CDKN1A, CFL2, PRKACB, RECK, RELA, VEGFA	ER-ve BC patients	ER-ve BC	indicative of lymph node metastasis	[94]
	miR-155	RhoA	ARFIP2, CCND1, CEBPB, CTNNB1, ETS1, FADD, FGF7, GNA13, IKBKE, INPP5D, MET, MYD88, PDE3A, PRKCI, PTPRJ, RAB5C, RHEB, RHOA, RIPK1, SMAD2, TAB2, TCF7L2	ND	BC	promoted EMT, cell migration and invasion	[98]
	miR-21	MMP-8, decorin, PCD4, TGF-β	ND	MDA-MB-231	BC	tumor suppressor and lung metastasis blockage	[107]
	miR-146a		CD40, CDKN3, CHUK, FADD, IL1R1, IL36B, IL36G, IRAK1, MMP16, STAT1, TLR10, TLR4, TLR9, TRAF6	ND	ND	ND	
	miR-200c, miR-210, miR-21		ND				
	miR-373, miR-151, miR-10b	ND	ND	ND	BC	metastasis promoters	[89]
	miR-520		ARHGEF3, CCND1, CDKN1A, CFL2, PRKACB, RECK, RELA, VEGFA				
	miR-143		BCL2, KRAS, MAPK12, MDM2				
	miR-9		ND				
	miR-139		FOXO1, IGF1R, SHC1				
	miR-335		PTPN11, PXN				
	miR-125	ND	BMPR1B, CDC25A, ELAVL1, H3F3A/H3F3B, ID2, IL1RN, IL1RN, MAP2K7, MYD88, SMO, TP53	ND	BC	metastasis suppressors	[89]
	miR-206		ARF3, ARF4, ARHGEF18, BCL2, EGFR, H3F3A/H3F3B, IGF1, INPP5F, ITGB4, LRP1, MET, NOTCH3, NRP1, PTPRF, TIMP3, TSPAN4, YWHAQ				
	miR-520/373 family	ND	ARHGEF3, CCND1, CDKN1A, CFL2, PRKACB, RECK, RELA, VEGFA	in vitro and in vivo	ER-ve BC cells	repressed invasion and intravasation	[94]
	miR-200	Sec23a	ND	BC cells	BC	contributes to BC colonization	[94]
	miR-22/SIRT1 (Sirtuin1) axis	SIRT1	ND	MCF-7 cells and (stage III-IV) BC tissues	mBC	BC growth and metastatic suppression and a potential therapeutic target against MBC	[96]
	miR-10b	TWIST	ND	mBC cells	mBC	increase in migration and invasion	[108]
	miR-199a		ETS1, HIF1A				
	miR-214, miR-141	ND	ND	ND	mBC	implicated in invasion	[11]
	miR-200a/b/c		PLCG1, PTEN, PTPN12, PTPN13, PTPRD, ZEB1, ZEB2				
	miR-429		PLCG1, PTEN, PTPN12, PTPN13, PTPRD, ZEB1, ZEB2				
	miR-31, miR-10b, miR-373, miR-214		ND				
	miR-20a	ND	BCL2, BMPR2, CCND1, CDKN1A, CREB1, JAK1, MAP3K12, MMP3, PTEN, STAT3, TGFBR2, TNF, VEGFA, VIM	ND	mBC	implicated in extravasation	[11]
	miR-10b, miR-34a, miR-155, miR-141	ND	ND	ND	mBC	implicated in prolifration	[11]
	miR-200a/b/c, miR-429		PLCG1, PTEN, PTPN12, PTPN13, PTPRD, ZEB1, ZEB2				
	miR-214	ITGA5 and ALCAM	ATF4, FGF16, PTEN	in vitro, in vivo, in primary BC patients	mBC	miR-214 downregulation &miR-148b upregulation blocked dissemination	[95]
	miR-148b		ND				
	miR-378		ND				
	miR-27a	ND	FADD, FOXO1, GRB2, IGF1, MMP13, NOTCH1, PDPK1, PXN, SMAD3, SMAD4	ND	BC	enhance angiogenesis & tumor survival	[105, 106]
	miR-31	RhoA, Fzd3,ITGA5, M-RIP, MMP16, RDX, PKCε, NF-κB	ND	MCF-10A and MDA-MB-231	BC	blocked metastasis, increase apoptosis and enhances radiosenaivity	[99, 100]
	miR-9	CDH1	ND	SUM149 breast cancer cells	BC	elevated cell motility and invasiveness	[93]
	miR-143	c-Myc and mucin, cyclin-D1, eIF4E	CLINT1, DDR1, EIF4E, IGF1R, IRS1, MDM2, MMP1, PPP3CA, RTKN	ND	BC	regulates cancer cell motility and cell cycle progression	[79]
	miR-140-5p	VEGF-A	SMAD3, VEGFA	in vitro and in vivo	BC and MBC	tumor suppressor, and possible novel anti-metastatic and anti-angiogenic agent	[104]

Within each cluster, upregulated miRNAs are highlighted in yellow, downregulated miRNAs in dark blue and dysregulated miRNAs (meaning miRNAs with conflicting dysregulation patterns between studies or dysregulation pattens not indicated in the study) in purple. The validated pathways selected in IPA included metastasis, NF-κB signalling, VEGF signalling and VEGF family ligands, inhibition of MMPs, JAK/STAT signalling, Pi3K/AKT signalling, Integrin signalling, epithelial adherens, remodelling of the epithelium and EMT pathways

ND Not Determined, *BC* Breast Cancer, *mBC* Metastatic Breast Cancer, *OS* overall survival, *DFS* disease-free survival, *PFS* progression-free survival, *TNBC* triple negative breast cancer, *DCIS* ductal carcinoma in situ, *CTCs* circulating tumor cells

Table 18.4 Summary of miRNAs implicated in both drug resistance and metastasis in BC and their dysregulation pattern, their target protein/pathway, validated targets from IPA, sample source, breast cancer type and function

Role	miRNA	target protein/pathway	validated targets from IPA	sample source (cell line vs patient samples)	breast cancer type	Function	Ref.
miRNAs implicated in both drug resistance and metastasis	miR-644a	CTBP1, p53, Noxa	ND	BC cell lines	various BC subtypes	sensitizes cells to targeted/chemotherapy and blocks metastasis	[26, 110]
	miR-9	E-cadherin , vimentin	ND	BC cell lines	BC	regulates EMT leading to endocrine resistance	[77, 93]
	miR-21	G5-PAMAM	ND	BC cell lines	BC	drive drug resistance and metastasis	[75]
	miR-7	KLF4	ND	breast CSCs	breast CSCs	CSC metastasize to the bone and brain	[111]
	miR-7	EMT	ND	BC cell lines	BC	EMT regulatory miRs that might lead to drug resistance	[92]
	miR-124		ARAF				
	miR-145		CLINT1, DDR1, EIF4E, IGF1R, IRS1, MDM2, MMP1, PPP3CA, RTKN				
	miR-200 family		PLCG1, PTEN, PTPN12, PTPN13, PTPRD, ZEB1, ZEB2				
	miR-205		ERBB3, INPPL1, MED1, PRKCE, PTEN, VEGFA				
	miR-375, miR-448		ND				
	miR-31	ND	ND	early/late postpartum BC patients	BC	correlation with differentially methylated regions	[113]
	miR-135b		APC				
	miR-138-1		RHOC, ROCK2				
	miR-124a-1/2/3	DNMT3b	ARAF, ARHGEF1, CDK2, CDK4, CDK6, CTGF, CTNND1, DRAM1, DVL2, E2F5, ELF4, ELK3, GNAI3, ITGB1, MAPK14, PRKD1, RARG, RELA, RHOG, SMAD5, SNAI2, SOX9, SP1, TLN1, TRIM29, TUBB6	ND	advanced BC	correlates aggressiveness and advanced BC with methylation patterns	[114]

Within each cluster, upregulated miRNAs are highlighted in yellow, downregulated miRNAs in dark blue and dysregulated miRNAs (meaning miRNAs with conflicting dysregulation patterns between studies or dysregulation pattens not indicated in the study) in purple. The validated pathways selected in IPA included cancer, drug resistance, metastasis, NF-κB signalling, VEGF signalling and VEGF family ligands, inhibition of MMPs, JAK/STAT signalling, Pi3K/AKT signalling, Integrin signalling, epithelial adherens, remodelling of the epithelium and EMT pathways
ND Not Determined, *BC* Breast Cancer, *mBC* Metastatic Breast Cancer, *OS* overall survival, *DFS* disease-free survival, *PFS* progression-free survival, *TNBC* triple negative breast cancer, *DCIS* ductal carcinoma in situ, *CTCs* circulating tumor cells

replication of hepatitis C virus, after it was proven effective in chimpanzees [65]. More than dozens of clinical trials are underway, testing the prognostic, metastatic and therapy predictive potential possessed by some candidate miRNAs, or alternatively, players in the biogenesis pathway of miRNAs (www.clinicaltrials.gov). Adams et al. [8] predicted the potential of using miR-34a for treatment of TNBC based on clinical studies investigating MRX34, an amphoteric liposome coupled with a synthetic miR-34a mimic, for its efficacy against hepatocellular carcinoma in phase I clinical trial. The rationale behind their prediction is that miR-34a was capable of sensitizing TNBC to dasatinib treatment by targeting c-SRC, and thus, administering miR-34a and dasatinib might be worth investigating in aggressive TNBC.

Finally, focus for BC understanding should be on the original molecular triggers for cellular transformation prior to cancer progression, drug resistance and metastasis. In other terms, it is essential to focus research on the basic molecular mechanisms that trigger cancer. Besides understanding the regulatory role of miRNAs in breast cancer, recent studies are focusing on circular RNAs (circRNAs) and their roles in "sponging" microRNAs. circRNAs are a large class of endogenous RNAs that originate from cellular splicing and play regulatory roles in mammalian cells. Sequencing analysis has also shown circRNAs to be dysregulated in cancers (cell lines, patient tissues, plasma and serum) and are characterized by their stability, conserved sequences and presence in the circulation. Thus, sequencing circRNAs along with their downstream miRNAs targets will add one more layer to better understand the drivers of cancer initiation, progression, drug resistance and metastasis and will bring us a step closer towards devising better breast cancer biomarkers [120]. Moreover, the commonly used integrative analysis approach for predicting miRNAs gene and protein targets and networks, known as the systems biology approach, is continuously being updated and developed to accommodate for better prediction of efficacy and activity of candidate miRNAs on a universal scale [89]. Improving the already available breast cancer miRNAs databases to elucidate details on sample sources, miRNAs expression profiles, extraction protocols, their diagnostic, prognostic, therapy predictive, therapeutic and metastatic potential, would lay grounds for better, more reproducible and more tumor-specific miRNAs studies [12]. This, of course, calls for a more integrative understanding of the miRNA–gene and miRNA-protein interaction networks through the development of multi-disciplinary systems biology approaches assimilating genomics, genetics, proteomics and bioinformatics, to better understand and combat cancer initiation, development, progression and recurrence.

Acknowledgments The authors would like to acknowledge Prof. Mounir AbouHaidar, Professor of Virology at the University of Toronto Dept. Cell & Systems Biology, for his critical reading of the manuscript and Ms. Nancy Nasr Al Deen for illustrating Fig. 18.1. The authors would also like to acknowledge the support of the Lebanese National Council for Scientific Research (CNRS-L), the University Research Board (URB-AUB) and the International Breast Cancer and Nutrition (IBCN) project. Dr. Rabih Talhouk and Dr. Rihab Nasr are both members of IBCN. Ms. Nataly Naser Al Deen is the recipient of the AUB-CNRS-L scholarship.

Conflict of Interest The authors declare no conflict of interest.

References

1. Siegel RL, Miller KD, Jemal A (2016) Cancer statistics, 2016. CA Cancer J Clin 66(1):7–30
2. Sørlie T, Perou CM, Tibshirani R, Aas T, Geisler S, Johnsen H et al (2001) Gene expression patterns of breast carcinomas distinguish tumor subclasses with clinical implications. Proc Natl Acad Sci 98(19):10869–10874
3. Liu Z, Zhang X-S, Zhang S (2014) Breast tumor subgroups reveal diverse clinical prognostic power. Sci Rep 4:4002
4. Prat A, Pineda E, Adamo B, Galván P, Fernández A, Gaba L et al (2015) Clinical implications of the intrinsic molecular subtypes of breast cancer. Breast 24:S26–S35
5. Spitale A, Mazzola P, Soldini D, Mazzucchelli L, Bordoni A (2008) Breast cancer classification according to immunohistochemical markers: clinicopathologic features and short-term survival analysis in a population-based study from the South of Switzerland. Ann Oncol 20(4):628–635
6. Bartel DP (2004) MicroRNAs: genomics, biogenesis, mechanism, and function. Cell 116(2):281–297

7. Bhattacharyya M, Nath J, Bandyopadhyay S (2015) MicroRNA signatures highlight new breast cancer subtypes. Gene 556(2):192–198
8. Adams BD, Wali VB, Cheng CJ, Inukai S, Booth CJ, Agarwal S et al (2016) miR-34a silences c-SRC to attenuate tumor growth in triple-negative breast cancer. Cancer Res 76(4):927–939
9. Fidler IJ (2003) The pathogenesis of cancer metastasis: the seed and soil hypothesis revisited. Nat Rev Cancer 3(6):453–458
10. Polyak K, Weinberg RA (2009) Transitions between epithelial and mesenchymal states: acquisition of malignant and stem cell traits. Nat Rev Cancer 9(4):265–273
11. McGuire A, Brown JA, Kerin MJ (2015) Metastatic breast cancer: the potential of miRNA for diagnosis and treatment monitoring. Cancer Metastasis Rev 34(1):145–155
12. Nassar FJ, Nasr R, Talhouk R (2017) MicroRNAs as biomarkers for early breast cancer diagnosis, prognosis and therapy prediction. Pharmacol Ther 172:34–49
13. Shao Y, Sun X, He Y, Liu C, Liu H (2015) Elevated levels of serum tumor markers CEA and CA15-3 are prognostic parameters for different molecular subtypes of breast cancer. PLoS One 10(7):e0133830
14. Dobbe E, Gurney K, Kiekow S, Lafferty JS, Kolesar JM (2008) Gene-expression assays: new tools to individualize treatment of early-stage breast cancer. Am J Health-Syst Pharm 65(1):23–28
15. Dai X, Li T, Bai Z, Yang Y, Liu X, Zhan J et al (2015) Breast cancer intrinsic subtype classification, clinical use and future trends. Am J Cancer Res 5(10):2929
16. BoydNF G (2007) Mammographic density and the risk and detection of breast cancer. N Engl J Med 356:227–236
17. Checka CM, Chun JE, Schnabel FR, Lee J, Toth H (2012) The relationship of mammographic density and age: implications for breast cancer screening. Am J Roentgenol 198(3):W292–W2W5
18. Singh SK, Pal Bhadra M, Girschick HJ, Bhadra U (2008) MicroRNAs–micro in size but macro in function. FEBS J 275(20):4929–4944
19. Winter J, Jung S, Keller S, Gregory RI, Diederichs S (2009) Many roads to maturity: microRNA biogenesis pathways and their regulation. Nat Cell Biol 11(3):228–234
20. Kutanzi KR, Yurchenko OV, Beland FA, Vasyl' FC, Pogribny IP (2011) MicroRNA-mediated drug resistance in breast cancer. Clin Epigenetics 2(2):171
21. Pink RC, Samuel P, Massa D, Caley DP, Brooks SA, Carter DRF (2015) The passenger strand, miR-21-3p, plays a role in mediating cisplatin resistance in ovarian cancer cells. Gynecol Oncol 137(1):143–151
22. He L, Hannon GJ (2004) MicroRNAs: small RNAs with a big role in gene regulation. Nat Rev Genet 5(7):522–531
23. Eulalio A, Huntzinger E, Nishihara T, Rehwinkel J, Fauser M, Izaurralde E (2009) Deadenylation is a widespread effect of miRNA regulation. RNA 15(1):21–32
24. Vasudevan S, Tong Y, Steitz JA (2007) Switching from repression to activation: microRNAs can up-regulate translation. Science 318(5858):1931–1934
25. Li M, Li J, Ding X, He M, Cheng S-Y (2010) microRNA and cancer. AAPS J 12(3):309–317
26. Raza U, Saatci Ö, Uhlmann S, Ansari SA, Eyüpoğlu E, Yurdusev E et al (2016) The miR-644a/CTBP1/p53 axis suppresses drug resistance by simultaneous inhibition of cell survival and epithelial-mesenchymal transition in breast cancer. Oncotarget 7(31):49859
27. Chim SS, Shing TK, Hung EC, Leung T-Y, Lau T-K, Chiu RW et al (2008) Detection and characterization of placental microRNAs in maternal plasma. Clin Chem 54(3):482–490
28. Lawrie CH, Gal S, Dunlop HM, Pushkaran B, Liggins AP, Pulford K et al (2008) Detection of elevated levels of tumour-associated microRNAs in serum of patients with diffuse large B-cell lymphoma. Br J Haematol 141(5):672–675
29. Weber JA, Baxter DH, Zhang S, Huang DY, Huang KH, Lee MJ et al (2010) The microRNA spectrum in 12 body fluids. Clin Chem 56(11):1733–1741
30. Lima LG, Chammas R, Monteiro RQ, Moreira MEC, Barcinski MA (2009) Tumor-derived microvesicles modulate the establishment of metastatic melanoma in a phosphatidylserine-dependent manner. Cancer Lett 283(2):168–175

31. Turchinovich A, Weiz L, Langheinz A, Burwinkel B (2011) Characterization of extracellular circulating microRNA. Nucleic Acids Res 39(16):7223–7233
32. Merkerova M, Vasikova A, Belickova M, Bruchova H (2010) MicroRNA expression profiles in umbilical cord blood cell lineages. Stem Cells Dev 19(1):17–26
33. Wu K, Feng J, Xing F, Liu Y, Sharma S, Watabe K (2017) Exosomal miR-19a: a novel communicator between cancer cell and osteoclast in osteolytic bone metastasis of breast cancer. AACR 77:4940–4940
34. Zhong S, Chen X, Wang D, Zhang X, Shen H, Yang S et al (2016) MicroRNA expression profiles of drug-resistance breast cancer cells and their exosomes. Oncotarget 7(15):19601–19609
35. Le MT, Hamar P, Guo C, Basar E, Perdigão-Henriques R, Balaj L et al (2014) miR-200–containing extracellular vesicles promote breast cancer cell metastasis. J Clin Invest 124(12):5109
36. Ma R, Jiang T, Kang X (2012) Circulating microRNAs in cancer: origin, function and application. J Exp Clin Cancer Res 31(1):38
37. Li Z, Peng Z, Gu S, Zheng J, Feng D, Qin Q et al (2017) Global analysis of miRNA–mRNA interaction network in breast cancer with brain metastasis. Anticancer Res 37(8):4455–4468
38. Mohammadi-Yeganeh S, Paryan M, Arefian E, Vasei M, Ghanbarian H, Mahdian R et al (2016) MicroRNA-340 inhibits the migration, invasion, and metastasis of breast cancer cells by targeting Wnt pathway. Tumor Biol 37(7):8993–9000
39. Madhavan D, Peng C, Wallwiener M, Zucknick M, Nees J, Schott S et al (2016) Circulating miRNAs with prognostic value in metastatic breast cancer and for early detection of metastasis. Carcinogenesis 37(5):461–470
40. Markou A, Zavridou M, Sourvinou I, Yousef G, Kounelis S, Malamos N et al (2016) Direct comparison of metastasis-related miRNAs expression levels in circulating tumor cells, corresponding plasma, and primary tumors of breast cancer patients. Clin Chem 62(7):1002–1011
41. Peng F, Tang H, Liu P, Shen J, Guan X, Xie X et al (2017) Isoliquiritigenin modulates miR-374a/PTEN/Akt axis to suppress breast cancer tumorigenesis and metastasis. Sci Rep 7:9022
42. Teoh S, Das S (2017) The role of MicroRNAs in diagnosis, prognosis, metastasis and resistant cases in breast cancer. Curr Pharm Des 23(12):1845
43. Miao Y, Zheng W, Li N, Su Z, Zhao L, Zhou H et al (2017) MicroRNA-130b targets PTEN to mediate drug resistance and proliferation of breast cancer cells via the PI3K/Akt signaling pathway. Sci Rep 7:41942
44. Cortez MA, Bueso-Ramos C, Ferdin J, Lopez-Berestein G, Sood AK, Calin GA (2011) MicroRNAs in body fluids—the mix of hormones and biomarkers. Nat Rev Clin Oncol 8(8):467–477
45. Roth C, Rack B, Müller V, Janni W, Pantel K, Schwarzenbach H (2010) Circulating microRNAs as blood-based markers for patients with primary and metastatic breast cancer. Breast Cancer Res 12(6):R90
46. Chen W, Cai F, Zhang B, Barekati Z, Zhong XY (2013) The level of circulating miRNA-10b and miRNA-373 in detecting lymph node metastasis of breast cancer: potential biomarkers. Tumor Biol 34(1):455–462
47. Schwarzenbach H, Milde-Langosch K, Steinbach B, Müller V, Pantel K (2012) Diagnostic potential of PTEN-targeting miR-214 in the blood of breast cancer patients. Breast Cancer Res Treat 134(3):933–941
48. Ahmad A, Sethi S, Chen W, Ali-Fehmi R, Mittal S, Sarkar FH (2014) Up-regulation of microRNA-10b is associated with the development of breast cancer brain metastasis. Am J Transl Res 6(4):384
49. Zhao F, Hu G, Wang X, Zhang X, Zhang Y, Yu Z (2012) Serum overexpression of microRNA-10b in patients with bone metastatic primary breast cancer. J Int Med Res 40(3):859–866
50. Madhavan D, Zucknick M, Wallwiener M, Cuk K, Modugno C, Scharpff M et al (2012) Circulating miRNAs as surrogate markers for circulating tumor cells and prognostic markers in metastatic breast cancer. Clin Cancer Res 18(21):5972–5982
51. Zhou W, Fong MY, Min Y, Somlo G, Liu L, Palomares MR et al (2014) Cancer-secreted miR-105 destroys vascular endothelial barriers to promote metastasis. Cancer Cell 25(4):501–515

52. Eichelser C, Flesch-Janys D, Chang-Claude J, Pantel K, Schwarzenbach H (2013) Deregulated serum concentrations of circulating cell–free microRNAs miR-17, miR-34a, miR-155, and miR-373 in human breast cancer development and progression. Clin Chem 59(10):1489–1496

53. Gasparri ML, Casorelli A, Bardhi E, Besharat AR, Savone D, Ruscito I et al (2017) Beyond circulating microRNA biomarkers: urinary microRNAs in ovarian and breast cancer. Tumor Biol 39(5):1010428317695525

54. Zheng R, Pan L, Gao J, Ye X, Chen L, Zhang X et al (2015) Prognostic value of miR-106b expression in breast cancer patients. J Surg Res 195(1):158–165

55. Sahlberg KK, Bottai G, Naume B, Burwinkel B, Calin GA, Borresen-Dale A-L et al (2015) A serum microRNA signature predicts tumor relapse and survival in triple negative breast cancer patients. Clin Cancer Res 21:1207–1214

56. Halvorsen AR, Helland Å, Gromov P, Wielenga VT, Talman MLM, Brunner N et al (2017) Profiling of microRNAs in tumor interstitial fluid of breast tumors–a novel resource to identify biomarkers for prognostic classification and detection of cancer. Mol Oncol 11(2):220–234

57. Lánczky A, Nagy Á, Bottai G, Munkácsy G, Szabó A, Santarpia L et al (2016) miRpower: a web-tool to validate survival-associated miRNAs utilizing expression data from 2178 breast cancer patients. Breast Cancer Res Treat 160(3):439–446

58. Guestini F, McNamara KM, Ishida T, Sasano H (2016) Triple negative breast cancer chemo-sensitivity and chemoresistance: current advances in biomarkers indentification. Expert Opin Ther Targets 20(6):705–720

59. Chen X, Lu P, Wang D-D, Yang S-J, Wu Y, Shen H-Y et al (2016) The role of miRNAs in drug resistance and prognosis of breast cancer formalin-fixed paraffin-embedded tissues. Gene 595(2):221–226

60. Erbes T, Hirschfeld M, Rücker G, Jaeger M, Boas J, Iborra S et al (2015) Feasibility of urinary microRNA detection in breast cancer patients and its potential as an innovative non-invasive biomarker. BMC Cancer 15:193

61. Pecot CV, Rupaimoole R, Yang D, Akbani R, Ivan C, Lu C et al (2013) Tumour angiogenesis regulation by the miR-200 family. Nat Commun 4:2427

62. Sarkar FH, Li Y, Wang Z, Kong D, Ali S (2010) Implication of microRNAs in drug resistance for designing novel cancer therapy. Drug Resist Updat 13(3):57–66

63. Ellis LM, Hicklin DJ (2009) Resistance to targeted therapies: refining anticancer therapy in the era of molecular oncology. Clin Cancer Res 15(24):7471–7478

64. Sorrentino A, Liu C-G, Addario A, Peschle C, Scambia G, Ferlini C (2008) Role of microR-NAs in drug-resistant ovarian cancer cells. Gynecol Oncol 111(3):478–486

65. Allen KE, Weiss GJ (2010) Resistance may not be futile: microRNA biomarkers for chemo-resistance and potential therapeutics. Mol Cancer Ther 9:3126–3136

66. Liang Z, Wu H, Xia J, Li Y, Zhang Y, Huang K et al (2010) Involvement of miR-326 in chemotherapy resistance of breast cancer through modulating expression of multidrug resistance-associated protein 1. Biochem Pharmacol 79(6):817–824

67. Kovalchuk O, Filkowski J, Meservy J, Ilnytskyy Y, Tryndyak VP, Vasyl' FC et al (2008) Involvement of microRNA-451 in resistance of the MCF-7 breast cancer cells to chemothera-peutic drug doxorubicin. Mol Cancer Ther 7(7):2152–2159

68. Yang S-J, Wang D-D, Li J, Xu H-Z, Shen H-Y, Chen X et al (2017) Predictive role of GSTP1-containing exosomes in chemotherapy-resistant breast cancer. Gene 623:5–14

69. Wu Q, Yang Z, Nie Y, Shi Y, Fan D (2014) Multi-drug resistance in cancer chemotherapeu-tics: mechanisms and lab approaches. Cancer Lett 347(2):159–166

70. Zhao J-J, Lin J, Yang H, Kong W, He L, Ma X et al (2008) MicroRNA-221/222 negatively regulates estrogen receptorα and is associated with tamoxifen resistance in breast cancer. J Biol Chem 283(45):31079–31086

71. Lau L-Y, 劉麗儀 (2011) Identification of microRNAs associated with tamoxifen resistance in breast cancer. HKU Theses Online (HKUTO)

72. Hong L, Han Y, Zhang Y, Zhang H, Zhao Q, Wu K et al (2013) MicroRNA-21: a therapeutic target for reversing drug resistance in cancer. Expert Opin Ther Targets 17(9):1073–1080

73. Wang Z-X, Lu B-B, Wang H, Cheng Z-X, Yin Y-M (2011) MicroRNA-21 modulates che-mosensitivity of breast cancer cells to doxorubicin by targeting PTEN. Arch Med Res 42(4):281–290

74. Bourguignon LY, Earle C, Wong G, Spevak CC, Krueger K (2012) Stem cell marker (Nanog) and Stat-3 signaling promote MicroRNA-21 expression and chemoresistance in hyaluronan/CD44-activated head and neck squamous cell carcinoma cells. Oncogene 31(2):149–160

75. Mei M, Ren Y, Zhou X, Yuan X-B, Han L, Wang G-X et al (2010) Downregulation of miR-21 enhances chemotherapeutic effect of taxol in breast carcinoma cells. Technol Cancer Res Treat 9(1):77–86

76. Zhou M, Zhao Y, Ding Y, Liu H, Liu Z, Xi Y et al (2010) Mir-125b confers the resistance of cancer cells to Taxol through suppression of Bak1. AACR 70, abstract 2109

77. Luqmani YA, Alam-Eldin N (2016) Overcoming resistance to endocrine therapy in breast cancer: new approaches to a nagging problem. Med Princ Pract 25(Suppl. 2):28–40

78. Joshi T, Elias D, Stenvang J, Alves CL, Teng F, Lyng MB et al (2016) Integrative analysis of miRNA and gene expression reveals regulatory networks in tamoxifen-resistant breast cancer. Oncotarget 7(35):57239–57253

79. Sachdeva M, Mo Y-Y (2010) miR-145-mediated suppression of cell growth, invasion and metastasis. Am J Transl Res 2(2):170

80. Rehman SK, Huang W-C, Yu D (2010) MiR-21 upregulation in breast cancer cells leads to PTEN loss and Herceptin resistance. AACR 70, abstract 4033

81. Gong C, Yao Y, Wang Y, Liu B, Wu W, Chen J et al (2011) Up-regulation of miR-21 mediates resistance to trastuzumab therapy for breast cancer. J Biol Chem 286(21):19127–19137

82. Scott GK, Goga A, Bhaumik D, Berger CE, Sullivan CS, Benz CC (2007) Coordinate sup-pression of ERBB2 and ERBB3 by enforced expression of micro-RNA miR-125a or miR-125b. J Biol Chem 282(2):1479–1486

83. del Pilar Camacho-Leal M, Sciortino M, Cabodi S (2017) ErbB2 receptor in breast cancer: implications in cancer cell migration, invasion and resistance to targeted therapy. In: Breast cancer-from biology to medicine. InTech

84. Lowery AJ, Miller N, Devaney A, McNeill RE, Davoren PA, Lemetre C et al (2009) MicroRNA signatures predict oestrogen receptor, progesterone receptor and HER2/neure-ceptor status in breast cancer. Breast Cancer Res 11(3):R27

85. Mattie MD, Benz CC, Bowers J, Sensinger K, Wong L, Scott GK et al (2006) Optimized high-throughput microRNA expression profiling provides novel biomarker assessment of clinical prostate and breast cancer biopsies. Mol Cancer 5(1):1–14

86. Breunig C, Pahl J, Küblbeck M, Miller M, Antonelli D, Erdem N et al (2017) MicroRNA-519a-3p mediates apoptosis resistance in breast cancer cells and their escape from recogni-tion by natural killer cells. Cell Death Dis 8(8):e2973

87. Anastasov N, Höfig I, Vasconcellos IG, Rappl K, Braselmann H, Ludyga N et al (2012) Radiation resistance due to high expression of miR-21 and G2/M checkpoint arrest in breast cancer cells. Radiat Oncol 7(1):206

88. Liang Z, Ahn J, Guo D, Votaw JR, Shim H (2013) MicroRNA-302 replacement therapy sen-sitizes breast cancer cells to ionizing radiation. Pharm Res 30(4):1008–1016

89. Raza U, Zhang JD, Şahin Ö (2014) MicroRNAs: master regulators of drug resistance, stem-ness, and metastasis. J Mol Med 92(4):321–336

90. Gupta GP, Massagué J (2006) Cancer metastasis: building a framework. Cell 127(4):679–695

91. Ma L, Teruya-Feldstein J, Weinberg RA (2008) Tumour invasion and metastasis initiated by microRNA-10b in breast cancer. Nature 455(7210):256

92. Luqmani YA, Khajah MA (2015) MicroRNA in breast cancer—gene regulators and targets for novel therapies. In: A concise review of molecular pathology of breast cancer. InTech

93. Ma L, Young J, Prabhala H, Pan E, Mestdagh P, Muth D et al (2010) miR-9, a MYC/MYCN-activated microRNA, regulates E-cadherin and cancer metastasis. Nat Cell Biol 12(3):247–256

94. Korpal M, Ell BJ, Buffa FM, Ibrahim T, Blanco MA, Celià-Terrassa T et al (2011) Direct targeting of Sec23a by miR-200s influences cancer cell secretome and promotes metastatic colonization. Nat Med 17(9):1101–1108
95. Orso F, Quirico L, Virga F, Penna E, Dettori D, Cimino D et al (2016) miR-214 and miR-148b targeting inhibits dissemination of melanoma and breast cancer. Cancer Res 76(17):5151–5162
96. Zou Q, Tang Q, Pan Y, Wang X, Dong X, Liang Z et al (2017) MicroRNA-22 inhibits cell growth and metastasis in breast cancer via targeting of SIRT1. Exp Ther Med 14:1009–1016
97. Li W, Li G, Fan Z, Liu T (2017) Tumor-suppressive microRNA-452 inhibits migration and invasion of breast cancer cells by directly targeting RAB11A. Oncol Lett 14(2):2559–2565
98. Kong W, Yang H, He L, Zhao J-J, Coppola D, Dalton WS et al (2008) MicroRNA-155 is regulated by the transforming growth factor β/Smad pathway and contributes to epithelial cell plasticity by targeting RhoA. Mol Cell Biol 28(22):6773–6784
99. Valastyan S, Reinhardt F, Benaich N, Calogrias D, Szász AM, Wang ZC et al (2009) RETRACTED: a pleiotropically acting MicroRNA, miR-31, inhibits breast cancer metastasis. Cell 137(6):1032–1046
100. Valastyan S, Chang A, Benaich N, Reinhardt F, Weinberg RA (2010) Concurrent suppression of integrin α5, radixin, and RhoA phenocopies the effects of miR-31 on metastasis. Cancer Res 70(12):5147–5154
101. Valastyan S, Weinberg RA (2010) miR-31: a crucial overseer of tumor metastasis and other emerging roles. Cell Cycle 9(11):2124–2129
102. Körner C, Keklikoglou I, Bender C, Wörner A, Münstermann E, Wiemann S (2013) MicroRNA-31 sensitizes human breast cells to apoptosis by direct targeting of protein kinase C ε (PKCε). J Biol Chem 288(12):8750–8761
103. Li H, Bian C, Liao L, Li J, Zhao RC (2011) miR-17-5p promotes human breast cancer cell migration and invasion through suppression of HBP1. Breast Cancer Res Treat 126(3):565–575
104. Lu Y, Qin T, Li J, Wang L, Zhang Q, Jiang Z et al (2017) MicroRNA-140-5p inhibits invasion and angiogenesis through targeting VEGF-A in breast cancer. Cancer Gene Ther 24:386–392
105. Mertens-Talcott SU, Chintharlapalli S, Li X, Safe S (2007) The oncogenic microRNA-27a targets genes that regulate specificity protein transcription factors and the G2-M checkpoint in MDA-MB-231 breast cancer cells. Cancer Res 67(22):11001–11011
106. Lee DY, Deng Z, Wang C-H, Yang BB (2007) MicroRNA-378 promotes cell survival, tumor growth, and angiogenesis by targeting SuFu and Fus-1 expression. Proc Natl Acad Sci 104(51):20350–20355
107. Soria-Valles C, Gutiérrez-Fernández A, Guiu M, Mari B, Fueyo A, Gomis R et al (2014) The anti-metastatic activity of collagenase-2 in breast cancer cells is mediated by a signaling pathway involving decorin and miR-21. Oncogene 33(23):3054–3063
108. Croset M, Goehrig D, Frackowiak A, Bonnelye E, Ansieau S, Puisieux A et al (2014) TWIST1 expression in breast cancer cells facilitates bone metastasis formation. J Bone Miner Res 29(8):1886–1899
109. Bishopric N, Speransky S, Kajan D, Laderian B, Iorns E, Clarke J et al. (2017) Abstract P4-07-03: dynamic regulation of a microRNA-mRNA network during breast cancer metastasis reveals an essential tumor-promoting role for miR-203. AACR 77, abstract P4-07-03
110. Blevins MA, Kouznetsova J, Krueger AB, King R, Griner LM, Hu X et al (2015) Small molecule, NSC95397, inhibits the CtBP1-protein partner interaction and CtBP1-mediated transcriptional repression. J Biomol Screen 20(5):663–672
111. Okuda H, Xing F, Pandey PR, Sharma S, Watabe M, Pai SK et al (2013) miR-7 suppresses brain metastasis of breast cancer stem-like cells by modulating KLF4. Cancer Res 73(4): 1434–1444
112. Zare M, Bastami M, Solali S, Alivand M (2017) Aberrantly miRNA promoter methylation and EMT-involving miRNAs in breast cancer metastasis: diagnosis and therapeutic implications. J Cell Physiol 233:3729–3744

113. Sasheva P, Grossniklaus U (2017) Differentially methylated region-representational difference analysis (DMR-RDA): a powerful method to identify DMRs in uncharacterized genomes. Plant Epigenetics: Methods Protocol 1456:113–125

114. Gacem RB, Abdelkrim OB, Ziadi S, Dhiab MB, Trimeche M (2014) Methylation of miR-124a-1, miR-124a-2, and miR-124a-3 genes correlates with aggressive and advanced breast cancer disease. Tumor Biol 35(5):4047–4056

115. Niu J, Xue A, Chi Y, Xue J, Wang W, Zhao Z et al (2016) Induction of miRNA-181a by genotoxic treatments promotes chemotherapeutic resistance and metastasis in breast cancer. Oncogene 35(10):1302–1313

116. Bai WD, Ye XM, Zhang MY, Zhu HY, Xi WJ, Huang X et al (2014) MiR-200c suppresses TGF-β signaling and counteracts trastuzumab resistance and metastasis by targeting ZNF217 and ZEB1 in breast cancer. Int J Cancer 135(6):1356–1368

117. Schwarzenbach H (2017) Clinical relevance of circulating, cell-free and exosomal microRNAs in plasma and serum of breast cancer patients. Oncol Res Treat 40(7–8):423–429

118. Pichler M, Calin G (2015) MicroRNAs in cancer: from developmental genes in worms to their clinical application in patients. Br J Cancer 113(4):569–573

119. Ohno S-i, Takanashi M, Sudo K, Ueda S, Ishikawa A, Matsuyama N et al (2013) Systemically injected exosomes targeted to EGFR deliver antitumor microRNA to breast cancer cells. Mol Ther 21(1):185–191

120. Huang G, Li S, Yang N, Zou Y, Zheng D, Xiao T (2017) Recent progress in circular RNAs in human cancers. Cancer Lett 404:8–18

Chapter 19
NEDD4 Family of E3 Ubiquitin Ligases in Breast Cancer: Spotlight on SMURFs, WWPs and NEDD4

Ghazala Butt, Ilhan Yaylim, Rukset Attar, Aliye Aras, Mirna Azalea Romero, Muhammad Zahid Qureshi, Jelena Purenovic, and Ammad Ahmad Farooqi

Abstract Massively parallel sequencing, genomic and proteomic technologies have provided near complete resolution of signaling landscape of breast cancer (BCa). NEDD4 family of E3-ubiquitin ligases comprises a large family of proteins particularly, SMURFs (SMURF1, SMURF2), WWPs and NEDD4 which are ideal candidates for targeted therapy. However, it is becoming progressively more understandable that SMURFs and NEDD4 have "split-personalities". These molecules behave dualistically in breast cancer and future studies must converge on detailed identification of context specific role of these proteins in BCa. Finally, we provide scattered clues of regulation of SMURF2 by oncogenic miRNAs, specifically

G. Butt
Department of Botany, GCU, Lahore, Pakistan

I. Yaylim (✉)
Department of Molecular Medicine, Aziz Sancar Institute of Experimental Medicine, Istanbul University, Istanbul, Turkey

R. Attar
Department of Obstetrics and Gynecology, Yeditepe University Hospital Istanbul, Istanbul, Turkey

A. Aras
Department of Botany, Faculty of Science, Istanbul University, Istanbul, Turkey

M. A. Romero
Facultad de Medicina, Laboratorio de Investigación Clínica, Universidad Autónoma de Guerrero, Acapulco, Guerrero México, Mexico

M. Z. Qureshi
Department of Chemistry, GCU, Lahore, Pakistan

J. Purenovic
Faculty of Technical Sciences, Cacak University of Kragujevac, Cacak, Serbia

A. A. Farooqi (✉)
Institute of Biomedical and Genetic Engineering (IBGE), Islamabad, Pakistan
e-mail: ammadfarooqi@rlmclahore.com

© Springer Nature Switzerland AG 2019
A. Ahmad (ed.), *Breast Cancer Metastasis and Drug Resistance*,
Advances in Experimental Medicine and Biology 1152,
https://doi.org/10.1007/978-3-030-20301-6_19

considering longstanding questions related to regulation of SMURF1 and WWPs by miRNAs in BCa. SMURFS, WWPs and NEDD4 are versatile regulators and represent a fast-growing field in cancer research and better understanding of the underlying mechanisms will be helpful in transition of our knowledge from a segmented view to a more conceptual continuum.

Keywords SMURF1 · NEDD4 · Cancer · Apoptosis · Signaling

19.1   Introduction

It was in early 1990s, when scientists made a landmark discovery and identified NEDD4 to be developmentally downregulated in central nervous system (CNS) of embryonic mouse [1]. Contemporary studies helped in the identification of additional proteins which resembled structurally with NEDD4 and contained different modular domains (reviewed by Rotin and Kumar [2]; Yang and Kumar [3]). Proteins of this family contained a catalytically active HECT domain at the C-terminus, and an N-terminal region involved in recognition of substrates. HECT ligases have characteristically unique features. Presence of a conserved Cys residue played central role in formation of an intermediate thio-ester bond with ubiquitin C terminus before catalyzing ubiquitylation of substrates. Intra-molecular association between the C2 domain of SMURF2 and a region present in proximity of the catalytic Cys of HECT inhibited activity of SMURF2 and mechanistically similar strategy had been proposed for the modulation of WWP2 and NEDD4. In this chapter we have comprehensively summarized most current knowledge related to role of SMURF1 and SMURF2 in BCa. It is relevant to mention that SMUF1 and SMURF2 context dependently behave either as a tumor suppressor or oncogenic protein in breast cancer. We also emphasized on role of WWPs in breast cancer. Our last segment of discussion will be devoted to NEDD4 role in breast cancer.

19.2   SMURF1: Is It a Double Edged Sword?

SMURF1 has been shown to play a dualistic role in BCa development and progression. In this section, we will strictly focus on role of SMURF1 both as an oncogenic protein and tumor suppressor.

19.3   Oncogenic Role

SMURF1 has attracted substantial attention because of its ability to post-translationally modify myriad of proteins in breast cancer. Staphylococcal nuclease domain-containing 1 (SND1) protein was reported to be frequently overexpressed in BCa [4]. SND1 was a positive regulator of SMURF1. Migratory potential of SND1-overexpressing MCF-7 and MDA-MB-231 BC cells was noted to be significantly enhanced. Promoter region of SND1 contained various SMAD-specific recognition elements which were recognized and used by the SMAD complex for transcriptional upregulation of SND1 [4]. Rho GTPases pleiotropically modulated cytoskeletal and cell adhesion dynamics and orchestrated wide ranging cellular processes, including cell migration [5]. Most Rho GTPases pendulously swing between an active state (GTP-bound) and an inactive state (GDP-bound) [5]. Rho GTPases are post-translationally modified by SMURF1 [4]. Ectopically overexpressed SND1 enhanced SMURF1 but simultaneously reduced RhoA whereas knockdown of SND1 decreased the SMURF1 protein level but induced an increase in RhoA in BCa cells. RhoA levels were reduced in SND1 overexpressing BCa cells but found to be increased with SMURF1 knockdown BCa cells [4].

Tropomyosins are actin-binding proteins reportedly involved in regulation of actin dynamics, cellular migration and tumor suppression [6]. Tropomyosin-2, an isoform encoded by the TPMα, blocked SMURF1-induced RhoA ubiquitination. RhoA ubiquitination was remarkably repressed in the cells which expressed Tm2 but not in the cells which expressed Tm1 or α-actinin-4 [6]. Synaptopodin also effectively sequestered SMURF1 away from GDP-bound RhoA and prevented its degradation [6].

Ubiquitin-specific peptidase 9, X-linked (USP9X/FAM) was found to be a unique interacting partner of SMURF1 [7]. Deletions of the two functionally important WW domains of SMURF1 (ΔWW) severely abrogated USP9X interactions. More importantly, deletion of the second (ΔWW2) WW domain considerably abrogated USP9X association. Carboxyl terminus of USP9X (C-2 domain) had a stronger ability to structurally associate with SMURF1 but C-1 domain which harbored deubiquitinating activity had weaker interactions with SMURF1. USP9X deubiquitinated SMURF1 and protected it from degradation [7]. There was a rapid degradation of SMURF1 in USP9X-depleted BCa cells. Migratory capacity of USP9X or SMURF1 silenced MDA-MB-231 BCa cells was observed to be remarkably reduced [7].

19.4   Tumor Suppressor

Type Iγ phosphatidylinositol phosphate kinase (PIPKIγ) was found to be frequently overexpressed in BCa tissues [8, 9]. SMURF1 structurally interacted with PIPKIγ in MDA-231 BCa cells. Functionally inactive SMURF1 catalytic mutant completely failed to degrade PIPKIγ which clearly suggested that SMURF1-driven degradation of PIPKIγ was dependent on its E3 ubiquitin ligase activity. Phosphorylation of SMURF1 at 306th threonine by Protein kinase-A (PKA) prevented SMURF1-induced ubiquitination and degradation of PIPKIγ [8, 9]. Data clearly suggested that targeted inhibition of PKA will be helpful in maximizing SMURF1 mediated control of oncogenic proteins.

19.5   Role of SMURF2 as a Tumor Suppressor

SMURF2 knockdown induced budding, outward growths and branching of breast cancer cell-derived organoids [10]. Protein inhibitor of activated STAT-3 (PIAS3), a SUMO E3-ligase triggered SMURF2 sumoylation at 26th and 369th lysine residues. Sumoylated-SMURF2 suppressed invasiveness of three-dimensional breast cell-derived multi-cellular architectures [10].

Ovatodiolide, a macrocyclic diterpenoid obtained from Anisomeles indica (L.) Kuntze was found to be effective against breast cancer cells [11]. There was a dose-dependent downregulation of stemness-related genes particularly, Nanog, octamer-binding transcription factor 4 (OCT4) and heat shock protein-27 (HSP27) in ovatodiolide-treated BCa cells. However, Ovatodiolide stimulated the expression of SMURF2 in mammospheric cells derived from BT-474 or AS-B145 BCa cells. HSP27 overexpression or SMURF2 knockdown in AS-B145 BCa cells severely impaired ovatodiolide–mediated repressive effects on formation of mammospheres [11].

Fucose-containing fraction of Ling-Zhi (FFLZ) worked synergistically with trastuzumab against trastuzumab-resistant BCa cells [12]. FFLZ triggered SMURF2-induced TGFR ubiquitination, promoted "re-localization" of the TGFR to the caveolae and facilitated TGFR degradation [12].

19.6   Cancer Promoting Role of SMURF2

SMURF2 inhibition substantially inhibited anchorage-independent growth of BCa cells [13]. WW2 domain of SMURF2 structurally associated with 'SPPPPY' motif of CNSRK2 and stabilized it. CNKSR2 degradation was more pronounced in SMURF2 depleted BCa cells. Comparatively higher expression levels of CNKSR2 and SMURF2 were observed in ER^{low} and PR^{low} samples as compared to HER2^{high} samples [13].

19.7   Degradation of SMURF1 by SMURF2 in Breast Cancer: Tug of War Between Two Main Actors of Story-Tale

SMURF2 interacted with SMURF1 and induced its degradation in MDA-MB-231 BCa cells [14]. There had been considerable formation of bone metastasis in mice inoculated with SMURF2 silenced BCa cells into the left cardiac ventricle. Area of bone metastasis in the tibiae of mice inoculated with SMURF2 silenced BCa cells was larger as compared to the mice inoculated with SMURF1 BCa cells [14].

19.8 microRNA Regulation of SMURF2 in Breast Cancer: Predator Becomes the Prey of Micro-hunters

Discovery of microRNAs has revolutionized "Central Dogma of Molecular Biology" and overwhelmingly increasing high-quality research has helped us to understand that miRNAs quantitatively controlled expression of myriad of protein-coding genes. miRNAs are categorically characterized into tumor suppressor and oncogenic miRNAs.

SMURF2 was found to be significantly reduced in BT549, DU-4475, MDA-MB-468 and MDA-MB-436 BCa cells [15]. Mechanistically, SMURF2 was directly targeted by miRNA-15a, miRNA-15b, miRNA-16 and miRNA-128 in BCa cells. miRNA-15 and miRNA-16 are transcriptionally controlled by E2F-transcription factors (shown in Fig. 19.1). Triple negative BCa had inactivating mutations of the retinoblastoma (RB) gene which resulted in hyper-activation of E2F. Therefore E2F stimulated the expression of different miRNAs. SMURF2 was notably higher in RB-transfected BT549 BCa ells [15]. Astonishingly, miRNA-424-503 cluster was remarkably upregulated in metastatically competent BCa cells [16]. miRNA-424 and miRNA-503 concomitantly targeted SMAD7 and SMURF2 and facilitated TGF-β-driven intracellular pathway and enhanced metastasizing ability of BCa cells [16].

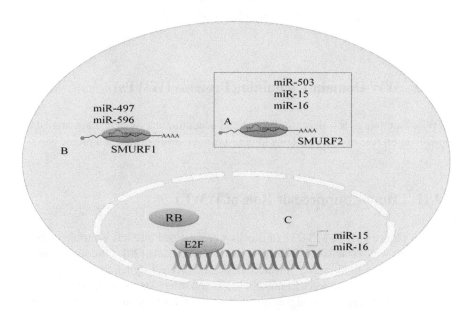

Fig. 19.1 shows regulation of SMURF1 and SMURF2 by miRNAs. (**a**) Oncogenic miRNAs regulate SMURF2. (**b**) Regulation of SMURF1 by tumor suppressor miRNAs. (**c**) E2F transcriptionally upregulated oncogenic miRNAs which directly targeted SMURF2

19.9   miRNA Regulation of SMURF1 in Breast Cancer: Missing Pieces of an Incomplete Jig-Saw Puzzle

There are no direct pieces of evidence related to miRNA regulation of SMURF1 in BCa. In this segment we have summarized certain clues which have been reported in ovarian and colorectal cancers.

Lower levels of miR-497 were found to be associated with tumor lymph node metastasis [17]. Silencing of SMURF1 markedly reduced migratory and invasive potential of SKOV-3 and OVCAR-3 cancer cells. Moreover, miR-497 was noted to directly target SMURF1 [17].

5-fluorouracil (5-FU) sensitivity was restored in SW480 cells reconstituted with miR-497 [18]. Moreover, miR-497 targeted SMURF1 in colorectal cancer cells and SMURF1 was significantly lower in treatment-sensitive patients as compared to neo-adjuvant therapy-resistant patients [18]. SMURF1 significantly extended Murine double minute-2 (MDM2) half-time and enhanced the MDM2 levels [19]. Thus, SMURF1 promoted degradation of p53. miR-596 overexpression attenuated SMURF1 to 26%. SMURF1 stabilized MDM2 and data clearly demonstrated that SMURF1 downregulation significantly lowered MDM2 levels [19].

It seems clear that SMURF1 regulation by miRNAs has not yet been convincingly explored in BCa. There is a need to identify different miRNAs which control SMURF1 levels in BCa. In the upcoming section we will discuss recent evidence related to WWP proteins and how they regulated different proteins in breast cancer.

19.10   WW Domain-Containing Proteins (WWPs)

WWPs function as E3-ubiquitin ligases and accumulating evidence has started to shed light on role of these proteins in breast cancer development and progression.

19.11   Tumor Suppressor Role of WWP1

WWP1-silenced MDA-MB-231 BCa cells were injected into left ventricle of nude mice using well-established BCa bone metastasis models [20]. Osteolytic lesions were noted to be significantly enhanced CXCL12/CXCR4 signaling axis had a central role in tumor metastases. Endothelial cells and osteoblasts within the bone marrow compartment produced higher quantities of CXCL12 which made bone an ideal site for tumor metastases. WWP1 silenced cells demonstrated higher rate of migration towards a CXCL12 gradient in a transwell assay [20].

First and third WW domains of WWP1 physically interacted with second PY motif of ERBB4 [21]. WWP1 knockdown markedly increased ERBB4 levels in

MCF7 and T47D BCa cells. HRG-mediated activation of ERBB4 induced upregulation of BRCA1 in MCF7 BCa cells. WWP1 overexpression decreased BRCA1 levels by ~30% in BCa cells. Findings clearly suggested that WWP1-triggered degradation of ERBB4 severely abrogated HRG-mediated upregulation of BRCA1 [21]. ERBB4-directed inhibitors have attracted attention [22] and WWP1 can be an ideal candidate as negative regulator of ERBB4.

19.12   Cancer Promoting Role of WWP1

Large Tumor Suppressor 1 (LATS1), a serine/threonine kinase was negatively regulated by WWP1 in BCa [23]. Overexpression of WWP1 dramatically increased cell proliferation in LATS1+ MCF10A mammary epithelial cells. Expectedly, only functionally active WWP1 rather than its ligase-dead or WW domain-lacking mutant degraded LATS1 in BCa cells [23].

Ataxin-3 like (ATXN3L) overexpression blocked WWP1-mediated degradation of KLF5 [24]. Whereas, ATXN3L knockdown reduced KLF5 levels both in SUM1315 and HCC1806 BCa cells. Furthermore, ATXN3L knockdown suppressed proliferation potential of BCa cells [24].

WWP 1 stabilized and protected ERBB2 and EGFR from degradation. WWP1 interacted with RING finger protein-11 (RNF11) and fueled proliferation and survival of BCa cells [25].

Apoptosis in WWP1-depleted cells was rescued by the overexpression of WWP1 (wild-type) but not by E3 ligase inactive WWP1-C890A mutant in MCF7 BCa cells [26]. WWP1 depletion and WWP1 (dominant negative) overexpression increased the TRAIL-driven apoptosis in BCa cells [26]. There is a need to deeply investigate different pro-apoptotic proteins degraded by WWP1 in BCa.

19.13   miRNA Regulation of WWP1 and WWP2 in Breast Cancer: More Questions Than Answers

It is astonishing to note that although regulation of WWP1 by miRNAs has been explored in different other cancers, however, we do not have a clear picture of miRNA regulation of WWP1 and WWP2 in BCa.

ΔNp63α is reportedly involved in interfering with trans-activities of p53 by formation of inhibitory heterogeneous complexes with p53 or competitively binding to promoters of its target genes [27]. DNA damage promoted degradation of ΔNp63α via WWP1 in MDA-MB-231 BCa cells. Knockdown of WWP1 abrogated ΔNp63α degradation and impaired apoptosis induced by DNA damage. miR-452 significantly reduced WWP1 and simultaneously upregulated ΔNp63α in miR-452-overexpressing MDA-MB-231 BCa cells [27].

MiR-584-5p directly interacted with a binding site present within 3′-UTR of WWP1 [8, 9]. MiR-584-5p effectively targeted WWP1, inhibited proliferation and induced apoptosis in gastric cancer cells. Tumor growth was drastically reduced in mice xenografted with miR-584-5p overexpressing SGC7901 cells. Immunohisto-chemically analyzed implanted tumors revealed remarkable downregulation of WWP1 in the miR-874-mimic-transfected group [8, 9].

In the upcoming section we will summarize significant role of NEDD4 in breast cancer.

19.14   NEDD4

Neural precursor cell-expressed developmentally downregulated gene-4 (NEDD4) an E3-ubiquitin protein ligase is reportedly involved in pleiotropic regulation of multiple proteins in different cancers. In this section we will emphasize on diametri-cally opposed roles of NEDD4 in BCa.

19.15   NEDD4 as a Tumor Suppressor

Protein kinase C-delta (PKCδ) inhibition resulted in higher contents of phosphorylated-ERK1/2 and lower expression of MKP3 (ERK1/2 phosphatase) [28]. MKP3 depletion led to higher levels of phosphorylated-ERK1/2 and conse-quent apoptotic death of BCa cells. Significantly higher levels of NEDD4 were noted in MKP3 silenced MDA-MB-231 BCa cells. Accordingly, MKP3 levels were found to be drastically enhanced in NEDD4 silenced MDA-MB-231 BCa cells [28].

Proline-rich tyrosine kinase-2 (PYK2) and FAK depletion severely impaired pro-liferation ability of basal-like TNBC cells [29]. PYK2 depletion enhanced degrada-tion of HER3 and concomitantly increased N-Myc Downstream-Regulated Gene-1 (NDRG1) levels. Increase in the quantity of NDRG1 also enhanced degradation of HER3. PYK2-knockdown increased NDRG1 and decreased HER3, whereas, NDRG1-knockdown increased HER3 in MDA-MB-468 BCa cells. Interestingly, stronger co-localizations were noted where HER3 co-existed with NEDD4-2 and also with NDRG1 in PYK2-depleted MDA-MB-468 BCa cells [29]. It was note-worthy that all HER3-positive structures co-stained with NEDD4-2 or NDRG1. However, astonishingly, NDRG1 depletion markedly inhibited co-localization of HER3–NEDD4-2, which clearly suggested that NDRG1 enhanced HER3–NEDD4-2 co-localization and their structural association. Mechanistically it was shown that PYK2-NDRG1-NEDD4 circuit played contributory role in degradation of receptor and development of resistance against various drugs [29]. Therefore targeting of PYK2/FAK may prove to be effective in overcoming the resistance against various drugs.

Estrogen ablation by letrozole and anastrozole dose-dependently decreased CX43 in both ER⁺ MCF7 and BT474 BCa cells [30]. 4-OH-tamoxifen and fulvestrant time-dependently enhanced phosphorylated levels of p38MAPK. Data clearly highlighted that ER inhibition by tamoxifen or fulvestrant significantly induced phosphorylation of p38 MAPK and simultaneously reduced CX43. Detailed mechanistic insights revealed that fulvestrant regulated reduction in CX43 was modulated by NEDD4 in BCa cells [30].

19.16   Tipping the Scales in the Favor of PI3K/AKT Pathway by NEDD4-1-Driven PTEN Degradation: Darker Side of NEDD4

It seems clear that there is a push and pull between PI3K/AKT pathway and PTEN. PI3K/AKT pathway fueled cancer cells whereas PTEN negatively regulated kinase-induced activation of oncogenic proteins. 34-KD protein encoded by the SEI-1 (p34SEI-1) was involved in repression of PTEN in BCa cells [31]. p34SEI-1 promoted NEDD4-1 E3 ligase-regulated degradation of PTEN. p34SEI-1 was observed to increase NEDD4-1 by increasing the level of nuclear factor kappa B (NF-κB). Expression levels of NEDD4-1 and p34SEI-1 were noticed to be low in normal breast tissues but strongly upregulated in BCa tissues [31].

Rak, a 54 kDa tyrosine kinase belonged to Src family of kinases and reportedly involved in protection of PTEN from NEDD4 [32]. Markedly enhanced association between endogenous PTEN and NEDD4-1 was noted in Rak knockdown MCF10A BCa cells. Moreover, polyubiquitination of PTEN was dramatically reduced in the absence of NEDD4-1. It was presumed that Rak mediated phosphorylation of PTEN at 336th tyrosine residue interfered with interaction of PTEN and NEDD4-1 [32].

19.17   Conclusion

It seems clear that we still insufficiently comprehend the context specific roles of SMURFs and NEDD4 in breast cancer. Detailed mechanistic studies are required to fully understand reasons for dualistic role of SMURFs and NEDD4. miRNA regulation of SMURF2 although has partially been explored but how SMURF1 is controlled by miRNAs in breast cancer needs in-depth research. Data obtained through functional studies, such as transgenic approaches and gene knockouts will be useful to develop a better understanding of the specificity of HECT E3 and network of proteins targeted by them for ubiquitylation. In accordance with this approach, systematically identified substrate/s and substrate specificity for E3 ligases using protein array and global proteomics approaches will be helpful. Our increasing knowledge related to deregulation of SMURFs WWPs and NEDD4 in BCa will undoubtedly inform the rational design of novel therapies.

References

1. Kumar S, Tomooka Y, Noda M (1992) Identification of a set of genes with developmentally down-regulated expression in the mouse brain. Biochem Biophys Res Commun 185(3):1155–1161
2. Rotin D, Kumar S (2009) Physiological functions of the HECT family of ubiquitin ligases. Nat Rev Mol Cell Biol 10(6):398–409. https://doi.org/10.1038/nrm2690
3. Yang B, Kumar S (2010) Nedd4 and Nedd4-2: closely related ubiquitin-protein ligases with distinct physiological functions. Cell Death Differ 17(1):68–77. https://doi.org/10.1038/cdd.2009.84
4. Yu L, Liu X, Cui K, Di Y, Xin L, Sun X, Zhang W, Yang X, Wei M, Yao Z, Yang J (2015) SND1 acts downstream of TGFβ1 and upstream of Smurf1 to promote breast cancer metastasis. Cancer Res 75(7):1275–1286. https://doi.org/10.1158/0008-5472.CAN-14-2387
5. Hodge RG, Ridley AJ (2016) Regulating Rho GTPases and their regulators. Nat Rev Mol Cell Biol 17(8):496–510. https://doi.org/10.1038/nrm.2016.67
6. Wong JS, Iorns E, Rheault MN, Ward TM, Rashmi P, Weber U, Lippman ME, Faul C, Mlodzik M, Mundel P (2012) Rescue of tropomyosin deficiency in Drosophila and human cancer cells by synaptopodin reveals a role of tropomyosin α in RhoA stabilization. EMBO J 31(4):1028–1040. https://doi.org/10.1038/emboj.2011.464
7. Xie Y, Avello M, Schirle M, McWhinnie E, Feng Y, Bric-Furlong E, Wilson C, Nathans R, Zhang J, Kirschner MW, Huang SM, Cong F (2013) Deubiquitinase FAM/USP9X interacts with the E3 ubiquitin ligase SMURF1 protein and protects it from ligase activity-dependent self-degradation. J Biol Chem 288(5):2976–2985. https://doi.org/10.1074/jbc.M112.430066
8. Li H, Xiao N, Wang Y, Wang R, Chen Y, Pan W, Liu D, Li S, Sun J, Zhang K, Sun Y, Ge X (2017) Smurf1 regulates lung cancer cell growth and migration through interaction with and ubiquitination of PIPKIγ. Oncogene 36(41):5668–5680. https://doi.org/10.1038/onc.2017.166
9. Li Q, Li Z, Wei S, Wang W, Chen Z, Zhang L, Chen L, Li B, Sun G, Xu J, Li Q, Wang L, Xu Z, Xia Y, Zhang D, Xu H, Xu Z (2017) Overexpression of miR-584-5p inhibits proliferation and induces apoptosis by targeting WW domain-containing E3 ubiquitin protein ligase 1 in gastric cancer. J Exp Clin Cancer Res 36(1):59. https://doi.org/10.1186/s13046-017-0532-2.
10. Chandhoke AS, Chanda A, Karve K, Deng L, Bonni S (2017) The PIAS3-Smurf2 sumoylation pathway suppresses breast cancer organoid invasiveness. Oncotarget 8(13):21001–21014. https://doi.org/10.18632/oncotarget.15471
11. Lu KT, Wang BY, Chi WY, Chang-Chien J, Yang JJ, Lee HT, Tzeng YM, Chang WW (2016) Ovatodiolide inhibits breast cancer stem/progenitor cells through SMURF2-mediated down-regulation of Hsp27. Toxins (Basel) 8(5):E127. https://doi.org/10.3390/toxins8050127
12. Tsao SM, Hsu HY (2016) Fucose-containing fraction of Ling-Zhi enhances lipid rafts-dependent ubiquitination of TGFβ receptor degradation and attenuates breast cancer tumorigenesis. Sci Rep 6:36563. https://doi.org/10.1038/srep36563
13. David D, Surendran A, Thulaseedharan JV, Nair AS (2018) Regulation of CNKSR2 protein stability by the HECT E3 ubiquitin ligase Smurf2, and its role in breast cancer progression. BMC Cancer 18(1):284. https://doi.org/10.1186/s12885-018-4188-x
14. Fukunaga E, Inoue Y, Komiya S, Horiguchi K, Goto K, Saitoh M, Miyazawa K, Koinuma D, Hanyu A, Imamura T (2008) Smurf2 induces ubiquitin-dependent degradation of Smurf1 to prevent migration of breast cancer cells. J Biol Chem 283(51):35660–35667. https://doi.org/10.1074/jbc.M710496200
15. Liu X, Gu X, Sun L, Flowers AB, Rademaker AW, Zhou Y, Kiyokawa H (2014) Downregulation of Smurf2, a tumor-suppressive ubiquitin ligase, in triple-negative breast cancers: involvement of the RB-microRNA axis. BMC Cancer 14:57. https://doi.org/10.1186/1471-2407-14-57
16. Li Y, Li W, Ying Z, Tian H, Zhu X, Li J, Li M (2014) Metastatic heterogeneity of breast cancer cells is associated with expression of a heterogeneous TGFβ-activating miR424-503 gene cluster. Cancer Res 74(21):6107–6118. https://doi.org/10.1158/0008-5472.CAN-14-0389

17. Wang W, Ren F, Wu Q, Jiang D, Li H, Peng Z, Wang J, Shi H (2014) MicroRNA-497 inhibition of ovarian cancer cell migration and invasion through targeting of SMAD specific E3 ubiquitin protein ligase 1. Biochem Biophys Res Commun 449(4):432–437. https://doi.org/10.1016/j.bbrc.2014.05.053
18. Liu L, Zheng W, Song Y, Du X, Tang Y, Nie J, Han W (2015) miRNA-497 enhances the sensitivity of colorectal cancer cells to neoadjuvant chemotherapeutic drug. Curr Protein Pept Sci 16(4):310–315
19. Ma M, Yang J, Wang B, Zhao Z, Xi JJ (2017) High-throughput identification of miR-596 inducing p53-mediated apoptosis in HeLa and HCT116 cells using cell microarray. SLAS Technol 22(6):636–645. https://doi.org/10.1177/2472630317720870
20. Subik K, Shu L, Wu C, Liang Q, Hicks D, Boyce B, Schiffhauer L, Chen D, Chen C, Tang P, Xing L (2012) The ubiquitin E3 ligase WWP1 decreases CXCL12-mediated MDA231 breast cancer cell migration and bone metastasis. Bone 50(4):813–823. https://doi.org/10.1016/j.bone.2011.12.022
21. Li Y, Zhou Z, Alimandi M, Chen C (2009) WW domain containing E3 ubiquitin protein ligase 1 targets the full-length ErbB4 for ubiquitin-mediated degradation in breast cancer. Oncogene 28(33):2948–2958. https://doi.org/10.1038/onc.2009.162
22. Sahu A, Patra PK, Yadav MK, Varma M (2017) Identification and characterization of ErbB4 kinase inhibitors for effective breast cancer therapy. J Recept Signal Transduct Res 37(5):470–480. https://doi.org/10.1080/10799893.2017.1342129
23. Yeung B, Ho KC, Yang X (2013) WWP1 E3 ligase targets LATS1 for ubiquitin-mediated degradation in breast cancer cells. PLoS One 8(4):e61027. https://doi.org/10.1371/journal.pone.0061027
24. Ge F, Chen W, Qin J, Zhou Z, Liu R, Liu L, Tan J, Zou T, Li H, Ren G, Chen C (2015) Ataxin-3 like (ATXN3L), a member of the Josephin family of deubiquitinating enzymes, promotes breast cancer proliferation by deubiquitinating Krüppel-like factor 5 (KLF5). Oncotarget 6(25):21369–21378
25. Chen C, Zhou Z, Liu R, Li Y, Azmi PB, Seth AK (2008) The WW domain containing E3 ubiquitin protein ligase 1 upregulates ErbB2 and EGFR through RING finger protein 11. Oncogene 27(54):6845–6855. https://doi.org/10.1038/onc.2008.288
26. Zhou Z, Liu R, Chen C (2012) The WWP1 ubiquitin E3 ligase increases TRAIL resistance in breast cancer. Int J Cancer 130(7):1504–1510. https://doi.org/10.1002/ijc.26122
27. Chen J, Shi H, Chen Y, Fan S, Liu D (2017) Li C. DNA damage induces expression of WWP1 to target ΔNp63α to degradation. PLoS One 12(4):e0176142. https://doi.org/10.1371/journal.pone.0176142
28. Lønne GK, Masoumi KC, Lennartsson J, Larsson C (2009) Protein kinase Cdelta supports survival of MDA-MB-231 breast cancer cells by suppressing the ERK1/2 pathway. J Biol Chem 284(48):33456–33465. https://doi.org/10.1074/jbc.M109.036186
29. Verma N, Müller AK, Kothari C, Panayotopoulou E, Kedan A, Selitrennik M, Mills GB, Nguyen LK, Shin S, Karn T, Holtrich U, Lev S (2017) Targeting of PYK2 synergizes with EGFR antagonists in basal-like TNBC and circumvents HER3-associated resistance via the NEDD4-NDRG1 Axis. Cancer Res 77(1):86–99. https://doi.org/10.1158/0008-5472.CAN-16-1797
30. Tsai CF, Cheng YK, Lu DY, Wang SL, Chang CN, Chang PC, Yeh WL (2018) Inhibition of estrogen receptor reduces connexin 43 expression in breast cancers. Toxicol Appl Pharmacol 338:182–190. https://doi.org/10.1016/j.taap.2017.11.020
31. Jung S, Li C, Jeong D, Lee S, Ohk J, Park M, Han S, Duan J, Kim C, Yang Y, Kim KI, Lim JS, Kang YS, Lee MS (2013) Oncogenic function of p34SEI-1 via NEDD4-1-mediated PTEN ubiquitination/degradation and activation of the PI3K/AKT pathway. Int J Oncol 43(5):1587–1595. https://doi.org/10.3892/ijo.2013.2064
32. Yim EK, Peng G, Dai H, Hu R, Li K, Lu Y, Mills GB, Meric-Bernstam F, Hennessy BT, Craven RJ, Lin SY (2009) Rak functions as a tumor suppressor by regulating PTEN protein stability and function. Cancer Cell 15(4):304–314. https://doi.org/10.1016/j.ccr.2009.02.012

Chapter 20
Emerging Novel Therapeutics in Triple-Negative Breast Cancer

Tomas G. Lyons and Tiffany A. Traina

Abstract The mortality from breast cancer has steadily decreased due in part to early detection and advances in therapy. The treatment options for breast cancer vary considerably depending on the histological subtype. There are a number of very effective targeted therapies available for estrogen receptor-positive disease and for human epidermal growth factor receptor 2-positive disease. However, triple-negative breast cancer is a particularly aggressive subtype. This subtype represents an unmet need for improved therapies. TNBC is a heterogenous subtype of breast cancer that is beginning to be refined by its molecular characteristics and clinical response to a targeted therapeutic approach. Here we review the recent advances in the treatment of TNBC with emphasis on the many emerging novel targeted therapies.

Keywords Triple-negative breast cancer · Targeted therapies · Androgen receptor · PARP inhibitor · Checkpoint inhibitor · Antibody-drug conjugate · AKT inhibitor

20.1 Introduction

In the United States, breast cancer (BC) is the most common cancer diagnosed in women and is the second most frequent cause of cancer death after lung cancer. In 2018, an estimated 266,120 women will be diagnosed with BC, with an estimated 40,920 deaths [1]. Triple-negative breast cancer (TNBC) is characterized by the

T. G. Lyons (✉)
Breast Medicine Service, Memorial Sloan Kettering Cancer Center, New York, NY, USA
e-mail: lyonst@mskcc.org

T. A. Traina
Breast Medicine Service, Memorial Sloan Kettering Cancer Center, New York, NY, USA

Department of Medicine, Weil Medical College of Cornell University, New York, NY, USA

© Springer Nature Switzerland AG 2019
A. Ahmad (ed.), *Breast Cancer Metastasis and Drug Resistance*,
Advances in Experimental Medicine and Biology 1152,
https://doi.org/10.1007/978-3-030-20301-6_20

absence of expression of the estrogen receptor (ER), progesterone receptor (PR) and human epidermal growth factor 2-receptor. TNBC represents approximately 15–20% of all breast cancers and generally has a more aggressive biology, with earlier onset of metastatic disease, visceral metastases, rapidly progressive disease, short response duration to available therapies and inferior survival outcomes [2]. While there are a number of very effective targeted therapies available for ER-positive disease and for human epidermal HER2 receptor-positive disease, TNBC lacks a standard of care approach guided by tumor biology. However, due to advances in both molecular classification of TNBC and genome sequencing we are identifying potential molecular targets in TNBC [3–5]. Numerous clinical studies are ongoing investigating a wide range of potential targets in TNBC including PARP inhibition, immune-directed therapy with checkpoint inhibitors, androgen receptor targeted agents, antibody-drug conjugates and targeting the AKT pathway (see Fig. 20.1). It is anticipated that many of these novel therapeutic approaches will result in a paradigm shift in how TNBC is treated in the future and lead to improved outcomes for patients. In this chapter we review the current data supporting the use of these emerging novel agents in TNBC.

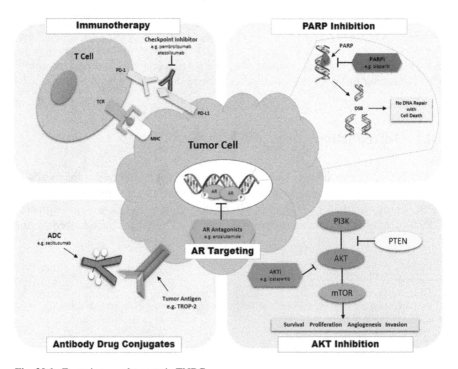

Fig. 20.1 Emerging novel targets in TNBC

20.2 PARP Inhibition

Poly (ADP-ribose) polymerase enzymes are essential for DNA damage repair. Cancers with defective homologous recombination DNA repair, such has BRCA1 and BRCA2 mutated breast cancer are targets for inhibition with PARP inhibitors (PARPi). The prevalence of a BRCA mutation is approximately 20% in an unselected TNBC population [6].

20.2.1 The Role of PARP in DNA Damage Repair

BRCA1 and BRCA2 are critical to the process of homologous recombination (HR) directed DNA repair. If HR repair is impaired by the loss of BRCA1 or BRCA2 function, then other DNA repair pathways may be engaged. The term synthetic lethality refers to cell survival in the presence of a defect in either of two genes, however a defect in both of the genes results in cell death [7]. Farmer et al. and Byrant et al. demonstrated synthetic lethality proof-of-concept with the PARPi olaparib in BRCA-mutated cells [8, 9]. This preclinical work led to clinical studies of PARP inhibition in BRCA mutation carriers. There are currently several PARPi in clinical development, including olaparib, veliparib, niraparib, rucaparib and talazoparib.

20.2.2 Olaparib

Early phase II studies of olaparib in gBRCAm-BC showed encouraging response rates [10–12]. OlympiAD was a randomized, open-label, phase III trial evaluating olaparib monotherapy compared with physician's choice conventional chemotherapy (capecitabine, eribulin or vinorelbine) [13]. Patients could have received neoadjuvant or adjuvant platinum chemotherapy if more than 12 months at elapsed since last dose. In addition, prior use of platinum in the metastatic setting was allowed if the patients had not progressed on platinum. In this study 302 patients having received no more than 2 prior therapies in the advanced setting were randomized in a 2:1 ratio to olaparib or chemotherapy. After a median follow-up of 14.5 months, progression-free survival (PFS) was significantly prolonged with olaparib vs. chemotherapy (7.0 months vs. 4.2 months; HR 0.58 [95% CI 0.43–0.8]; p < 0.001). The response rate in the olaparib group was also increased (59.9% vs. 28.8%). At planned interim analysis, there was no difference in overall survival (OS) between the two groups. There were no new safety signals observed. Health realted quality of life measures favored olapraib over treatment of physician's choice. Olaparib was the first PARPi to demonstrate superior efficacy and better tolerability compared with standard chemotherapy for gBRCAm-BC and has resulted in FDA approval in this patient subgroup.

20.2.3   Talazoparib

Talazoparib is another PARPi undergoing evaluation in breast cancer. The EMBRACA study tested talazoparib as monotherapy in patients with gBRCAm-BC compared to physician choice therapy (capecitabine, eribulin, gemcitabine, or vinorelbine) [14]. In this open-label, phase III study, 287 patients were randomized to talazoparib at 1 mg daily and 144 patients to chemotherapy. All patients had gBRCAm-BC, HER2-negative advanced disease and could have received no more than three prior lines of chemotherapy in the advanced setting. Patients could have received neoadjuvant or adjuvant platinum chemotherapy if more than 6 months at elapsed since last dose. In addition, patients could have received but not have progressed on a platinum in the metastatic setting. The median PFS, which was the primary endpoint, was significantly improved with talazoparib compared with the chemotherapy arm (8.6 months vs 5.6 months, HR = 0.542, $P < .0001$). In addition, the ORR was superior for talazoparib (62.6% vs 27.2%, HR = 4.99, $P < .0001$). An interim analysis of overall survival appeared to show a positive trend in favor of talazoparib, although these data are immature. Quality-of-life measurements revealed that in the talazoparib arm, patients had a significant delay in the time to clinical deterioration, which was 24.3 months for patients on talazoparib, vs 6.3 months for those on standard-of-care chemotherapy. Based on the results from the EMBRACA study, talazoparib has also been FDA approved for patients with gBRCAm-BC.

20.2.4   Veliparib

A phase II study of single agent veliparib demonstrated a PFS of 5.2 months with RR of 14% and 36% for BRCA1 and BRCA2 patients respectively [15]. Results of combining veliparib with carboplatin and paclitaxel in the randomized phase II BROCADE study in patients with gBRCAm-BC have been published in abstract form [16]. The combination resulted in a significantly improved ORR compared with carboplatin/paclitaxel and placebo (77.8% vs. 61.3% p = 0.027). The PFS was 14.1 months for the veliparib arm vs. 12.3 months for placebo, which was not statistically significant. There was no increase in toxicity reported between the two arms. A confirmatory phase III 'BROCADE 3' study is currently ongoing (NCT02163694).

20.2.5   PARP Inhibition in Early Stage Breast Cancer

The OlympiA trial (NCT020032823), is a phase III randomized study, evaluating olaparib at a dose of 300 mg twice daily for 1 year in patients with gBRCA1/2 mutation with residual disease post neoadjuvant chemotherapy or patients with node positive TNBC or node-negative TNBC with a tumor measuring ≥2 cm following adjuvant chemotherapy or ER+ patients with ≥4 nodes following surgery and adjuvant chemotherapy.

Veliparib in combination with neoadjuvant chemotherapy was evaluated in unselected TNBC patients as part of the I-SPY 2 study [17]. The predicted pathological complete response rate (pCR) was 51% versus 26% in the control arm. However, results of the phase III BRIGHTNESS study, of the addition of veliparib to carboplatin vs. carboplatin vs. placebo followed by standard chemotherapy in the neoadjuvant setting in patients with TNBC failed to show an improvement in pCR for the combination of veliparib and carboplatin vs. carboplatin (53% and 58% respectively) [18].

Lastly, talazoparib was tested as monotherapy in the neoadjuvant setting for patients with a gBRCAm-BC (NCT02282345). This phase II study enrolled 20 women with stage I–III gBRCAm-BC [19]. Seventeen of the women had triple-negative disease. Patients were treated with 6 months of talazoparib followed by surgery and with appropriate adjuvant chemotherapy (1 patient withdrew consent after 5 months of therapy). The study's primary endpoint was residual cancer burden (RCB) or pCR. Results showed that 53% of patients (10 of 19) achieved a pCR, or a score of RCB0; combined, 63% (12 of 19) received a score of RCB0 and RCB1. A larger single arm Phase II study is currently ongoing (NCT03499353).

Neoadjuvant PARP inhibition is promising given the encouraging results and the fact that these agents appear to be better tolerated than cytotoxic chemotherapy. However, larger confirmatory randomized studies will be required to validate these findings. In addition, if a patient achieves a pCR (which is a surrogate endpoint) with single agent PARP inhibition - can adjuvant chemotherapy be omitted? Additional studies to address this clinical scenario.

20.2.6 PARP Inhibitors Combined with Other Therapies

A number of trials attempted to combine PARPi with chemotherapy but toxicity has been a significant issue. Combining PARPi with immunotherapy is an attractive scientific approach with minimal additional toxicity expected and may result in enhanced clinical activity given the greater genomic instability in BRCA mutated cancers.

The MEDIOLA trial is a phase I/II open-label basket study of olaparib and durvalumab (anti-PD-L1 checkpoint inhibitor) in patients with advanced solid tumors [20]. The cohort with HER2 negative and gBRCAm-BC was recently presented. Patients could not have received a PARP inhibitor or immunotherapy, prior anthracycline and taxane was required and prior platinum therapy was allowed. Patients received single agent olaparib for 4 weeks with the addition of durvalumab 1.5 g IV every 4 weeks introduced at week 4. A total of 25 patients were enrolled, 12 (48%) having ER positive disease and 13 (52%) having TNBC. The ORR was 67% in patients with no prior therapy (n = 6/9), 67% in patients with one prior therapy (n = 6/9), 20% in patients with two prior therapies (n = 1/5) and 0% patients with 3+ prior therapies (n = 0/2). The median PFS had not been reached, with data cutoff at 6 months. The combination was generally well tolerated with no unexpected toxicity observed. Of note, there is uncertainty about the incremental contribution from durvalumab because this degree of clinical activity is not significantly different from single agent olaparib in OlympiAd.

The DORA study is a phase II trial evaluating olaparib plus durvalumab as a maintenance therapy following response to platinum chemotherapy in unselected TNBC (NCT03167619).

Lastly, there are early phase studies investigating PARPi as a single agent in patients with somatic BRCA mutations and/or germline or somatic mutations in other DNA repair genes (e.g. ATM, CHEK2, PALB2, RAD51, BRIP1 and NBM). Combination studies of PARPi with inhibitors of cell cycle checkpoints and DNA repair are also underway, e.g. ATR, WEE1 and CHEK1/2 inhibitors.

20.3   Immunotherapy

The clinical activity of immune checkpoint inhibitors – cytotoxic T lymphocyte antigen-4 (CTLA-4) and programmed death-1 (PD-1) and/or programmed death-ligand 1 (PD-L1) has dramatically changed the treatment landscape for many cancers. BC has not been regarded as an immunogenic tumor. However, tumor-infiltrating-lymphocytes (TILs) have been shown to be present in BC tissues, with a positive association in outcome in both the early-stage and the advanced disease setting in TNBC [21–25]. In addition, tumors with a high mutational burden have superior responses to checkpoint inhibition. TNBC has a higher mutational burden than other BC subtypes [26]. Early phase studies in addition to the first phase III study of a checkpoint inhibitor in TNBC have demonstrated evidence of activity (see Tables 20.1 and 20.2).

20.3.1   Checkpoint Inhibitors in Metastatic TNBC

Pembrolizumab, a PD-1 inhibitor, was evaluated in the phase II KEYNOTE-086, single arm study, in advanced TNBC [27]. Cohort A of KEYNOTE-086, evaluated the efficacy and safety of pembrolizumab in 170 patients with previously treated TNBC, regardless of PD-L1 expression. Forty-four percent of patients had three prior lines of chemotherapy in the advanced setting. Sixty-two percent had PD-L1 positive tumors (n = 105). The ORR was low at only 4.7%, with 1 patient achieving a complete response (CR) and 7 patients a partial response (PR), in addition to 35 patients having SD. The PFS was similar in both the PD-L1 positive and negative cohorts (2.7 and 1.9 months respectively). There was no significant difference in OS, being 8.9 months in all patients and 8.3 vs 10 months in the PD-L1 positive and negative cohorts respectively.

Table 20.1 Published results of anti PD-1 and PD-L1 monoclonal antibodies in TNBC

Drug	Trial	Phase	Disease setting	BC subtype	Patients (n)	ORR
Pembrolizumab	KEYNOTE-012	Ib	Metastatic	TNBC PD-L1+	27	18.5%
	KEYNOTE-086	II	Metastatic	TNBC PD-L1+	105	4.7%
	Cohort A			TNBC PD-L1-	64	4.8%
	KEYNOTE-086	II	Metastatic	TNBC PD-L1+	84	23.1%
	Cohort B					
	ENHANCE-1	Ib/II	Metastatic	TNBC total population	106	26.4%
	Pembro + Eribulin			PD-L1+	49	30.6%
				PD-L1-	49	22.4%
				1st line	65	29.2%
				1–2 prior lines	41	22%
	KEYNOTE-173	Ib	Neoadjuvant	TNBC		pCR
	Cohort A			Pembro + NP-AC	10	60%
	Pembro + NP-AC					
	KEYNOTE-173	Ib	Neoadjuvant	TNBC		pCR
	Cohort B			Pembro + NP+C-AC	10	90%
	Pembro + NP+C-AC					
	I SPY-2	II	Neoadjuvant	TNBC		pCR
	Pembro + P-AC vs P-AC			Pembro + P-AC	29	60%
				P-AC	85	20%

(continued)

Table 20.1 (continued)

Drug	Trial	Phase	Disease setting	BC subtype	Patients (n)	ORR
Atezolizumab	Atezolizumab	I	Metastatic	TNBC total population	112	10%
				PD-L1+	71	13%
				PD-L1-	37	5%
				1st line		26%
				≥2nd line		12%
	Impassion130	III	Metastatic	TNBC total population	902	
	Atezolizumab+nab-paclitaxel vs nab-paclitaxel+placebo		1st line	Atezo+NP ITT	451	56%
				Atezo+placebo ITT	451	46%
				Atezo+NP PD-L1+	185	59%
				Atezo+placebo PD-L1+	184	43%
						OS results
				Atezo+NP ITT	451	21.3 months
				Atezo+placebo ITT	451	17.6 months
				Atezo+NP PD-L1+	185	25.0 months
				Atezo+placebo PD-L1+	184	15.5 months
Durvalumab	MEDIOLA	I/II	Metastatic	gBRCA BC		
	Durvalumab + Olaparib			1st line	9	67%
				2nd line	9	67%
				3rd line	5	20%
				≥4th line	2	0%

Pembro pembrolizumab, *BC* breast cancer, *NR* not reported, *NE* not evaluable, *TNBC* triple-negative breast cancer, *ER+* estrogen receptor positive, *HER2+* human epidermal receptor positive, *pCR* pathological complete response, *PD-L1* programmed death 1 ligand, *ORR* overall response rate, *mPFS* median progression free survival, *mOS* median overall survival, *OS* overall survival, *NP-AC* nab-paclitaxel followed by doxorubicin and cyclophosphamide, *NP+C-AC* nab-paclitaxel and carboplatin followed by doxorubicin and cyclophosphamide, *P-AC* paclitaxel followed by doxorubicin and cyclophosphamide, *gBRCA* germline BRCA mutated, *ITT* intention-to-treat

Table 20.2 Selection of ongoing phase II/III studies of anti PD-1 and PD-L1 monoclonal antibodies in TNBC

Drug	Trial identifier	Phase	BC subtype	Neoadjuvant	Adjuvant	1st line metastatic	≥2nd line metastatic	Target accrual status
Pembrolizumab	KEYNOTE-119 (NCT02555657)	III	TNBC				Pembrolizumab vs single agent chemotherapy of physicians choice[a]	600 Ongoing
	KEYNOTE-355 (NCT02819518)	III	TNBC			Pembrolizumab + P or NP or GC vs placebo + P or NP or GC		858 Recruiting
	KEYNOTE-522 (NCT03036488)	III	TNBC	Pembrolizumab + PC-AC or EC vs Placebo + PC-AC or EC				855 Recruiting
	(NCT02954874)	III	TNBC		Pembrolizumab in patients with residual disease (>1 cm and/or positive nodes) post standard NACT			1000 Recruiting
Atezolizumab	IMpassion131 (NCT03112590)	III	TNBC			Atezolizumab + P vs placebo + P		540 Recruiting
	Impassion031 (NCT0319793)	III	TNBC	Atezolizumab + NP-AC vs Placebo + NP-AC				204 Recruiting
	NCT03281954	III	TNBC	Atezolizumab + PC-AC or EC vs Placebo + PC-AC or EC				1520 Recruiting

(continued)

Table 20.2 (continued)

Drug	Trial identifier	Phase	BC subtype	Neoadjuvant	Adjuvant	1st line metastatic	≥2nd line metastatic	Target accrual status
Durvalumab	DORA (NCT03167619)	II	TNBC				Durvalum ab + olaparib vs olaparib in TNBC patients following response to platinum	60
								Planned

Pembro pembrolizumab, *BC* breast cancer, *TNBC* triple-negative breast cancer, *ER+* estrogen receptor positive, *HER2+* human epidermal receptor positive, *pCR* pathological complete response, *NP* nab-paclitaxel, *P* paclitaxel, *AC* doxorubicin and cyclophosphamide, *EC* epirubicin and cyclophosphamide, *GC* gemcitabine and carboplatin, *NACT* neoadjuvant chemotherapy

aChoice of chemotherapy incudes, capecitabine, eribulin, gemcitabine and vinorelbine

Cohort B of KEYNOTE-086 evaluated pembrolizumab as first line therapy for patients with PD-L1 positive TNBC [28]. The study enrolled 84 patients, 73 (87%) of which had received prior neoadjuvant or adjuvant chemotherapy. The ORR was 23.1%, with 3 patients achieving a CR and 16 a PR. Twelve of the 19 responses were ongoing at data cutoff, and the median DOR was 8.4 months (range 2.1+ to 13.9+). Median PFS was 2.1 months and median OS was 16.1 months.

Results from the phase I trial evaluating atezolizumab (PD-L1 inhibitor) in TNBC have been reported [29]. Of the evaluable 112 patients, 17% were treated in the first line setting, 24% as second-line, and 58% had received ≥2 prior therapies. The ORR was 10% in the total population, 13% for PD-L1 positive disease and 5% in PD-L1 negative tumors. In addition, patients treated in the first line setting had a higher response rate in comparison to those treated with ≥1 lines of therapy (26% vs 12% respectively). The median OS was 9.3 months (95% CI 7–12.6) and the median duration of response was durable at 21.1 months. Of note, among the 11 responders (CR and PR), all were alive at 2 years.

An important observation to note from both this study with atezolizumab and from the KEYNOTE-086 cohort A, is that while the ORR is low in this heavily pretreated population of TNBC, if patients do achieve a response, it is often durable.

20.3.2 Checkpoint Inhibition Combined with Chemotherapy in Metastatic TNBC

The phase Ib/II ENHANCE-1 trial of pembrolizumab and the chemotherapy agent eribulin mesylate enrolled 107 patients with metastatic TNBC, for which 66 (61.7%) patients had received no prior chemotherapy in the metastatic setting and 41 (38.3%) patients had received 1–2 prior lines of chemotherapy [30]. Of the 106 evaluable patients, the ORR for all patients was 26.4% (3 CR and 25 PR). The ORR was 29.2% in patients treated in the first-line setting and 22% in patients with 1–2 prior lines of therapy. The median DOR was 8.3 months with a PFS of 4.2 months and OS of 17.7 months.

Atezolizumab in combination with nab-paclitaxel was evaluated in a phase Ib study, that enrolled 32 patients with advanced TNBC [31]. Patients could have received 0–2 prior lines of therapy and PD-L1 positivity was not a required for enrollment. The ORR was 38% (95% CI, 21–56) in the total population and 46% (95% CI, 19–75) in patients treated as first-line. Historically, the reported response rate from first-line nab-paclitaxel in TNBC is in the range of 30–35%.

The Impassion130 (NCT02425891) is a phase III randomized study evaluating nab-paclitaxel plus atezolizumab vs nab-paclitaxel plus placebo in patients as first line therapy for metastatic or inoperable locally advanced TNBC [32]. Prior neoadjuvant or adjuvant therapy was allowed if >12 months from end of therapy. Patients were stratified by PD-L1 which was defined as positive if >1% staining on immune cells. The co-primary endpoints were PFS and OS in ITT and PD-L1+ population. The primary endpoint of PFS was to be assessed in both ITT and PD-L1+ population. First interim OS analysis was to be tested in ITT population and only if significant, would the investigators then test OS in the PD-L1+ population. In total 902 patients were randomized (1:1) with 41% of patients being PD-L1+ in both arms. The median follow-up was 12.9 months. The PFS was improved by just over 1.5 months in the ITT population with the combination of atezolizumab to nab-paclitaxel, 7.2 months vs 5.5 months (HR 0.80; CI 0.69–0.92; P = 0.002). In the PD-L1+ patients the PFS was improved by 2.5 months with atezolizumab. PFS was 7.5 months vs 5.0 months, respectively (HR, 0.62; 95% CI, 0.49–0.78; P < 0.001). OS in the ITT population was improved by approx. 4 months with atezolizumab. The median OS was 21.3 months with atezolizumab and 17.6 months with placebo (HR, 0.84; 95% CI, 0.69–1.02; P = 0.08). However, this was not statistically significant. In the PD-L1+ population the difference in OS was much greater at an impressive 10.5 months, with 54% of patients alive at 2 years. Median OS was 25.0 vs 15.5 months, respectively (HR, 0.62; 95% CI, 0.45–0.86). The HR was 0.62 but this could not be formally tested as the OS difference in ITT was not shown to be significant. No new safety signals were seen for either drug. Based on Impassion130, the FDA on March 8th 2019, granted accelerated approval for atezolizumab in combination with nab-paclitaxel for the treatemnt of pateints with unresectable locally advanced or metastaic PD-L1+ TNBC. This approval marks the first checkpoint inhibitor to be approved for use in breast cancer. In addition we await the outcome of Impassion131, a similar design phase III trial of atezolizumab + paclitaxel vs paclitaxel + placebo as first line therapy in TNBC, to see if a similar survival benefit is observed in the PD-L1+ population (NCT03125902).

20.3.3   Checkpoint Inhibition Combined with Chemotherapy in the Neoadjuvant Setting

Pembrolizumab has also been investigated in the neoadjuvant setting. The KEYNOTE-173, is a phase Ib study of pembrolizumab plus chemotherapy as neoadjuvant therapy for locally advanced TNBC [33]. Patients were enrolled into one of two cohorts; cohort A – pembrolizumab plus weekly nab-paclitaxel (125 mg/m^2) followed by pembrolizumab plus doxorubicin and cyclophosphamide (AC) every 3 weeks and cohort B – pembrolizumab plus weekly nab-paclitaxel (100 mg/m2) and carboplatin (AUC 6) followed by pembrolizumab plus AC. The pathological complete response (pCR) rate (defined as no invasive residual disease in the breast and lymph nodes; ypT0TisN0) was 60% (90% CI, 30–85) in cohort A (n = 10) and 90% (90% CI, 61–100) in cohort B (n = 10). There were no new safety signals observed with the combination of pembrolizumab and chemotherapy.

Pembrolizumab was also evaluated in the phase II, neoadjuvant, adaptively randomized, multicenter I-SPY2 trial [34]. The goal of this trial design is to efficiently identify promising agents to take to phase III with a high probability of success.

A total of 249 patients were randomized, 69 to receive pembrolizumab in combination with weekly paclitaxel and 180 patients to weekly paclitaxel alone in the control arm, and all patients then continued to receive neoadjuvant AC, followed by surgery. Pembrolizumab was not continued in the adjuvant setting. Forty patients in the pembrolizumab arm had ER+ disease and 29 had TNBC. It is worth noting that the results are estimated pCR rates, as raw pCR rates are biased due to the adaptive design of the trial. If the predicted probability of success in a phase III trial of 300 patients was >85%, then the drug would graduate from the trial. Findings showed that the estimated pCR rate (ypT0/Tis and ypN0) was significantly higher with the addition of pembrolizumab in patients with TNBC than in the control arm; (60% vs 20%; HR 0.60; 95% CI 0.43–0.78), with a >99% probability of success in a phase III study.

20.3.4 Future of Checkpoint Inhibition in TNBC

Single agent checkpoint inhibitor therapy is unlikely to be sufficient in BC unlike other cancers. Pretreated patients can expect a response rate of between 5% and 10% while response rates for untreated advanced TNBC is approx. 20–25%. However, in the small subset of patients who do respond, the response is often durable. The difficulty is in identifying these patients. Biomarkers are needed to inform better patient selection for treatment with checkpoint inhibition. Higher response rates are seen when checkpoint inhibitors are combined with chemotherapy in the first-line setting and the use of these agents at an earlier stage of the disease does show promise. The Impassion130 study is the first phase III study to report, with encouraging results in patients with PD-L1+ disease. and has lead to FDA approval. The immune related adverse events observed across the trials of checkpoint inhibitors in BC have been similar to published data in other disease types. However, in the I-SPY 2 trial the rate of adrenal insufficiency was higher than previously reported in other studies of pembrolizumab across different cancer types. Caution needs to be exerted with the use of these drugs in unselected and/or lower risk patients in the neo or adjuvant setting as toxicity is not insignificant, with patients exposed to potential lifelong toxicities (such as endocrinopathies) for as of yet no proven clinical benefit.

Strategies to enhance responses with immune-directed therapies in TNBC include combination studies of checkpoint inhibitors with other immune targets such as GITR, PIK3CA-gamma, adenosine, TIGIT are all enrolling cohorts of TNBC patients. Checkpoint inhibitors are also being evaluated in combination with local therapies such as radiation, cytotherapy, photodynamic therapy in an attempt to enhance responses. Lastly, the use of personalized cancer vaccines and cellular therapies such as adoptive T cell transfer and CAR-T cell therapy are also being investigated in TNBC (see Fig. 20.2).

Immunotherapy Combination Strategies

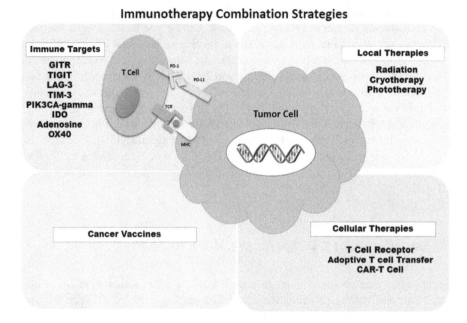

Fig. 20.2 Immunotherapy combination approaches

20.4   Androgen Receptor Directed Therapy

Emerging evidence has identified the androgen receptor (AR) pathway as a potential driver for BC carcinogenesis. Preclinical and clinical data support the activity of the anti-androgen bicalutamide and more recent, next-generation, AR-targeted agents such as enzalutamide, abiraterone acetate and seviteronel in targeting the AR in TNBC.

Androgen receptor expression varies across breast cancer subtypes. In TNBC the prevalence of AR by IHC is 12–55%. Preclinical work by Farmer et al. and Doane et al. identified a subpopulation of tumors that were ER− and AR+, which demonstrated an expression profile compatible with increased androgen signaling and dependence [35, 36]. More recently, Lehmann and colleagues, identified six distinct subtypes with unique gene-expression profiles [5]. One of the six molecular subtypes identified, luminal AR (LAR), was characterized by high AR mRNA and protein expression. The pre-clinical observations regarding the AR and its role in TNBC has led investigators to explore the AR as a therapeutic target.

20.4.1   Bicalutamide

Bicalutamide is an orally available nonsteroidal competitive AR inhibitor was evaluated in a proof of concept, multicenter, single-arm, phase II trial through the Translational Breast Cancer Research Consortium (TBCRC) [37]. The primary endpoint was clinical benefit rate (CBR) defined as CR, PR, or stable disease [5] >6 months. Bicalutamide resulted in a CBR of 19% (95% confidence interval [CI], 7–39%) with a median progression-free survival (PFS) of 12 weeks (95% CI, 11–22 weeks) in patients in this population. Treatment was well tolerated. These data offered the first signal of activity for androgen blockade in AR-driven ER/PR(−) breast cancer.

20.4.2   Enzalutamide

Enzalutamide is a pure AR antagonist that is thought to inhibit androgen receptor nuclear translocation, DNA binding, and coactivator mobilization. Enzalutamide was evaluated in a single-arm, nonrandomized phase II study in 118 patients with AR>0%, ER/PR<1%, HER2 negative metastatic breast cancer [38]. The primary endpoint of this study was CBR16 in the evaluable population, defined here as CR+PR+SD at 16 weeks rather than 24 weeks as in TBCRC011. Individuals with AR staining >10% and having a single post baseline assessment available were considered evaluable. Of the 75 evaluable patients, the CBR was 35% at 16 weeks and 29% at 24 weeks. Enzalutamide was well tolerated, with the most common adverse events observed being fatigue (34%), nausea (25%), and decreased appetite (13%).

As a preplanned exploratory substudy, a genomic signature was developed and internally validated which sought to serve as a biomarker. When the intention to treat population was analyzed for efficacy outcomes including PFS and OS, those patients who were diagnostic positive by this biomarker had improved outcomes as compared to those patients with biomarker negative tumors. For example, biomarker positive patients had a doubling of median OS (20 months [95% CI; 13–29] vs 8 months [95% CI; 5–11] as compared to biomarker negative patients.

Based on the encouraging data available in the metastatic setting, a phase II study has completed enrollment to evaluate the feasibility of enzalutamide therapy in patients with early stage, AR+ TNBC (NCT02750358).

20.4.3   Abiraterone Acetate

Abiraterone acetate is a potent, orally available, selective inhibitor of both 17α-hydroxylase and c17, 20-lyase, which targets adrenal and tumor intracrine androgen biosynthesis. A phase II multicenter trial was conducted through the French cooperative group UNICANCER in women with metastatic or inoperable locally advanced AR+ TNBC [39]. Overall, 138 patients with ER/PR(−) metastatic breast cancer were screened for AR of which 38.4% were positive. From July 2013 to December 2014, Bonnefoi and colleagues treated 34 women with metastatic AR+ TNBC. The primary endpoint, CBR24, measured 20.0% (95% CI: 7.7%–38.6%), including 1 CR and 5 SD ≥6 months. Median PFS was 2.8 months (95% CI: 1.7–5.4). The CBR24 rate and objective responses observed were similar to TBCRC011.

20.4.4   Seviteronel (VT-464)

Seviteronel is an oral, selective CYP17-lyase inhibitor and AR antagonist with activity in castrate-resistant prostate cancer. It is also under investigation in AR+ breast cancer. A phase I dose-escalation study in patients with advanced or metastatic breast cancer has been completed. A phase II, multi-cohort trial of seviteronel is actively recruiting patients with HER2 normal metastatic breast cancer; preliminary results have shown activity in AR+ TNBC and ER+ disease, with further investigation ongoing (NCT02580448).

20.4.5   Dual CDK4/6 and PI3K with AR Inhibition

Preclinical data have found that breast cancer cell lines with a luminal subtype were highly associated with sensitivity to palbociclib. A phase I/II evaluating the combination of bicalutamide and palbociclib in women with AR+ TNBC is currently enrolling patients (NCT02605486). A similar study of bicalutamide in combination with ribociclib in AR-positive TNBC is also open to accrual (NCT03090165). Activating mutations in PI3KCA have been described in association with AR positivity in breast tumors. A multicenter phase I/II trial of enzalutamide in combination with taselisib for the treatment of patients with advanced AR+ TNBC is ongoing (NCT02457910).

20.5   Antibody-Drug Conjugates

Antibody-drug conjugates (ADCs) are a novel anticancer treatment that permit the targeted delivery of a potent cytotoxic 'payload' to cancer cells through the specific binding of an antibody to a selective cancer cell surface molecule. ADCs have been under evaluation for many years, however, newer linker technology, along with more potent cytotoxic agents has resulted in the development of ADCs with superior efficacy and less toxicity. Currently, the only approved ADC in breast cancer is ado-trastuzumab emtansine (T-DM1) for HER2 positive disease. However, recent years have seen a number of ADCs enter clinical studies across many cancer types including TNBC.

20.5.1   Antibody-Drug Conjugates: Mechanism of Action

An ADC is comprised of three components – an antibody, a cytotoxic agent and a linker. The antibody should be specific for a cell surface molecule, which is specifically expressed on the cancer cell or more highly expressed on cancer cells relative to normal cells. The cytotoxic payload must be highly potent so that it can kill tumor cells at the intracellular concentration achieved. And the linker needs to be sufficiently stable in the circulation to allow the payload to stay attached to the antibody while in the circulation but permit efficient release of the payload when the antibody is internalized into the cancer cell. In short, the antibody binds to the tumor-associated target molecule on the cancer cell. The compound becomes internalized into the cancer cell. In the cytosol the linker is cleaved and the cytotoxic payload is released, leading to cell apoptosis. If a tumor does not homogenously express the tumor-associated target, the ADC may still result in tumor cell killing by the bystander effect. In this process membrane-permeable free cytotoxic payload can induce cell death in the surrounding cancer cells after being internalized and cleaved from the linker. However, this bystander effect can also lead to off-target systemic toxicity from the ADCs.

20.5.2 Antibody-Drug Conjugates in Development in TNBC

A number of ADCs are being investigated in TNBC (see Fig. 20.3). Early results are encouraging with confirmatory studies ongoing or planned.

20.5.2.1 Sacituzumab Govitecan

Sacituzumab govitecan is an ADC that combines a fully human IgG1 monoclonal antibody against the tumor-associated trophoblast antigen 2 (Trop-2) and SN-38 (7-ethyl-10-hydroxycamptothecin), which is a topoisomerase I–inhibiting drug.

	Sacituzumab Govitecan	Ladiratuzumab Vedotin	Trastuzumab Deruxtecan
Target	TROP-2	LIV-1	HER2 low
Cytotoxic 'payload'	SN-38 topoisomerase I inhibitor	MMAE microtubule inhibitor	Exatecan topoisomerase I inhibitor
Response Rate	30%	25%	50%*
Ongoing Trials	Phase III ASCENT NCT02574455	Phase 1 NCT01969643	Phase 1 NCT02564900

*Includes ER+ and TNBC patient cohort

Fig. 20.3 Antibody drug conjugates in TNBC

Irinotecan is the prodrug of SN-38, and is used in many solid tumors. However, SN-38 has a 100- to 1000-fold higher potency than irinotecan. Therefore, sacituzumab govitecan can deliver higher levels of SN-38 to the cancer cells. Trop-2 is overexpressed in many epithelial cancers and has been shown to be expressed in >80% of TNBC. A phase I dose-finding trial in advanced solid cancers, including metastatic TNBC showed encouraging activity. The single arm phase II study of sacituzumab govitecan enrolled 69 patients with heavily pretreated (median 5 lines) TNBC [40]. Results demonstrated an ORR of 30% (19 PRs and 2 CRs). Median PFS was 6.0 months, and median OS was 16.6 months. Trop-2 expression was positive in 88% (48/69) of patients. Grade $\geq$3 adverse events included neutropenia (39%), leukopenia (16%), anemia (14%), and diarrhea (13%); the incidence of febrile neutropenia was 7%. Based on these results the phase III randomized ASCENT trial has commenced and is accruing patients with TNBC who have progressed on $\geq$2 lines of therapy (NCT02574455). Patients are randomized to sacituzumab govitecan vs physicians' choice chemotherapy (capecitabine, eribulin, gemcitabine and vinorelbine).

20.5.2.2   Ladiratuzumab Vedotin

Ladiratuzumab vedotin is an ADC composed of a humanized IgG1 and monoclonal antibody targeting LIV-1 and the microtubule inhibitor MMAE. LIV-1 is a transmembrane protein with zinc transporter and metalloproteinase activity. LIV-1 is expressed in more than 90% of breast tumors and has limited expression in normal tissues. A phase 1 study consisted of a dose escalation phase (n = 81) and a phase 1b expansion phase (n = 63) with metastatic TNBC [41]. The recommended dose for the expansion phase was 2.5 mg/kg, with a maximum dose of 200 mg per cycle. Patients enrolled had received $\geq$2 cytotoxic regimens (with a median of 4) in the metastatic setting. Ninety percent of metastatic breast tumor samples screened were LIV-1 positive, including moderate to high in 68% of screened TNBC patients. The most frequent toxicities observed included alopecia (40.7%), neutropenia (24.7%) and peripheral neuropathy (19.8%). In the TNBC cohort the ORR was 25.0%, SD rate of 33%, CBR of 28%, and DCR of 58% and median PFS was 13 weeks. Enrollment in the TNBC cohort is ongoing and further evaluation of ladiratuzumab vedotin as monotherapy and in combination with checkpoint inhibitor in TNBC is planned.

20.5.2.3   Trastuzumab Deruxtecan (DS-8201a)

Trastuzumab deruxtecan is an ADC that targets HER2. It consists of an antibody component which is a humanized immunoglobulin G1 (IgG1) monoclonal antibody produced with reference to the amino acid sequence of trastuzumab, and a cytotoxic payload exatecan derivative – which is a topoisomerase I inhibitor. This ADC is being investigated in HER2 positive breast cancer and is showing very promising results in patients with refractory HER2+ disease despite prior trastuzumab and T-DM1 based therapy. The phase I study of trastuzumab deruxtecan also enrolled patients with HER2-low breast cancer (defined as IHC 1+/ISH negative or 2+/ISH negative) [42]. Results of this cohort have been presented in abstract form and demonstrated impressive results in heavily pretreated HER2 low breast cancer. TNBC patients were also eligible for enrollment in the study. Thirty-four patients with HER2 low tumors were enrolled. The ORR was 50% (17/34), DCR was 85.3% (29/34) and median PFS had not been reached. The drug is generally well tolerated with GI and hematologic adverse events being the most frequently reported. This drug is generating great excitement not only for HER2 positive disease but also as potential therapeutic option for HER2 low tumors of which TNBC patient may be candidates. Enrollment in the HER2 low cohort is ongoing (NCT02564900) and larger monotherapy studies in HER2 low breast cancer are planned.

Future work with ADCs may allow re-examination of prior cytotoxics that failed in development due to toxicity. This delivery mechanism may open new opportunities for old drugs.

20.6 Inhibition of the PIK3/AKT/mTOR Pathway

Activation of the PIK3/AKT/mTOR pathway is a relatively frequent event in TNBC, through activation of *PIK3CA* or *AKT1* and loss of *PTEN*, which can result in hyperactivation of AKT pathway [43]. Targeting the AKT pathway is an attractive option in TNBC. The phase II LOTUS trial randomized patients with advanced TNBC to first line treatment with paclitaxel in combination with the AKT inhibitor ipatasertib (n = 62) or placebo (n = 62) [44]. The combination of paclitaxel/ipatasertib demonstrated an improvement in median PFS 6.2 months vs 4.9 months in the paclitaxel/placebo arm (HR 0.60, 95% CI: 0.37–0.98, p = 0.037). In the subset of patients with *PIK3CA/AKT1/PTEN*-altered tumors (n = 42), the benefit of ipatasertib was even greater - PFS 9.0 months vs. 4.9 months (HR, 0.44; 95% CI, 0.20–0.99). Interim survival data from the study was recently presented in abstract form and showed a trend in improved median OS of 23.1 months with paclitaxel/ ipatasertib vs 18.4 months with paclitaxel/placebo [45]. Ipatasertib has been generally well tolerated, with diarrhea being the most frequent treatment-related adverse event. The randomized phase III placebo controlled study IPATunity130 is currently enrolling patients with *PIK3CA/AKT1/PTEN*-altered TNBC to first line paclitaxel +/− ipatasertib.

The Phase II PAKT study with a similar design to the LOTUS study, investigated the addition of the AKT inhibitor capivasertib to paclitaxel as first-line therapy in 140 patients with metastatic TNBC [46]. The addition of capivasertib resulted in significantly longer PFS (median PFS 5.9 months vs 4.2 months; HR 0.74) and OS (median OS 19.1 months vs 12.6 months; HR 0.61). The most common grade ≥3 adverse events were diarrhea, infection, neutropenia, rash, and fatigue.

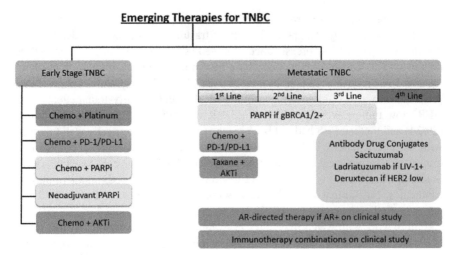

Fig. 20.4 Potential target driven treatment paradigm for TNBC

Lastly, the combination of paclitaxel and ipatasertib is also being evaluated as neoadjuvant therapy in the randomized placebo controlled phase II FAIRLINE study for stage I-III TNBC (NCT02301988).

20.7 Conclusions

Until recently the backbone of therapy against TNBC has been cytotoxic chemotherapy. However, the breast oncology community is now seeing encouraging clinical activity from novel targeted approaches to TNBC including; PARP inhibition, immunotherapy, AR-targeted therapy, ADCs and AKT inhibition. The expanding armamentarium of efficacious novel therapies is cause for optimism about the future of TNBC treatment (see Fig. 20.4). The term TNBC may in fact become redundant in the coming years as this heterogenous subtype of breast cancer is further refined by its molecular characteristics and clinical response to a targeted therapeutic approach. Results of ongoing and future clinical research in TNBC will validate the efficacy of such novel treatment strategies.

References

1. Siegel RL, Miller KD, Jemal A (2018) Cancer statistics, 2018. CA Cancer J Clin 68(1):7–30
2. Dent R, Trudeau M, Pritchard KI, Hanna WM, Kahn HK, Sawka CA et al (2007) Triple-negative breast cancer: clinical features and patterns of recurrence. Clin Cancer Res 13(15 Pt 1):4429–4434
3. Perou CM, Sorlie T, Eisen MB, van de Rijn M, Jeffrey SS, Rees CA et al (2000) Molecular portraits of human breast tumours. Nature 406(6797):747–752

4. Prat A, Perou CM (2011) Deconstructing the molecular portraits of breast cancer. Mol Oncol 5(1):5–23

5. Lehmann BD, Bauer JA, Chen X, Sanders ME, Chakravarthy AB, Shyr Y et al (2011) Identification of human triple-negative breast cancer subtypes and preclinical models for selection of targeted therapies. J Clin Invest 121(7):2750–2767

6. Gonzalez-Angulo AM, Timms KM, Liu S, Chen H, Litton JK, Potter J et al (2011) Incidence and outcome of BRCA mutations in unselected patients with triple receptor-negative breast cancer. Clin Cancer Res 17(5):1082–1089

7. Lord CJ, Ashworth A (2017) PARP inhibitors: synthetic lethality in the clinic. Science 355(6330):1152–1158

8. Bryant HE, Schultz N, Thomas HD, Parker KM, Flower D, Lopez E et al (2005) Specific killing of BRCA2-deficient tumours with inhibitors of poly(ADP-ribose) polymerase. Nature 434(7035):913

9. Farmer H, McCabe N, Lord CJ, Tutt AN, Johnson DA, Richardson TB et al (2005) Targeting the DNA repair defect in BRCA mutant cells as a therapeutic strategy. Nature 434(7035):917–921

10. Fong PC, Boss DS, Yap TA, Tutt A, Wu P, Mergui-Roelvink M et al (2009) Inhibition of poly(ADP-ribose) polymerase in tumors from BRCA mutation carriers. N Engl J Med 361(2):123–134

11. Tutt A, Robson M, Garber JE, Domchek SM, Audeh MW, Weitzel JN et al (2010) Oral poly(ADP-ribose) polymerase inhibitor olaparib in patients with BRCA1 or BRCA2 mutations and advanced breast cancer: a proof-of-concept trial. Lancet 376(9737):235–244

12. Kaufman B, Shapira-Frommer R, Schmutzler RK, Audeh MW, Friedlander M, Balmaña J et al (2015) Olaparib monotherapy in patients with advanced cancer and a germline BRCA1/2 mutation. J Clin Oncol 33(3):244–250

13. Robson M, Im SA, Senkus E, Xu B, Domchek SM, Masuda N et al (2017) Olaparib for metastatic breast cancer in patients with a germline BRCA mutation. N Engl J Med 377(6):523–533

14. Litton JK, Rugo HS, Ettl J et al (2018) Talazoparib in patients with advanced breast cancer with a germline bRCA mutation. N Engl J Med 379(8):753–763

15. Puhalla SBJ, Pahuja S et al (2014) Final results of a phase 1 study of single-agent veliparib (V) in patients (pts) with either BRCA1/2-mutated cancer (BRCA+), platinum-refractory ovarian, or basal-like breast cancer (BRCA-wt). J Clin Oncol 32(Suppl):abstract 2570

16. Han HS, Sook DV, Robson ME, Palácová M et al (2017) Efficacy and tolerability of veliparib (V; ABT-888) in combination with carboplatin (C) and paclitaxel (P) vs placebo (Plc)+C/P in patients (pts) with BRCA1 or BRCA2 mutations and metastatic breast cancer: a randomized, phase 2 study. Cancer Res 77(4 Supplement):S2-05-02. SABCS16-s2-05

17. Rugo HS, Olopade OI, DeMichele A, Yau C, van 't Veer LJ, Buxton MB et al (2016) Adaptive randomization of veliparib–carboplatin treatment in breast cancer. N Engl J Med 375(1):23–34

18. Loibl S, O'Shaughnessy J, Untch M et al (2018) Addition of the PARP inhibitor veliparib plus carboplatin or carboplatin alone to standard neoadjuvant chemotherapy in triple-negative breast cancer (BrightNess): a randomized, phase 3 trial. Lancet Oncol 19(4):497–509

19. Litton JK, Scoggins M, Hess KR, Adrada B, Barcenas CH, Murthy RK et al (2018) Neoadjuvant talazoparib (TALA) for operable breast cancer patients with a BRCA mutation (BRCA+). J Clin Oncol 36(15_suppl):508

20. Domchek SM P-VS, Bang Y-J, et al. (2017) An open-label, multitumor, phase II basket study of olaparib and durvalumab (MEDIOLA): results in germline BRCA-mutated (gBRCAm) HER2-negative metastatic breast cancer (MBC). San Antonio Breast Cancer Symposium. Abstract PD6–11

21. Savas P, Salgado R, Denkert C, Sotiriou C, Darcy PK, Smyth MJ et al (2015) Clinical relevance of host immunity in breast cancer: from TILs to the clinic. Nat Rev Clin Oncol 13:228

22. Loi S, Michiels S, Salgado R, Sirtaine N, Jose V, Fumagalli D et al (2014) Tumor infiltrating lymphocytes are prognostic in triple negative breast cancer and predictive for trastuzumab benefit in early breast cancer: results from the FinHER trial. Ann Oncol: Off J Eur Soc Med Oncol 25(8):1544–1550

23. Denkert C, von Minckwitz G, Darb-Esfahani S, Lederer B, Heppner BI, Weber KE et al (2018) Tumour-infiltrating lymphocytes and prognosis in different subtypes of breast cancer: a pooled analysis of 3771 patients treated with neoadjuvant therapy. Lancet Oncol 19(1):40–50

24. Adams S, Gray RJ, Demaria S, Goldstein L, Perez EA, Shulman LN et al (2014) Prognostic value of tumor-infiltrating lymphocytes in triple-negative breast cancers from two phase III randomized adjuvant breast cancer trials: ECOG 2197 and ECOG 1199. J Clin Oncol 32(27):2959–2966
25. Loi S DD, Adams S, et al. (2015) Pooled individual patient data analysis of stomal tumor infiltrating lymphocytes in primary triple negative breast cancer treated with anthracycline-based chemotherapy. San Antonio Breast Cancer Symposium. p S1–03
26. Alexandrov LB, Nik-Zainal S, Wedge DC, Aparicio SA, Behjati S, Biankin AV et al (2013) Signatures of mutational processes in human cancer. Nature 500(7463):415–421
27. Adams S, Schmid P, Rugo HS, Winer EP, Loirat D, Awada A et al (2017) Phase 2 study of pembrolizumab (pembro) monotherapy for previously treated metastatic triple-negative breast cancer (mTNBC): KEYNOTE-086 cohort A. J Clin Oncol 35(15_suppl):1008
28. Adams S LS, Toppmeyer DL, et al. (2017) KEYNOTE-086 cohort B: pembrolizumab monotherapy for PD-L1–positive, previously untreated, metastatic triple-negative breast cancer (mTNBC). San Antonio Breast Cancer Symposium. Abstract PD6–10
29. Schmid P, Cruz, C, Braiteh, FS, et al. (2017) Atezolizumab in metastatic triple-negative breast cancer: long-term clinical outcomes and biomarker analyses. American Association for Cancer Research (AACR Annual Meeting). Abstract 2986
30. Tolaney S, Kalinsky K, Kaklamani V et al. (2017) Phase 1b/2 study to evaluate eribulin mesylate in combination with pembrolizumab in patients with metastatic triple-negative breast cancer. San Antonio Breast Cancer Symposium. Abstract PD6-13
31. Adams S, Diamond JR, Hamilton EP et al (2016) Phase Ib trial of atezolizumab in combination with nab-paclitaxel in patients with metastatic triple-negative breast cancer (mTNBC). J Clin Oncol 34:1009. suppl; abstr 1009
32. Schmid P, Adams S, Rugo HS et al (2018) Atezolizumab and nab-paclitaxel in advanced triple-negative breast cancer. N Engl J Med 379:2108–2121
33. Schmid P, Park YH, Munoz-Couselo E et al (2017) Pembrolizumab + chemotherapy as neoadjuvant treatment for triple negative breast cancer (TNBC): preliminary results from KEYNOTE-173. J Clin Oncol 35:556. suppl; abstr 556
34. Nanda R, Liu MC, Yau C et al (2017) Pembrolizumab plus standard neoadjuvant therapy for high risk breast cancer (BC): results from I-SPY 2. J Clin Oncol 35:506. suppl; abstr 506
35. Farmer P, Bonnefoi H, Becette V, Tubiana-Hulin M, Fumoleau P, Larsimont D et al (2005) Identification of molecular apocrine breast tumours by microarray analysis. Oncogene 24(29):4660–4671
36. Doane AS, Danso M, Lal P, Donaton M, Zhang L, Hudis C et al (2006) An estrogen receptor-negative breast cancer subset characterized by a hormonally regulated transcriptional program and response to androgen. Oncogene 25(28):3994–4008
37. Gucalp A, Tolaney S, Isakoff SJ, Ingle JN, Liu MC, Carey LA et al (2013) Phase II trial of bicalutamide in patients with androgen receptor-positive, estrogen receptor-negative metastatic breast cancer. Clin Cancer Res 19(19):5505–5512
38. Traina TA, Miller K, Yardley DA, Eakle J, Schwartzberg LS, O'Shaughnessy J et al (2018) Enzalutamide for the treatment of androgen receptor–expressing triple-negative breast cancer. J Clin Oncol 36(9):884–890
39. Bonnefoi H, Grellety T, Tredan O, Saghatchian M, Dalenc F, Mailliez A et al (2016) A phase II trial of abiraterone acetate plus prednisone in patients with triple-negative androgen receptor positive locally advanced or metastatic breast cancer (UCBG 12-1). Ann Oncol 27(5):812–818
40. Bardia A, Mayer IA, Diamond JR, Moroose RL, Isakoff SJ, Starodub AN et al (2017) Efficacy and safety of anti-trop-2 antibody drug conjugate sacituzumab govitecan (IMMU-132) in heavily pretreated patients with metastatic triple-negative breast cancer. J Clin Oncol 35(19):2141–2148
41. Modi S, Tsurutani J, Takahashi S, et al. (2017) Safety and efficacy results from a phase 1 study of DS-8201a in patients with HER2 expressing breast cancers. Presented at: 2017 San Antonio Breast Cancer Symposium. San Antonio, Texas. Abstract PD3–07

42. Iwata H, Tamura K, Doi T, Tsurutani J, Modi S, Park H et al (2018) Trastuzumab deruxtecan (DS-8201a) in subjects with HER2-expressing solid tumors: long-term results of a large phase 1 study with multiple expansion cohorts. J Clin Oncol 36(15_suppl):2501
43. Zardavas D, Marvelde Lt, Milne RL, Fumagalli D, Fountzilas G, Kotoula V, et al. Tumor PIK3CA genotype and prognosis in early-stage breast cancer: a pooled analysis of individual patient data. J Clin Oncol 0(0):JCO.2017.74.8301
44. Kim S-B, Dent R, Im S-A, Espié M, Blau S, Tan AR et al (2017) Ipatasertib plus paclitaxel versus placebo plus paclitaxel as first-line therapy for metastatic triple-negative breast cancer (LOTUS): a multicentre, randomised, double-blind, placebo-controlled, phase 2 trial. Lancet Oncol 18(10):1360–1372
45. Dent R, Im S-A, Espie M, Blau S, Tan AR, Isakoff SJ et al (2018) Overall survival (OS) update of the double-blind placebo (PBO)-controlled randomized phase 2 LOTUS trial of first-line ipatasertib (IPAT) + paclitaxel (PAC) for locally advanced/metastatic triple-negative breast cancer (mTNBC). J Clin Oncol 36(15_suppl):1008
46. Schmid P, Abraham J, Chan S, Wheatley D, Brunt M, Nemsadze G et al (2018) AZD5363 plus paclitaxel versus placebo plus paclitaxel as first-line therapy for metastatic triple-negative breast cancer (PAKT): a randomised, double-blind, placebo-controlled, phase II trial. J Clin Oncol 36(15_suppl):1007

Chapter 21
Breast Cancer: Proteolysis and Migration

Kingsley O. Osuala, Kyungmin Ji, Raymond R. Mattingly,
and Bonnie F. Sloane

Abstract Understanding breast cancer cell proteolysis and migration is crucial for
developing novel therapies to prevent local and distant metastases. Human cancer
cells utilize many biological functions comparable to those observed during embryogenesis conferring the cancer cells with survival advantages. One such advantage is
the ability to secrete proteases into the tumor microenvironment in order to remodel
the extracellular matrix to facilitate migration. These proteases degrade the extracellular matrix, which initially functions as a barrier to cancer cell escape from their
site of origin. The extracellular matrix also functions as a reservoir for growth factors that can be released by the secreted proteases and thereby further aid tumor
growth and progression. Other survival advantages of tumor cells include: the ability to utilize multiple modes of motility, thrive in acidic microenvironments, and the
tumor cell's ability to hijack stromal and immune cells to foster their own migration
and survival. In order to reduce metastasis, we must focus our efforts on addressing
the survival advantages that tumor cells have acquired.

Keywords Proteolysis · Tumor cell motility · Modeling breast cancer · Tumor
microenvironment · 3D cell culture · Extracellular matrix · Live-cell imaging ·
Breast cancer

21.1 Introduction

Breast cancer remains the most common cancer among women and the second leading cause of cancer-related death [57]. Breast cancer-related deaths are most often a
result of cancer cell metastasis to major organs including bone, lung, brain, and liver
[24, 62]. Proteases have been identified as primary players in tumor cell migration,
extravasation, and invasion [37, 40, 51, 59]. The cysteine cathepsins and matrix

K. O. Osuala (✉) · K. Ji · R. R. Mattingly · B. F. Sloane
Department of Pharmacology and Barbara Ann Karmanos Cancer Institute, Wayne State
University School of Medicine, Detroit, MI, USA

© Springer Nature Switzerland AG 2019
A. Ahmad (ed.), *Breast Cancer Metastasis and Drug Resistance*,
Advances in Experimental Medicine and Biology 1152,
https://doi.org/10.1007/978-3-030-20301-6_21

metalloproteinases are notable proteases involved in the development and progression of breast cancer [20, 44]. Here, we will review the roles that some proteases play in breast tumor cell proteolysis and motility and in the breaking down of physical barriers that tumor cells encounter in the context of *in vivo* and *in vitro* 4D (3D over a measure of time) studies.

Proteolytic enzymes play a significant role in the development and functions of all organisms. From the nascent stages of human development [33] to the slowed and aberrant proteolytic activity associated with age-related neurodegeneration [48], proteolysis is a crucial aspect of life. There are roughly 600 proteases in the human genome, which have been divided into five major families. These are: metalloproteases, which account for the majority of all proteases; cysteine proteases; threonine proteases; aspartic proteases; and serine proteases [41].

Being an essential aspect of cellular functions, proteolysis provides a considerable contribution to cell motility [25, 32, 35, 63].When examining motility of individual cells on a two-dimensional plane, such as that of cells cultured on plastic surfaces, we can visualize the utilization of cellular membrane protrusions that extend outward from the cell body and attach to the flat surface. This adhesion to the target surface is followed by a de-adhesion of the trailing end of the cell and retraction towards the frontward attachment point. Cell membrane protrusions, called lamellipodia, along with fingerlike extensions that reach beyond the lamellipodia, called filopodia, are regulated by proteases [13, 42].

Increased study of cellular functions in 3D cultures have led to a better understanding of the multitude of processes that cells use to achieve motility [13, 15]. Modes of motility have been subdivided by the type of pseudopodium or false feet that protrude from the cell membrane. Many of these modalities involve the use of proteases to generate, activate, and recycle protein components necessary for motility [8, 13, 14, 64]. Some modes of motility have been shown to be regulated by a signaling axis involving RhoA [43]. Additionally, researchers have shown that the use of either lamellipodia or blebbing during migration can change quickly dependent upon environmental cues, and that the use of one form of migration over another is independent of cell morphology during migration [1].

21.2   Barriers of the Tumor Microenvironment

Breast tissue is made up of specialized structures that all play a crucial role in the proper development and function of the breast. The mammary gland is a classic example of an organ in which structure is dynamically involved in its function. For example, if the cells that make up the mammary gland do not form normal lobes and ducts, or properly align their cell polarity in regard to the basement membrane, the gland will not produce or secrete milk.

The breast is comprised of ducts, lobes and lobules, adipose tissue, nerves, blood vessels with lymphatic drainage, and fibrous connective tissues (Fig. 21.1a).

Breast tissue organization

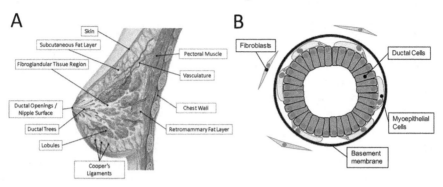

Fig. 21.1 Organization of human breast tissue. (**a**) Midsagittal view of the human breast showing the configuration of adipose tissue, muscles, vasculature, connective tissue, lobes, and ducts that form ductal trees leading to the ductal openings at the nipple. (**b**) Cross-sectional illustration of a single duct. The lumen of the duct is lined by a single layer of ductal cells that are encompassed by a layer of myoepithelial cells. The basement membrane separates the ductal and myoepithelial cells from the surrounding stroma in which fibroblasts reside. (Illustration provided by Patrick J. Lynch, Yale University (**a**), and Christopher A. Jedeszko, Wayne State University (**b**))

In humans, each breast contains approximately 10–20 ducts, and 15–25 lobes. Each of these lobes is further divided into many small lobules, which are the functional units for breast milk production. Lobes, lobules and ducts are surrounded by adipose tissue and held together by connective tissues that attach the breast to the chest wall. The lobules are bi-layered structures consisting of a layer of luminal epithelial cells, which secrete milk during lactation, and a layer of myoepithelial cells, which lie between the luminal epithelial cells and the basement membrane and are responsible for the contraction of the lobules resulting in the excretion of milk from the lobe to the ducts (Fig. 21.1b) [17]. Myoepithelial cells secrete tumor suppressor proteins such as laminin, a specialized extracellular matrix (ECM) protein [18, 55] and protease inhibitors such as; tissue inhibitor of metalloproteinase 1, protease nexin-II, alpha-1 antitrypsin, stefin A and maspin [10, 60]. The ducts of the breast are tube-like structures that facilitate the drainage of milk from each lobe to the nipple (Fig. 21.1a).

Adipose tissue makes up the majority of the volume of the human breast. Adipose tissue is composed of mature adipocytes, preadipocytes, and stem cells [2]. Adipose cells, mainly white fat cells, secretebiomolecules such as; hormones, growth factors (e.g., adipokines) [2], and pro-inflammatory cytokines (e.g., tumor necrosis factor-alpha, and interleukins -1beta and -6) [7], many of which are necessary for normal development and function of the neighboring ductal cells [30]. Many of the secreted factors from adipose tissue also support breast tumor growth by increasing the stabilization of pro-oncogenic factors such as beta-catenin and CDK6, through positive feedback loops [22].

Connective tissue, primarily collagen, helps maintain structural integrity of the breast and aids in attachment to the chest wall. As cancer progresses, collagen progressively thickens and stiffens, a process known to promote metastasis by increasing cell migration [3, 11, 21]. Identifying alterations in breast collagen density and/or arrangement has become a valuable tool in our efforts to improve the accuracy of breast cancer patient prognosis.

Extracellular matrix (ECM)of the breast is a complex network composed of various polysaccharides and proteins including collagens, elastin, fibronectin, tenascin, laminin, proteoglycans, glycoproteins, and ECM remodeling enzymes, all of which contribute to structural integrity and biological function of the breast. These components of the ECM have a role in: (1) maintenance of support tissue architecture and its integrity as a scaffold; (2) development; (3) homeostasis; (4) cell migration; (5) anchorage site for cell division; (6) cell polarity; and (7) cell-cell communication [29, 34]. Alteration of ECM homeostasis via aberrant secretion of proteases or activation of proteases in ECM stores can contribute to tumor growth and metastasis [29]. Release of stored ECM growth factors can activate surrounding tumor stromal, endothelial, and immune cells, which in turn further modify the ECM promoting tumor progression.

The basement membrane (BM), located between epithelia and stroma, is a thin sheet-like assembly that supports the breast epithelial structure by surrounding the lobules and ducts. The BM is predominantly composed of type IV collagen, laminins, proteoglycans, and glycoproteins, which act as a physical barrier separating epithelia from the surrounding stroma. The stroma contains various cell types including fibroblasts, adipocytes, endothelial cells, and innate immune cells embedded in type I collagen and other ECM proteins. In addition to its role as a structural barrier, the BM has a dynamic role as a communication bridge between epithelia and stroma. Signals sent across the BM regulate cell behavior and the activation of signaling pathways such as integrin and non-integrin (e.g., dystroglycan and syndecan) [65]. Loss of BM integrity is a detrimental shift in tumor progression [36]. Collectively, the constituents of the ECM act as an initial barrier suppressing breast tumor progression.

21.3 Proteolysis in 4D

Since the seminal work of Bissell and colleagues showing the importance of environmental context to cell growth and organization [61], the scientific community has examined various aspects of tumor microenvironments, one aspect being extracellular proteolysis. Proteolysis is a ubiquitous process in biology and its role in cancer development and progression is yet to be fully understood. In an effort to better understand the progression of breast cancer, we have optimized an *in vitro* 3D model that closely mimics *in vivo* cell growth and organization [54].This avatar has been named *mammary architecture and microenvironment engineering* or MAME.

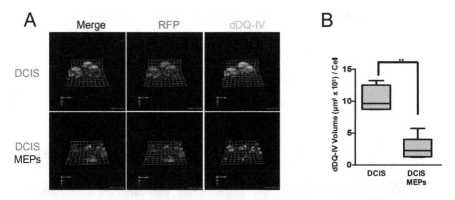

Fig. 21.2 Proteolysis of DQ-collagen IV in MAME cultures of human ductal carcinoma *in situ* cells. (**a**) MCF10.DCIS cells transduced with red fluorescent protein (RFP) were grown alone or in co-culture with myoepithelial cells (MEPs) for 21 days. Degradation products of DQ-collagen IV (dDQ-IV, green) indicating proteolysis are observed. (**b**) The graph illustrates quantification of fluorescent degradation products per cell in the entire volume of 3D reconstructions of 18 contiguous fields of optical sections for 6 independent experiments. (Figure adapted from Sameni et al. [55])

By adding a dye-quenched (DQ) ECM substrate, in this case DQ-collagen IV, to the matrix in which MAME cultures are grown, we can visualize proteolysis in 3Dand over periods of time (i.e., in 4D) [53]. This proteolysis (Fig. 21.2) can be both localized and quantified, providing data pertaining to directional movement, intra- vs. extracellular proteolysis and rate of ECM degradation [6, 31, 49]. Such data aid in the interpretation of cellular functions under various conditions and/or therapeutic treatments. In order to evaluate the contribution of individual proteases or protease classes to ECM degradation by breast tumor cells in co-culture with carcinoma-associated fibroblasts, we selectively inhibited several classes of proteases in MAME co-cultures of the BT549 human triple negative breast carcinoma cell line and WS-12Ti human breast carcinoma-associated fibroblasts (CAFs). Proteolysis was increased threefold in the co-cultures and was reduced ~ninefold by blocking activity of either MMPs, cysteine cathepsins or serine proteases (Fig. 21.3). As mentioned previously, myoepithelial cells act as tumor suppressors by inhibiting these same classes of proteases [60]. Careful identification of which protease or which protease class to inhibit, and in some cases which cell type is the source of the protease, are crucial aspects to consider when targeting proteases. There is extensive preclinical data that demonstrates causal roles for MMPs in cancer. For recent reviews, please see articles in the special issue of Biochimica et Biophysica Acta on MMPs [12, 45, 52]. Nonetheless, broad spectrum MMP inhibitors failed in clinical trials in part due to failure to achieve levels in tumors that would inhibit MMPs, yet at the same time achieving levels that resulted in side-effects such as development of peritonitis and skeletomuscular toxicities [9, 50]. Subsequently, researchers found that some MMPs are tumor suppressors, e.g., MMP-8, which is highly expressed in neutrophils and in normal breast myoepithelial cells, but lost with progression to DCIS [19, 28, 56]. Thus, efforts to develop inhibitors that are

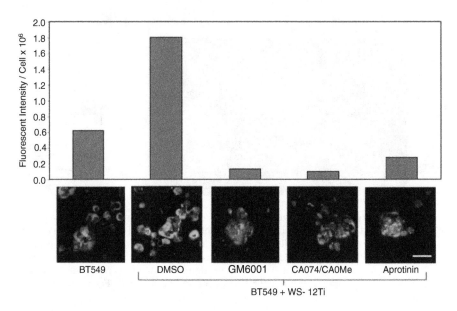

Fig. 21.3 Abrogation of proteolysis of DQ-collagen IV in MAME co-cultures of human BT549breast carcinoma cells and human WS-12Ti breast CAFs. CAFs markedly increase proteolysis and this is reduced by the broad spectrum MMP inhibitor GM6001, the cysteine cathepsin inhibitors CA074 and CA074Me, or the serine protease inhibitor aprotinin. Scale bar, 10 μm. (Figure from Sameni et al. [54])

selective for particular MMPs are ongoing as our efforts to identify which MMPs should be targeted; see [12].

Targeting proteases in specific cell types may be an ideal way to utilize protease inhibitors. For example, when cultured in 3D culture systems and *in vivo*, CAFs have been shown to lead invasion of tumor cells from several tumor types, e.g., squamous cell carcinoma, breast carcinoma and salivary gland adenoid cystic carcinoma [16, 27, 38]. It might be possible to use a highly specific fibroblast antibody such as TE-7, directed against a fibroblast surface protein and shown to control fibroblast overgrowth in cultures, in an antibody/drug-conjugated micelle or nanosphere to target proteases in fibroblasts. Having the capability to target proteases in fibroblasts or other tumor-associated cells such as macrophages may significantly improve the efficacy of protease inhibitor therapies.

21.4 Tumor Cell Motility in 4D

During embryogenesis neural crest cells migrate throughout the body [4]. Such migration continues at various rates in multiple cell types throughout adulthood [26]. In the neoplastic state, epithelial cells lose proper signaling clues that guide cell polarity and adhesion to one another and the basement membrane [46]. These changes in the cellular microenvironment may lead to cell adaptation and a reversion to a state

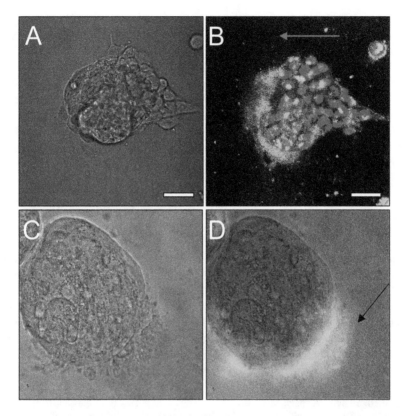

Fig. 21.4 Migratory phenotype of human breast DCIS cell lines grown in MAME cultures with DQ-collagen IV. (**a**) Differential interference contrast image of 3D structures formed by MCF10. DCIScells at 8 days of culture. (**b**) Fluorescent confocal image of panel A showing degradation products of DQ-collagen IV (green) and cell nuclei (blue). Note the extensive proteolysis at the leading edge of the collective migration. Arrow (red) indicates direction of migration. Scale bar for A and B, 100 μm. (**c**) DIC image of a single cell of the SUM102 cell line grown in 3D overlay culture for 8 days. (**d**) Fluorescent confocal image overlay of panel (**c**). Note the blebbing at the cell surface and the associated proteolysis (arrow). Images represent a single confocal section taken at the equatorial plane of the 3D structures. Magnification of C and D, 100X

similar to that during embryogenesis. This process of reversion has commonly been referred to as an epithelial to mesenchymal transition or EMT [23, 58]. During this cellular transition, epithelial cells upregulate genes needed for motility and cell: cell communication, e.g., vimentin, beta-catenin [66]. Having the ability to proliferate and migrate, tumor cells can escape acidic or hypoxic microenvironments and invade various nutrient rich organ systems. Therefore, a tumor cell's ability to migrate is an indispensable target in our efforts to reduce metastasis and cancer related deaths.

We and others have shown in 3D and 4D *in vitro* models that ECM degradation permits tumor cell motility and that inhibiting protease activity broadly or specifically can significantly reduce ECM degradation and cell motility [39, 55]. On flat surfaces cells tend to utilize protrusions such as lamellipodia with filopodia extensions [47], whereas cells grown in 3D or visualized *in vivo* show the use of cytoplasmic blebbing (Fig. 21.4) [47]. Tumor cells can also attach to stromal cells and/or macrophages, which then assume the task of matrix degradation [31]. The mechanisms that guide these interactions are not fully understood. However, in some studies, blocking cytokine communication, i.e. interleukin-6/IL-6 receptor signaling, inhibited interaction between tumor cells and stromal cells and reduced matrix degradation [38]. Furthermore, tumor cells have been shown to migrate through ECM microtracks previously scored by stromal and/or immune cells, providing a path of low resistance for tumor cells to migrate [5]. Treatment of cells in 3D culture with protease inhibitors or small molecule cytokine inhibitors has shown significant decreases in extracellular proteolysis and cell motility/invasion into the surrounding matrix [38].

21.5   Concluding Remarks

Examining tumor proteolysis and motility in 4D will enable scientists and clinicians to more clearly understand and visualize how tumors develop an invasive phenotype. These methodologies will open the door to new therapeutic targets that may prevent ECM degradation and confine solid tumors to their site of origin. Such therapies could be used in conjunction with surgical tumor excision to cure cancers before life threatening metastases ever occur. Looking forward, we will continue to pursue a more comprehensive knowledge of protease substrates and both proteolytic and non-proteolytic roles of proteases in tumors.

Acknowledgments We thank M. Sameni, C. Jedeszko and P. Lynch for the contribution of figures. We would like to thank laboratory members for their discussions and contributions to the development of 3D/4D cultures and co-cultures. This work was supported in part by R01 CA131990 (RRM and BFS) and R21 CA175931 (BFS) from the National Institutes of Health and Congressionally Directed Medical Research ProgramW81XWH-12-1-0024(KOO) from the Department of Defense. Imaging was performed in the Microscopy, Imaging and Cytometry Resources Core, which is supported, in part, by NIH Center grant P30 CA022453 to the Karmanos Cancer Institute at Wayne State University, and the Perinatology Research Branch of the National Institutes of Child Health and Development at Wayne State University.

References

1. Bergert M, Chandradoss SD, Desai RA, Paluch E (2012) Cell mechanics control rapid transitions between blebs and lamellipodia during migration. Proc Natl Acad Sci USA 109(36):14434–14439
2. Berry DC, Stenesen D, Zeve D, Graff JM (2013) The developmental origins of adipose tissue. Development 140(19):3939–3949
3. Boyd NF, Li Q, Melnichouk O, Huszti E, Martin LJ, Gunasekara A, Mawdsley G, Yaffe MJ, Minkin S (2014) Evidence that breast tissue stiffness is associated with risk of breast cancer. PLoS One 9(7):e100937
4. Bronner-Fraser M, Stern CD, Fraser S (1991) Analysis of neural crest cell lineage and migration. J Craniofac Genet Dev Biol 11(4):214–222

5. Carey SP, Rahman A, Kraning-Rush CM, Romero B, Somasegar S, Torre OM, Williams RM, Reinhart-King CA (2015) Comparative mechanisms of cancer cell migration through 3D matrix and physiological microtracks. Am J Physiol Cell Physiol 308(6):C436–C447

6. Chalasani A, Ji K, Sameni M, Mazumder SH, Xu Y, Moin K, Sloane BF (2017) Live-cell imaging of protease activity: assays to screen therapeutic approaches. Methods Mol Biol 1574:215–225

7. Coppack SW (2001) Pro-inflammatory cytokines and adipose tissue. Proc Nutr Soc 60(3):349–356

8. Cortesio CL, Chan KT, Perrin BJ, Burton NO, Zhang S, Zhang ZY, Huttenlocher A (2008) Calpain 2 and PTP1B function in a novel pathway with Src to regulate invadopodia dynamics and breast cancer cell invasion. J Cell Biol 180(5):957–971

9. Coussens LM, Fingleton B, Matrisian LM (2002) Matrix metalloproteinase inhibitors and cancer: trials and tribulations. Science 295(5564):2387–2392

10. Duivenvoorden HM, Rautela J, Edgington-Mitchell LE, Spurling A, Greening DW, Nowell CJ, Molloy TJ, Robbins E, Brockwell NK, Lee CS, Chen M, Holliday A, Selinger CI, Hu M, Britt KL, Stroud DA, Bogyo M, Moller A, Polyak K, Sloane BF, O'Toole SA, Parker BS (2017) Myoepithelial cell-specific expression of stefin A as a suppressor of early breast cancer invasion. J Pathol 243(4):496–509

11. Fang M, Yuan J, Peng C, Li Y (2014) Collagen as a double-edged sword in tumor progression. Tumour Biol 35(4):2871–2882

12. Fridman R (2017) Preface – matrix metalloproteinases. Biochim Biophys Acta 1864(11 Pt A):1925–1926

13. Friedl P, Sahai E, Weiss S, Yamada KM (2012) New dimensions in cell migration. Nat Rev Mol Cell Biol 13(11):743–747

14. Friedl P, Wolf K (2009) Proteolytic interstitial cell migration: a five-step process. Cancer Metastasis Rev 28(1–2):129–135

15. Friedl P, Wolf K (2010) Plasticity of cell migration: a multiscale tuning model. J Cell Biol 188(1):11–19

16. Gaggioli C, Hooper S, Hidalgo-Carcedo C, Grosse R, Marshall JF, Harrington K, Sahai E (2007) Fibroblast-led collective invasion of carcinoma cells with differing roles for RhoGTPases in leading and following cells. Nat Cell Biol 9(12):1392–1400

17. Gudjonsson T, Adriance MC, Sternlicht MD, Petersen OW, Bissell MJ (2005) Myoepithelial cells: their origin and function in breast morphogenesis and neoplasia. J Mammary Gland Biol Neoplasia 10(3):261–272

18. Gudjonsson T, Ronnov-Jessen L, Villadsen R, Rank F, Bissell MJ, Petersen OW (2002) Normal and tumor-derived myoepithelial cells differ in their ability to interact with luminal breast epithelial cells for polarity and basement membrane deposition. J Cell Sci 115(Pt 1):39–50

19. Gutierrez-Fernandez A, Fueyo A, Folgueras AR, Garabaya C, Pennington CJ, Pilgrim S, Edwards DR, Holliday DL, Jones JL, Span PN, Sweep FC, Puente XS, Lopez-Otin C (2008) Matrix metalloproteinase-8 functions as a metastasis suppressor through modulation of tumor cell adhesion and invasion. Cancer Res 68(8):2755–2763

20. Hillebrand LE, Bengsch F, Hochrein J, Hulsdunker J, Bender J, Follo M, Busch H, Boerries M, Reinheckel T (2016) Proteolysis-a characteristic of tumor-initiating cells in murine metastatic breast cancer. Oncotarget 7(36):58244–58260

21. Indra I, Beningo KA (2011) An in vitro correlation of metastatic capacity, substrate rigidity, and ECM composition. J Cell Biochem 112(11):3151–3158

22. Iyengar P, Combs TP, Shah SJ, Gouon-Evans V, Pollard JW, Albanese C, Flanagan L, Tenniswood MP, Guha C, Lisanti MP, Pestell RG, Scherer PE (2003) Adipocyte-secreted factors synergistically promote mammary tumorigenesis through induction of anti-apoptotic transcriptional programs and proto-oncogene stabilization. Oncogene 22(41):6408–6423

23. Kalluri R, Weinberg RA (2009) The basics of epithelial-mesenchymal transition. J Clin Invest 119(6):1420–1428

24. Kimbung S, Loman N, Hedenfalk I (2015) Clinical and molecular complexity of breast cancer metastases. Semin Cancer Biol 35:85–95

25. Kumar S, Kulkarni R, Sen S (2016) Cell motility and ECM proteolysis regulate tumor growth and tumor relapse by altering the fraction of cancer stem cells and their spatial scattering. Phys Biol 13(3):036001
26. Kurosaka S, Kashina A ̇ (2008) Cell biology of embryonic migration. Birth Defects Res C Embryo Today 84(2):102–122
27. Li J, Jia Z, Kong J, Zhang F, Fang S, Li X, Li W, Yang X, Luo Y, Lin B, Liu T (2016) Carcinoma-associated fibroblasts lead the invasion of salivary gland adenoid cystic carcinoma cells by creating an invasive track. PLoS One 11(3):e0150247
28. Lopez-Otin C, Bond JS (2008) Proteases: multifunctional enzymes in life and disease. J Biol Chem 283(45):30433–30437
29. Lu P, Takai K, Weaver VM, Werb Z (2011) Extracellular matrix degradation and remodeling in development and disease. Cold Spring Harb Perspect Biol 3(12):a005058
30. Mathew H, Castracane VD, Mantzoros C (2017) Adipose tissue and reproductive health. Metabolism 86:18–32. pii: S0026-0495(0017)30309-30308
31. Moin K, Sameni M, Victor BC, Rothberg JM, Mattingly RR, Sloane BF (2012) 3D/4D functional imaging of tumor-associated proteolysis: impact of microenvironment. Methods Enzymol 506:175–194
32. Mu W, Rana S, Zoller M (2013) Host matrix modulation by tumor exosomes promotes motility and invasiveness. Neoplasia 15(8):875–887
33. Nandadasa S, Foulcer S, Apte SS (2014) The multiple, complex roles of versican and its proteolytic turnover by ADAMTS proteases during embryogenesis. Matrix Biol 35:34–41
34. Nelson CM, Bissell MJ (2006) Of extracellular matrix, scaffolds, and signaling: tissue architecture regulates development, homeostasis, and cancer. Annu Rev Cell Dev Biol 22:287–309
35. Neurath H, Walsh KA (1976) Role of proteolytic enzymes in biological regulation (a review). Proc Natl Acad Sci USA 73(11):3825–3832
36. Nguyen-Ngoc KV, Cheung KJ, Brenot A, Shamir ER, Gray RS, Hines WC, Yaswen P, Werb Z, Ewald AJ (2012) ECM microenvironment regulates collective migration and local dissemination in normal and malignant mammary epithelium. Proc Natl Acad Sci USA 109(39):E2595–E2604
37. Olson OC, Joyce JA (2015) Cysteine cathepsin proteases: regulators of cancer progression and therapeutic response. Nat Rev Cancer 15(12):712–729
38. Osuala KO, Sameni M, Shah S, Aggarwal N, Simonait ML, Franco OE, Hong Y, Hayward SW, Behbod F, Mattingly RR, Sloane BF (2015) Il-6 signaling between ductal carcinoma in situ cells and carcinoma-associated fibroblasts mediates tumor cell growth and migration. BMC Cancer 15:584
39. Packard BZ, Artym VV, Komoriya A, Yamada KM (2009) Direct visualization of protease activity on cells migrating in three-dimensions. Matrix Biol 28(1):3–10
40. Pal A, Donato NJ (2014) Ubiquitin-specific proteases as therapeutic targets for the treatment of breast cancer. Breast Cancer Res 16(5):461
41. Perez-Silva JG, Espanol Y, Velasco G, Quesada V (2016) The Degradome database: expanding roles of mammalian proteases in life and disease. Nucleic Acids Res 44(D1):D351–D355
42. Perrin BJ, Amann KJ, Huttenlocher A (2006) Proteolysis of cortactin by calpain regulates membrane protrusion during cell migration. Mol Biol Cell 17(1):239–250
43. Petrie RJ, Yamada KM (2012) At the leading edge of three-dimensional cell migration. J Cell Sci 125(Pt 24):5917–5926
44. Radisky ES, Radisky DC (2015) Matrix metalloproteinases as breast cancer drivers and therapeutic targets. Front Biosci (Landmark Ed) 20:1144–1163
45. Radisky ES, Raeeszadeh-Sarmazdeh M, Radisky DC (2017) Therapeutic potential of matrix metalloproteinase inhibition in breast cancer. J Cell Biochem 118(11):3531–3548
46. Rejon C, Al-Masri M, McCaffrey L (2016) Cell polarity proteins in breast cancer progression. J Cell Biochem 117(10):2215–2223
47. Ridley AJ, Schwartz MA, Burridge K, Firtel RA, Ginsberg MH, Borisy G, Parsons JT, Horwitz AR (2003) Cell migration: integrating signals from front to back. Science 302(5651):1704–1709

48. Ristic G, Tsou WL, Todi SV (2014) An optimal ubiquitin-proteasome pathway in the nervous system: the role of deubiquitinating enzymes. Front Mol Neurosci 7:72
49. Rothberg JM, Bailey KM, Wojtkowiak JW, Ben-Nun Y, Bogyo M, Weber E, Moin K, Blum G, Mattingly RR, Gillies RJ, Sloane BF (2013) Acid-mediated tumor proteolysis: contribution of cysteine cathepsins. Neoplasia 15(10):1125–1137
50. Rothenberg ML, Nelson AR, Hande KR (1999) New drugs on the horizon: matrix metalloproteinase inhibitors. Stem Cells 17(4):237–240
51. Roy DM, Walsh LA (2014) Candidate prognostic markers in breast cancer: focus on extracellular proteases and their inhibitors. In: Breast cancer, vol 6. Dove Med Press, pp 81–91
52. Sakamoto T, Seiki M (2017) Integrated functions of membrane-type 1 matrix metalloproteinase in regulating cancer malignancy: beyond a proteinase. Cancer Sci 108(6):1095–1100
53. Sameni M, Anbalagan A, Olive MB, Moin K, Mattingly RR, Sloane BF (2012) MAME models for 4D live-cell imaging of tumor: microenvironment interactions that impact malignant progression. J Vis Exp (60):3661
54. Sameni M, Cavallo-Medved D, Dosescu J, Jedeszko C, Moin K, Mullins SR, Olive MB, Rudy D, Sloane BF (2009) Imaging and quantifying the dynamics of tumor-associated proteolysis. Clin Exp Metastasis 26(4):299–309
55. Sameni M, Cavallo-Medved D, Franco OE, Chalasani A, Ji K, Aggarwal N, Anbalagan A, Chen X, Mattingly RR, Hayward SW, Sloane BF (2017) Pathomimetic avatars reveal divergent roles of microenvironment in invasive transition of ductal carcinoma in situ. Breast Cancer Res 19(1):56
56. Sarper M, Allen MD, Gomm J, Haywood L, Decock J, Thirkettle S, Ustaoglu A, Sarker SJ, Marshall J, Edwards DR, Jones JL (2017) Loss of MMP-8 in ductal carcinoma in situ (DCIS)-associated myoepithelial cells contributes to tumour promotion through altered adhesive and proteolytic function. Breast Cancer Res 19(1):33
57. Siegel RL, Miller KD, Jemal A (2017) Cancer statistics, 2017. CA Cancer J Clin 67(1):7–30
58. Sikandar SS, Kuo AH, Kalisky T, Cai S, Zabala M, Hsieh RW, Lobo NA, Scheeren FA, Sim S, Qian D, Dirbas FM, Somlo G, Quake SR, Clarke MF (2017) Role of epithelial to mesenchymal transition associated genes in mammary gland regeneration and breast tumorigenesis. Nat Commun 8(1):1669
59. Sloane BF, K L, Fingleton B, Matrisian L (2013) Proteases in cancer: significance for invasion and metastasis. In: Stöcker W, Brix K (eds) Proteases: structure and function. Springer, Vienna. Springer, Vienna
60. Sternlicht MD, Kedeshian P, Shao ZM, Safarians S, Barsky SH (1997) The human myoepithelial cell is a natural tumor suppressor. Clin Cancer Res 3(11):1949–1958
61. Weaver VM, Fischer AH, Peterson OW, Bissell MJ (1996) The importance of the microenvironment in breast cancer progression: recapitulation of mammary tumorigenesis using a unique human mammary epithelial cell model and a three-dimensional culture assay. Biochem Cell Biol 74(6):833–851
62. Witzel I, Oliveira-Ferrer L, Pantel K, Muller V, Wikman H (2016) Breast cancer brain metastases: biology and new clinical perspectives. Breast Cancer Res 18(1):8
63. Wolf K, Te Lindert M, Krause M, Alexander S, Te Riet J, Willis AL, Hoffman RM, Figdor CG, Weiss SJ, Friedl P (2013) Physical limits of cell migration: control by ECM space and nuclear deformation and tuning by proteolysis and traction force. J Cell Biol 201(7):1069–1084
64. Xu Y, Bismar TA, Su J, Xu B, Kristiansen G, Varga Z, Teng L, Ingber DE, Mammoto A, Kumar R, Alaoui-Jamali MA (2010) Filamin A regulates focal adhesion disassembly and suppresses breast cancer cell migration and invasion. J Exp Med 207(11):2421–2437
65. Yurchenco PD (2011) Basement membranes: cell scaffoldings and signaling platforms. Cold Spring Harb Perspect Biol 3(2):a004911
66. Zeisberg M, Neilson EG (2009) Biomarkers for epithelial-mesenchymal transitions. J Clin Invest 119(6):1429–1437

Chapter 22
Current and Emerging 3D Models to Study Breast Cancer

Sophie Roberts, Sally Peyman, and Valerie Speirs

Abstract For decades 2D culture has been used to study breast cancer. In recent years, however, the importance of 3D culture to recapitulate the complexity of human disease has received attention. A breakthrough for 3D culture came as a result of a Nature editorial 'Goodbye Flat Biology' (Anonymous, Nature 424:861–861, 2003). Since then scientists have developed and implemented a range of different and more clinically relevant models, which are used to study breast cancer. In this chapter multiple different 3D models will be discussed including spheroids, microfluidic and bio-printed models and *in silico* models.

Keywords Breast cancer · 3D · Spheroids · Microfluidics · Primary culture · Bio-printing · Virtual pathology

22.1 Introduction

Significant progress has been made in our understanding of the biology of breast cancer and much of this has come from laboratory models. Mindful of the diversity and complexity of breast cancer, scientists have gradually recognised the inadequacy of simple 2D culture models as experimental tools. Innovative work by the Bissell laboratory has contributed enormously to our understanding of the tumour microenvironment in breast cancer and has advocated the use of more advanced 3D culture models [1–4]. As a result of a 2003 Editorial in Nature 'Goodbye Flat Biology' [5], such models are gradually being adopted and implemented by breast cancer biologists, with an exponential rise in the number of

S. Roberts · V. Speirs (✉)
Leeds Institute of Cancer and Pathology, University of Leeds, Leeds, UK
e-mail: v.speirs@leeds.ac.uk; valerie.speirs@abdn.ac.uk

S. Peyman
School of Physics and Astronomy, University of Leeds, Leeds, UK

© Springer Nature Switzerland AG 2019
A. Ahmad (ed.), *Breast Cancer Metastasis and Drug Resistance*,
Advances in Experimental Medicine and Biology 1152,
https://doi.org/10.1007/978-3-030-20301-6_22

papers reporting 3D cell culture, which is now overtaking those reporting 2D models [6]. This chapter describes some of the current and emerging 3D models and how these are being used in breast cancer research.

22.2   Why 3D?

Cancer is a heterogeneous disease whose progression relies on the complex interactions between multiple cell types and the surrounding extracellular matrix (ECM). Collectively this forms the tumour microenvironment, a complex milieu of cellular and non-cellular components including tumour cells, cancer associated fibroblasts (CAFs) and ECM proteins such as collagen (Fig. 22.1b). Within this environment, cancer cells have the ability to become polarised allowing effective interaction with components of their microenvironment, which can contribute towards tumour growth and metastasis. This is hard to replicate in 2D models where cells are maintained on flat plastic substrates and often in isolation from other cell types (Fig. 22.1a). 3D modelling allows cell-cell and cell-ECM interactions to be studied [7] that direct tissue structure [4] and ultimately contribute to tumour formation and progression.

Animal models of breast cancer, notably rodent models [8], have been used extensively to address tumour complexity and to provide microenvironmental cues, however there are limitations. For example mouse disease does not always mirror human disease and it is difficult to retain human CAFs in mouse models. This is a concern as CAFs are the main cell type in the tumour microenvironment and have tumour promoting ability [9]. The development of increasingly complex 3D *in vitro* models can address some of these issues.

22.2.1   3D Spheroid Models

These were developed initially in the 1970s and used in irradiation studies [10]. Subsequent improvements and modifications have led to their use in other aspects of cancer research. Spheroids show similarities to tumours *in vivo*. If grown large enough they can have a quiescent and/or necrotic centre surrounded by actively proliferating cells at the periphery (Fig. 22.2) [11]. The necrotic cores are a result of oxygen and nutrient deprivation much like in cancerous tumours [11]. Furthermore, drug delivery to cells grown as 3D spheroids often differs to those grown in 2D [12]. This is important and indicates that in order to successfully mimic drug penetration to a solid tumour, 3D models would be beneficial in drug discovery programmes.

Early spheroid culture was monotypic, meaning that a single cell type was cultured in 3D e.g. 3D culture of the MCF-10A breast cell line to investigate luminal development in the normal mammary gland [13]. However, such culture makes studies of the microenvironment challenging as the heterogeneous nature observed

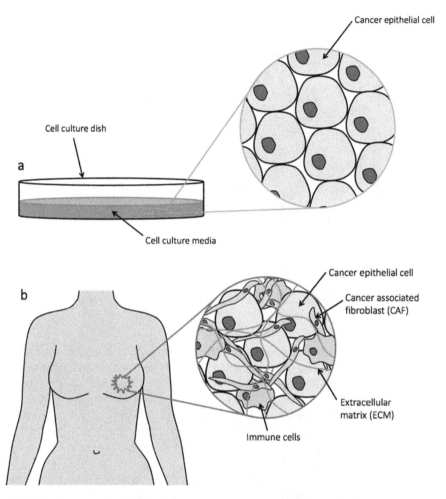

Cancer epithelial cell

Cell culture dish

a

Cell culture media

Cancer epithelial cell

Cancer associated
fibroblast (CAF)

b

Extracellular
matrix (ECM)

Immune cells

Fig. 22.1 Diagram to show how simple 2D culture of cancer cells (**a**) differs from the complex interrelationships of multiple cell types found in cancer in vivo (**b**). Such complex interactions are recognised to influence cell behaviour

in tumours *in vivo* is not captured. More advanced spheroid culture has since been employed in breast cancer using co-culture of different cell types to recapitulate aspects of human disease [14, 15].

A number of different approaches have been used to generate spheroid cultures. These include the spinner flask technique where cells are seeded as single cell suspension which is continuously stirred and thus encourages cells to aggregate forming spheroids [16]. In the liquid overlay technique, cells are cultured on a non-adhesive surface that encourages cell aggregation rather than adherence to the culture flask [17].

The addition of carboxymethyl cellulose to cell culture medium increases viscosity, preventing cells from being able to adhere to the culture surface and encour-

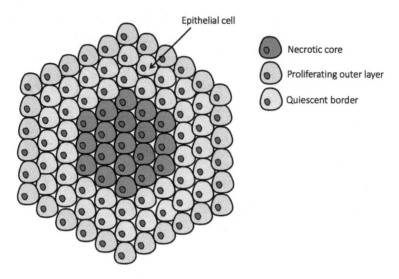

Fig. 22.2 Schematic of epithelial cells growing as a 3D spheroid. Generally if spheroids grow to >0.5 mm the centre of the spheroid becomes necrotic (red) due to limited oxygen supply. This core is surrounded by quiescent cells (cream) and then an actively proliferating outer (blue)

aging aggregation [17]. In the hanging drop technique cells are cultured as droplets of media on a petri dish lid, the lid is turned over and placed on the bottom petri dish and cells are cultured until spheroids of desired size are reached [18]. The type of cell culture medium used can also encourage spheroid formation e.g. modification of FibroLife™ medium, originally developed to promote fibroblast culture, to epiFL by the exclusion of fibroblast growth factor and transforming growth factor β, encourages breast cancer epithelial cells to lift off the surface of culture flasks and form viable 3D spheroids [15].

Cells cultured in 3D usually require a supportive matrix or scaffold to mimic the ECM [19]. Various methods have been employed. Collagen-I is the primary basement membrane protein in breast tissue [20] and has been used in 3D culture of primary breast cells [14] however, has the drawback of being animal derived, which can be an issue if looking to develop fully humanised culture systems. Matrigel™ is a commercially available reconstituted basement membrane derived from Englebreth-Holm-Swarm tumour [21] and has been used in many 3D breast models showing to be effective in recreating the basement membrane [22]. However, Matrigel™ contains animal components too, and these are not well-defined leading to batch to batch variability. Hydrogels are an alternative to collagen-I and Matrigel™ and have been used in the culture of primary breast cells also [23]. A scaffold free *in vitro* model was generated by Jaganathan and colleagues using breast cancer epithelial cells lines and fibroblasts cultured using magnetic levitation [19]. The characteristics and behaviour of the 3D structures formed was consistent with *in vivo* studies. Fibroblasts were found more at the periphery of 3D structures while epithelial cells were in the centre [19]. Another aim of the model was to assess its ability to mimic drug responses seen *in vivo*. Treatment of the 3D tumour with Doxorubicin, a commonly used chemotherapeutic agent in breast cancer, resulted in a decrease in its size mimicking what is observed *in vivo* [19]. This suggested that these types of 3D models could be useful in drug discovery.

A drawback of spheroid culture is that it can be difficult to produce spheroids that are homogeneous in size, which may impact on response to treatment, potentially limiting their use in high-throughput drug screens and subsequent translatability of results to the clinic [24]. Of note, two HER2 overexpressing breast cancer cell lines behave differently when grown in 3D in epiFL. While BT-474 cells form spherical aggregates, SKBr3 cells form grape-like arrangements [15].

In breast cancer 3D monoculture spheroids are often referred to as mammospheres and since there is evidence that breast cancer cells with a stem cell-like phenotype are the cell type most likely to go on to form metastases [25, 26], mammosphere culture is often used to study breast cancer stem cells.

22.3 Primary Culture Models

A number of specialist breast tissue banks exist [27]. Such biobanks allow scientists to develop experimental models that incorporate patient samples. These are attractive since using human tissue to address a human problem offers a more clinical angle for developing stratified medicine approaches. Organoids (Fig. 22.3), multicellular tissue pieces which mimic the tissue they are derived from, both through the components it contains and its cellular organisation are used frequently [28]. Human breast cancer organoids have been generated [28, 29]. Multiple organoids can be derived from single tissue biopsies which leads to the potential for testing of multiple drugs using a small amount of tissue [29]. Drugs have been tested on

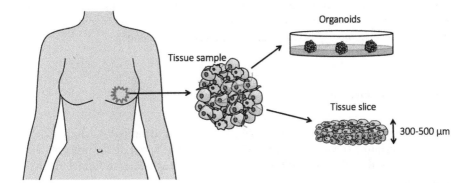

Fig. 22.3 Example of how patient derived tissue can be used in cell culture. Resected tissue can be dispersed into organoids or maintained as tissue slices to study different aspects of breast cancer biology. This has the advantage of retaining the tissue in its native state

mammary organoids and growth was inhibited as anticipated illustrating their potential as predictors for *in vivo* drug studies [29].

Furthering the use of primary patient samples, the tissue slice model (Fig. 22.3) has been applied to breast cancer [30]. Here slices of tissue are retained tissue in their native state, thus preserving cell-cell and cell-ECM communications [31, 30]. Tissue slices are thin enough (300–400 µm) to allow the diffusion of media through the tissue [31, 30]. Breast cancer tissue slices have been used to analyse the gene profiles of breast cancer subtypes after treatment with rapamycin [32] and also to look at infectivity by oncolytic viruses observing a higher rate of virus infectivity in tumour opposed to normal tissue [33]. Tissue slices have been cultured for up to 7 days with no signs of regression, suggesting there is potential to grow longer which may allow their implementation in personalised medicine [34].

However, the main disadvantage of using tissue slices is the delicate nature of the sample which can make downstream analysis challenging [30].

22.4   Modelling Metastatic Disease

Metastasis accounts for the majority of cancer related deaths. The process of metastasis is complex and modelling it using *in vitro* cancer models is challenging. Metastasis is a multi-step process involving extravasation of tumour cells from the primary tumour site into the blood and then intravasation into a distant site. This process is, therefore, impossible to fully mimic using 2D culture and so 3D models have been employed. One of the most common sites for breast cancer metastasis is to the bone. Bone has a complex environment that requires 3D modelling to mimic (reviewed in [35]). One study compared 2D and 3D culture to model bone metastasis and found that only breast cancer cells grown in 3D were able to capture events, such as tissue penetration, observed *in vivo* [36]. Another study showed the importance of a supportive microenvironment for the growth of dormant breast cancer cells by co-culturing cells in a 3D collagen bio-matrix and repeating this experiment in SCID mice *in vivo* to confirm the results [37] suggesting that 3D modelling can potentially bridge the gap between 2D culture and mouse models.

22.5   Bio-printing

A new generation of 3D modelling is beginning to emerge through the development of 3D bio-printing (reviewed in [38, 39]). Much like 3D printing the process relies on the successive printing of 2D structures on top of each other to form a 3D scaffold (Fig. 22.4).

Bio-printers print using biomaterials that are both able to be printed and also promote the growth and survival of cells. A major advantage of bio-printing over other approaches is the ability to create complex but controlled 3D structures of

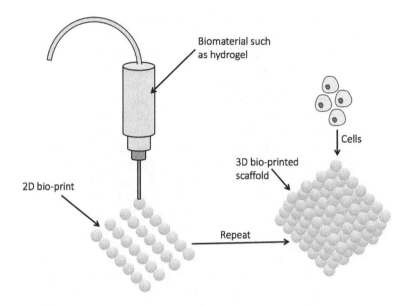

Fig. 22.4 Cartoon to show how biomaterials, such as hydrogels, can be printed to form 3D scaffold structures in which cells can then be seeded into to form a 3D cellular environment

heterogeneous tissue in a manner that recapitulates that of *in vivo* tumours [38]. 3D bio-printing has been used to model breast cancer in recent years. One model utilised bio-printing to promote the self-assembly of MDA-MB- 231 spheroids seeded within a scaffold of fibroblasts [40]. Another used bio-printing to investigate breast cancer metastasis to bone; the bio-printer created matrices of bone in hydrogels and the effects of adding breast cancer cells was observed [41]. Bio-printing is a new field that holds promise for the future of 3D cell culture modelling. 3D bio-printing holds many advantages over previously used models such as the ability to model small complex structures as blood capillaries, potentially more accurate drug studies and the ability to recreate tissue structures [39]. However, a disadvantage of using bio-printing is that a biological material must be chosen that both supports the growth of cells and is also able to be printed effectively [39].

22.6   Microfluidics in 3D Modelling

Microfluidics is an emerging technology that is proving to be revolutionary in the biomedical sciences, from clinical diagnostics to modelling and biomimetic systems [42]. Microfluidic technology involves the fabrication of micron sized fluidic channels in a polymer or glass substrate to which tubing and pumping peripherals are attached and through which fluid is pumped. Fluidic handling on the micron scale reduces the volume of reagents required for an assay, and the waste produced and thus the overall cost of an assay. Fluid flow inside micron sized channels is predominantly laminar in behaviour, so fluid can be described as highly controllable and predictable. In addition to flow being easily controlled, objects that are in flow inside a microchannel, such as particles or single cells, can also be easily manipulated and microfluidic based single cell analysis is one area of microfluidics that has become very popular [43]. Further advantages of precision control over fluid flow is the ability to pattern ECM and cells in to specific areas within a single device, allowing for the fabrication of stratified tissue structures and interfaces that more closely resemble those found *in vivo*.

Consequently, one area that is currently utilising the advantages of microfluidic technology is that of tissue and organ modelling on chip [44, 45]. The microscale dimensions and precise control over fluid dynamics allows *in vivo* microenvironments to be recapitulated more meaningfully than current *in vitro* methods. Fluid flow rate, shear forces, interstitial pressures, reagent and temperature gradients and mechanical stresses can be easily controlled in these systems, making it possible to mimic *in vivo* physical and biochemical environments in a way that has not been realised previously. In addition, continuous perfusion of media and removal of waste, similar to what tissues experience *in vivo*, allows for stable, long term cell culture. As well as improving current *in vitro* models, the advancements of microfluidic technology in 3D cell cultures and disease modelling may help to reduce the cost and risk associated with in vivo animal models and drug screening.

Due to the increasing popularity of microfluidics as diagnostic and modelling tools, there is a wealth of material now published on various disease models, device designs and applications; this chapter will focus on examples from culturing of cells inside microfluidic devices for breast cancer models for high-throughput screening and modelling of disease progression. The following are a collection of relevant examples to give a feel for what microfluidics can offer to the future of 3D breast cancer modelling, rather than an exhaustive review of the current literature and also excludes literature on single cells or 2D-only models.

22.6.1   Drug Screening and Therapy Assessment On-chip

The ability to culture multiple cell types in microchannels, and the small volumes associated with the internal volumes along with the optical transparency of the devices makes microfluidics an ideal platform for rapid drug screening *in vitro* [46, 47, 48]. In addition to the intrinsic predictability of laminar flow in microchannels, on and off-chip valve components add an extra layer of controllability to an assay as reagents can be pumped, stopped, switched and washed out a channel in a reproducible and automated fashion. In addition, by designing multiple screening channels on one device, high-throughput parallelisation of experiments becomes relatively easy, reducing time and associated costs. For instance a multi-cellular, 3D tissue model was cultured inside a chamber for assessing the effect of photodynamic therapy was developed in which eight chambers were parallelised on a single device, creating eight independent, reproducible models to evaluate new therapeutics [49].

There are many examples of the co-culturing of multiple cell types in close proximity in microfluidic devices for mimicking in vivo tissue interfaces and assessing a range of therapeutic agents, from more commonly known chemotherapy drugs to new nanoparticle based therapies [50, 51, 52]. In these examples, hydrogels are introduced into the channels that have been designed in a side-by-side geometry. The drug of interest is usually pumped through a channel parallel to those containing cell cultures so the diffusion and uptake of the drug through the tissue interfaces and microenvironments can be analysed. For example, a tumour-microenvironment-on-chip or TMOC was developed to recapitulate the complex transport of nanoparticles to a tumour. The multi-cellular model used MCF-7 and human microvascular endothelial cells to mimic a vasculature-tumour-lymphatic structure in order to simulate the microenvironment and interstitial pressures that nanoparticles would interact with during in treatments. The model was used to inform on nanoparticle behaviour and future nanoparticle design considerations [53].

Spheroids have already been introduced above (Sect. 22.2.1) and these are now being applied to microfluidic platforms as one of the simplest forms of on-chip 3D culture systems. Here, spheroids are either physically trapped or cultured inside microfluidic channels, over which fluid can be pumped. For example the on-chip encapsulation and seeding of LCC6/HER2 breast cancer cells inside droplets of alginate produced inside a microfluidic device was demonstrated [54]. After off-chip gelation, the droplets were injected into a second microfluidic device and captured in small sieves fabricated in the channel so the beads were retained and spheroids grown within the beads under a continuous flow of media. By encapsulating the cells inside the alginate bead, the growing cells were protected from the effects of shear stress. The resultant spheroids were then in a fixed position, and in parallel to one another and were used to assess the effect of differing doses of Doxorubicin [54]. In a more recent example, droplets of alginate containing MCF-7 cells or a co-culture of MCF-7 and HS-5 fibroblasts were formed and retained on the same microfluidic device and could form an array of 1000 spheroids for high-throughput, multiplexed drug screening. Spheroids were grown in the alginate droplets and maintained for 2 weeks before exposure to varying dosages of Doxorubicin ± Paclitaxel and cytotoxicity analysis. This example highlights the advantages of microfluidic based systems for large-scale, parallel models for drug screening [55].

22.6.2   Disease Modelling and Progression On-chip

Another emerging area for 3D culturing of breast tissue models in microfluidics is the investigation of disease progression. Monitoring and assessing how the early stages of cancers progress is particularly difficult and advanced animal models are often very costly and time consuming. As it is becoming clear that the microenvironment of tissues plays a central role in how the disease develops, being able to study meaningful models on the microscale, in the correct environment and in a controlled way, is becoming increasingly important. The metastatic cascade is an area that has found benefits from microfluidic models. The movement of cells from one physiological environment into another can be studied on the single cell level in specially designed microfluidic channels. Due to the optical transparency of these devices, cells can be imaged and analysed in real time as they traverse between different microenvironments and tissues. In addition, factors influencing metastases and invasion, such as chemokines, can be finely controlled in order to try to understand the process and the phenotypical changes these cells undergo into order to become invasive.

22.6.3   On-chip Models of Tumour Growth and Invasion

Grafton et al. developed an on-chip model of the breast ductal system by cultivating human mammary epithelial cells in laminin 111-coated branched, curved channels of defined sizes to mimic the branched nature and decreasing lumen size of ductal system in the breast. The branched channel system decreased in size from 120 to 30 μm [56]. Non-neoplastic epithelial monolayers grown on the laminin-111 functionalised surface of these channels underwent phenotype differentiation to display basoapical polarity. Impressively, the authors later went on to develop a 'disease-on-a-chip' model in which HMT3522-T4-2, from the HMT3522 breast cancer progression series were introduced to the on-chip ductal model system, where they attached and thrived. Interestingly, those developed in channels showed differences in circularity and other shape descriptors compared with those grown on a flat surface. The co-cultured, disease-on-a-chip system was used to test chemotherapeutic agents, with cells on flat surfaces showing differences sensitivity to therapies compared to those grown in curved channels, high-lighting the importance of the microenvironment of the tissue models in in vitro drug screening.

A model of the transformation of non-invasive ductal cell carcinoma in situ (DCIS) into the invasive form, invasive ductal carcinoma (IDC) and the effect fibroblasts had on this transition was developed by the Beebe group in Wisconsin, USA. The microfluidic model consisted of a normal mammary duct mimic which featured a central channel fabricated in a collagen I matrix and lined with a thin layer of Matrigel™ acting as the basement membrane of the lumen structure. A monolayer of human mammary epithelial cells (MCF10a) featuring basoapical polarity was cultured on the internal Matrigel™ surface. MCF10aDCIS cells were then seeded in high concentrations and cultured inside the internal bore of the lumen to model an advanced stage of DCIS. The lumen-DCIS mimic was fabricated centrally to two side channels in which human mammary fibroblasts (HMFs) were cultured. Specifically designed diffusion distances between the central lumen and side channels allowed for the relationship between the DCIS model and the fibroblasts to be investigated. Invasion from the inside of the lumen to the surrounding ECM was observed after 5 days only in the presence of the HMF cells and was validated by numerous analysis on the invasive legions, the breakdown of adherens junctions and changes in the structure of the collagen matrix, which acted as the stroma. This model is an excellent example of the potential of microfluidics for advanced in vitro models for studying disease progression and could be adapted to investigate the relationship between DCIS and other stromal cell types [57, 58].

22.6.4 On-chip Models of Metastases

Factors that influence metastases are of great interest in cancer research as the majority of cancer related deaths are due to development of metastatic disease. Microfluidics provides an environment in single, circulating tumour cells can be pumped through model tissues and exposed to various factors that affect their site-specific adhesion and subsequent invasion.

Song et al. built a vascularised on-chip model for investigating the adhesion of circulating breast cancer cells in site-specific regions by exposure of the endothelium of the model vasculature to the chemokine CXCL12. The device featured a straight 'upper' channel intersecting two perpendicular 'bottom' chambers. A monolayer of endothelium cells (HDMECs) was grown along the straight channel which was separated by a polyester membrane from the two bottom chambers. The two chambers had were filled with CXCL12 so only two regions of the endothelium were exposed to the chemokine. Circulating breast cancer cells (MDA-MB-231) were pumped along the top channel and adhesion was monitored in the regions exposed to CXCL12 and regions that were not. The device was used to investigate the interaction of CXCL12 with CXCR4 and CXCR7 receptors on the cancer cells, and on the endothelia cells. A preference of adhesion of circulating cancer cells to regions of endothelium exposed to CXCL12 was observed. In addition, inhibiting the signalling between the chemokine and cells significantly reduced adhesion of circulating cells, suggesting a possible therapeutic route to blocking a key step in metastases [59].

In another excellent example an on-chip vascularized osteo-microenvironment was developed to investigate bone microenvironment preference in metastatic breast cancer cells [60]. The authors described a tri-culture system in a specially designed microfluidic device featuring three cell culture chambers, interconnected by short hydrogel regions. In the central chamber, a bone-like matrix was generated by seeding and cultivating osteo-differentiated human bone marrow-derived mesenchymal stem cells (hBM-MSCs) into a collagen matrix. In one of the side channels, a model vasculature was created using human umbilical vein endothelial cells (HUVECs) to line the channel. As a model circulating metastatic cell, human mammary adenocarcinoma cells (MDA-MB-231) were pumped down the model vasculature. The MDA-MB-231 cells were observed to migrate across the endothelial monolayer of the vasculature model and into the osteo-cell microenvironment of the bone mimic. Extravasation of MDA-MB-231s across the endothelia barrier to the central channel was significantly higher in the presence of the hBM-MSCs osteo-cell microenvironment than a control of collagen only. In addition, the migration distance of MDA-MB-231 was also significantly higher into the central channel in the presence of the osteo-cell microenvironment. The model was then used to investigate the effect of the osteoblast chemokine CXCL5 and the CXCR2 receptor on the breast cancer cells extravasation and migration distances [60]. A more recent adaptation of this model, modified the microfluidic design so different ECM regions with different cell compositions could be aligned directly in a continuous, side-by-side manner to mimic better the interconnected tumour and stroma regions found *in vivo*. The model was used to study the effect of EGF gradients on the speed and persistence of breast cancer cell invasion into the stroma from a high cell density, tumour region [61].

22.7 Virtual Tissue Models

Advances in digital pathology has allowed the creation of virtual 3D models of early, pre-invasive breast cancer, DCIS [62]. Using in silico methods, DCIS has been reconstructed by creating image stacks of up to 100 serial sections of virtual slides. Using custom 3D software, 3D tissue volumes can be created and annotated to highlight distinct features which may help in studying the biology of DCIS.

22.8 Conclusions

This chapter has outlined a range of 3D *in vitro* and in silico models that are now available to study breast cancer. Increasing the complexity of these models is now possible and the explosion of interest in using microfluidic devices provide a micro-structure and micro-flow environment that is highly suitable to the culturing of 3D tissue models for drug screening and in studying disease behaviour. The ability to recapitulate multi-cellular tissue structures in a device where fluid flow, temperature and chemical gradients can be finely controlled, allows more complex and more representative *in vitro* models to be fabricated compared to current *in vitro* methodologies. The advancements in tissue-on-chip models is predicted to accelerate drug discovery, reduce the need for animal models and provide a new and versatile route towards personalised medicine. These can be complemented with virtual in silico models. The complexities of systems generated is ever increasing with the acceptance of multidisciplinary approaches to create the best models possible. Whilst it is unlikely that any one model will be better than the rest, a combined approach to improve disease modelling should help towards improving patient outcome in breast cancer.

Acknowledgements Sophie Roberts is supported by a studentship from the NC3Rs (NC/N00325X/1).

References

1. Bissell MJ, Radisky DC, Rizki A et al (2002) The organizing principle: microenvironmental influences in the normal and malignant breast. Differentiation 70:537–546
2. Bissell MJ, Rizki A, Mian IS (2003) Tissue architecture: the ultimate regulator of breast epithelial function. Curr Opin Cell Biol 15:753–762
3. Bissell MJ, Weaver VM, Lelievre SA et al (1999) Tissue structure, nuclear organization, and gene expression in normal and malignant breast. Cancer Res 59:1757–1763s; discussion 1763s–1764s
4. Weaver VM, Fischer AH, Peterson OW et al (1996) The importance of the microenvironment in breast cancer progression: recapitulation of mammary tumorigenesis using a unique human mammary epithelial cell model and a three-dimensional culture assay. Biochem Cell Biol 74:833–851
5. Anonymous (2003) Goodbye, flat biology? Nature 424:861–861
6. Roberts S, Speirs V (2017) Advances in the development of improved animal-free models for use in breast cancer biomedical research. Biophysical Rev 9:321–327
7. Kim JB, Stein R, O'hare MJ (2004) Three-dimensional in vitro tissue culture models of breast cancer – a review. Breast Cancer Res Treat 85:281–291
8. Holen I, Speirs V, Morrissey B et al (2017) In vivo models in breast cancer research: progress, challenges and future directions. Dis Model Mech 10:359–371
9. Orimo A, Gupta PB, Sgroi DC et al (2005) Stromal fibroblasts present in invasive human breast carcinomas promote tumor growth and angiogenesis through elevated SDF-1/CXCL12 secretion. Cell 121:335–348
10. Sutherland RM, Inch WR, Mccredie JA et al (1970) A multi-component radiation survival curve using an in vitro tumour model. Int J Radiat Biol Relat Stud Phys Chem Med 18:491–495
11. Mehta G, Hsiao AY, Ingram M et al (2012) Opportunities and challenges for use of tumor spheroids as models to test drug delivery and efficacy. J Control Release 164:192–204
12. Torisawa YS, Takagi A, Shiku H et al (2005) A multicellular spheroid-based drug sensitivity test by scanning electrochemical microscopy. Oncol Rep 13:1107–1112
13. Debnath J, Mills KR, Collins NL et al (2002) The role of apoptosis in creating and maintaining luminal space within normal and oncogene-expressing mammary acini. Cell 111:29–40
14. Nash CE, Mavria G, Baxter EW et al (2015) Development and characterisation of a 3D multi-cellular in vitro model of normal human breast: a tool for cancer initiation studies. Oncotarget 6:13731–13741
15. Roberts GC, Morris PG, Moss MA et al (2016) An evaluation of matrix-containing and humanised matrix-free 3-dimensional cell culture systems for studying breast cancer. PLoS One 11:e0157004
16. Achilli TM, Meyer J, Morgan JR (2012) Advances in the formation, use and understanding of multi-cellular spheroids. Expert Opin Biol Ther 12:1347–1360
17. Metzger W, Sossong D, Bachle A et al (2011) The liquid overlay technique is the key to formation of co-culture spheroids consisting of primary osteoblasts, fibroblasts and endothelial cells. Cytotherapy 13:1000–1012
18. Foty R (2011) A simple hanging drop cell culture protocol for generation of 3D spheroids. J Vis Exp 51:e2720
19. Jaganathan H, Gage J, Leonard F et al (2014) Three-dimensional in vitro co-culture model of breast tumor using magnetic levitation. Sci Rep 4:6468
20. Booth ME, Nash CE, Roberts NP et al (2015) 3-D tissue modelling and virtual pathology as new approaches to study ductal carcinoma in situ. Altern Lab Anim 43:377–383
21. Kleinman HK, Mcgarvey ML, Hassell JR et al (1986) Basement membrane complexes with biological activity. Biochemistry 25:312–318
22. Lee GY, Kenny PA, Lee EH et al (2007) Three-dimensional culture models of normal and malignant breast epithelial cells. Nat Methods 4:359–365

23. Sokol ES, Miller DH, Breggia A et al (2016) Growth of human breast tissues from patient cells in 3D hydrogel scaffolds. Breast Cancer Res 18:19
24. Zanoni M, Piccinini F, Arienti C et al (2016) 3D tumor spheroid models for in vitro therapeutic screening: a systematic approach to enhance the biological relevance of data obtained. Sci Rep 6:19103
25. Charafe-Jauffret E, Ginestier C, Iovino F et al (2009) Breast cancer cell lines contain functional cancer stem cells with metastatic capacity and a distinct molecular signature. Cancer Res 69:1302–1313
26. Croker AK, Goodale D, Chu J et al (2009) High aldehyde dehydrogenase and expression of cancer stem cell markers selects for breast cancer cells with enhanced malignant and metastatic ability. J Cell Mol Med 13:2236–2252
27. Wilson H, Botfield B, Speirs V (2015) A global view of breast tissue banking. Adv Exp Med Biol 864:69–77
28. Walsh AJ, Cook RS, Sanders ME et al (2016) Drug response in organoids generated from frozen primary tumor tissues. Sci Rep 6:18889
29. Walsh AJ, Cook RS, Sanders ME et al (2014) Quantitative optical imaging of primary tumor organoid metabolism predicts drug response in breast cancer. Cancer Res 74:5184–5194
30. Holliday DL, Moss MA, Pollock S et al (2013) The practicalities of using tissue slices as preclinical organotypic breast cancer models. J Clin Pathol 66:253–255
31. Davies EJ, Dong M, Gutekunst M et al (2015) Capturing complex tumour biology in vitro: histological and molecular characterisation of precision cut slices. Sci Rep 5:17187
32. Grosso SH, Katayama ML, Roela RA et al (2013) Breast cancer tissue slices as a model for evaluation of response to rapamycin. Cell Tissue Res 352:671–684
33. Pennington K, Chu QD, Curiel DT et al (2010) The utility of a tissue slice model system to determine breast cancer infectivity by oncolytic adenoviruses. J Surg Res 163:270–275
34. Naipal KA, Verkaik NS, Sanchez H et al (2016) Tumor slice culture system to assess drug response of primary breast cancer. BMC Cancer 16:78
35. Salamanna F, Contartese D, Maglio M et al (2016) A systematic review on in vitro 3D bone metastases models: a new horizon to recapitulate the native clinical scenario? Oncotarget 7:44803–44820
36. Krishnan V, Shuman LA, Sosnoski DM et al (2011) Dynamic interaction between breast cancer cells and osteoblastic tissue: comparison of two- and three-dimensional cultures. J Cell Physiol 226:2150–2158
37. Marlow R, Honeth G, Lombardi S et al (2013) A novel model of dormancy for bone metastatic breast cancer cells. Cancer Res 73:6886–6899
38. Albritton JL, Miller JS (2017) 3D bioprinting: improving in vitro models of metastasis with heterogeneous tumor microenvironments. Dis Model Mech 10:3–14
39. Charbe N, Mccarron PA, Tambuwala MM (2017) Three-dimensional bio-printing: a new frontier in oncology research. World J Clin Oncol 8:21–36
40. Jiang T, Munguia-Lopez JG, Flores-Torres S et al (2017) Directing the self-assembly of tumour spheroids by bioprinting cellular heterogeneous models within alginate/gelatin hydrogels. Sci Rep 7:4575
41. Zhou X, Zhu W, Nowicki M et al (2016) 3D bioprinting a cell-laden bone matrix for breast cancer metastasis study. ACS Appl Mater Interfaces 8:30017–30026
42. Sackmann EK, Fulton AL, Beebe DJ (2014) The present and future role of microfluidics in biomedical research. Nature 507:181–189
43. Prakadan SM, Shalek AK, Weitz DA (2017) Scaling by shrinking: empowering single-cell 'omics' with microfluidic devices. Nat Rev Genet 18:345–361
44. Bhatia SN, Ingber DE (2014) Microfluidic organs-on-chips. Nat Biotechnol 32:760–772
45. Van Duinen V, Trietsch SJ, Joore J et al (2015) Microfluidic 3D cell culture: from tools to tissue models. Curr Opin Biotechnol 35:118–126
46. Bhise NS, Ribas J, Manoharan V et al (2014) Organ-on-a-chip platforms for studying drug delivery systems. J Control Release 190:82–93

47. Esch EW, Bahinski A, Huh D (2015) Organs-on-chips at the frontiers of drug discovery. Nat Rev Drug Discov 14:248–260
48. Han B, Qu CJ, Park K et al (2016) Recapitulation of complex transport and action of drugs at the tumor microenvironment using tumor-microenvironment-on-chip. Cancer Lett 380:319–329
49. Yang YM, Yang XC, Zou J et al (2015) Evaluation of photodynamic therapy efficiency using an in vitro three-dimensional microfluidic breast cancer tissue model. Lab Chip 15:735–744
50. Hwang H, Park J, Shin C et al (2013) Three dimensional multicellular co-cultures and anti-cancer drug assays in rapid prototyped multilevel microfluidic devices. Biomed Microdevices 15:627–634
51. Lee JM, Seo HI, Bae JH et al (2017) Hydrogel microfluidic co-culture device for photothermal therapy and cancer migration. Electrophoresis 38:1318–1324
52. Yildiz-Ozturk E, Gulce-Iz S, Anil M et al (2017) Cytotoxic responses of carnosic acid and doxorubicin on breast cancer cells in butterfly-shaped microchips in comparison to 2D and 3D culture. Cytotechnology 69:337–347
53. Kwak B, Ozcelikkale A, Shin CS et al (2014) Simulation of complex transport of nanoparticles around a tumor using tumor-microenvironment-on-chip. J Control Release 194:157–167
54. Yu LF, Chen MCW, Cheung KC (2010) Droplet-based microfluidic system for multicellular tumor spheroid formation and anticancer drug testing. Lab Chip 10:2424–2432
55. Sabhachandani P, Motwani V, Cohen N et al (2016) Generation and functional assessment of 3D multicellular spheroids in droplet based microfluidics platform. Lab Chip 16:497–505
56. Grafton MMG, Wang L, Vidi PA et al (2011) Breast on-a-chip: mimicry of the channeling system of the breast for development of theranostics. Integr Biol 3:451–459
57. Bischel LL, Beebe DJ, Sung KE (2015) Microfluidic model of ductal carcinoma in situ with 3D, organotypic structure. BMC Cancer 15:12
58. Sung KE, Yang N, Pehlke C et al (2011) Transition to invasion in breast cancer: a microfluidic in vitro model enables examination of spatial and temporal effects. Integr Biol 3:439–450
59. Song JW, Cavnar SP, Walker AC et al (2009) Microfluidic endothelium for studying the intra-vascular adhesion of metastatic breast cancer cells. PLoS One 4:e5756
60. Bersini S, Jeon JS, Dubini G et al (2014) A microfluidic 3D in vitro model for specificity of breast cancer metastasis to bone. Biomaterials 35:2454–2461
61. Truong D, Puleo J, Llave A et al. (2016) Breast cancer cell invasion into a three dimensional tumor-stroma microenvironment. Sci Rep 6:3404–3412
62. Booth ME, Treanor D, Roberts N et al (2015) Three-dimensional reconstruction of ductal carcinoma in situ with virtual slides. Histopathology 66:966–973

CPSIA information can be obtained
at www.ICGtesting.com
Printed in the USA
BVHW010813250919

559360BV00002B/2/P